Phlebology '95

Phlebology '95

Proceedings of the XII World Congress
Union Internationale de Phlébologie

London 3 – 8 September 1995

Editors

David Negus
Georges Jantet
Philip D. Coleridge-Smith

Volume 2

ISBN 978-3-540-19999-1   ISBN 978-1-4471-3095-6
DOI 10.1007/978-1-4471-3095-6

First Published in two volumes by Springer-Verlag London Ltd as
Supplement 1 (1995) to the journal *Phlebology*.

Originally published by the Venous Forum of the Royal Society of Medicine and
Societas Phlebologica Scandinavica in 1995

Printed by The Alden Press, Osney Mead, Oxford, UK
28/3830-543210 Printed on acid-free paper

Contents - Volume 2

Thrombo-embolic Disorders

Diagnosis of Thrombo-embolism

Prevention of Thrombo-embolism

Treatment of Thrombo-embolism

Deep Venous Reflux and Occlusion/Venous Ulcers

Natural History

Clinical Research

Treatment of Deep Venous Disorders and Venous Ulceration

Conservative Treatment

The Surgical Treatment of Deep Venous Disorders and Leg Ulcers

Venous Dysplasias

Axillary, Subclavian and Arm Venous Disorders

Gynaecology, Hormones and Pelvic Disorders

Lymphoedema

Miscellaneous Topics

Satellite Symposia

Servier

Thuasne

Thrombo-embolic Disorders

TOGETHER

Successful compression therapy is a combined reward for the doctor, the patient and good compression stockings.

With our experience, research and innovative manufacturing procedures, we produce high-quality, medically effective compression stockings in which you feel comfortable, that you enjoy wearing – a vital condition for optimum patient compliance.

Let us make our contribution to human well-being – together.

medi UK   **medi** Bayreuth   **medi** Austria   **medi** Danmark   **medi** France   **medi** Italia   **medi** Nederland   **medi** USA

...and in thirty other countries

medi Bayreuth · D-95448 Bayreuth · Germany

Thrombo-embolic Disorders

Epidemiology/Pathology

Phlebology '95, D. Negus et al. (eds.). Phlebology (1995) Suppl. 1: 658-660

OP/10.6

Free Floating Thrombus and Embolic Risk in Patients with Angiographically Established Proximal Deep Venous Thrombosis. A Prospective Study

G. Pacouret[1], D. Alison[2], B.Charbonnier[1], M.P. Augusseau[1] and J.M. Pottier[3]

1 Cardiology D and Coronary Care Unit, 2 Radiology Department and 3 Nuclear Medicine Department, University Hospital Trousseau, Tours, France

INTRODUCTION

The primary aim of this descriptive trial was to evaluate the short term risk of pulmonary embolism in patients with proximal deep venous thrombosis treated with anticoagulants with or without free floating thrombus.The secondary aims were first to assess the value of a non invasive test, color venous duplex scanning, in the diagnosis of free floating thrombus, and secondly to evaluate the long term risk of symptomatic pulmonary embolism according to the presence or the absence of free floating thrombus.

METHODS

During a 2 year recruitment period in our department, patients were considered for inclusion when having symptoms of acute phlebitis and/or pulmonary embolism and when a proximal deep venous thrombosis diagnosis was angiographically established.

Exclusion criteria were as follows : contra-indication to heparin treatment, history of vena cava filtering, curative heparin treatment for more than 24 hours, life threatening pulmonary embolism requiring thrombolysis or embolectomy, allergy to x-ray dye, delay between invasive and non invasive tests for the diagnosis of venous thrombosis or pulmonary embolism over 24 hours.

Venography, color venous duplex scanning and perfusion lung scan were performed on admission. In case of abnormal perfusion lung scan, pulmonary angiography had to be performed within 24 hours. Perfusion lung scan was repeated on day 10 ± 1 or earlier in case of clinically suspected pulmonary embolism, despite anticoagulant treatment. At this stage, pulmonary angiography was mandatory only in patients with abnormal baseline lung scan and follow up lung scan showing impairment. A clinical evaluation was scheduled at 3 months.

All venograms were reviewed by one experienced radiologist blinded to the clinical and ultrasound data. The thrombus was considered as being free floating if its greater proximal segment was outlined by contrast material. All films were antero-posterior views. In the same way, color venous duplex scannings were performed by co-investigators blinded to the angiographic data and the thrombus was considered as being free floating if its greater proximal segment visualized was unattached to the vein wall and outlined by the color signal in both long axis and short axis views.

STUDY POPULATION

276 patients with proximal deep venous thrombosis were screened and 95 patients were finally included. Out of these 95 patients, 5 were retrospectively excluded because the angiographic diagnosis of free floating or occlusive thrombus was doubtful. Thus 90 patients were considered for the comparison of color venous duplex scanning with venography. During the in-hospital course, 2 patients (one in each group) underwent vena cava filtering : one because of a major bleeding and the other one because an emergency cholecystectomy had to be performed. Therefore, 88 patients were considered for the epidemiologic part of the study.

Out of the 90 patients with suitable venogram, 62 were considered as having a free floating thrombus and 28 as having an occlusive thrombus. Baseline characteristics of the 2 groups are listed in table 2. Both groups were balanced accord to age, sex and delay between onset of symptoms to admission. A statistically significant difference was observed between the 2 groups according to the deep vein thrombosis location which was more proximal in the group of patients with an occlusive thrombus. Conversely, bilateral deep venous thrombosis was more frequent in the group of patients with a free floating thrombus. Admission pulmonary embolism prevalence was comparable in the 2 groups. Massive pulmonary embolisms were equally distributed and mean Miller index was comparable in the 2 groups.

Table 1. Baseline characteristics of the 2 study groups.

	FFT + n = 62	FFT - n = 28	p
Age (yrs)	69 ± 15	66 ± 17	ns
Sex (M/F)	35/27	14/14	ns
Onset of symptoms (days)	12 ± 14	7 ± 7	ns
Deep vein thrombosis :			
- caval	1	0	
- iliac	4	11	0.001
- femoral	38	12	
- popliteal	19	5	
- unilateral/bilateral	50/12	27/11	0.04
- floating segment length (cm)	12 ± 10	-	
Pulmonary embolism :			
- n	40 (65)	14 (50)	ns
- massive (n)	9	4	ns
- Miller index	15 ± 5	15 ± 5	ns

FFT + : free floating thrombus ; FFT - : occlusive thrombus.

89 patients out of 90 were treated with subcutaneous twice daily administered low molecular weight heparin and the remaining patient was treated with intravenous unfractionated heparin. Treatment characteristics of both groups are listed in table 2.

Table 2. Treatment characteristics of the study population

	FFT + n = 62	FFT - n = 28	p
Heparin :			
- unfractionated	1	0	
- low molecular weight heparin	61	28	ns
Warfarin			
- n (%)	56 (90)	23 (82)	ns
- onset of treatment (d)	4 ± 2	3 ± 1	ns
Immobilization (d)	3 ± 1	3 ± 2	ns

RESULTS

Pulmonary Embolism and Mortality (table 3)

Pulmonary embolism occured in 3 patients during the in-hospital course : 2 symptomatic FFT + and 1 silent FFT- . All these 3 events were minor and did not result in any modification of the treatment of the concerned patients. No symptomatic pulmonary embolism occured in either of the 2 groups between discharge and 3 month follow-up. During this period, 4 patients died from evolutive neoplasms without symptoms in favor of pulmonary embolism.

Table 3. Pulmonary embolism and mortality rates

	FFT + n = 61	FFT - n = 27	p
Pulmonary embolism n (%) :			
- day 10 ± 1	2 (3.3)	1 (3.8)	ns
- 3 months	0	0	
Death n (%) :			
- day 10 ± 1	0	0	
- 3 months	3 (4.9)	1 (3.7)	ns

Color venous duplex scanning

Sensitivity and specificity of color venous duplex scanning in the diagnosis of free floating thrombus were respectively 68 and 86 % and positive and negative predictive values were respectively 91 and 55 %, as compared to venography.

Conclusion

In this series of 90 patients with proximal deep venous thrombosis, we observed a high prevalence of free floating thrombi. Color venous duplex scanning revealed to have a high positive predictive value in the diagnosis of such thrombi but negative predictive value of this test was low. Pulmonary embolism incidence, despite adequate anticoagulant therapy was below 5 % whatever the type of venous thrombosis was, free floating or occlusive. Therefore, we can assert that the identification of deep venous thrombosis greater proximal segment should not be mandatory in patients with proximal deep venous thrombosis and moreover vena cava filtering of patients with a free floating thrombus should be most often avoided unless anticoagulant therapy is contra-indicated.

Phlebology '95, D. Negus et al. (eds.). Phlebology (1995) Suppl. 1: 661–663

P007

Deficiency of Protein C, Protein S and Antithrombin III in Venous Diseases

P.L. Antignani, A.R. Todini, T. Di Fortunato, M.L. Paiella and M. Bartolo

Department of Angiology, s.Camillo Hospital, Rome, Italy

INTRODUCTION

Many episodes of phlebothrombosis of lower limbs can be framed in those forms of hypercoagulability that include a whole of syndromes characterized by an hereditary deficiency of many proteins involved in the control of coagulation, such as the antithrombin III and the proteins C and S.

On the base of the suggestion of literature [1,2,3,4,5], the deficit of proteins C, protein S and antithrombin III can be a factor which predisposes to the development of venous thrombosis. We valued, in other studies [6,7,8], which was the real incidence of this lack in a group of subjects arrived at our observation owing to an acute phlebothrombosis and presenting a familiar positive anamnesis for phlebopathies, without a clear etiologic factors. We present, in this paper, a review and an updating of our casuistics.

METHODS

96 consecutive patients (72 men and 24 women; average age 39,7 years) were selected since January 1989 to December 1994, according to the peculiarity of the clinical condition. 33 relatives were also examined.

The diagnosis was based on clinical and instrumental data such as Doppler, duplexscanner and color Doppler evaluations.

The assays of protein C, protein S and Antithrombin III were carried out.

For the protein S we used the ACL coagulative method (Centrifugal analyzer; I.L.; the normal values fall between 60 % and 140%); for the protein C and the Antithrombin III we used the chromogenic method (Baxter; the normal values fall, respectively, between 70% and 120% and between 80% and 120%).

We also evaluated several hemocoagulative and immunological parameters such as hemochrome, protidogram, fibrinogenemia, plasminogenemia, APT, PTT, LE phenomenon, reactive protein C, immunoglobulinemia, FDP, Dimer test and antibody assays for ANA, ASMA, ACA, ANA and LAC.

RESULTS

Of the 96 patients, 38 showed a deficiency of protein S (39,58% of cases; mean value: 37,46%), 12 cases a deficiency of protein C (12,5%; mean value: 53,7%) and 7 a deficiency of Antithrombin III (7,29%; mean value: 59,5%). In the group of the 33 relatives, we found 18 cases which presented a deficiency of protein S and 4 subjects with a deficiency of protein C. We followed, at present, 41 patients and we confirmed the deficiency in 37 cases.

DISCUSSION

This study confirm the importance of the deficiency of examined proteins in the patients with acute phlebothrombosis.

The prevalence and above all the clinical importance of lacking of anticoagulant proteins vitamin-K dependent has not been completely defined. In a study of U.S.A. on the blood of givers, the heterozygote deficiency of protein C has resulted to be of one case on 300 [5]. In a further policentric italian study executed on 253 subjects, has emerged that the deficit of antithrombin III is the most frequent (36%) followed by the deficiency of protein C (32%) and of protein S (18%) [9].

In particular way, the deficit of type I (relative to a reduction of antigenic activity) reaches the 74% of the kinds of deficit of antithrombin III, to the 75% for the protein C and to the 84% for the protein S.

From a clinical point of view the 51% of the subjects has presented a venous thrombosis and the 49% was asymptomatic.

In another study executed in the urban area of Frankfort [10] the deficit of type I heterozygous protein S was present in 5% of subjects examined while the deficit of type I heterozygous protein C in the 4% of subjects.

From such data we cannot draw a conclusion on the real incidence of the lacking of proteins C and S and of antithrombin III, because the percentages are very different; in any case all the data, included ours, state the importance of deficit of such substances in the determinism of phlebothrombosis, above all the venous ones, in young subjects.

The high percentage noticed in our case-report of deficiency of protein S as regards as the deficiency of protein C, that is a datum that doesn't agree with the results of literature [11], could be connected with the selection particularly careful of the subjects both for what concerns the familiarity and the absence of etiologic factors that are commonly at the base of thrombotic events.

This fact could be also due to the used method which tends towards to give low levels of protein S activity in presence of resistence to Activated Protein C (APC). Therefore, a lot of these patients could have a resistance to APC. We surmised that plasma-based protein S functional assays might be sensitive to resitance to APC, mimicking low levels of protein S activity. To evaluate this possibility, we are reinvestigating all positive patients by means of a new method.

In conclusion we think that the determination of the proteins C, protein S and Antithrombin III must be now effected on all the young subjects with phlebitic episodes and it is essential even in asymptomatic cases with familiarity for phlebopathy in order to carry out a fair prophylactic protocol both for the prevention of the relapses and in particularly risk conditions for thrombosis such as surgical operations, pregnancy, delivery, etc.

In all the symptomatic patients with deficiency there was been established according to the protocols of literature an initial therapy with sodium-heparin in the acute phase followed by a therapy for a long period with oral anticoagulant.

Such a scheme should be applied even to the asymptomatic subjects if it is necessary, in order to avoid collateral effects such as dermal necrosis due to the administration in the first request of the oral anticoagulant.

REFERENCES

1) Comp PC. Hereditary disorders predisponing to thrombosis. Prog Haemost Thromb 1986; 8:71-102.

2) Glodson CL, Shaner I, Hach V, Beck KH, Griffin JH. The frequency of type I .heterozygous protein S and protein C deficiency in 141 unrelated young patients with venous thrombosis. Thromb Haemost 1988; 59:18-22.

3) Gruppo RA, Leimer P, Frencis RB, Marler RA, Gilbestein E. Protein C deficiency resulting from possible double heterozygosity and its response to Danazol. Blood 1988; 71:370-74.

4) Millaire A, Jude B, Petetin N, Marquand A, Watel A, Ducloux G. Maladie thromboembolique veineuse et arterielle familiale par deficit en protein C. J Mal Vasc 1988; 13:292-93.

5) Rick ME. Protein C and protein S vitamin-K dipendent inhibitors of blood coagulation. JAMA 1990; 263:701-03.

6) Antignani PL, Di Fortunato T, Franzè A. Incidenza del deficit di proteine C ed S in soggetti con flebotrombosi. Atti VII congresso della Società Italiana di Flebologia Clinica e Sperimentale. Bologna: Monduzzi Ed, 1990:67-70.

7) Antignani PL, Di Fortunato T, Sotira A, Grassi F, Ricci A, Bartolo M. The incidence of protein C, protein S and Antithrombin III deficiency in the phlebothrombotic subjects. In: Raymond-Martinbeau P, Prescott R, Zummo M, editors. Phlebology 92. London: John Libbey, 1992:442-44.

8) Antignani PL, Di Fortunato T, Sotira A., Grassi F, Ricci A, Bartolo M. Deficit di proteina C, proteina S ed Antitrombina III in soggetti con flebotrombosi. Min Angio 1993; 18:113-15.

9) Tripodi A, Mannucci PM. A survey of inherited thrombotic syndromes in Italy. Res Clin Lab 1989; 19:67-74.

10) Tollefson DBJ, Friedman KD, Marlar RA, Bondyk DF, Towne JB. Protein C deficiency. Arch Surg 1988; 123:881-84.

11) Wiesel ML, Grunebaum L, Freyssinet JM, Cazaneve JP. La proteine C: interet de son dosage en pathologie. Presse Med 1988; 26:1333-37.

Phlebology '95, D. Negus et al. (eds.). Phlebology (1995) Suppl. 1: 664-666

OP/8.7

Deaths from Pulmonary Embolism Amongst Surgical Patients in Scotland

T.E. Gillies and C.V. Ruckley

Scottish Audit of Surgical Mortality, Royal College of Surgeons, and Vascular Surgery Unit, Royal Infirmary, Edinburgh

INTRODUCTION

Deaths amongst inpatients from thromboembolic disease are preventable by the use of prophylaxis, either mechanical or pharmacological. The Scottish Audit of Surgical Mortality is a national audit group, based in four regional offices - Glasgow, Edinburgh, Dundee and Aberdeen. Details of all surgical inpatient deaths in Scotland, excluding those with terminal malignancy, are received at one of these offices. This study set out to look at all deaths from pulmonary embolism during 1994, to identify common factors and the extent of prophylaxis against thromboembolic disease used in each case.

METHODS

All deaths where thromboembolic disease was cited as the cause of death were identified. The circumstance of the surgical admission and diagnosis, management, risk factors for thromboembolic disease, and the use of prophylaxis were recorded. Patients in the care of the following health boards were assessed; Lothian, Fife, Forth Valley, Borders, Dumfries and Galloway, Tayside, Grampian, Highlands and Islands and Orkney, Shetland and the Western Isles. All deaths under the care of general surgeons were included. Orthopaedic cases were only considered for Grampian and Highlands and Islands regions. Obstetric and gynaecological patients were not included.

RESULTS

1893 deaths during 1994 were reported to the Scottish Audit of Surgical Mortality and in 57 of these, pulmonary embolism was stated as the cause of death. Trauma and orthopaedic conditions were the reasons for admission in 18 of these and further subspecialties, including vascular surgery (6 cases), and urology (3 cases) accounted for another 13 deaths.

Elective admissions or transfers accounted for 18 (32%) of the cases. 41 patients (72%) had a surgical procedure, with 4 undergoing a second procedure. Benign disease was the indication for operative intervention in 17, malignancy in 14 and orthopaedic conditions and trauma in 14 (45 procedures). The median length of procedure was 60 minutes (range 10-260 minutes). General anaesthesia was used in 25 procedures, regional anaesthesia in 14 and a combination in 5. The remaining 16 cases were treated conservatively. Of these cases, the reason for admission was benign disease in 9.

Pre-admission immobility was the most commonly identified risk factor, present in 32 cases, malignant disease had been diagnosed in 23 cases, and obesity in 8. Only 6 patients were noted to have had a previous episode of thromboembolic disease or a history suspicious of this.

The length of inpatient stay prior to a surgical procedure was greater than 48 hours in 17 cases (median 7 days, range 3-60 days), and involved a transfer from another hospital or unit in 8. In the nonoperative group, the median stay before the first clinical manifestation of the thrombo-embolic event was 6.5 days (range 1-44 days).

The mode of presentation was sudden death in 16 patients, collapse in 21 and a subacute episode in 20.

The form of prophylaxis used is shown in the table below.

	orthopaedic/trauma n=18	general surgery/specialities n=39
subcut. heparin	2	6
subcut. heparin and stockings	0	9
stockings	4	1
aspirin	1	2

In the group treated by operation, and with a preoperative inpatient stay of greater than 48 hours , 9/17 received no prophylaxis at all. Six of these were emergency admissions, although in four the operation was carried out on an elective list.

The diagnosis was made on clinical grounds with supporting investigations such as chest X-ray, Blood gases and ECG in all but 6 cases. Arterial blood gases were helpful in making the diagnosis in 90% of cases where they were done. An autopsy was carried out in 24 cases, and a clinically unsuspected deep venous thrombosis was a common finding.

DISCUSSION

All studies of thrombo-embolic disease are limited by the method of diagnosis and by cases which are excluded because the diagnosis is not considered. This is further hampered by the low autopsy rate [1]. The numbers reported here are, without doubt, an underestimate, but a number of important points are raised. Despite the generally accepted view that all patients should be assessed as to their risk for thromboembolic disease and receive appropriate prophylaxis [2,3], this does not happen [4]. More than half the patients (32/57) received no prophylaxis of any sort. Two groups of patients are particularly involved; those admitted as emergencies, many of whom do not undergo a surgical procedure but who are unwell and possibly in bed for some time; and those admitted to another unit or ward and transferred to the surgical team for further management. The very low use of prophylaxis preoperatively suggests that the consideration of prophylaxis is triggered in the peri or post operative period. Many patients will therefore have been at increased risk for some time before prophylaxis is started.

The use of pharmacological prophylaxis is sometimes delayed by the consideration of regional anaesthesia, dependent on individual practice [5]. It is questionable whether this such delay can be justified, and in any case this should not prevent the use of mechanical means, such as intermittent compression and anti-thromboembolism stockings. Documentation of the use of mechanical means is often poor but is important for medico-legal reasons.

Pulmonary embolism continues to be an important cause of death amongst surgical patients. Prophylaxis should be extended to all inpatients from the time of admission if it is to be effective. When surgical patients present with thromboembolic disease, an aggressive policy of investigation and intervention should be considered.

REFERENCES

1. Sandler D A, Martin J F. Autopsy proven pulmonary embolism in hospital patients : are we detecting enough deep venous thrombosis? J Roy Soc Med 1989;82:203-5
2. MacLeod D C. Lessons from a symposium on thromboembolic disease. Proc R Coll Physicians Edinb. 1994;24:548-553.
3. Thromboembolic Risk Factors (THRIFT) Consensus Group. Risk of and prophylaxis for venous thromboembolism in hospital patients. Br Med J 1992;305:567-574.
4. Caprini J A, Arcelus J I, Hoffman K, et al. Prevention of venous thromboembolism in North America: results of a survey among general surgeons. J Vasc Surg 1994;20:751-758.
5. Wildsmith J A W, McClure J H. Anticoagulant drugs and central nerve blockade. Anaesthesia 1991;46:613-614.

Phlebology '95, D. Negus et al. (eds.). Phlebology (1995) Suppl. 1: 667-670

PI/8.4

Suivi Echo - Doppler a Court et Moyen Terme des Thromboses Veineuses Profondes des Membres Inférieurs

J.M. Baud[1], L. Stephas[1], C. Ribadeau-Dumas[1], F. Chleir[1], D. Louvet[1], Ph. Lemasle[1] and J.L. Bosson[2]

1 Unite d'Angiologie. Service de chirurgie vasculaire, CH Versailles
2 Service Communication médicale et informatique, CHU Grenoble

Short and Medium Term Echo-Doppler Follow-Up of Deep Vein Thrombosis of the Lower Limbs

SUMMARY

The authors describe a Doppler follow-up study of the fate of the thrombus over 1 year following deep vein thrombosis.

SUIVI ECHO - DOPPLER A COURT ET MOYEN TERME DES THROMBOSES VEINEUSES PROFONDES DES MEMBRES INFERIEURS.

JM Baud *, L.Stephas* , C.Ribadeau-Dumas*, F. Chleir *, D. Louvet *, Ph. Lemasle*, JL Bosson**.

* : Unite d'Angiologie. Service de chirurgie vasculaire . CH Versailles
**: Service Communication médicale et informatique. CHU Grenoble .

INTRODUCTION :

Lorsqu'il existe un signe clinique d'appel de TVP au niveau des membres inférieurs , le diagnostic de thrombose par l'Echo Doppler pulsé est fiable comparée à la phlébographie (entre 93 et 100% selon les auteurs et selon les territoires). Le devenir et l'évolution du thrombus est mal connu en raison de l'impossibilité de pratiquer en routine des phlébographies répétitives. Depuis quelques années , l'echo-doppler pulsé s'impose progressivement comme un méthode de choix pour suivre les TVP mais il nécessite de définir des critères quantitatifs ou semi quantitatifs reproductibles et fiables pour permettre de mettre au point une standardisation de l'examen et de limiter le plus possible le caractère opérateur dépendant des ultrasons .
Notre étude a pour objectifs d'étudier par echo-doppler la régression ou l'extension du thrombus à court et moyen terme (1 an) , ainsi que de définir des critères échographiques prédictifs d'un potentiel emboligène.

MATERIEL ET METHODE

75 patients présentant une thrombose veineuse profonde récente avec ou sans embolie pulmonaire ont été inclus dans cette étude .
Un examen echo-doppler pulsé a été pratiqué systématiquement à J0 , J2 , J5 , J10 et J30 pour le suivi à court terme et J90 et au bout d'un an pour le suivi à moyen terme .
Une scintigraphie pulmonaire de perfusion a été réalisée chez tous les patients le premier et le dixième jour . En cas de positivité une angiographie a complété le bilan . 5 % des sujets ont dû subir une phlebocavographie en raison d'incertitude diagnostique .
Tous les patients ont reçu le même traitement debuté par de l'héparine à la dose de 500 UI/kg/j pendant 10 jours . Le relais par du Préviscan a été entrepris au 4è jour et prolongé pendant 3 mois minimum .
La surrélévation des pieds et le port d'une contention classe 3 ont été systématiques et tous les patients ont été levés précocément , dès le deuxième jour .

Plusieurs éléments ont été consignés à l'examen echo-doppler : la topographie et l'aspect de la thrombose , l'état de la veine et sa compressibilité , et enfin , le caractère mobile ou non du pôle supérieur du thrombus .

Pour pouvoir suivre l'évolution de la thrombose , des scores ont été établis : un score local concernant la veine atteinte : 0 en l'absence de TVP , 1 pour une TVP partielle et 2 pour une oblitération compléte . Un score global correspondant au score précédent multiplié par le nombre de segments atteints. La régréssion a été définie par la baisse du score global , l'extension par son augmentation et la recanalisation par la réduction du score local.

RESULTATS :

Sur les 75 patients , agés en moyenne de 62 ans , 1275 segments veineux ont été étudiés (17 segments par patient). 343 segments étaient thrombosés (27%). La répartition selon le coté était à peu près comparable (44,6% à droite et 55,4% à gauche). 11 patients avaient une embolie pulmonaire symptomatique (14,7%) et 16 une embolie pulmonaire asymtomatique (21,3%). La distribution topographique de la thrombose est résumé dans le tableau 1 . 33 patients avaient une thrombose suro-popliteo - femorale. L'évolution du score échographique global montre un faible taux de régréssion dans les 10 premiers jours et surtout une extension ou une augmentation de la thrombose in situ dans 8 % des cas entre J0 et J2. Une régression du score global était de 51 % à un mois, de 72% à 3 mois et 84% au bout d'un an (tableau 2) .Au total 28 TVP ont complétement régréssé. L'évolution du score échographique veine par veine a permis de définir des profils évolutifs différents en fonction du site de la TVP : Les thromboses surales , poplitees et femorales superficielles avaient des scores de base identiques et une vitesse de régréssion comparable et importante . Les atteintes de la fémorale commune s'accompagnait d'un score de base plus bas , mais la vitesse de régréssion était similaire . En revanche , les thromboses iliaques avaient des scores de base significativement plus bas et leur vitesse de régression était plus lente (tableau 4). L'évolution de la thrombose selon le coté atteint montrait un score échographique significativement plus bas à droite , mais la vitesse de régression était comparable des 2 cotés.

53,6% des sujets qui présentaient un pôle supérieur de thrombus mobile avaient une embolie pulmonaire symptomatique ou asymptomatique contre 23% chez ceux qui avaient un pôle supérieur de thrombus immobile (p<0,01). Ce critère peut être retenu comme un facteur emboligène . A J10 , la deuxième scintigraphie a mis en évidence 4 (5,5%) nouvelles embolie pulmonaire sous traitement héparinique bien conduit , 2 sur thrombus mobiles et 2 sur thrombus immobiles. Sur les 28 thrombi mobiles initialement , 50% étaient adhérents à J5 et 70% à J10. A J30 , on ne retrouvait plus qu'un seul thrombus mobile . Le rapport entre l'existence d'une embolie pulmonaire (EP) et la topographie du thrombus montrait 43% d'EP pour les thromboses surales , 43% à partir de la poplitée et 45% pour les femorales. A l'inverse , sur les 19 TVP iliaques (17 gauches et 3 extension cave), on dénombrait 12% d'EP. Enfin , il n'y avait pas de liaison entre l'embolie pulmonaire et le score échographique .

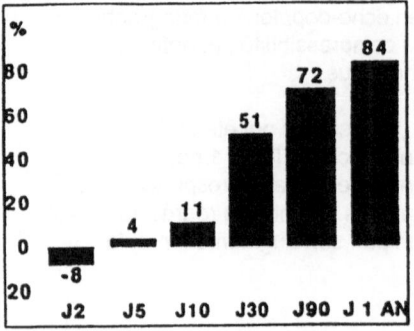

Tableau 2.
POURCENTAGE DE REGRESSION DU SCORE GLOBAL

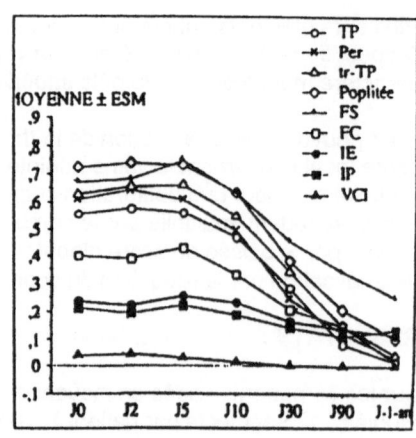

Tableau 4.
EVOLUTION DU SCORE ECHOGRAPHIQUE
VEINE PAR VEINE

REFERENCES

1. Baldridge ED , Martin MA , Welling RE
   Clinical significance of free floating venous thrombi.
   J.Vasc Surg 1990; 11:62-69.

2. Barrelier MT
   Echographie veineuse des membres inférieurs dans le diagnostic des
   thromboses. Méthodologie d'examen et de présentation des résultas.
   Artères et veines , 1991 ,10, 6,440–446

3. Berry RE , Georges JE , Shaver WO
   Free floating deep venous thrombosis : a retrospective study
   Ann Surg 1990; 211 ;719-23

4. Bosson JL , Djedidi M , Pichot O , Carpentier PH
   Quantification des thromboses veineuses profondes en echographie. Etude
   de reproductibilité . Communication ANGIO GENEVE 94 . Octobre 1994.

5. Elias A
   Detection par échographie Doppler des thromboses veineuses profondes des
   membres inférieurs : Techniques , valeur diagnostique, avantages et limites
   JEMU , 1992 ; 13;4, 195-206.

6. Heuboer H , Jongbloets LM , Buller HR , Lensing AWA , Ten cate JW
   Clinical utility of real time compression ultrasonography for diagnostic
   management of patients with recurrent venous thrombosis
   Acta Radiologica 33 , 1992 , Fasc 4

7. Koopman MMW , Buller HR , Ten cate JW
   The disgnosis of recrrent deep vein thrombosis
   Haemostasis 1994 , in press.

8. Krupski WC ,Ralph B , Bernstein E, Shirley M
   Propagation of deep venous thrombosis identified by duplex ultrasonography.
   J. Vasc Surg ,1990 ;12;4;467-75

9. Prandoni P , Cogo A , Bernadi E , Villalta S,Polistena P and al
   A simple ultrasound approach for detection of reccurent proximal vein
   thrombosis. Circulation 1993;88;4 1730-1735

10. Ramshorst B , Bemmelen P , Hoeneveid H, Faber J ,Eikelboom B
    Thrombus regression in deep venous thrombolysis with duplex scanning
    Circulation ;86 ;2 ;1992 :414-19

Phlebology '95, D. Negus et al. (eds.). Phlebology (1995) Suppl. 1: 671-673

P264

Femoral Artery Flow During Slow Versus Acute Peripheral Vein Occlusion

J. Iwinski, T. Petelenz, A. Gruszka and P. Weiss

IIIrd Clinic of Cardiology, Silesian Medical Academy Katowice, Poland

INTRODUCTION

Deterioration of results were observed in arterial reconsrtuctive surgery for peripheral artery diseases,in the event of peripheral deep vein thrombosis of the limb /PDVT/, even though the affected veins have recanalized[1..4].Based on the experimental model of acute vein occlusion PDVT has been implicated as the decisive factor in graft patency. Shifrin[5] Wright[6] again using an acute model of venous obstruction have shown 50-60% reduction of femoral artery flow during the first few minutes followed by slight increase during the following 2 hours. Hemodynamic characteristic of PDVT is totally different from experimental acute occlusion[7,8].Our study was designed to test the hemodynamics of femoral artery during gradual prolonged calf vein occlusion of the femoral vein /FV/, which leads to reduction of flow in the femoral artery /FA/.

METHODS

Subjects were healthy male volunteers ranging in age from 18 to 32 years,mean 26 +/- 6 who volunteered for the study.The protocol was explained and written consent was obtained from each subject.The study was approved by the Ethical Committee for Human Investigation at our institution.The study was done with subjects in a supine position an identical manner in an air-conditioned room with room temperature of about 25ºC to 26ºC. Vein pressure were measured by High-Fidelity micromanometer/Simonsen -Biazet Denmark Inc./introduced into the femoral vein.The systemic arterial pressure,collateral blood pressure was measured noninvasively using narrow pressure cuff /Red Cuff II Biomet Inc.,Warsaw,Ind. Poland / and strain-gauge transducer /Tycos Instruments Co .USA./ All variables were simultaneously recorded an a multi-channel recorder /Siemens,Inc. Germany / Following a 30 min.period during which baseline measurements of all parameters were made slow occlusion of the calf had begun.All parameters were measured every 60 min. for a period of 3 hours.After total occlusion had been achieved the cuff was deflated all parameters were again measured every 10 min. for 30 min.In acute occlusion of the calf the variables were measured continuously during occlusion as well as 5 min.after release of the cuff.. The following parameters were determined; arterial resistance (A.r), systemic blood pressure (BPS), collateral blood pressure (CBP), volume of femoral artery flow (FAF), venous resistance (V.r), femoral vein pressure (FVP), volume of femoral vein flow (FVF). Study was divided in two parts;

1) 15min.acute occlusion /AC/ of the CV
2) 3 hours slow occlusion /SO/ of the CV

Statistics :

comparison of continuous variables between groups were made by Student's unpaired two-tailed t-test. The relation between continuous variables was evaluated by linear regression. Independence of association was assessed by Stepwise multiple regression. A p value $< 0,05$ was considered significant.

RESULTS

All the experimental results are summarised in table. I and tablel.II.AC of the CV resulted in decrease of FAF 46,2%, $p<0,01$, CBP 40,0% $p<0,01$, A.r 24,1%, FVF 15,4%, and increase of RV 3,7%,FVP 40,0%.Release of the occlusion wasn't followed by reversion of all the parameters to baseline level during 5 min.SC of CV produced after 3 hours maximal drop of FAF 34,7% $p<0,05$, FVF 48% $p<0,01$, A.r 66,6% $p<0,01$, FVP 100,0%, V.r 285,0% $p<0.01$. 30 min after deflation of the venous occluder the parameters tested returned to the baseline value.

Hemodynamics of acute occlusion of peripherial vein
Tab(1)

Indicators	0	15 min. after occlusion		5 min. after deflation	
FAF ml/min	100 %	53,8 p<0,05	-46,2 ⇊	77,9	-22,1 ⇊
CBP mm Hg	100 %	60,0 p<0,05	-40,0 ⇊	80,0	-20,0 ⇊
%					
FVF ml/min	100 %	84,6	-15,4 ⇊	108,3	+8,3 ⇑
FVP mm/Hg	100 %	60	+40 ⇑	120,0	+20,0 ⇑
%					
A.r.	100 %	75,9	+24,1 ⇊	110,3	+10,3 ⇑
V.r.	100 %	103,7	+3,7 ⇑	104,8	+4,8 ⇑

Hemodynamics of prolonged gradual occlusion of peripheral vein.
Tab (2)

Indicators	0	1hour		2 hours		3 hours		after occlusion	
FAF ml/min	100 %	83,8	-16,2 ⇊	69,9 p<0,01	-30,1 ⇊	65,3 p<0,01	-34,7 ⇊	84,0	-16,0 ⇊
CBP mm Hg	100 %	89,2	-10,8 ⇊	140,7 p<0,01	+40,7 ⇑	160,4 p<0,01	+60,4 ⇑	122,0	+22,0 ⇑

%								
FVF ml/min	100 %	72,2	-27,8 ⇓	70,0 p<0,01	-30,0 ⇓	52,0 p<0,01	-48,0 ⇓	121,0	+21,0 ⇑
FVP ml/min	100 %	115,0	+15,0 ⇑	166,5 p<0,01	+66,5 ⇑	200,0 p<0,01	+100,0 ⇑	187,5 p<0,01	+87,5 ⇑
%								
A.r.	100 %	96,0	-4,0 ⇓	42,9 p<0,01	-57,1 ⇓	33,4 p<0,01	-66,6 ⇓	91,5	-8,5 ⇓
V.r.	100 %	159,5 p<0,01	+59,5 ⇑	238,2 p<0,01	+138,2 ⇑	385,0 p<0,01	+285,0 ⇑	155,1	+55,1 ⇑

LEGEND   Table 2 -continued

FAF - Femoral artery flow   A.r. - Arterial resistance
CBP - Collateral blood pressure   V.r. - Venous resistance
FVF - Femoral vein flow   ⇑ – Arise
FVP - Femoral vein pressure   ⇓ – Fall

CONCLUSION:
 both AO and SO of CV cause a significant reduction in FA flow. Decrease in FA flow under SO FV have different pathological mechanism than that responsible for acute vein occlusion. PDVT may change hemodynamic effects of arterial reconstructive surgery.

REFERENCES
1/Eickhoff J.H.,Engell H.C.:Local regulation of blood flow and the occurrence of oedema after arterial reconstruction of the lower limbs.Ann.Surg.195;474-8 1982.
2/Coburn M.,Ashwort Ch.,Francis W.,Morin Ch.,Broukhim M.,-Venous stasis complications of the use of the superficial femoral and popliteal veins for lower extremity bypass.J.Vasc.Surg.1993;17:1005-9.
3/Callam M.J.,Harper DR,Dale JJ,Ruckley CV.Arterial disease in chronic leg ulceration;an underestimated hazard? Lothian and Forth Valley leg ulcer study.BMJ 1987;294:929-31.
4/Morgan RH,Psaila JV,Stone J,Carolan G,Woodcock JP.Postural changes in femoral artery blood flow in normal subjects,patients with peripheral vascular occlusive disease and patients undergoing lumbar sympathectomy,measured by duplex ultrasound flowmetry.Eur.J.Vasc.Surg.1992;6:408-15.
5/Wright CB,Swan KG,Hemodynamics of venous occlusion in the canine hind limb.Surg.73:141-6,1973.
6/Shifrin EG,Femoral artery flow in Deep Vein Thrombosis.Hemodynamics of Slow Versus Acute Femoral Vein Occlusion.Angiology 1985,3:154-159.
6/Neglerz P,Raju S.Detection of outflow obstruction in chronic venous insufficiency J.Vasc.Surg.1993;17:583-9.
7/Raju S.A pressure-based technique for the detection of acute and chronic venous obstruction.Phlebology 1988;3:207-16.
8/Whyman MR,Hockins PR,Gillan CL,Allan PL,Donnan PT,Ruckley V,Fowkes GR.Accuracy and reproducibility of duplex ultrasound imaging in a phantom model of femoral artery stenosis.J.Vasc,Surg.1993;17:524-30. /

Phlebology '95, D. Negus et al. (eds.). Phlebology (1995) Suppl. 1: 674-676

OP/19.3

The Incidence of Activated Protein C Resistance in Deep Vein Thrombosis (DVT) Patients

M. Ojiro[1], M. Takenoshita[2], K. Yamazumi[2], R. Toshinaga[2] and M. Kazama[3]

[1] Department of Surgery, Kagoshima Prefectural Ohshima Hospital, Naze, Japan
[2] First Department of Surgery, Faculty of Medicine, Kagoshima University, Kagoshima, Japan
[3] First Department of Internal Medicine, Teikyo University Hospital, Tokyo, Japan

INTRODUCTION

Recently Dahlback[1], Griffin[2], Koster[3], Svensson[4] and Halbmayer[5] described Activated Protein C resistance (APC-R) was founded as many as 20-40% of patients with thrombophilia and this abnormality was main cause of deep vein thrombosis (DVT). Therefore, we investigated how many incidence of APC-R was in DVT patients in Japan.

MATERIALS & METHODS

On 60 cases of DVT patients, 25 cases of ischemic heart diseases (IHD) patients and 32 healthy adults, the APC ratio which was calculated by dividing the clotting time obtained with the APC-calcium chloride solution by the clotting time obtained with calcium chloride alone, was measured by Coatest APC-resistance® (Chromogenix, Sweden) and also Factor-V, proteins S (PS), protein C (PC), anti thrombin III (AT-III) and plasminogen (plg) activity were determined with commercially available function assay; a Factor V clotting assay was performed with factor V deficient plasma, Staclot Protein S® (Boehringer Mannheim, Germany), Testzyme Protein C® (Daiichi, Japan), Testzyme AT-III® (Daiichi, Japan) and Testzyme PLG® (Daiichi, Japan).
The abnormality of Factor V, PS, PC, AT-III and plg was estimated by below 50% of factor V activity, 60%, 65%, 70% and 70% respectively.

RESULTS

The APC ratio of healthy adult plasma was 2.61 ± 0.58 and the lowest level of APC ratio which included 95% of healthy adults was 2.2 (Fig.1). Therefore, although the abnormal range was below 2.0 APC ratio which an explanatory leaflet of this kit showed, we estimated below 2.2 APC ratio was abnormal and suggested these cases had APC-R. Six cases of 60 DVT patients were abnormal (10%) and in 25 cases of IHD patients, 3 cases were suggested APC-R (12%). However, if the abnormal range was based on below 2.0 APC ratio, only three cases of 60 DVT patients (5%) and one case of 25 IHD patients (4%) were APC-R positive. At the same time, in these abnormal APC ratio cases, Factor V and PS activity were normal without one case (Table 1). Although all families of these APC-R cases were not investigated APC ratio, one family line was suggested APC-R was hereditary. On the simultaneously measured PC, PS, AT-III and plg activity, the abnormality was founded in 4 cases (6.7%), 2 cases (3.3%), one case (1.7%) and 0 respectively (Table 2).

DISCUSSION

Dahlback et al. showed a poor anticoagulant response to APC, a anticoagulant serine protease known to inactivated Factor Va and VIIIa in plasma and this APC-R was shown to be inherited and associated with familial thrombophilia. Also, Griffin et al. described this defect was present in 52-64% of thrombophilic patients and Koster et al. recognized 64 patients of 301 DVT patients (21%) who were above 70 years old. Svensson et al. showed high proportion of this APC-R in DVT patients, especially in familial thrombophilic patients. Halbmayer et al. reported 20% of young patients with stroke had APC-R. The prevalence of APC-R in general population is unknown, but its high prevalence in patients with thrombosis suggests that it may be common.

However, our investigated prevalence of APC-R in DVT patients was six cases of 60 DVT patients (10%). Furthermore, even if the abnormal range was based on below 2.0 APC ratio, only three cases was abnormal (5%). Therefore the incidence of APC-R in DVT patients in our study was not so many. This discrepancy might be due to nation, age, recurrence and familial thrombosis. However, this assay method is influenced by low PS level, by reduced level of Factor V, VIII and IX and by platelet[6], therefore these factors must be checked at the same time. Furthermore the range of APC ratio may be depend on not only the measuring instruments, but also various nations. Although de Ronde et al. proposed one possible solution of this problem was the use of the "normalized-APC-SR"[7], the estimate depended on APC ratio is not accurate and this assay method is only a screening test. Therefore it should be necessary to develop a new accurate assay method.

CONCLUSION

Although the assay of APC-R is still now not definite, our study suggested the prevalence of APC-R in DVT patients was not so many (10%).

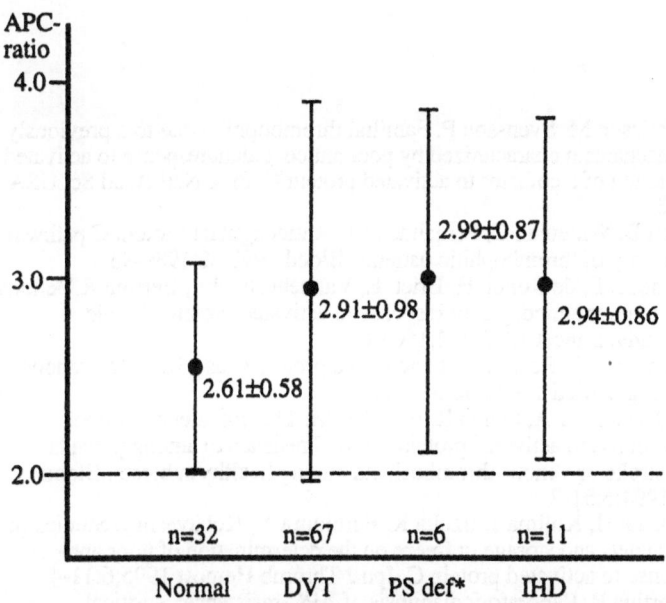

Fig.1. The deviation of APC-ratio in healthy adults, DVT patients, PS deficient patients (PS def*) and IHD patients

Table 1. The details of the cases of abnormal APC-ratio in DVT patients

Case	Sex	Age	DVT	Trigger	APC-R	F-V	PS	PC	AT	plg	LAC
KN§	F	58	Lt Leg	Delivery	2.0	117	69	112	90	96	n.d.
HK	F	33	Lt Leg*	Delivery	2.0	69	68	135	104	99	+
MY	M	48	Rt Leg	Trauma	2.16	113	84	89	95	98	-
EH	F	74	Rt Leg	Unknown	2.04	132	91	110	98	110	n.d.
MK	M	44	Lt Leg	Unknown	2.16	154	199	122	103	128	n.d.
SK	M	57	Lt Leg*	Unknown	2.18	82	44↓	90	92	106	+

§; This patient (KN) was suspected to be familial APC-R, *; Recurrence
F-V; Factor V, AT; AT-III, LAC; Lupus anticoagulant, n.d.; not done

Table 2. The prevalence of APC-R, PS, PC, AT-III and plg abnormality among patient with DVT

Factors		No.	%
APC-R		6	10.0
PS	(<50%)	4	6.7
PC	(<60%)	2	3.3
AT-III	(<70%)	1	1.7
Plg	(<70%)	0	0
Total (n=60)		13	21.7

REFERENCES

1. Dahlback B, Carlsson M, Svensson P. Familial thrombophilia due to a previously unrecognized mechanism characterized by poor anticoagulant respense to activated protein C; prediction of a cofactor to activated protein C. Proc Natl Acad Sci USA 1993;90:1004-8
2. Griffin JH, Evatt B, Wideman C, Fernandez JA. Anticoagulant protein C pathway defective in majority of thrombophilic patients. Blood 1993;82:1989-93
3. Koster T, Rosendaal F, de Ronde H, Briet E, Vandenbrouck J, Bertina R.Venous thrombosis due to poor anticoagulant response to activated protein C; Leiden thrombophilia study. Lancet 1993;342:1503-6
4. Svensson P, Dahlback B. Resistance to activated protein C as a basis for venous thrombosis. N Engl J Med 1994;330:517-22
5. Halbmayer W, Haushofer A, Schon R, Fishcher M. The prevalence of poor anticoagulant response to activated protein C (APC resistance) among patients suffering from stroke or venous thrombosi and among healthy subjects. Blood Coag Fibrinol 1994;5:51-7
6. Shizuka R, Amagai H, Kojima J, Iizuka K, Furumura Y, Kobayashi I. Studies on the effects of platelets and storage in freeze on the determination of poor anti-coagulant response to activated protein C. Jpn J Thromb Hemost 1995;6:11-4
7. de Ronde H, Bertina R. Laboratory diagnosis of APC-resistance; a critical evaluation of the test and the development of diagnostic criteria. Thromb Haemost 1994;72:880-6

Phlebology '95, D. Negus et al. (eds.). Phlebology (1995) Suppl. 1: 677-678

P266

Cold as a Cause of Superficial Thrombophlebitis

R. Benoit

Angiology Practice, Beau-Soleil 12, 1206 Geneve, Switzerland

Introduction

Cold is a well known cause of a number of vascular deseases such as Raynaud phenomenon, chilblain, frostbite, trench foot...

Cold is also becoming an important therapeutic aid in sports medicine and traumatology. Nerve injury and skin frostbite are recognised side effects of cold application. For the first time we report 3 cases of superficial thrombophlebitis due to cold therapy.

Case reports

Case 1. Man 53 y. A regular jogger, one day he feels an unusual pain around the left knee at the infero-medial side, and treats himself with a (very) cold pack for long periods that same day. However, he can't walk better the following days and he must see a physician after a week. There is a typical appearance of a dermo-hypodermitis by the inner side of the knee, but the echography reveals an extended thrombus in the vena saphena magna (VSM) from mid-calf to mid-thigh. He was treated by subcutaneous low molecular weight heparin(LMWH) only, and was fine after 5 days already. Months later, the vein was normal, there was no reflux at echo-doppler test.

Case 2. Female 50 y. Spending holidays in Antillas Islands, she twisted her left knee during a hard walk in a forest. She was given diclofenac gel and a cold pack, but next day already she could feel a cord above the inner side of the distal half of the thigh. The local treatment of that pseudohypodermitis didn't help and 3 weeks later the correct diagnosis was made only when she was eventually seen by the angiologist. The inflammation was still obvious but disappeared in ten days with compression and s.c. LMWH. At 6 months follow up the thrombus was still occluding the vein.

Case 3. Female 38 y. She feels a sharp pain in her left knee when playing football with her children. As soon as she can she applies a cold pack on the inner side of her knee. Hours later, the area is swollen, reddish an painful. The physician consulted prescribes an antibiotic because of the infectious appearance of the lesion. After a week, beeing still disabled, she was seen by the angiologist and the diagnosis of VSM thrombophlebitis was made at echography only because it was clinically impossible, owing to the importance of the inflammation.

Discussion

The 3 cases reported are didactic because they are similar. In all 3 there is a knee traumatism, not too serious, of the medial side. The patients are treated with cold for long periods (hours) and an extensive inflammation occurs rapidly (skin frostbite appearing as dermo-hypodermitis or even as infectious dermatitis). Only days or weeks later, for lack of amelioration, the patients were referred to the specialist and the extended thrombophlebitis of the VSM could be diagnosed thanks the duplex scan.
Since the thrombus may approach the cross we believe that it is safer to give these patients an anticoagulant treatment. In one case the vein was varicose but the most delayed recovery was not that one.

Conclusion

Cold packs or ice bags have to be used carrefully in patients with knee lesions of the medial side, because the freezing cold may harm the skin, causing frostbite and may harm the VSM too, causing thrombophlebitis, a difficult diagnosis in this case owing to the extensive skin inflammation overlying the phlebitis.

Reference

Kaul MP, Herring SA. Superficial Heat and Cold. The physician and sportsmedicine. 1994;22(12):65-74.

Phlebology '95, D. Negus et al. (eds.). Phlebology (1995) Suppl. 1: 679-680

OP/8.6

Deaths from Pulmonary Embolism in the United States

G. Johnson Jr. and J. Ligush Jr.

Department of Surgery, University of North Carolina at Chapel Hill, 210 Burnett-Womack, CB# 7210, Chapel Hill, NC 27599, USA

INTRODUCTION

"If estimates of deaths from pulmonary embolism include both those cases in which pulmonary embolism was the sole cause of death and those in which it was a major contributory cause, both Coon and Willis and Hume, Sevitt, and Thomas arrive at a figure between 142,000 and approximately 200,000 deaths per year."[1] This statement, made 20 years ago after a community population study was done in Tecumseh, Michigan, has been cited as an accurate estimate of the number of people who die each year in the United States from pulmonary embolus (PE). Yet statistics from the Department of Health and Human Resources (DHHR) in 1990 reported this figure to be 9,472 [2]. The wide variation is probably due to the difficulty in making an accurate diagnosis of pulmonary embolism. This paper will be an attempt to estimate the number of deaths from PE in the USA using several different data bases.

METHODS

The data bases used include: 1) the well-documented population based study from Worcester, MA, USA [3] for 1985, which was extended to the US population; 2) the North Carolina Medical Database (NCDB) [4] for 1993, which records all hospital discharges by diagnostic related codes (DRG), and was extended to the US population; and 3) mortality for the US population from the DHHR [2] statistical data for ICD-9 code 415.1, which is based on death certificates.

Realizing the latter two data bases depend on the clinical diagnosis of pulmonary embolus, the accuracy of the clinical diagnosis at the University of North Carolina Hospitals, based on autopsy data, was used as a "correction factor" (UNC-CF).

RESULTS

In the Worcester study there were 23 PE per 100,000 population for the year 1985. The USA population was 238 million, suggesting 54,740 people had a PE that year. There was a 23% immediate mortality (an unusually high mortality) in Worcester, or 12,590 in the USA.

For the 195 clinical diagnoses of PE on the death certificate of 5,682 autopsies done at UNC hospitals from 1972 to 1989, there were a total of 143 or 0.73 (UNC-CF) patients who had a major PE (one the prosector thought substantially contributed to the patient's death).

Using the NCDB, there were 450 deaths reported due to PE in a population of 6.7 million people. Correcting it for errors in clinical diagnosis based the UNC-CF (0.73 x 450 = 329) and extrapolating to the USA population of 254 million for 1992, the mortality for PE in the USA for 1992 was predicted to have been 12,254.

The 9,472 deaths reported by the DHHR for 1990 after being corrected by the UNC-CF became 6,914 (9,472 x 0.73).

SUMMARY: Deaths in the USA from PE

DATABASE
Worcester	12,590
NCDB	12,254
DHHR	6,914

DISCUSSION

None of these databases estimates the number of deaths from PE in the USA to be near the numbers previously reported.

The Worcester population is not representative of the United States population as a whole. For example, the Worcester population is mostly white. Mortality for PE among whites according to the data from the DHHR is 4.1/100,000 compared with the mortality in blacks, which is 6.2 (51% higher). Because blacks make up 15.2% of the USA population, this would increase the estimated USA mortality.

On the other hand, the mortality for PE in the Worcester series was reported to be 23%, approximately 10 times greater than the 2.5% recently reported in 1992 by Carson et al.[5] from a multicenter experience. This might overestimate the number of deaths in the USA.

The inaccuracy of death certificate reporting has been studied. In 1983, Dismuke [6] reported after reviewing 2,398 autopsies that the sensitivity and specificity of the death certificates were 37.2% and 94.9% respectively. This may be misleading. Another way of looking at their data is that, of the 169 death certificates with PE listed as a major cause of death, 54 (32.0%) in fact proved to have had a major PE; of the 145 patients who had a major PE at autopsy, 54 (37.2%) had been predicted on the death certificate.

Although the data derived from DRGs is relatively accurate because reimbursement depends on it, it reflects only in-hospital deaths.

All of the estimates based on hospital autopsy data (UNC-CF) will undoubtedly overestimate the deaths from PE. Because this is primarily an in-hospital disease, the hospital incidence will be high and cannot be extrapolated to the population at large.

The UNC-CF is based on diagnoses from a referral center with ready access to all the current diagnostic modalities. Thus the data probably overestimate the accuracy of the clinical diagnosis. This would tend to underestimate the deaths from PE in the USA.

Despite the above mentioned flaws, the authors consider this to be very provocative information. It suggests that the number of deaths from PE in the USA has been tremendously overestimated. The correct number will be impossible to determine until the accurate diagnosis of PE can be made in a simple manner.

This study should not detract from the efforts toward prophylaxis against a lethal hospital disease that can potentially be prevented.

REFERENCES

1. Coon WW, Willis III PW, Keller JB. Venous thromboembolism and other venous disease in the Tecumseh Community Health Study. Circulation 1973;48:839-46.
2. Vital Statistics of the United States 1990, Volume II, Mortality, Part A, U.S. Department of Health and Human Services.
3. Anderson Jr FA, Wheeler HB, Goldberg RJ, Hosmer DW, Patwardhan JA, Jovanovic B, Forcier A, Dalen JE. A population-based perspective of the hospital incidence and case-fatality rates of deep vein thrombosis and pulmonary embolism. Arch Int Med 1991;151:933-8.
4. North Carolina Medical Database Commission. North Carolina Hospital Discharge Data, January 1, 1988-September 30, 1993.
5. Carson JL, Kelley MA, Duff A, Weg JG, Fulkerson WJ, Palevsky HI, Schwartz JS, Thompson BT, Popovich Jr J, Hobbins TE, Spera MA, Alavi A, Terrin ML. The clinical course of pulmonary embolism. N Engl J Med 1992;326:1240-5.
6. Dismuke SE, VanderZwaag R. Accuracy and epidemiological implications of the death certificate diagnosis of pulmonary embolism. J Chron Dis 1984;37:67-73.

Phlebology '95, D. Negus et al. (eds.). Phlebology (1995) Suppl. 1:681-683

OP/2.6

Air Plethysmography versus Venography and/or Duplex Scanning in the Diagnosis of Acute Deep Vein Thrombosis

Evi Kalodiki, S.K. Volteas and A.N. Nicolaides

Academic Surgical and Vascular Unit, St Mary's Hospital Medical School, London, UK

INTRODUCTION

Air plethysmography (APG) is highly accurate in vein reflux studies [1-3], for the assessment of the calf muscle pump function [4] and for the detection of outflow fraction (OF) in chronic venous insufficiency (CVI) [5-7]. Studies that tested the ability of APG in the detection of acute deep vein thrombosis (DVT) however, failed to demonstrate the full potential of the method, especially in the calf; this was due to the use of OF in the first second without, (OF_1), or with occlusion of the superficial veins (OF/SO_1) as the only crierion [8]. We tested the hypothesis that the calculation of the OF not only at the 1st second (OF_1) but also at the 2nd and 3rd second, without (OF_2, OF_3) or with superficial occlusion $(OF/SO_2, OF/SO_3)$, could improve the efficacy of APG in the detection of the suspected acute DVT; we also took into account the venous volume (VV) as it reduces in the presence of an haemodynamically significant thrombus.

MATERIALS AND METHODS

The normal values of $OF_{1,2,3}$, $OF/SO_{1,2,3}$ and VV were established in the first part of this study using 200 volunteers (200 legs). All subjects were first examined with venography and/or colour flow Duplex imaging (CFDI) to exclude thrombosis of the leg examined; APG examination was then performed, using the standard technique as developed in our institution [7]. In part II of our study we applied these normal values on 300 legs of patients referred to us to be investigated for suspected acute DVT; patients were first examined with venography and/or CFDI followed by APG.

RESULTS

As normal we considered $OF_{1,2,3}$ values greater than 31%, 50% and 61% respectively, $OF/SO_{1,2,3}$ values greater than 25%, 40% and 48% and VV values greater than 70ml.
   Thrombosis was detected in 134 out of the 300 patients (45%). It was proximal in 67, proximal and distal (extended) in 41 and distal (calf) in 26 patients. Using only OF_1 and

OF/SO$_1$ APG identified 99 DVTs (74%). It also gave 17 false positive and 6 false negative results. The sensitivity was 74%, the specificity 90%, the positive predictive value 85%, the negative predictive value 81% and the overall accuracy 83%.

When we applied our additional criteria by calculating OF$_{2,3}$, OF/SO$_{2,3}$ and VV, APG was diagnostic (positive identification or suspicion) in 122 DVTs (91%). Overall APG missed 12 DVTs: in 6 the thrombosis was proximal with a small thrombus partially occluding the vein lumen and in 6 it was distal caused by isolated calf thrombi. In the 17 patients in whom APG, using OF$_1$ or OF/SO$_1$ gave false positive results, the values of OF$_{2,3}$, OF/SO$_{2,3}$ and VV were all normal. By applying the additional criteria the sensitivity improved from 74% to 91%, the specificity from 90% to 100%, the positive predictive value from 85% to 100%, the negative predictive value from 81% to 93% and the overall accuracy from 83% to 96%. (Table 1).

DISCUSSION

The demand for CFDI is today remarcably high because of its accuracy [9]: the necessity of simple screening tests, like APG, has become therefore evident. If a method can efficiently identify the legs that do or do not have DVT this will result in important savings in scanning time, as only the suspicious cases will need further investigation with CFDI.

The reported relatively low accuracy of APG in the detection of calf DVT [8] can probably be explained by the fact that only OF$_1$ or OF/SO$_1$ and not the whole outflow curve was taken into account so far (Figure 1). In the present study we analyzed up to the 3rd second of the outflow curve (figure 1).

On analyzing our results, 149 out of the 166 negative patients had all tested values negative on APG. The remaining 17 patients with abnormal OF$_1$ and/or OF/SO$_1$ values (although very close to normal), had the OF$_{2,3}$, OF/SO$_{2,3}$ and VV values normal. These patients should be considered suspicious and CFDI is needed to exclude DVT. CFDI was also needed in 10 DVT patients; 3 with extended (with abnormal VV values) and 7 with calf DVT (2 with OF/SO$_2$ and 5 with VV abnormal values). Using APG as a screening test, only these 27 patients (9%) who had either OF/SO$_1$ and/or VV abnormal would need CFDI to establish the diagnosis; this is both cost-effective and screening time preserving, while the danger of missing a significant thrombosis is low (4%). Further diagnostic improvement could be achieved by combining APG with other quick and sensitive screening methods, and liquid crystal thermography looks promising in this field [9].

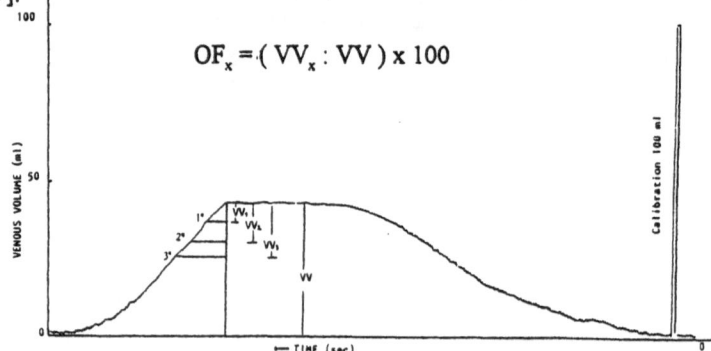

$$OF_x = (VV_x : VV) \times 100$$

Figure 1. Recording of the outflow curve and calculation of OF with APG.

We conclude that additional criteria should be applied when using APG in the detection of the suspected acute DVT, especially when using the computerised version of the traditional instrument that can easily adopt and calculate them; we also conclude that APG, a reliable, accurate, easy-to-perform and inexpensive diagnostic tool, could be used as a screening test for the diagnosis of acute DVT.

Table 1. The diagnostic value of APG using the standard and the additional criteria

		Standard Criteria OF_1 or OF/SO_1			Additional criteria $OF_{1,2,3}$ or $OF/SO_{1,2,3}$ and VV		
		+	-	TOTAL	+	-	TOTAL
Venography	+	99	35	134	122	12	134
and/or							
CFDI	-	17	149	166	0	166	166
	TOTAL	116	184	300	122	178	300

Sensitivity	74%	91%
Specificity	90%	100%
Positive predictive value	85%	100%
Negative predictive value	81%	93%
Overall accuracy	83%	96%

REFERENCES

1. Christopoulos D, Nicolaides AN, Szendro G. Venous reflux: quantification and correlation with the clinical severity of chronic venous disease. Br J Surg 1988; 75:352-6.
2. Katz ML, Comerota AJ, Kerr R. Air plethysmography (APG): a new technique to evaluate patients with chronic venous insufficiency. J Vasc Technol 1991;15: 23-7.
3. Neglen P, Raju S. A rational approach to detection of significant reflux with duplex Doppler scanning and air plethysmography. J Vasc Surg 1993;17:590-5.
4. Tierney S, Burke P, Fitzegerald P et al. Venous pump function is impaired after ankle fractures. Br J Surg 1992; 79(4):368 (Abst).
5. Christopoulos D, Nicolaides AN, Duffy P, Georgiou I. Noninvasive diagnosis and quantification of outflow obstruction in venous disease. J Cardiovasc Surg 1989;30:72-3 (Abst).
6. Neglen P, Raju S. Detection of outflow obstruction in chronic venous insufficiency. J Vasc Surg 1993;17:583-9.
7. Christopoulos D, Nicolaides AN, Belcaro G. Air plethysmography. Phlebology Digest 1992; 4(3):4-11.
8. Nicolaides AN, Kalodiki E, Christopoulos D, Leon M, Volteas N. Diagnosis of deep vein thrombosis by air-plethysmography. In: Vascular diagnosis, EF Bernstein editor, Mosby-Year book Inc 1993; 830-1.
9. Kalodiki E, Marston R, Volteas N et al. The combination of liquid crystal thermography and duplex scanning in the diagnosis of deep vein thrombosis. Eur J Vasc Surg 1992; 6: 311-16.

OP/19.2

FIBRINOLYTIC DISTURBANCES IN PATIENTS WITH KLINEFELTER SYNDROME COMPLICATED BY ULCERATION OF THE LEG.

J C J M Veraart[1], C E G Pernot[2], K Hamulyak[2], H A M Neumann[1]
From the Department of Dermatology and Haematology[2], Academisch Ziekenhuis, Maastricht, the Netherlands

Objective: To investigate fibrinolytic parameters in patients with Klinefelter's syndrome (sexual differentiation in men, with two or more X-chromosomes, affecting 1 in 500 males). Leg ulcers, especially in combination with hyperpigmentation, have been reported in association with Klinefelter's syndrome and are usually attributed to venous disease in these patients.

Design: Open clinical investigation.

Patients: 8 patients with Klinefelter's syndrome were studied. 4 of them had leg ulcers and skin changes on both legs resembling CVI. All patients with ulceration had these manifestations since they were about 25 years of age. The other 4 had no ulceration nor skin changes.

Measurement: Patients were investigated with the aid of a light reflection rheography, Doppler ultrasonography, Duplex scanning and phlebography for venous diseases. Furthermore routine and specialised hemostatic investigations were performed.

Results: We could exclude venous abnormalities in most of the patients. Routine blood investigations were without abnormalities. Fasting levels of plasminogen activator inhibitor 1 (PAI-1) activity were markedly increased (mean 28.25 U/L) in the ulcer group, also after 10 minutes of venous occlusion. Klinefelter patients without ulceration had normal fibrinolytic parameters (mean: 13 U/L). Treatment with testosterone did not influence these parameters.

Conclusions: The results suggest a disturbed fibrinolysis and diminished response to venous occlusion. The inhibitors of fibrinolysis may therefore play a role in the pathogenesis of the skin alterations seen in venous insufficiency. Patients with Klinefelter's syndrome, especially if complicated with skin changes and ulceration on the leg, can be used a study model for the skin alterations that occur in chronic venous insufficiency.

P254

PULMONARY EMBOLISM RISK AND CORRELATION WITH SITING AND ECHOGRAPHIC ASPECT OF THROMBUS

Todini A.R., Antignani P.L., Paiella M.L., Bartolo M.
Department of Angiology, s.Camillo Hospital, Rome, Italy

Objective: It is difficult to discern the danger in a case of thrombophlebitis without the direct identification of the thrombus. In these cases we prefer ecography to phlebography. The most important datum from this method is the masurement of the condition of risk and embolization of the venous thrombus. We wanted to differentiate the cases at risk from those not at risk of pulmonary embolism and the causes which determine it.

Design: We used the Acuson 164 colour Doppler daily to study the superficial and deep venous system of the lower limbs and abdomen.

Patients: 184 consecutive subjects affected by phlebothrombosis of the lower limbs, admitted to our Department of Angiology.

Results: Alongside the already known aspects of the floating, peduncolate and mobile thrombus, the most significant appearce of the thrombus we found to be the "cutting off" the same with a typical appearance of "the mouthpiece of a flute" when the vein is joined by a collateral vein at an angle and fully charged with blood (killer vein). This scenario is a sign of an embolism that has already occured (35,5%) in our case histories of which 8,1% are without symptoms. The most frequent siting of embolisms is the area of convergence of the important veins: the femoral vein, the popliteal vein, the iliac veins and the cava vein.

Conclusions: The eco Doppler undertaken daily aids us significantly and includes the evolution of the thromboembolism which until now was impossible to evaluate eith the traditional invasive methods.

P256

PULMONARY EMBOLISM AND VENOUS PATHOLOGIES CORRELATED.

Eleuteri P; Manni C.; Villeggia P.

Private Laboratory, Rome, Italy

Objective:To compare the venous diseases and pulmonary embolism (P.E.),investigated by Radionuclide Venography(R.N.V.) and Perfusional Pulmonary Scintigraphy (P.P.S.).
Design: Retrospective review.
Patients: 1095 patients with varios venous pathologies.
Method:All patients were submitted to R.N.V. and contemporary to P.P.S.
Measurements:P.P.S. were examinated by PIOPED criteria and the RNV utilizing the method described by Eleuteri ,1985. (1)
Results:The multisegment obstructions of venous system shows the greatest incidence of PE,with 25 cases of High Probability(HP) and 25 cases of Intermediate P. a total of 112 and only 2 cases were knowed in anamnesis. Then follows the obstruction of left iliac vein with 17 cases of HP and 18 of IP a total of 117 cases, and only 4 cases were acquainted in anamnesis.
Conclusions:The RNV and the PPS offer high reliability in the diagnosis of venous diseases especially where the clinical symptoms are difficult to interprete.

1)Eleuteri P,Villeggia P,Manni GB in Phlebology 85, London 1985,pg. 428-432;

P258

VEIN THROMBOSIS PROPHYLAXIS AFTER RECTAL AND SIGMOID CANCER SURGERY IN CLINICAL EXPERIENCE.

Zbroński R, Pardela M, Urbaniak A, Lemieszewski A, Kozłowski A, Piecuch J,
2nd Department and Clinic of General Surgery and Vessels, Zabrze, Poland

Objective:To evaluate the efficiacy and safety of applying a low-molecular-weight heparin in the perioperative prophylaxis of lower limbs deep thrombosis.
Design:Prospective evaluation of a homogenous group of patients.
Patients:102 patients after operation caused cancer of sigmoid and rectum.
Intervention:Prior to and following the surgical treatment the deep vein condition was determined by physical and Doppler examinations. All patients were adminstered treatment included low-molecular-weight heparin /Fraxiparine,Clexane/,physiotherapy and earlier mobilisation. Safety of this management was evaluated on the basis of haemorrhage complications. On the average heparin was administered for five days.
Measurements:Before and after surgery essential parameters of the coagulation were determined. Incidence of deep vein thrombosis was estimated.
Results:Deep vein thrombosis was found in eight patients but did not cause any deaths,which was confirmed by autopsies.
Conclusion:Low-molecular-weight heparins are efficacious agents in prophylaxis of lower limbs deep vein thrombosis. This is a safe,simple method of prophylaxis of lower limbs deep vein thrombosis.

OP/8.2

THE INCIDENCE OF ACUTE DEEP LEG VEIN THROMBOSIS IN DIFFERENT GROUPS OF AGES

Björgell O, Nylander G
Dept of Radiology, University Hospital MAS, University of Lund, Malmö, Sweden

Objective: To determine the incidence of deep vein thrombosis (DVT) in different groups of ages.

Design: Retrospective review of a consecutive series.

Patients: 2069 acute phlebographies, performed in a two-year period on query thrombosis.

Measurements: Ascending phlebography was performed as a two-step procedure in vertical and supine position allowing most patients to be examined. All phlebographies were reviewed and classified as normal or with DVT.

Results: 72 (3,5%) examinations failed. Three files were lost. 1994 examinations were possible to classify, corresponding to 1838 patients. In 847 (46%) patients a DVT was found. 44% were males and 56% females. The total incidence of DVT was 1.83/1000 (in females 1.94/1000, in males 1.71/1000). No one of the thrombosis was found below the age of 20, and thrombosis was uncommon below the age of 40, less than 0.2/1000.

From the age of 40 the incidence increased in both sexes. 86% (67/78) of all females below the age of 36, who underwent phlebography, did not suffer from DVT.

Conclusions: In about half of all phlebographies a DVT was found. Few patients below the age of 40 had thrombosis and no one below the age of 20. Of the patients without DVT there was a predominance of females below the age of 36.

P025

FACTOR V ANOMALIES: ASSOCIATED THROMBOEMBOLIC EVENTS (STUDY OF TWO FAMILIES).

Cattabiani MI., Bernardi F*, Ieran M, Moratti A.
Dept Medical Angiology, Arcispedale S. Maria Nuova
Reggio Emilia, Italy
*Dept Molecular Biochemistry and Biology, University of Ferrar, Italy

Objective: To study the frequent thromboembolic events in two families with factor V anomalies.

Patients: Neri's family had 4 thromboembolic events (the prospositus, the parents and a son). Among the studied subjects the prospositus and her son presented with factor V deficiency. In Bartoli's family 6 subjects presented with thromboembolic events (prospositus, parents and three sons); three of them had factor V deficiency.

Methods and Results: The presence of the FV Leiden (R506Q), found to be associated with inherited thrombophilias (APC resistance), was excluded in both prospositi and in two members of their families by PCR amplification and restriction analysis of exon 10.
Novel F.V gene polymorphisms, investigated in the same subjects, indicate that a different genetic background is associated with the F V deficiency in the two families. FV platelet mRNA was studied by reverse transcription and PCR. The nucleotide sequence of the amplified products is under investigation.

Conclusions: F.V Leiden is not responsible for the inherited thrombophilia in these subjects.
Different F.V gene defects are probably responsible for the F.V deficiency in the two families.

P261

VENOUS THROMBOSIS OF THE EXTREMITIES.

Pollice F., Salerno F.

Institute of Cardiovascular Surgery, University of Bari, Italy.

Objective: To evaluate differences in late sequelae between patients with subclavian and iliofemoral vein thrombosis.

Design: Retrospective review of a consecutive series.

Patients: The chart of all patients with a diagnosis of iliofemoral venous thrombosis or subclavian vein thrombosis over a 6-year period were reviewed.There were 59 patients with iliofemoral venous thrombosis and 18 patients with subclavian vein thrombosis. Iliofemoral venous thromboses were three times more common, showed the classic leftside predominance and were more likely to be idiopathie.Subclavian vein thromboses showed no side or sex predilection and were due to anatomic abnormalities,intra-venous lines, or radiation.

Intervention: Those patients without contraindications were treated with lytic agents in appropriate doses for 24 to 72 hours.There were six patients in the subclavian vein thrombosis group who only had removal of a central line or refused all treatment.All remaining patients were treated with intravenous heparin to increase the partial thromboplasmin time to 1½ times normal for 7 to 10 days.

Results: Lytic therapy was used in six cases of subclavian vein thromboses and was successful in all six.Iliofemoral venous thrombosis,however, was successfully treated with lytic therapy in only 4 of 14 patients. In-travenous heaprin was successful in ameliorating the acute symptoms in both groups.

Conclusions: We see that massive venous thromboses of the extremities,al-though similar in their acute effect of venous hypertension,swelling, do not manifest the same long-term sequelae.They should be viewed as separa-te and distinct entities that must be diagnosed early and treated effe-ctively in order to minimize the long-term effects of venous disease.

P263

LONG TERM EFFECTS OF DEEP VENOUS THROMBOSIS

Robb G M

New Westminster Vein Clinic, 501 - 625 5th Avenue, New Westminster, BC, Canada V3M 1X4

Objective: To review the long term effects of deep vein thrombosis on venous function, and assess the importance of a history of DVT on subsequent symptoms.

Design: A retrospective study to review the long term effects of deep venous thrombosis in the 6% of patients presenting with such a history between 1970 and 1980 as evidenced by subsequent follow up.

Results: Aching in the leg was experienced by most patients. In 47% swelling was a problem; 34% presented with ulceration.

Conclusions: Prior to DVT will usually lead to significant symptoms. These can be helped significantly by the methods employed to deal with the superficial venous problem. Results are compared to a group of patients aged over 80 years and another group presenting with severe ankle swelling.

P265

PROBLEMS OF THE DEEP VEIN THROMBOSIS IN THE GASTROENTEROLOGICAL SURGERY

Oczkowicz, Lorenc Z, Kusmierski A, Caban A, Malczyk M

I Department of Surgery, Silesian Medical Academy in Katowice Szpital Górniczy, 41-200 Sosnowiec, Poland

The purpose of the study was to assess the efficacy of perioperational prophylaxis during the last 20 years.
The risk factors assumed were: age above 60 years, obesity, heart diseases, malignant neoplasm of the alimentary duct, varicose veins of the lower limbs or past deep vein thrombosis, long term immobilisation - allowing 1 point for each factor. In the high-risk group of patients with the occurrence of thrombotic and embolic complications, who has surgical treatment because of neoplastic diseases of alimentary duct, and received 3 points in the aforenamed scale, 1038 patients were subjected to retrospective analysis.
In this group perioperational prophylaxis was applied to 316 patients, making up 30.4% of the total number of operated patients, whereas thrombotic and embolic complications occurred in 32 patients (10.1%). In a group of 722 patients not subjected to prophylaxis complications occurred in 154 patients, i.e. 21.3%.
Results: Without prophylaxis – in 722 patients, thrombosis in 154 patients (21.3%); Aspirin - in 76 patients, thrombosis in 13 patients (17.1%), risk reduction - 19.7%; Heparin - in 95 patients, thrombosis in 9 patients (9.5%), risk reduction - 55.4%; LMW heparin - in 81 patients, thrombosis in 6 patients (7.4%), risk reduction - 65.3%; f.p* + haemodilution – in 64 patients, thrombosis in 4 patients (6.25%), risk reduction - 71%.
f.p* - pharmacological prophylaxis
Conclusions: In the high-risk group the application of pharmacological prophylaxis reduces the frequency of thrombotic and embolic complications. Haemodilution, apart from the possibility of protecting the patient's own blood for surgery, is also a prevention factor for patients threatened with occurrence of complications.

OP/8.4

FREQUENCY OF PULMONARY EMBOLISM (PE) IN PATIENTS PRESENTING WITH PROXIMAL DEEP VEIN THROMBOSIS (DVT).

Hull R.D., Elliott C.G., Pineo G.F., Brant R.F.

The Canadian-American Thrombosis Group and the University of Calgary, Alberta, Canada.

Objective: To determine the frequency of PE in patients presenting with documented proximal DVT.

Design: A randomized clinical trial comparing the efficacy and safety of once daily subcutaneous low-molecular-weight heparin (LMWH) with continuous intravenous heparin (IVH) (with warfarin starting on Day 2) in patients with proximal DVT. All patients had baseline ventilation perfusion (V/Q) lung scans and chest x-rays at entry, and signs and symptoms of PE were recorded on the clinical report forms.

Patients: 213 patients received LMWH and 219 received IVH. Adequate V/Q scans and chest x-rays were available on 289 patients; 150 (70.4%) on LMWH and 139 (63.5%) on heparin. The lung scans were interpreted by two experts without knowledge of the patient's treatment group or clinical outcomes, and were interpreted as high probability (HP), nondiagnostic (ND) or a normal (N) according to the PIOPED and Biello specifications.

Results: Signs and symptoms of PE were present in 18 (12.0%) of patients on LMWH and 20 (14.4%) on IVH. For asymptomatic patients on LMWH, the lung scan patterns were HP-63, ND-64, and N-5; while on IVH they were HP-64, ND-53, and N-2. In the total group the incidence of HP and ND patterns was 96.9%.

Conclusion: Asymptomatic PE occurs frequently in patients presenting with proximal DVT. Our findings support the use of baseline lung scans in patients presenting with proximal DVT.

Thrombo-embolic Disorders

Diagnosis of Thrombo-embolism

Phlebology '95, D. Negus et al. (eds.). Phlebology (1995) Suppl. 1: 690-692

OP/10.8

Color Doppler Evidence of Temporary Vena Cava Filters' Embolism

A. Pieri[1], G. Santoro[2], A. Duranti[3], F. Mori[1], G. Squillantini[2], G. Corti[2],
S. Michelagnoli[1], F. Marcelli[1], A. Dolara[2], G.C. Berni[4] and G. De Saint Pierre[1]

[1] III Cardiology Unit, Diagnostic Angiology Module (Dir. Prof. G. de Saint Pierre), [2] II Cardiology Unit II,
Invasive and Interventional Module (Dir. Dott. A. Dolara), [3] General and Vascular Surgery Unit (Dir. Prof.
G. Borrelli), [4] General Medicine Unit (Dir. Prof. C.G. Berni)
Azienda Ospedaliera, Careggi, Firenze, Italy

INTRODUCTION

Deep Vein Thrombosis (DVT) of the lower limbs represents a life threatening disease owing to its potential evolution into Pulmonary Embolism (PE). Natural history of DVT provides thrombus' progression and fragmentation, with consequent PE in an high percentage of cases (often asymptomatic). Primary and secondary prevention of PE methods are still under discussion. Classic heparin therapy shows no significant action in avoiding neither PE nor thrombus' progression. Thrombolythic therapy may result in a further facilitation of thrombi's fragmentation with consequent PE. Oral anticoagulation allows a good protection for the follow-up period but no acute action. Surgical thrombectomy represents an alternative choice face to temporaneous contra-indications to thrombolysis. Definitive Vena Cava Filters do not offer sure long term safety qualifications and must be reserved to clinically selected patients.

Temporary Vena Cava Filters (TVCF) were used in this study to perform a protected Urokinase Thrombolysis (UKT) or a protected surgical thrombectomy during heparin infusion. Color Doppler (CD) ultrasounds demonstrated to be a complete and reliable diagnostic tool for DVT ascertainment, therapy's control and follow-up.

AIMS OF THE STUDY

a) To assess TVCF usefulness during prolonged high dose UKT and after surgical thrombectomy, in the prevention of primary or recurrent PE.

b) To validate CD investigation both in the diagnosis and follow-up of DVT.

MATHERIALS and METHODS

Routinary CD essays in risk patients (mainly surgical and orthopedical) and elective CD essays in patients that showed clinical evidence or suspicion of DVT or PE, demonstrated the presence of a floating thrombus (life threatening) of the lower limbs and/or abdominal veins in 72 consecutive patients.

49 (68%) patients (aged 18-75 years, mean age 42,7 y.) who presented floating common femoral, iliac or inferior vena cava DVT, were selected for a filter protected high dose (3.200 - 4.400 I.U./kg/h) UKT therapy (44 cases) or surgical thrombectomy (5 cases).

Filcard devices were used in 41 cases and Lysofilter in 8 cases. All the filters were placed into infra-renal vena cava or in the neighborhood of the thrombi.

Filcard devices (7 F) were introduced via basilic vein while Lysofilter ones were introduced via right jugular vein owing to their larger size (9 F).

Patients' selection criterias were as follows: 1) absence of absolute contra-indications to thrombolithic therapy; 2) proximal level of floating thrombus in common femoral, iliac or inferior cava veins; 3) presumable DVT onset up to three months. Temporaneous contra-indications to thrombolysis (e.g. major trauma or surgery <15 days) leaded to a filter protected surgical thrombectomy.

Floating DVT of the lower limbs and of the abdominal veins was always detected by CD: the demonstration of a complete or a quasi complete colour halo all around the thrombus (between the thrombus and the vein's wall) was considered the reference standard. CD also pointed out the thrombus' proximal level in all but two cases owing to abdominal metheorism (AngioTC was performed in these cases). The latter was confirmed in all the cases by cavo-iliac retrograde venography (CIV) that was performed during TVCF implantation. Ascendent venography was never performed because of the evidence of CD findings. CD ultrasounds were also useful in demonstrating pulmonary hypertension and/or functional heart involvment in clinical or suspected PE.

DVT's evolution during UKT was controlled daily by CD to avoid to repeat contrast medium essays and further radiological exposures. UKT also required daily assessment of various biological parameters (mainly fibrinogen rate).

Almost all the patients underwent a pulmonary scintigram before and after thrombolysis.

RESULTS

CD demostrated TVCF obstruction in 11 (22%) patients (9 in the primary thrombolysis group and 2 in the primary thrombectomy group) and the findings were always confirmed by CIV.

CD findings showed a quasi constant pattern: distal veins dilatation with P.W. doppler continuous flow and further slowing of flow velocity below the filter; a colour acceleration mosaic was evident in a tiny (semilunar shaped) lateralized part of inferior vena cava corresponding to filter's allocation.

In 9 patients prolonged UKT (till a plasmatic fibrinogen lowering of 100 mg/100 ml) resulted in a full lysis of the TVCF clots. The 2 patients that underwent surgical thrombectomy were treated by newly onset thrombolysis with the same good results. Maximum UKT duration time was of 14 days (mean duration of 4,3 days: 3-14 days).

TVCF obstructions were always of **embolic origin**. Filter's primary thrombosis was excluded according to CIV findings because retrograde contrast medium injection, through filter's relied catheter, frequently produced thrombus' dislocation distal to the filter. Thrombus' lack of adherence to inferior vena cava walls was considered as a sure proof of embolism. Moreover full lysis both of floating thrombi and TVCF clots was considered a supplementary proof of filter's embolism.

Full lysis of the floating thrombi was always achieved while occlusive DVT of superficial or deep femoral veins, from which DVT originated, did never show any change according to the hypothesis of an external lysis for the thrombolithic agents.

8 of the 11 patients who presented TVCF embolism had clinical symptoms or strumental evidence of DVT from at least 15 days up to three months.

All the patients did not show any new clinical or scintigraphic evidence of primary or recurrent PE after the therapy.

ADVERSE REACTIONS

Minor bleeding and mild anemia were a quasi constant pattern.Two patients (4%), died for cerebral haemorrhage during thrombolysis, although no preliminary clinical contra-indications to thrombolysis were referred. Two patients (4%) showed right basilic vein thrombosis (in the site of introduction of Filcard filter's catheter) and one patient (2%) presented acute abdominal pain owing to left ileo-psoas muscle haemorrhage. TVCF did never cause any other serious complications that were all related to UKT.

CONCLUSIONS

TVCF usefulness in preventing PE is still under examination. TVCF embolism, in absence of primary or recurrent PE, can be a proof of their usefulness expecially in the cases of "older" DVT.

CD investigation both in the diagnosis and follow-up of life threatening DVT has proven its efficacy in this study. Patients' selection for floating DVT was always achieved by CD and the findings were always confirmed.

CD ability to detect floating DVT and its low examination cost, can make this diagnostic tool the new gold standard in life threatening thrombosis' diagnosis.

REFERENCES

1 - Pieri A., Santoro G., Duranti A., Mori F., Vannuzzi A., Benelli L.: Filtres caves temporaires, notre experience. Analyse preliminaire de 24 cas. Phlebologie 1993; 46 (3): 457-466

2 - Pieri A., Santoro G., Duranti A., Acquafresca M., Mori F., Vannuzzi A., Benelli L., Squillantini G.: La diagnostica con ecocolor doppler nelle indicazioni e nel follow-up dei filtri cavali temporanei e definitivi. Atti del III International Workshop: What's new in prophylaxis and therapy of venous thromboembolism. Medical, surgical and radiological aspects. Monza 14-15 Sett. 1993, 112 (abstr.)

3 - Santoro G., Pieri A., Zuppiroli A., Mori F., Corti G., Duranti A., Vannuzzi A., Benelli L., Gori A.: Trombosi venosa profonda e rischio di embolia polmonare: utilita' dei filtri cavali temporanei. Atti del III International Workshop: What's new in prophylaxis and therapy of venous thromboembolism. Medical, surgical and radiological aspects. Monza 14-15 Sett. 1993, 111 (abstr.)

4 - Santoro G., Pieri A., Zuppiroli A., Mori F., Corti G., Duranti A., Gori A., Gensini G.F., Dolara A.: Trombosi venosa profonda e rischio di embolia polmonare: utilita' dei filtri cavali temporanei. Atti del Convegno Angiologia '93 - Pisa 3-4 Nov. 1993, 157 (abstr.)

5 - Théry C., Asseman P., Becquart J., Bauchart J.J., Jabinet J.L., Marache P.: Filtre cave temporaire permettant le diagnostic et la fibrinolyse chez les patients supects d' embolie pulmonaire massive. Arch. Mal. Coeur 1991; 84: 525-30

6 - Théry C., Asseman P., Amrouni N., Becquart J., Pruvost P., Lesenne M., Marache P.: Use of a new removable vena cava filter in order to prevent pulmonary embolism in patients submitted to thrombolysis. Eur. Heart J. 1990; 11: 324-341.

7 - Winchell R.J., Hoyt D.B., Walsh J.C., Simons R.K., Eastman A.B.: Risk factors associated with pulmonary embolism despite routine prophylaxis: implications for improved protection. J.Trauma 1994; (37) 4: 600-5.

8 - (REVUE) Filtre cave temporaire et thrombolyse. Artères et Veines 1991; (X) 7: 496-7

Phlebology '95, D. Negus et al. (eds.). Phlebology (1995) Suppl. 1: 693-695

OP/12.4

The Cost Effectiveness and Clinical Impact of Deep Vein Thrombosis Detection using Duplex Sonography

A.D. Fox, M.S. Whiteley, G. Evison[1], J.S. Budd and M. Horrocks

University Department of Surgery and the 1 Department of Radiology, Royal United Hospital, Combe Park, Bath, United Kingdom

INTRODUCTION

Venous duplex sonography has been shown to be accurate for evaluation of symptomatic patients [1-3] with deep vein thrombosis (DVT) and is considered by many to be the new gold standard. Venography is sometimes difficult to interpret [4] and remains invasive, painful and may be associated with complications of using contrast media [5,6]. Following introduction of the duplex scanner (ATL,Ultramark 9,USA), referrals were shared between Xray and the vascular studies unit (VSU). Greater awareness of the direct access facilities within the VSU by all specialities, including general practice, has resulted in a greater demand for non-invasive assessment for DVT. Demand now exceeds the capability of the VSU to provide the service and further expansion, both in staff and equipment, is required.

To determine ways to secure this and future expansion, a prospective comparison was performed between venography and duplex assessment in patients suspected of having DVT.

PATIENTS AND METHODS

All patients referred for investigation between May 1992 and May 1993 were recruited. A standard proforma was used for data collection at the time of request for venography and was completed by the radiologist after reviewing the results. The collective patients' data was then entered into a large database facility (Statistical Package for Social Sciences, SPSS (UK) Ltd, SPSS House, 5 London Street, Chertsey, Surrey. KT16 8AP) for analysis. All duplex examination results were recorded at the time of the scan, copies of the results being filed in the VSU, the patient's notes, and discussed at the time with the referring physician. The presence of occlusive or non-occlusive thrombus within the popliteal, femoral or iliac venous system was recorded but no attempt was made to assess the calf vessels. Information was easily retrieved from these sources for direct comparison. The referral patterns, delays, outcome and costs were analysed and compared with the last 6 months of 1994 now that the service is fully established.

RESULTS

Two hundred and forty five consecutive patients were referred for venography. The median ages were; females 55.5 years, males 57.6 years. There were seven cases of failed vessel cannulation due to excessive oedema and 23 other cancellations. As a result, 215 completed examinations were performed. The results demonstrated 121(56.5%) normal venograms, 86 (40.2%) positive DVT's, 4 (3.3%) Baker's cysts and 4 incomplete records. Only 17.1% (42) of patients were investigated within the first 24 hours following admission. Normal venograms were reported in 23 of these patients but they remained in hospital for at least 24 hours prior to discharge. The majority (62.9%) of venograms were performed after an average delay of 3.3 days. Only 52 (43%) patients with normal venograms were discharged on the same day of investigation. A further 39 (32%) were discharged within 1 - 6 days and the remainder were accounted for by post-operative convalescence.

During the same period 187 duplex examinations were performed in the vascular studies unit. The sex distribution was 74 (39.6%) males and 113 (60.4%) females with a median age 57 years (range 16 - 89 years). The results demonstrated 103 (55%) normal venograms, 67 (36%) positive DVT's, 2 (1%) Baker's cysts and 15 (8%) equivocal scans. There was no significant difference between the two sets of results (Mann Whitney U Test).

Examining the pattern of referral it is evident that throughout the initial study period the number of referrals for non-invasive assessment was increasing monthly with a significant increase ($p < 0.05$. Mann Whitney U Test) in the number of scans being performed (Figure 1). During the last 6 months of 1994 287 patients were referred for non-invasive assessment but only 30 patients were referred for venography (ratio 10.6:1). Three of these were referrals from the VSU rather than de novo problems for contrast imaging.

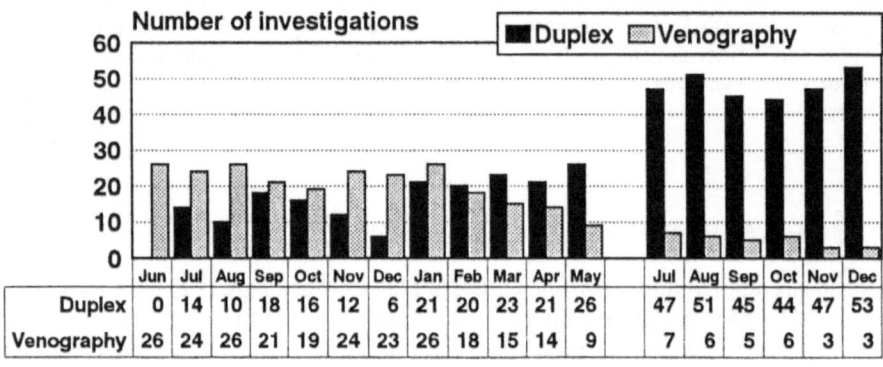

Time in months

Fig.1 Changing trends duplex versus venography
Comparison 1992 - 1993 versus last 6 months 1994

DISCUSSION

The 'cumulative delay cost' involved with venography has been assessed and summated (Table 1) with the presumptive cost of running a duplex service for the study population. Assuming that the current (last 6 months of 1994) ratio of duplex and venography (10.6:1) is reflective of an established practice it is evident that a potential saving slightly in excess of £90000 may be achieved.

Table 1   Cost analysis: Duplex and Venography

| Medical bed | £150 | Surgical bed | £200 | Venogram | £278 | Duplex Scan | £90 |

Bed occupancy		**TOTAL**
24 hour delay to discharge (23 patients normal venogram)	£3558	
Average delay to venography 3.3 days	£53864	£57422
Cost of investigations		
Venography (215)	£59770	
Duplex scanning (187)	£16830	
Total cost DVT detection (402 investigations)	£76600	
Cost of 402 duplex scans	£36180 -	£40420
Current ratio of venography versus duplex 10.6:1		
Therefore 38 patients would have had venography	£10564	
Cost of 38 duplex scans	£3420 -	
Additional cost for venography		£7140 -

Total potential saving	**£90702**

Duplex sonography has replaced venography as the method of choice for the detection of proximal DVT in our institute. Provision of an outpatient service prevents avoidable bed usage and the unnecessary risks of anticoagulation. We feel that we can justify the policy of not routinely assessing the calf veins for thrombus providing patients with continuing symptoms are rescanned within 48 hours or sent for venography. The direct access policy for all specialities has resulted in a large increase in the number of requests for DVT detection, perhaps greater than would have been anticipated by the reduction in the number of venograms. As a result it has been necessary to expand the vascular studies unit both in terms of staff and equipment but this cost is easily off-set by the savings that can be made by the introduction of duplex sonography.

REFERENCES

1   Quintavalla R, Larini P, Miselli A, Mandrioli R, Ugolotti U, Pattacini C, Pini M. Duplex ultrasound diagnosis of symptomatic proximal deep vein thrombosis of the lower limbs.European Journal of Radiology 1992; 15: 32 - 36.
2   Lensing AWA, Prandoni P, Brandjes D, Huisman PM, Vigo M, Tomasella G, Krekt J, ten Cate JW, Huisman MV, Bueller HR. Detection of deep-vein thrombosis by real time B-mode ultrasonography.
     Intern Med 1989; 111: 297 - 304
3   Schindler JM, Kaiser M, Gerber A, Vuilliomenet A, Popovic A, Bertel O. Colour coded duplex sonography in suspected deep vein thrombosis of the leg. BMJ 1990; 301: 1369 - 1370.
4   McLachlan MSF, Thomson JG, Taylor DW, Kelly ME, Sackett DL. Observer variation in the interpretation of lower limb venograms.
     American Journal of Radiology 1979;132: 227 - 229.
5   Albrechtsson U, Olsson CG:Thrombotic side effects of lower limb venography. Lancet 1976; 1: 723 - 724.
6   Thomas ML, MacDonald LM: Complications of ascending phlebography of the leg. Br Med J 1978; 2: 317 - 318.

Phlebology '95, D. Negus et al. (eds.). Phlebology (1995) Suppl. 1: 696-698

OP/8.1

Co-Existing Findings in DVT Patients

S.K. Volteas, N. Labropoulos, M. Leon, E. Kalodiki and A.N. Nicolaides

Academic Surgical and Vascular Unit, St Mary's Hospital Medical School, London, UK

INTRODUCTION

Although previous reports identified pathologies that co-exist with deep vein thrombosis (DVT) [1,2], their incidence is unknown. The aim of this prospective study was to identify the magnitude and incidence of conditions that co-exist with DVT and may lead to a false diagnosis.

MATERIALS AND METHODS

A total of 1000 unselected patients with clinically suspected DVT entered the study. Patients were referred from medical and surgical wards, casualty and general practitioners. They were all investigated with the ATL Ultramark 9 Duplex Scanner (Advanced Technology Laboratories, Bothell, Washington) using a 5 MHz linear array scanhead. The examination technique has been previously described in detail [3].

RESULTS

From these 1000 patients 663 (66.3%) were found negative for DVT, in 32 the examination was inconclusive and 305 were positive (30.5%.). In 52 of these 305 patients we found other pathologies as well (n=57): an unruptured Baker's cyst in 3, a ruptured in 1, superficial thrombophlebitis in 14, an arteriovenous (AV) fistula in 3, deep venous reflux in 11, superficial venous reflux in 12, a thigh cyst in 1, while inflammatory skin disease was recorded in 7 patients. Five of these 52 patients, 3 with deep venous reflux and 2 with inflammatory skin disease, in addition had superficial venous reflux.

DISCUSSION

There are some important issues that should be kept in mind while examining patients with suspected DVT. Baker's cysts, AV fistulae, superficial thrombophlebitis and inflammatory skin changes are usually obvious and easily detected; it is therefore common to attribute the patient's symptoms to these conditions and overlook the

be around 3% [1]. There was also no case of haematoma co-existing with DVT in our series; however the theoretical possibility cannot be excluded and the danger of haemorrhage during anticoagulation exists. [6]. Haematomata on Duplex scanning appear as black and usually circular structures that have well defined borders and are localized between the muscles. They show no flow and produce no Doppler signal during augmentation. A haematoma is compressible when not thrombosed, but this manoeuvre is occasionally very painful or impossible to perform.

Finally, inflammatory skin changes due to lymphangiitis or cellulitis were recorded in 2.3% of DVT cases. These patients should always be scanned, as symptoms can easily be attributed to the skin disease and, as the compression manoeuvre is very painful, co-existing DVT can be missed.

CONCLUSIONS

The results of this study show that the clinical diagnosis of DVT can be unreliable in two thirds of the symptomatic cases. They also show that important pathologies, co-existing with DVT, can be found in 17% of cases. Baker's cysts, AV fistulae, superficial thrombophlebitis and inflammatory skin diseases must attract increased attention as they may conceal DVT, while the presence or absence of deep venous reflux must also be recorded in order to study the natural history of DVT.

REFERENCES

1.   Buchbinder D, McCullough GM, Melick CF. Patients evaluated for venous disease may have other pathologic conditions contributing to symptomatology. Am J Surg 1993;166:21-5.
2.   Jorgensen JO, Hanel KC, Morgan AM, Hunt JM. The incidence of deep venous thrombosis in patients with superficial thrombophlebitis of the lower limbs. J Vasc Surg 1993;18:70-3.
3.   Labropoulos N, Leon M, Kalodiki E, Al -Kutoubi A, Chan P, Nicolaides AN. Colour flow duplex scanning in suspected acute deep vein thrombosis; Experience with routine use. Eur J Vasc Endovasc Surg 1995;9:49-52.
4.   Renton S, Crofton M, Nicolaides A. Impact of duplex scanning on vascular surgical practice. Br J Surg 1991; 78: 1203-7.
5.   Chaudhuri R, Salari R. Baker's Cyst Simulating Deep Vein Thrombosis. Clin Radiol 1990;41:400-4.
6.   Wigley RAD, Paterson DE. Calf haematoma following anticoagulants in synovian rupture. N Z Med J 1982; 95: 630-2.
7.   Blattler W, Frick E. Complications of superficial thrombophlebitis. Sweitz Med Worchenschr 1993; 123: 223-8.
8.   Stradness D.E. The clinical spectrum of venous disease. In: Vascular diagnosis, 4th Ed, E.F. Bernstein Editor, Mosby-Year book Inc, 1993; 772-8.
9.   Rutherford RB. Noninvasive testing in the diagnosis and assessment of arteriovenous fistula. In: Vascular diagnosis, 4th Ed, E.F. Bernstein Editor, Mosby-Year book Inc, 1993;608-19.

thrombosis. Duplex scanning is highly accurate for the anatomic location and extend of thrombi [4] but if the above mentioned pathologies are missed, the study of suspected re-thrombosis or thrombus propagation becomes difficult: the rupture of a previously unseen Baker's cyst or the development of superficial thrombophlebitis (acute or recurrent-previously undetected) may lead to unnecessary medical actions if the patient is not re-scanned and the diagnosis is only clinical. A further problem is the post-thrombotic chronic venous insufficiency (CVI) that the patient is most likely to develop; if reflux in the deep system is not detected at the time of the DVT diagnosis, then a follow-up study of the natural history of DVT could be biased. The same is true if a significant, previously unseen, AV fistula is present.

A Baker's cyst, present in 1.3% of our DVT cases, is visualized as an hypoechoic structure emerging from the knee joint. It enlarges progressively and usually dissects through the muscles, above and -mainly- below the knee [5]. Echolucent material can occasionally be identified inside the cyst while no flow is seen during the augmentation manoeuvre. The cyst is easily compressible when full of fluid, but when it contains material (crystals) the compression is only partial. A ruptured Baker's cyst produces swelling and acute pain that worsens with the compression manoeuvre; a misdiagnosis of DVT may lead to bleeding complications following anticoagulation [6]. The experienced examiner should not rely upon compression only but should perform the augmentation manoeuvre as well, finding the adjacent veins -when free of thrombus- with normal cephalic flow. It is routine in our laboratory to look for a Baker's cyst in the other extremity, but only one contralateral cyst, smaller and asymptomatic, has been found so far.

Superficial thrombophlebitis was seen in 4.6% of our DVT cases. It's co-existence with DVT however has been reported to occur in 23-44% of cases [2,7]. It can conceal DVT, especially when localized in the calf [8]. Calf DVT can also be missed, as the compression manoeuvre becomes very painful; the augmentation manoeuvre is therefore very important. The diagnosis of superficial thrombophlebitis on Duplex is easy by superficial scanning and gentle compression of the painful area that identifies thrombi within the superficial veins.

An AV fistula was present in 1% of our DVT cases. For it's diagnosis the use of colour is essential: arterialized flow is seen in the affected vein, with the colour showing a pattern of high speed typical of a shunt [9]. There is no previous report of co-existence with DVT. On the other hand, AV fistulae can cause symptoms similar to DVT (moderate pain and increased local temperature) with the extent of both the local and distal symptoms related to the size of the fistula and the degree of the venous hypertension [9]; patients symptoms therefore can easily be attributed to an AV fistula and DVT can be missed.

Deep venous insufficiency was identified in 3.6% of DVT cases. In the identification of reflux with Duplex scanning the Doppler signal is more sensitive than the colour change. Depending on it's severity, CVI may produce swelling, discomfort and pain [8] and may even be thought responsible for the patients symptoms. The most important issue, however, as stated before, is the post-thrombotic assessment of patients with previously unseen CVI.

Superficial venous reflux was detected in 3.9% of DVT cases; it was recorded as an incidental finding, however, as it does not appear to have any major significance.

There was only one thigh cyst identified, while no soft tissue tumors were found. The incidence of these tumors, that can either produce or mimic DVT, has been reported to

OP/8.5

THE LOW PROBABILITY LUNG SCAN: A NEED FOR CHANGE IN NOMENCLATURE.

Hull R.D., Pineo G.F., Raskob G.E.

University of Calgary.

Objective: To determine the prognosis of patients with suspected pulmonary embolism (PE) who present with a low probability lung scan pattern and poor cardiorespiratory reserve (CRR).

Design: A cohort analytic study using long-term follow-up for three months in patients with poor CRR, who presented with suspected PE. Poor CRR was defined as: pulmonary edema, right ventricular failure, hypotension, syncope, acute tachyarrhythmia, abnormal spirometry ($FEV_1 < 1.0$ or $VC < 1.5$) or abnormal arterial blood gases ($PO_2 < 50$ or $PCO_2 > 45mmHg$).

Results: The outcomes of 117 consecutive patients with suspected PE and poor CRR were compared with those in 586 consecutive patients with normal lung scans who were entered over the same period of time. 77 of the 117 patients with poor CRR had low probability lung scans and six (7.8%) died within days of entry of fatal PE proven by autopsy compared with none with normal lung scans (p<0.00001).

Conclusion: Our findings indicate that the term low probability lung scan, which has been synonymous historically with a good prognosis, is clearly a misnomer and should be abandoned particularly in patients with severe cardiac and pulmonary disease.

PI/83

PHLEBOGRAPHIC PATTERN OF ASYMPTOMATIC DEEP VEIN THROMBOSIS 4 WEEKS AFTER TOTAL HIP REPLACEMENT

Björell Q*, Nilsson P*, Nylander G*, Benoni G**, Bergqvist D***, Fredin H**, Hedlund U**,

Depts of Diagnostic Radiology* and Ortopedics**, University Hospital MAS, Malmö. Dept of Surgery***, University Hospital, Uppsala, Sweden.

Objective: To describe the phlebographic pattern of asymptomatic deep vein thrombosis (DVT) 4 weeks after total hip replacement and compare it to a group of patients with symptomatic DVT.

Design: Combined prospective and retrospective study.

Patients: 251 consecutive patients of whom 224 without symptoms underwent bilateral ascending phlebography 28 days postoperatively. The remaining 27 had symptomatic DVT verified at phlebography 3-46 days (median 17) postoperatively. Low molecular weight heparin was used as thromboprophylaxis.

Measurements: All phlebographies were reviewed by three radiologists. The location, frequency of subfascial edema, extension and affected side of DVT were noted.

Results: Asymptomatic DVT was found in 53 (24%) patients. Of these 15 (28%) had bilateral DVT, 35 (66%) only on the operated side and 3 (6%) only on the non operated side. In 40 patients (75%) there was minor isolated DVT located at the junction of the superficial and deep femoral veins, the posterior tibial, or in the arcade veins of the soleus muscle. A subfascial edema was found in 1 (2%) patient.
In the group of 27 symptomatic patients 5 (19%) had this type of DVT appearance (the remaining had widespread DVT) and 15 (56%) had a subfascial edema.

Conclusions: The incidence of asymptomatic DVT 4 weeks after total hip replacement is rather high (24%). However, they appear as minor DVT, quite different from those seen in acute symptomatic patients which are extensive, with multiple location and with subfascial edema.

Thrombo-embolic Disorders

Prevention of Thrombo-embolism

Phlebology '95, D. Negus et al. (eds.). Phlebology (1995) Suppl. 1: 701-703

OP/10.5

Venous Hemodynamic Alteration Induced by the Venopress (A New Intermittent Compression Pneumatic Device for Prevention of Deep Vein Thrombosis

A. Zelikovski, I. Ben-Tov, A. Koren, E. Stelman and M. Haddad

Department of Vascular Surgery, Beilinson Medical Center, Petah Tiqva, Sackler Faculty of Medicine, Tel Aviv University, Israel

ABSTRACT

The hemodynamic effect of general anesthesia on the venous velocity of the lower limbs was investigated in 20 patients who volunteered to undergo venous compression with the use of a new pneumatic device, the Venopress. Venous velocity in the common femoral vein was monitored by a duplex device before and after induction of general anesthesia. Results indicated that prior to general anesthesia, venous velocity was increased two- to fourfold by the Venopress and when anesthesia was induced, a further augmentation of 10 to 30% was achieved. We conclude that, the Venopress is a very efficient device for venous velocity augmentation, especially during general anesthesia.

INTRODUCTION

Postoperative deep vein thrombosis (DVT) remains an important medical problem which continues to endanger patients despite the use of such prophylactic methods as anticoagulants, pneumatic devices, elastic support, and electrical stimulation [1].

The use of pneumatic devices is based on the assumption that intraoperative augmentation of venous velocity in the lower limbs will prevent the formation of DVT. There are also reports indicating an elevation in fibrinolytic activity due to the release of fibrinolytic substances from the compressed venous wall during pneumatic compression [2]. However, no information on variations in compressed venous velocity under general anesthesia has been published.

Thirteen years ago, we reported our findings on the preoperative prevention of DVT in neurosurgical patients with the Lymph-Press device, designed for reduction of lymphedema) [3]. Using marked fibrinogen to monitor DVT, we noted a reduction in the frequency of DVT in the control group from 50% to 4.3% [4]. These excellent results, together with the introduction of the noninvasive vascular duplex device, prompted us to develop a new pneumatic device the Venopress (manufactured by Mego Afek, Israel), for the prevention of postoperative DVT. The present work investigates the affect of the Venopress on the compressed venous blood velocity before and after induction of general anesthesia.

OPERATION OF THE VENOPRESS
The venopress has two parts:

1. **The sleeve** consists of five independent overlapping cells, connected to form a boot. Each cell is fed independently by an air tube from the pneumatic machine. Two sleeves are used, one for each leg, during operation of the device.

2. **The pneumatic machine** consists of a compressor and distributor. Air pressure may be set at 50 or 60 mmHg. The distributor divides the air sequentially among the ten cells of the two sleeves, at 2 seconds per each pair of cells. When all ten cells are full, they are emptied simultaneously. The air insufflation cycle lasts 10 seconds, followed by a 1-minute pause.

PATIENTS AND METHODS

Patients
Twenty patients (12 men, 8 women, mean age 64 years) undergoing surgery unrelated to the lower limbs (cholecystectomy, hemicolectomy, gastrectomy) gave their informed consent for this study.

Methods
Each patient was investigated in three stages while on the operating table:
1. Prior to undergoing anesthesia, baseline venous velocity was measured using a duplex device (Elscint, Israel) placed on the common femoral vein (6.5 MHz probe, 60°angle).
2. With the duplex device still monitoring venous velocity in the same place and at the same angle as in stage 1, the Venopress was applied to both legs.
3. Five minutes after general anesthesia was induced venous velocity in the common femoral vein was again measured.

Twenty-four hours after surgery all patients underwent investigation of the deep vein in the lower limb for the presence of postoperative DVT.

RESULTS

The results can be seen in Figure 1.

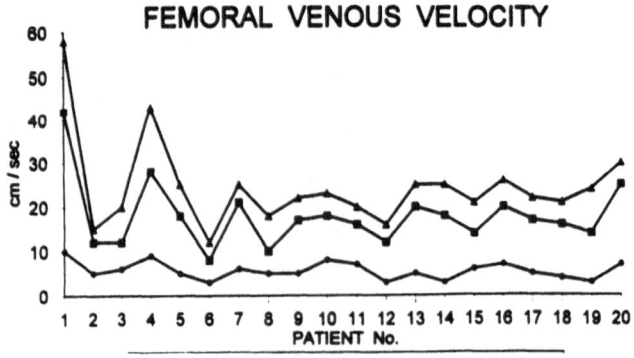

The mean baseline venous flow velocity in the lower limbs in all patients was 6.6 cm/sec. After application of the Venopress, venous velocity increased to a mean of 17.8 cm/sec. When general anesthesia was induced, a further augmentation was noted, to a mean of 24.5 cm/sec. In addition, the duplex device indicated a 30% enlargement of the common femoral vein after general anesthesia was induced [5]. Twenty-four hours after surgery, a control deep vein duplex examination revealed no DVT in any of the patients.

DISCUSSION

Of the many methods used today to prevent DVT, the pneumatic devices are the safest and, in the long run, have the highest cost-benefit ratio. We tested a new pneumatic device, the Venopress, before and after induction of anesthesia, and found it to be much more effective during general anesthesia, presumably because of the attendant muscle relaxation, which, in turn, led to enlargement of the veins. This factor most probably contributes to the reduction in venous flow during anesthesia and the consequent of intraoperative DVT. Since the enlarged veins contain a greater amount of venous blood in the lower limbs, their compression was more prominent during general anesthesia, as shown by the increase in the velocity wave detected over the common femoral vein.

In high risk patients, i.e., those with a past history of DVT, or a hypercoagulation state, undergoing long operations (neurosurgery) or with contraindications to prophylactic heparin, the pneumatic compression device is the best method for prevention of DVT [6].

The Venopress proved to be a very efficient device for augmentation of intraoperative venous blood flow velocity.

REFERENCES

1. Laveric MD, McGivern RC, Crone MD, Mollan RAD. A comparison of the effects of electrical calf stimulation and the venous foot pump of the venous blood flow in the lower leg. Phlebology 1990;5:285-90.
2. Ah-See AK, Arfors A, Bergquist D, Dahlgren S. The haemodynamic and antithrombotic effects of intermittent pneumatic compression on femoral vein blood flow. Acta Chir Scand 1976;142:381-5.
3. Zelikovski A, Haddad M, Reiss R. The "Lympha-Press" intermittent sequential pneumatic device for the treatment of lymphoedema: five years of clinical experience. J Cardiovasc Surg 1986;27:288-90.
4. Zelikovski A, Zucker G, Eliashiv A, Reiss R, Shalit M. A new sequential pneumatic device for the prevention of deep vein thrombosis. J Neurosurg 1981;54:652-4.
5. Comerota AJ, Stewart GJ, Alburger PD, Smalley K, White JV. Operative venodilatation: a previously unsuspected factor in the cause of postoperative deep vein trhrombosis. Surgery 1988;106:301-9.
6. Hamilton MG, Hull RD, Pineo GF. Venous thromboembolism in neurosurgery and neurology patients: a review. Neurosurgery 1994;34:280-6.

Phlebology '95, D. Negus et al. (eds.). Phlebology (1995) Suppl. 1: 704-706

OP/20.2

Is Routine Heparin Prophylaxis Justified in Varicose Vein Stripping?

K. Böhler[1], M. Baldt[2] and H. Watzke[3]

[1] Department of Dermatology, Div. of General Dermatology, [2] Department of Radiology and
[3] Department of Internal Medicine I, Div. of Hematology and Hemostaseology, University of Vienna,
Medical School, Vienna, Austria

INTRODUCTION

Insufficiency of epifascial veins promotes venous ulceration and increases thromboembolic risk in general surgery patients. Epifascial varicose vein stripping (VVS) is therefore considered the most effective prophylactic procedure. According to the literature the thrombotic risk of patients undergoing this surgical procedure is low (1.1 to 2.6 %) (1,2), but has not yet been evaluated prospectively. Elevation of activation markers of blood coagulation is not only found in overt thrombosis but any prethrombotic state (3). This study was conducted to prospectively investigate the thrombotic risk of stripping operations (Part I) and to evaluate whether VVS induces a prethrombotic state (Part II).

METHODS

Part I: 100 consecutive patients referred to the Department of Dermatology for primary varicose vein surgery were entered into the study. For detailed clinical diagnosis see Table 1. Patients with secondary varicosis due to postthrombotic syndrome were excluded. Mean age of the patients treated was 45 years. Operations were performed under general anaesthesia with the operating table in the Trendelenburg position. 87 patients underwent saphenofemoral junction ligation with stripping of the long saphenous vein. The short saphenous vein was stripped in three limbs and a saphenopopliteal junction ligation was performed in the remaining three patients. Ligation of the saphenofemoral junction in addition to an avulsion of major side branches was performed in two patients. In one patient the mid-thigh perforator vein was ligated and the distal part of the long saphenous vein was stripped. The six patients with recurrent varicose veins underwent multiple avulsions in addition to ligation of perforator veins. Elastic bandages were applied immediately after vein surgery for the consecutive eight weeks. Patients were encouraged to walk immediately after operation but no anticoagulatory medication was given peri- or postoperatively. Ascending pressure phlebography (APP) was performed according to Hach (4) in the affected legs of the 100 patients pre- and 10 to 21 days postoperatively. Preoperatively we looked for signs of deep vein thrombosis and for postthrombotic changes of the deep venous system; postoperatively APP was employed to detect deep vein thrombosis.

Part II: 15 consecutive patients with a mean age of 50 years, who were referred to the Department of Dermatology for primary varicose vein surgery were studied. Preoperative work up and peri- and postoperative handling of the patients was as described in Part I. 13 patients (mean age: 61 years), who underwent operative procedures without major soft tissue trauma served as a control. All patients included in the study were operated under general anaesthesia and had no anticoagulant treatment throughout the investigation. Plasma samples for the determination of thrombin-antithrombin complex (TAT), prothrombin fragment1+2 (F1+2) and D-Dimer were obtained before the stripping operation and on the first postoperative day. Blood was collected via vacutainer system into a 3.8% sodium citrate solution (1:9) and was then centrifuged at 2000x g for 15 minutes. TAT, F1+2 and D-Dimer were determined using commercially available test kits (Enzygnost TAT and F1+2 Behringwerke, Stago Diagnostica, Boehringer Mannheim, Germany). The mean biological change of the three variables within one group was expressed as the ratio of the pre-and postoperative mean values. To compare the pre-and postoperative values within the two groups (VVS, Control) we used the Wilcoxon matched pairs signed rank test. To compare changes in the three variables between the respective groups we used the Wilcoxon rank sum test for independent samples. All patients gave informed consent to the study (Part I and II).

RESULTS

Part I: No case of postoperative deep vein thrombosis was noted by APP in all of the 100 legs investigated (95 % CI: 0 to 2.95). In one patient APP outlined a flotating thrombus in the first Cockett's perforator vein after saphenofemoral junction ligation with stripping of the long saphenous vein. Minor thrombi in residual epifascial tributaries were observed in three patients.

Part II: In the VVS group the operation induced increase of TAT was 2.6 fold of F1+2 1.6 fold and of D-Dimer 1.8 fold. A highly significant postoperative elevation was observed for all three variables in the VVS group (TAT: $p<0.0001$, F1+2: $p<0.002$, D.Dimer: $p<0.001$). In the control group postoperative increase of the three variables was statistically not significant.(Table II). Comparison of changes in TAT, F1+2 and D-Dimer between the VVS and the control group revealed a median change of 3.2 versus - 0.5 for TAT, 0.3 versus 0 for F1+2 and 230 versus 29 for D-Dimer (Table III). Changes were significantly higher in the VVS group.

CONCLUSION

According to the results of Part I of our study we emphasize that VVS is a safe procedure provided patients are properly selected and surgical and postoperative procedures are optimized to prevent thromboembolic events. Therefore we discourage routine prophylactic anticoagulation. This conclusion exclusively applies to a patient selection as outlined in our study, and should not be generalized for a heterogenous unselected population.

According to the results of Part II of our study a marked and highly significant postoperative elevation of TAT, F1+2 and D-Dimer occurs in patients undergoing VVS. Anaesthesia-related effects could be excluded. It thus seems likely that coagulation activation is caused by the surgical procedure. Although we showed a marked peroperative activation of coagulation in VVS actual thromboembolic risk is low. These findings emphasize that the immediate postoperative period has major implications on the development of deep vein thrombosis. On the basis of the results of Part II heparin prophylaxis must be reconsidered.

Table 1: Epifascial varicose vein pathology among 100 patients investigated.

Condition	Number
Long saphenous vein insufficiency	85
Long and short saphenous vein insufficiency	2
Short saphenous vein insufficiency	4
Recurrent varicose veins after stripping	6
Mid-thigh perforator incompetence	1
Side branch varicosis	2

Table 2: Pre-and postoperative values of the three variables (TAT, F1+2, D-Dimer) in the VVS and control group. Mean biological change are estimated by the quotient of pre- and postoperative mean values. Pre- and postoperative values were compared by the Wilcoxon sign test.

Variable	Group	Preop	Postop	Change	p value
TAT*	VVS	2,7 (2,6±0,7)	6,2 (6,8±2,6)	2,6	< 0,0001
	Control	2,9 (4,1±3,2)	3,3 (3,5±1,3)	0,8	n.s.
F1+2**	VVS	0,9 (1,0±0,4)	1,4 (1,6±0,7)	1,6	< 0,002
	Control	0,9 (1,0±0,2)	0,9 (0,9±0,3)	0,9	n.s.
D-Dimer°	VVS	330 (334±120)	635 (602±208)	1,8	< 0,001
	Control	410(496±228)	574 (559±203)	1,1	n.s.

The values are expressed as median (mean $\pm$ SD)
*ng/ml; **nmol/l; °ng/ml

Table 3: Comparison of changes in the three variables (TAT, F1+2, D-Dimer) between the VVS and Control group.

Variable	Change in Control	Change in VVSG	p value (Wilcoxon)
TAT	- 0,5 (- 0,61±3,00)	3,2 (4,21±2,43)	0,0001
F1+2	0 (- 0,09±0,34)	0,3 (0,54±0,66)	0,0023
D-Di	29 (63,4±150)	230 (267,7±185,2)	0,0053

the values are expressed as median (mean±SD)

REFERENCES

1. Mc Namara MF, Takaki HS, Yao JST, Venous disease. Surg Clin North Am 1977;57:1201-20.
2. Lofgren EP, Coates HLC, O'Brien PC, Clinically suspect pulmonary embolism after vein stripping. Mayo Clin Proc 1976;51:77-80.
3. Bauer KA, Laboratory Markers of coagulation activation. Arch Pathol Lab Med 1993;117:71-7.
4. Hach W, Phlebographie der Bein- und Beckenvenen. 1985 Schnetztor, Konstanz

Phlebology '95, D. Negus et al. (eds.). Phlebology (1995) Suppl. 1: 707-709

PI/8.1

Current Status of Thromboembolism Prophylaxis

D. Bergqvist

Department of Surgery, Academic Hospital, Uppsala, Sweden

INTRODUCTION

The immediate threat of deep venous thrombosis (DVT) in connection with surgery is pulmonary embolism which may be fatal and it has been - and without prophylaxis still is - one of the major causes of death postoperatively. Today it is possible to significantly decrease the risk of DVT and fatal pulmonary embolism. It is therefore important to identify various risk factors to be able to institute prophylaxis in an optimal way. There is consensus among the majority of surgeons dealing with high risk operations to use some form of prophylaxis [1].

RISK FACTORS

In a large number of investigations risk factors for the development of postoperative venous thromboembolism have been evaluated, also in groups of patients who develop thromboembolism despite adequate prophylaxis. There are great variations in design between the studies, and in quite a few multivariate analysis has been used in an attempt to weigh the relation between various factors and their relative importance. The construction of a number of risk factor indices has been of limited practical value and, except for research, they are hardly used in the clinical routine to select patients for prophylaxis. Without going into details some clinical factors have come out as dominating in the risk factor profiles:

- age, after 40-45 years of age there is a rapid increase in risk.
- type of surgery, from low risk hernial surgery to high risk orthopaedic.
- malignant disease.
- previous thromboembolism.
- varicose veins.
- immobilization.
- reoperation.

In surgical patients a special high risk group has been defined where the risk to develop proximal DVT is above 10% and the risk of fatal pulmonary embolism is 1-5%: general and urological surgery in patients over 40 years with recent history of venous thromboembolism, extensive pelvic or abdominal surgery for malignant disease and major orthopaedic surgery of the lower limbs.

There is also an increased risk in some non-surgical situations such as stroke, myocardial infarction with heart failure, spinal cord lesion and alterations within the haemostatic system (APC-resistance, deficiency in antithrombin, protein C and protein S, antiphospolipid antibodies, hyperhomocysteinemia). The importance of APC-resistance in the development of postoperative thromboembolism is still to be established [2].

PROPHYLACTIC OPTIONS

In addition to general prophylaxis (such as atraumatic surgery, early mobilization, optimal fluid balance) there are a number of specific methods, which also can be combined in various ways:

Mechanical methods
- electrical calf muscle stimulation
- intermittent calf muscle compression
- intermittent pedal compression
- graduated elastic compression.

Pharmacological methods
- oral anticoagulation
- dextran
- unfractionated low dose heparin
- low molecular weight heparins
- other glucosaminoglucans
- thrombin inhibitors
- antiplatelet substances.

Except for graduated elastic compression the mechanical methods have been considered somewhat impractical and have therefore not gained widespread use. Elastic stockings, on the other hand, have been fairly extensively used, often in combination with pharmacological methods and also in situations where there is no scientific proof that there is a potentiating effect. The effect of mechanical methods to prevent fatal pulmonary embolism has not been evaluated in large studies.

Of the pharmacological methods oral anticoagulants are rarely used because the need of laboratory control and the bleeding risk. Dextran, although effective against fatal pulmonary embolism, has a limited prophylactic effect against deep vein thrombosis. Until recently, unfractionated low dose heparin has dominated and the effect is without doubt [3]. The problems with haemorrhagic complications and less effect in orthopaedic surgery have been largely overcome with the low molecular weight heparins. There are many commercially available low molecular weight heparins and besides being effective and safe they are also practical to use with only one injection daily and start in the evening before surgery. There are several reviews and metaanalyses which are consistent in their conclusions [4,5,6,7]. They are also effective in nonsurgical situations such as stroke, spinal cord injury and plaster cast treatment for leg injuries. Other glucosaminoglucans such as dermatan sulphate are still under evaluation as are thrombin inhibitors such as recombinant hirudin, but data so far indicate efficacy. The large metaanalysis performed by the Antiplatelet Trialists' Collaboration [8] makes it probable that acetylsalicylic acid may have a preventive effective on postoperative fatal pulmonary embolism and prospective studies to verify this are under way.

CONCLUSION

Today it is possible to identify patients with risk for DVT and fatal pulmonary embolism and there are several effective preventive alternatives which must be considered in risk situations. There are several important questions to be answered by future research: is postoperative start of prophylaxis as effective as preoperative start, are there groups of patients where prolonged prophylaxis is indicated, what is the need for prophylaxis in the rapidly increasing group of patients undergoing laparoscopic surgery?

REFERENCES

1. Nicolaides AN, Arcelus J, Belcaro G et al. Prevention of venous thromboembolism. Int Angiol 1992:11:151-59.
2. Dahlbäck B. Physiological anticoagulation. Resistance to activated Protein C and venous thromboembolism. J Clin Invest 1994;94:923-927.
3. Collins R, Scrimgeour A, Yusuf S, Phil D, Peto R. Reduction in fatal pulmonary embolism and venous thrombosis by perioperative administration of subcutaneous heparin. Overview of results of randomized trials in general, orthopaedic, and urologic surgery. N Engl J Med 1988;318:1162-73.
4. Bergqvist D. Review of clinical trials of low molecular weight heparins. Eur J Surg 1992;158:67-78.
5. Nurmohammed MT, Rosendaal FR, Büller HR, et al. Low-molecular-weight heparin versus standard heparin in general and orthopaedic surgery: a meta-analysis. Lancet 1992;340:152-156.
6. Leizorovicz A, Haugh MC, Chapuis F-R, Samama MM, Boissel J-P. Low molecular weight heparin in prevention of perioperative thrombosis. Br Med J 1992;305:913-920.
7. Jørgensen LN, Wille-Jørgensen P, Hauch O. Prophylaxis of postoperative thromboembolism with low molecular weight heparins. Br J Surg 1993;80:689-704.
8. Antiplatelet Trialists' Collaboration. Collaborative overview of randomized trials of antiplatelet therapy-III: Reduction in venous thrombosis and pulmonary embolism by antiplatelet prophylaxis among surgical and medical patients. Br J Med 1994;308:235-246.

Phlebology '95, D. Negus et al. (eds.). Phlebology (1995) Suppl. 1: 710-713

PI/8.2

Pre-Clinical Evaluation of a Percutaneous Greenfield Stainless Steel Filter

L.J. Greenfield, M.C. Proctor and E.A. James

Department of Surgery, University of Michigan, USA

The titanium Greenfield filter (TGF) has made percutaneous insertion of the device possible but at the sacrifice of guidewire centering of the carrier. The latter is believed to be the cause of occasional asymmetry of the filter when it is discharged against the wall of the vena cava. Therefore, a percutaneous stainless steel Greenfield filter with an over-the-wire delivery system has long been an objective. The initial design change involved decreasing the apex angle of the limbs from 17.5 to 0 ° thus reducing the profile of the device and making it more flexible. Additionally, the nosebead was welded rather than swaged to the limb. The filter was composed of the same 316 stainless steel wire as the original Greenfield filter with the same curved hook design. However, early animal studies indicated poor stability within the cava. [1] The hook configuration was then changed to that used with the TGF-modified hook(TGF-MH).[2] Performance improved but was still not comparable to the TGF-MH. A four step research plan was then initiated to improve the design development process. The plan included

    1. Identification of design factors significantly associated with filter performance.

    2. Development of in vitro models to allow rapid evaluation of filter prototypes.

    3. Evaluation of the best prototypes in in vivo studies testing characteristics unable to be assessed in the in vitro models.

    4. Clinical trials.

This development plan was successfully used in evaluating the current version, the SGF-alternating hook (SGF-AH), awaiting approval by the Food and Drug Administration (FDA).

Materials and Methods

In order to determine design characteristics associated with resistance to migration and caval penetration we employed a mathematical modeling program, ECHIP (1989, Hockessin, DE). Sixteen prototypes were subjected to testing. Filters were positioned in 20 mm silastic cava and submitted to sufficient downward force to move them three inches at a compression rate of 5"/min. The data were entered into the modeling program and the variables analyzed.

Having identified the factors significantly associated with superior resistance to displacement, additional prototypes were prepared. Four in vitro tests were developed which allowed devices to be ranked with respect to stability, clot capture and flow obstruction. Norms for these tests were established after multiple repetitions with the currently marketed Greenfield filters. The testing procedures were modified until reproducible results were obtained and correlated with the known performance of the marketed devices. All tests were conducted using the Embolic Capture Unit (ECU) previously described.[3] This device is used for evaluation of clot capture, filter stability and resistance to flow.

A limited number of the SGF-AH filters were prepared for animal studies. The purpose of these studies was to validate the fixation data, determine the incidence of caval penetration and determine whether the presence of the filter resulted in a tissue reaction. Two filters were placed in each of five sheep with follow-up consisting of AP, lateral and angled radiographs immediately, seven and thirty days post placement. Cavagrams were obtained at thirty days and animals were sacrificed.

In all instances, the new design proved superior to the earlier versions thus an IDE was obtained and the clinical trial was undertaken.

Results

The ECHIP analysis indicated that the angle of the hook was the most significant factor in determining filter stability and that the association was linear. In addition, the hook width and the interaction of hook width and height with hook width and angle were found to have a minor effect ($p<0.05$). Based upon the results, filter prototypes differing with respect to hook angle, orientation and length were developed. These models were tested in the in vitro system.

The in vitro tests established that the prototype with two downward directed hooks, the SGF-AH was comparable to the original and titanium filters and superior to all of the other prototypical devices..

The SGF-AH demonstrated superior performance to the earlier SGF-MH with respect to fixation and the incidence and extent of caval penetration.

There was no evidence of any inflammatory reaction and the filter hooks were well incorporated. This device had corrected the problems associated with the two earlier percutaneous stainless steel filters. An IDE was issued by the FDA. The clinical trial involving 75 patients was initiated in March of 1994 and completed January 20, 1995. FDA approval is pending.

Discussion

The Food and Drug Administration is requiring healthcare industries to provide a higher level of evidence to support claims of safety and efficacy. At the same time, there is stiff intra and extramural competition for research and development funds. In order to compete in this arena, those involved in biomedical device development are being forced to work more efficiently to bring devices to market. The development of the 12 Fr percutaneous stainless steel Greenfield vena caval filter reflects this effort.

During the process of developing this device a research plan was initiated that decreased the time required to bring a model from concept to market. Computer-generated mathematical models were used to identify design characteristics associated with filter performance. Standardized in vitro models were developed that allowed early decisions regarding prototype filter performance. The filter with the highest probability of success then underwent in vivo studies prior to initiation of clinical trials. The mathematical modeling focused development on those characteristics shown to be associated with filter stability. The standardized in vitro testing system allowed multiple prototypes to be evaluated in a short period of time preventing delays from pursuit of inferior designs. The in vivo studies provided confirmation of the data obtained from the modeling and in vitro studies and allowed investigation of the histologic effects of the device on the vena cava.

This process enabled us to move from a mathematical model to completion of the clinical study in less than two years. Our level of confidence in the results of the first three steps was confirmed by the data from the recent clinical trial which demonstrated a low incidence of movement and caval penetration.

1. Greenfield LJ, Tauscher J, Marx V, Evaluation of a new percutaneous stainless steel Greenfield filter by intravascular ultrasonography. Surg 1991;109:722-729.

2. Greenfield LJ, Cho KJ, Proctor M, et al, Results of a multicenter study of the modified hook titanium Greenfield filter. J Vasc Surg 1991;14:253-257.

3. Greenfield LJ, Proctor M, Experimental embolic capture by asymmetric Greenfield filters. J Vasc Surg 1992;16(3):436-444.

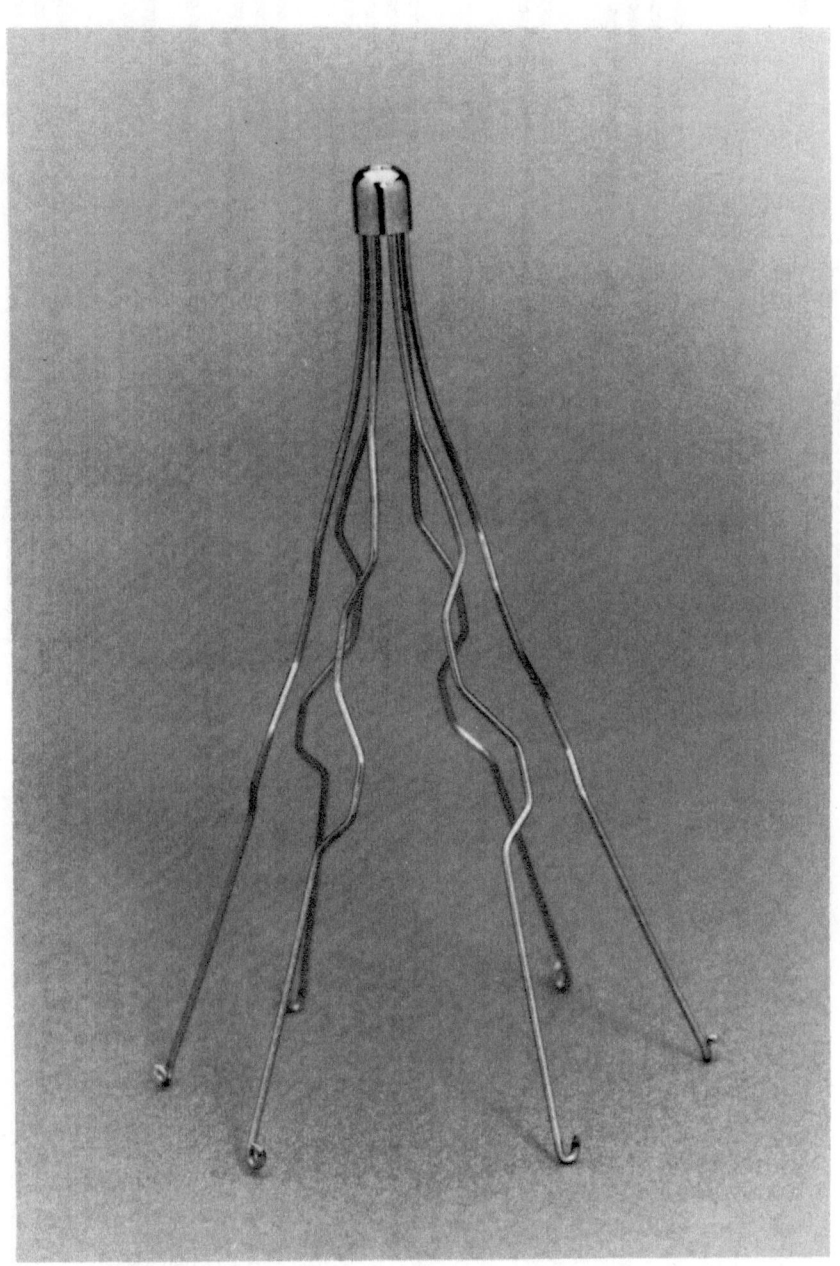

OP/10.3

The Low-Molecular-Weight Heparin, for the prevention of deep venous thrombosis after elective Surgery.

Gutierrez V, Carpintero LA, Alvarez JL, Fernandez L, Agundez I, Abejon A, Carrera S and Vaquero C.

c/García Morato 23 5° Ñ Valladolid 47007 (SPAIN)
Hospital Universitario. c/ Ramón y Cajal s/n Valladolid 47002 (SPAIN)

A randomized, parallel-group, open label clinical trial, was conducted, between January 1989 and September 1994, to compare the safety and efficacy of enoxaparin, a low-molecular-weight, with the safety and efficacy of unfractionated heparin for the prevention of deep venous thrombosis after elective Surgery.

PATIENTS AND METHODE:

410 patients were randomized. The evaluation of efficacy included contrast-media venography, non invasive vascular examination, and clinical examination. For 410 patients had been assigned three groups:

- ❶ Twenty milligrams of enoxaparin every twelve hours (128 patiens)
- ❷ Forty milligrams of enoxaparin once daily (189 patiens)
- ❸ 5000 units of unfractionated heparin every eight hours (93 patiens)

All drugs were administered subcutaneously. Dosages were not adjusted on the basis of the results of coagulation test or the body weight of the patient. Treatment was iniciated within twenty-four hours after the operation and continued for a maximun of seven days. The primary safety outcome waas the occurrence of bleeding episodes.

RESULTS:

An intent-to-treat patient analysis revealed that deep venous thrombosis occurred in 19 (14.8 per cent) of the 128 patients of the first group, in 9 (4.7 per cent) of the 189 patients of the second group and in 16 (17.2 per cent) of the 93 patients of the third group.

The rate of deep venous thrombosis was significantly lower in the second group, group that received forty milligrams of enoxaparin once daily.

No clinically symptomatic pulmonary embolism was observed during the treatment or follow-up phase of this study in the group that received forty milligrams of enoxaparin once daily.

CONCLUSSIONS:

This study demonstrated that enoxaparin, administered postoperatively in a dosage of forty milligrams once daily, is more effective than, and as safe as, unfractionated heparin in the prevention of deep venous thrombosis in patients who have had an elective surgery.

OP/10.4

Assessment of the Effects of the Footpump and Graduated Elastic Compression Stockings

A Abu-Own, J H Scurr and P D Coleridge Smith

Department of Surgery, The Middlesex Hospital, London, UK.

Pneumatic compression of the foot using an AVI (arterio-venous impulse) footpump device is effective in prophylaxis of deep vein thrombosis and treatment of post-traumatic swelling. The purpose of this study was to assess whether there is an advantage in the application of both graduated elastic (TED) stockings and footpump (FP) simultaneously. Twenty healthy volunteers were studies in the supine, 45° recumbent and sitting positions. Strain gauges were attached at the mid-calf region of both legs and connected to a computer recording system. A footpump was attached to the right foot. Continuous strain gauge plethysmography recordings were made from both limbs for a period of 10 minutes in each of the three study positions. The same protocol was repeated after the application of TED stockings.

RESULTS

In the 45° head-elevated position the net decrease in calf volume was significantly greater with the combined use of FP and TED stocking compared to either of the two methods alone. Moving to the sitting position caused a significant increase in calf volume. This increase was less with the combined use of FP and TED stocking (p = 0.04). In the supine position there was no significant change in calf volume.

Net change in calf volume in the 45° head-elevated position (ml%): M (IQR)			
No TED or FP	TED alone	FP alone	TED+FP
0.27 (0.05, 0.53)	0.25 (0.07, 0.50)*	0.03 (0.26, 0.25)†	0.22 (0.90,0.04)*†

M (IQR) = median (interquartile range);* p , 0.01, † p = 0.03 (Wilcoxon matched-pairs signed-ranks test); TED = Thrombo Embolic

We conclude that the combined use of AVI footpump and TED stockings is more effective in preventing leg swelling compared to either of the two methods alone.

OP/19.6

DECREASED MORTALITY IN CANCER PATIENTS TREATED FOR PROXIMAL DEEP VEIN THROMBOSIS (DVT) WITH LOW-MOLECULAR-WEIGHT HEPARIN (LMWH) AS COMPARED WITH UNFRACTIONATED HEPARIN

Pineo GF, Hull RD, Raskob GE, Brant RF, Green D; the Canadian-American Thrombosis Group, Calgary

Objective: To compare all cause mortality rate in cancer patients with proximal DVT being treated with LMWH compared with classic intravenous heparin (IVH).

Design: A multicentre clinical trial comparing the efficacy and safety of initial therapy with once-daily subcutaneous LMWH and dose adjusted continuous IVH with warfarin started on Day 2 and continued for three months in both groups. Deaths were classified as abrupt or insidious.

Results: Cancer was present in 49 of 219 patients (21.0%) of patients on IVH and 46 of 213 (21.6%) of patients on LMWH. Death occurred in 14 of 49 (28.3%) of patients on IVH (8 abrupt and 6 insidious) compared with 7 of 46 (15.2%) of patients on LMWH (2 abrupt and 5 insidious). The observed difference in mortality between the 2 groups was 13.4%; 95% confidence interval (CI), on this difference in mortality ranges between -3% and 29.7% favouring LMWH. The most common sites of cancer were: colon*, prostate, breast, skin, brain*, lung* pancreas*, ovary, cervix, lymphoma, myeloma and bladder* (*-associated with most deaths). With the exception of pancreatic cancer, all other cancers associated with death showed a lower mortality with LMWH.

Conclusion: The mortality rate (particularly due to abrupt causes) was lower in patients receiving initial LMWH compared with initial IVH. This surprise survival advantage of LMWH warrants further study in those cancer patients with the highest mortality rate whether or not they present with venous thromboembolism.

Thrombo-embolic Disorders

Treatment of Thrombo-embolism

Phlebology '95, D. Negus et al. (eds.). Phlebology (1995) Suppl. 1: 717-719

P201

The Surgical Treatment of Thrombophlebitis of Varicose Veins of the Lower Limbs

J. Mazuch, K. Géc, L. Machan and V. Kovàcs

The Department of Surgery, NsP Hospital Regional, Lucenec, Slovakia

INTRODUCTION

Thrombophlebitis of varicose veins is an inflammatory process resulting from insufficient superficial vein, followed by thrombosis, that could partly or completely close the lumen of a vein and spread accordingly. Thrombophlebitis of varicose veins is a complication of the lower limbs extended varicose veins. At the most frequent localisation is the great saphenous vein and its branches, sometimes also the short saphenous vein.

It is identified by signs of inflammation on the skin, oedema, rubor and pain in the thrombophlebitic vein. Periphlebitis is developed and the vein can be palpably seen like a hard line. Local signs of inflammation are usual, but sometimes there is also an overall reaction including fever, high FW, and leucocytosis present.

The causes of thrombophlebitis of varicose veins are numerous: stasis of blood in the vein system, activation of coagulation, trauma or previous surgery. However we think the most important cause of thrombophlebitis of varicose veins is the degenerative damage of vein wall with damaged endothelium. Further factors are: the age of patients, higher level of lipoproteins, infection (interdigital mycosis, pyodermia) and toxic damage of the vein wall by bacterial or other toxins.

MATERIAL AND METHODS

At the Department of Surgery, NsP Lucenec we operated (from 1.1.1984 to 1.10.1994) on 1205 patients with varicose veins of the lower limbs. From these 58 patients (4.8%) were operated on for thrombophlebitis of varicose veins. In this period we treated 4 patients with thrombophlebitis of varicose veins without surgery.

Mean age of these patients was 53.8 years (from 24 to 87 years) the oldest operated patient was 78 years. There were 19 male (30.6%) and 43 female (69.4%) in our study. One patient had thrombophlebitis on both lower limbs. After localisation of thrombosis of varicose veins we recognise 3 forms: (1) crural form 37 (58.7%), (2) femoral form 7 (11.1%), and (3) combined femoro-crural form 19 (30.2%).

Ascending thrombosis of the great saphenous vein we found in 6 patients, where there was thrombosis in the siphon of the great saphenous vein discovered during dissection in inguinal region. Thrombosis did not extend to v. femoralis any time. The trunk of great saphenous vein was thrombosed 19 times and the trunk of the short saphenous vein 3 times.

TREATMENT OF THROMBOPHLEBITIS OF VARICOSE VEINS

The treatment of thrombophlebitis could be conservative or surgical. Conservative treatment is used usually used in out patient departments. It is local application of antiflogistics (Heparoid, Hirudoid gel) analgesics and elastic bandaging. Anticoagulants are used to treat thrombosis into the deep veins system. We use antibiotics only in sepsis with the signs of cellulitis on the lower limbs.

From 63 cases of thrombophlebitis of varicose veins of lower limbs in our study we treated 4 (6.3%) conservatively and 59 (93.7%) surgically. We did 59 radical surgical extirpations of thrombosed varicosities, we added stripping of great saphenous vein 3 times and subfascial ligation of incompetent perforators 25 times. By delicate preparation we can remove the whole thrombosed trunk of great saphenous vein and all thrombosed varicosities. After this surgical procedure the patient soon becomes much better, is without pain and soon mobilised. Part of the treatment is an elastic compression bandage. When thrombophlebitis is advanced or the patient neglected there is also subcutaneous infiltration and periphlebitis. Here we perform dissection of thrombosed veins, and express the thombus incising the vein and applying compression. The healing of the incision is usually good.

Mean hospital stay was 11.05 days. We had 13 (21%) complications. Four cases of suppuration, 4 patients with superficial inflammation of the wound, 3 haematomas, 1 seroma and 1 case of pleuritis exudative. Long term results are excellent, patients are without signs of relapse. Mean time after operation is 5 years. Our surgical procedure is radical, because in one procedure we remove all incompetent veins as well as those without thrombophlebitis, and incompetent perforators.

DISCUSSION

Thrombophlebitis of varicose veins of the lower limbs is the disease of elderly patients with trophic skin changes. We observed 6 cases of thrombosis of the great saphenous vein extending to the saphenofemoral junction but we did not see thrombosis of femoral vein at any time. Delicate dissection of thrombosis in the siphon of the great saphenous vein is very important, because squeezing of the thrombus into the femoral vein could cause pulmonary embolus.

Thrombophlebitis of the great saphenous vein could have ascended into the deep venous system with the risk of pulmonary embolus. We decided in favour of anticoagulant rather than thrombolytic therapy (Mazuch and all, 1993).

We recommend the conservative treatment of thrombophlebitis or varicose veins which are smaller in their extent. We use antiflogistics, ointments, compressive elastic bandages, venotonic drugs, antiagregants and antibiotics, exceptionally anticoagulants or evacuation of the thrombus (Plettner, 1993).

In thrombophlebitis of extensive varicose veins conservative treatment is not sufficient, and allows periphlebitic infiltration, induration and hyperpigmentation of the skin. Conservative treatment is slow. Surgical treatment is more efficient, faster and more radical. We remove whole varicose thrombotic veins, other incompetent veins and perforators.

In thrombophlebitis of minor varicose veins it is possible to remove thrombosed veins through small incisions followed by elastic compression bandages and antiflogisitc therapy.

At the Department of Surgery NsP Lucenec we use the following process: the patient is admitted immediately, and after standard preoperative investigations subjected to operation. The operative procedure is the same as planned operations on varicose veins. If there is ascending of thrombophlebitis, we dissect out the siphon of great saphenous vein and observe the extent of the thrombosis. When thrombosis of the sapheno-femoral junction is present, we ligate all the veins of the junction. Then we ligate the great saphenous veins at the saphenofemoral junction. After this we extirpate all thrombosed varicose veins and do the stripping. When there is inflammation or trophic changes in the skin, we excise the vein in this area and suture. If we find incompetent perforators, then we use subfascial ligation and suture of fascia. Surgical treatment of thrombophlebitis of varicose veins is widely accepted (Lohr et al 1992, Rettori, 1986 Karadzos 1993). After operation we apply elastic bandages. Surgical treatment is completed by antiflogistics, venotonics or antibiotics. Anticoagulants we give if the deep venous system is involved. Surgical treatment of extended thrombophlebitis of varicose veins is the most effective and the fastest way of treatment with excellent results.

Phlebology '95, D. Negus et al. (eds.). Phlebology (1995) Suppl. 1: 720-721

P253

Venous Thromboembolism Treatment. Viewpoint Proposal

C. Pereira Alves, J. Neves, A. Formiga, J. Domingos and C. Alves Pereira

Hospital Stº Antonio dos Capuchos, Serviço 6, Unidade Vascular, Lisboa, Portugal

STATEMENTS

Clinical picture of venous thrombosis is unreliable and elusive.
Diagnostic confirmation with complementary methods is mandatory before starting active treatment .Venography, ecodoppler and haemodynamic plethysmographic studies are the main used methods (1) .
Usualy patients with venous thrombosis are first seen by general practitioners or in hospitals where this methods or technicians are not available , and in a significant number of cases diagnostic confirmation will take 2 or 3 days.
Delay in starting treatment will be the possible consequence , mainly because standard accepted treatment is still intravenous heparin , with three important problems : 1 - route of administration with the need of six daily administrations or perfusion ; 2 - need of laboratory controls ; 3 - danger of haemorrhage .
The possibility of treatment with the low molecular weight heparins twice daily subcutaneous seems as efective as unfractionated heparins and without the three previous problems (2) .
Moreover it seems that "heparins are able to act as scavengers of the first traces of thrombin which are formed at the initial phase of blood coagulation , delaying or preventing factor V and factor VIII activation : inhibition of the so called thrombin feed-back loops " (Michel M Samama - chapter 13 in Prevention of venous thromboembolism Med-Orion 1994) (3) .
Early start of tratment will then be linked with the best benefits . "The earlier the best " Extension of thrombus will be limited and even a complete resolution of the thrombotic process could be achieved , and this is the gold objective of any form of treatment (1) .

PROPOSAL

Considering the previous statements we propose :

1 - Facing a clinical suspition of venous thrombosis doctors should start subcutaneous low molecular weight heparin using treatment doses .

2 - Patients should be refered as soon as possible to a center where it is possible to confirm the diagnosis of venous thrombosis and show its location , the extension and the age characteristics of the thrombus .

3 - Acording to data of venous thrombosis , treatment should be :
- maintained
- changed
- stopped

4 - To confirm influence of this early start practice we consider a protocol using coloured ecodoppler as follow-up method.

REFERENCES

(1) - Anthony J.Comerota, M.D. Samuel C. Aldridge, M.D. Appropriate Therapy for Acute Lower-Extremity Venous Thrombosis . Advances in Vascular Surgery , vol 1 , pags 213-224, Mosby Year Book , Inc. 1993

(2) - Low Molecular Weight Heparins in Prophylaxis and Treatment of Thromboembolic Diseases . edited by Henry Bounameaux , Marcel Dekker , Inc. 1994

(3) - Michel M Samama . Low molecular weight heparins : mode of action and dosage in Prevention of Venous Thromboembolism . chapiter 13 . Med - Orion 1994

Phlebology '95, D. Negus et al. (eds.). Phlebology (1995) Suppl. 1: 722-723

PI/8.5

Venous Thrombectomy. 10-Year Results of a Prospective Randomised Study

G. Plate[1], B. Eklöf[1], J.A. Dahlström[2], H. Åkesson[1] and L. Norgren[3]

[1] Department of Surgery and [2] Clinical Physiology, Central Hospital, Helsingborg, Sweden
[3] Lund University, Sweden

INTRODUCTION

Controversy still exists regarding the value of venous thrombectomy in the treatment of deep venous thrombosis. This procedure has not been shown to reduce the incidence of pulmonary embolism but is occasionally limbs saving in severe cases of phlegmasia coerulea dolens. Whether venous thrombectomy reduces late postthrombotic sequelae is also controversial [1]. The present study presents 10-year results in a prospective randomised study, comparing venous thrombectomy combined with a temporary arteriovenous fistula and conventional anticoagulation to the results obtained with anticoagulation treatment alone.

METHODS

Initially, 58 patients with acute iliofemoral venous thrombosis extending above the inguinal ligament but not into the vena cava and a history of leg swelling not exceeding seven days were included in the study. Thirteen surgically treated and 17 conservatively treated patients were available for follow-up ten years later. This included evaluation of clinical outcome, venous patency and physiological function. The late postthrombotic sequelae were graded according to "Reporting standards in venous disease" by the Ad Hoc Committee [2]. Patency of the iliac vein was assessed by radionuclide angiography. Duplex ultrasound examination was performed as described by Bemmelen et al [4] using a reflux time of 0,5 sec as cut-off level between normal and abnormal reflux. Overall venous function was assessed by foot volumetry [5,6] and ambulatory venous pressure measurements [7].

RESULTS

One (8%) surgically treated patient and 3 (18%) conservatively treated patients developed leg ulcers during the ten years after the initial thrombosis. At follow-up, one (8%) surgically treated and 2 (12%) conservatively treated patients experienced leg pain during exercise (=venous claudication). Moderate or severe postthrombotic sequelae were present in 4 (31%) surgically and in 10 (59%) conservatively treated patients. Radionuclide angiography demonstrated a patent iliac vein in 10 (77%) of the surgically and in 8 (47%) of the conservatively treated patients. Duplex ultrasound demonstrated venous reflux at the femoral level in 6 of 9 (67%) surgically and in 12 of 14 (86%) conservatively treated patients. At the popliteal level, venous reflux was present in 2 of 9 (22%) surgically treated and in 8 of 14 (57%) conservatively treated patients. Foot volumetry demonstrated no difference in calf muscle pump function (EVrel) or venous reflux (Q/EVrel). Venous hypertension (ambulatory venous pressure > 50 mm Hg) was present in 4 (40%) of the surgically treated and in 11 (69%) of the conservatively treated patients. None of these differences were significant using Fisher exact probability test and Mann Whitney U-test for statistical analysis.

CONCLUSION

Most examined parameters were in favour of surgical treatment, but the small number of obseravtions may be responsible for the lack of statistical difference between the two treatment groups. Still, the long-term results following anticoagulation treatment alone are acceptable. Venous thrombectomy should probably be reserved for younger patients with a fresh iliofemoral thrombosis and without a history of previous deep venous thrombosis.

REFERENCES

1. Solis MM, Ranval TJ, Thompson BW, Eidt JF. Results of venous thrombectomy in the treatment of deep vein thrombosis. Surg Gyn Obstet 1993;177:633-9.
2. Porter JM, Rutherford RB, Clagett GP et al. Ad Hoc Committee. Reporting standards in venous disease. J Vasc Surg 1988;8:172-81.
3. Åkesson H, Cwikiel W, Dahlström JA, Eklöf B, Ohlin P, Plate G. Radionuclide angiography in the evaluation of iliofemoral venous patency. Inter Angiol 1989;8:22-7.
4. Bemmelen PS, Bedford G, Beach K, Strandness DE. Quantitative segmental evaluation of venous valvular reflux with duplex ultrasound scanning. J Vasc Surg 1989;10:425-31.
5. Norgren L. Functional evaluation of chronic venous insufficiency by foot-volumetry. Acta Chir Scand 1974;Suppl 444.
6. Brudin L, Landgren IM, Bengtsson M, Ohlin P. A modified method of curve analysis in foot-volumetry and its reference values. Clin Physiol 1989;9:189-97.
7. Nicolaides AN, Zukowski AJ. The value of dynamic venous pressure measurements. World J Surg 1986;10:919-24.

Phlebology '95, D. Negus et al. (eds.). Phlebology (1995) Suppl. 1: 724-726

P255

Permanent or Temporal Vena Cava Filter Devices in Deep Venous Thrombosis: Which and When?

M. Pocek[1], Mr Guazzaroni[1], G. Sodani[1], R. Gloria[2], R. Pepe[2], E. Marchitelli[2] and G. Simonetti[1]

[1] Department of Radiology, S.Eugenio Hospital, Tor Vergata University of Rome and [2] Department of Angiology, S.Eugenio Hospital of Rome, Italy

INTRODUCTION

Pulmonary embolysm (PE) is a dramatic complication of deep venous thrombosis (DVT), and it represents the third cause of exitus in hospitalized patients [1].

Anticoagulant prophylaxis and praecox mobilization are able to reduce effectively PE incidence, while absence of prophylaxis raises to 50% this incidence[2].

Nowadays an emergent alternative to surgical procedures (venous thrombectomy, caval ligation and caval clips) is the deployment of vena cava filters. These devices prevent cranial migration of embolic material, trapping it within its net.

Hemodinamics of vena caval district is not significantly modified as a result of the deployment of the vena cava filter.

MATERIAL AND METHODS

From January 1987 to April 1995 we deployed 53 permanent vena cava filters (PF) and 16 temporary filters (TF) in 69 patients: the average was 56 in P.F. and 45 in T.F.

In all of these patients a DVT of lower limbs was diagnosed, and of these, 56 also presented a DVT extended to the iliac-caval district.

We performed color-flow-Doppler (Apogeex Cx Interspect) that detected the emboligen thrombi such as: fluctuating clots, thrombi characterized by slow organization, thrombi tending towards new appositions, or blood clots situated in superficial vein confluence.

If DVT was developed over the inguinal ligament, we performed a CT of abdomen and pelvis (Philips Tomoscan LX) for a better diagnostic definition; patients with a clinical suspect of PE, or patients presenting some ultrasonographic patterns of occurred embolism (beheaded thrombus or wedge shaped clot) underwent high resolution pulmonary CT.

Phlebography of iliac-caval district was performed before the deployment of the vena caval filter, to confirm the extension and the peculiar features of the thrombus.

The access site was trans-jugular in 42 patients, in order to deploy the permanent devices. The carrier system calibre has made venotomy mandatory 21 times. The transfemoral venous via was used in 11 patients.

We implanted Kimray-Greenfield PF [3,4,5] in 35 cases (21 Kimray-Greenfield PF of 24 Fr. and 14 titanium Kimray-Greenfield PF of 12 Fr.), 7 L.G.M. Bruneau PF, 5 Filcard PF, 5 Antheor PF, and only in one case we deployed a Gunther filter.

To introduce TF the brachial access was used 8 times, the trans-jugular via 3 times, and the trans-femoral via, contra lateral to thrombosis, 5 times. In particular we introduced Filcard TF, L.G.M. Bruneau, and Antheor TF respectively in 12,2 and 2 cases.

The follow-up was based on coagulation tests, because the failure of the deployment of the vena cava filter, especially with TF, is generally due to the inadequate fibrinolytic and eparinic therapy. Therefore we used rTPA bolus of 30 mg finally to reaching a total of 100 mg. We also gave 35,000-40,000 UI for a 24-48 hours period, through a local trans-catether therapy.

We fixed the pletismographic [6] and clinical evaluation of treated patients every six months and we valued thrombus involution or evolution, in order to decide anticoagulant therapy duration.

Radiological follow-up varied from 2 to 42 months: every patient underwent Rx-abomen with two projections evaluating possible mobilization of device, color-flow-Doppler examining the caval lumen, and Angio-CT if we suspected filter thrombosis.

RESULTS

64 out of the 69 patients observed had a DVT in action, and 16 of these manifested clinically a PE episode; in 8 patients PE represented the first manifestation of DVT, that was confined to the popliteal district in 4 of then and to the femoral-popliteal district in the remaining 4. Other localizations of DVT were more cranial: we observed 40 DVT extending to the iliac-caval district, and 16 isolated iliac-caval DVT. Only 10 patients manifested a bilateral DVT.

Our criteria for choosing between temporal and permanent devices (Table 1), depended on different parameters: patient age, thromboembolic risk entity and its duration, preoperative risk of PE presence, and fibrinolytic therapy effectiveness.

Table 1

DVT: causal factors	53 Permanent Filters	16 Temporal Filters
Coagulopathies:		
- deficit AT III	3	1
- deficit Prot C	3	2
- deficit Prot S	1	-
Neoplasms:	9	-
Surgical interventions:		
- orthopaedic	9	2
- urological	3	3
- oncological	7	2
- gynaecologic	2	-
- other	5	2
Immobilization:	7	1
Trauma:	4	1
Pregnancy:	-	2

The occurred complications were all minor with no long-term sequelae: filter thrombosis in 3 patients; cranial migration with two pliers in renal vein and with consensual angulation in one case, detachment of a lateral plier during deployment of a L.G.M. Bruneau filter in a patient and, finally, the detachment of Antheor filter from its carrier system with a following angulation one time.

DISCUSSION

Vena cava filter placement should be reserved to subjects suffering DVT with high risk of PE such as in the following situations:

1. DVT extended to the iliac-caval district in immobile and thrombophilic patients [7];
2. DVT with associated serious pulmonary hypertension;
3. insufficient anticoagulant or fibrinolytic treatment for preventing PE;
4. controindicated thrombolytic therapy;
5. after embolectomy;
6. documented fluctuating blood clot, wherever it is located.

We prefer TF to PF for patients with high life prospective, for surgical cases to prevent embolic episodes or in association with a local fibrinolytic therapy [4,5]. TF devices offer different advantages: facility of introduction, small dimensions and possibility of trans-catheter fibrinolytic treatment. Little motions shoud be imparted to these filters every day, in order to avoid device endothelialization. Diagnosis, therapy and follow of patients with DVT need multidisciplinary collaboration between angiologist, angioradiologist, haematologist and vascular surgeon. If a correct management of TF fails, we suggest to deploy PF, that involves a minor management difficulty [8] .

REFERENCES

1. Alexander JJ, Zarins CK. The diagnosis of pulmonary embolism. In: Bergan JJ, editor. Surgery of the veins. New York: G&S, 1985.
2. Rohrer MJ, Scheidler MG, Brownell W, Citler B. Extended indications for placement of an inferior vena cava filter. J Vasc Surg 1989; 1-44.
3. Greenfield LJ, Kyung JC, Tauscher JR. Limitations of percutaneous insertion of Greenfield filters. J Cardiov Surg 1990; 31:344.
4. Greenfield LJ, Proctor MC, Williams DM, Wakefield TW. Long term experience with transvenous catheter pulmonary embolectomy. J Vasc Surg 1993; 18(3):450-7.
5. Denny DF, Cronan JJ, Dorfman GS, Esplin C. Percutaneous Kimray-Greenfield placement by femoral vein puncture. AJR 1985; 145: 827-9.
6. Cardella JF, Young AT, Smith TP, et al. Lower extremity venous thrombosis: comparison of venography impedance pletismography and intravenous manometry. Radiology 1988; 168: 109-112.
7. Rosen MP, Porte DH, Kim D. Reassessment of vena cava filter use in patients with cancer. JVIR 1994; 5:501.
8. Simonetti G, Fava C, Urigo F, Grosso M, Carpanese L, Guazzaroni Mr, et al. Filtri cavali: indicazioni e tecnica di posizionamento.In Simonetti G, Pistolese R editors. La flebografia quando e perché. Rome: Delfino A, 1990.

Phlebology '95, D. Negus et al. (eds.). Phlebology (1995) Suppl. 1: 727-730

OP/10.7

Prevalence and Incidence of Pulmonary Embolism in Deep Vein Thrombosis Treated by Compression, Ambulation and Low Molecular Weight Heparin

B. Kechavarz[1], H. Köhn[2], A. Mostbeck[3] and H. Partsch[1]

[1] Department of Dermatology, [2] Department of Nuclear Medicine and [3] L. Boltzmann-Institute for Nuclear Medicine, Wilhelminen Hospital, Vienna, Austria

INTRODUCTION

Several randomized trials have demonstrated that low molecular weight heparin (LMWH) is at least as effective and safe as unfractioned i.v. heparin in the treatment of DVT (1,2,3). The frequency of new pulmonary emboli (PE) seems to be a valuable parameter concerning therapeutic quality control.

This study reports on a total of consecutive 370 patients with DVT treated by LMWH, firm compression bandages and avoidance of bed rest in whom lung scans were performed before and after 7-11 days of treatment.

Patients and Methods

Between 2/1992 and 12/1994 all 370 consecutive patients who were admitted to our department because of acute DVT of the lower extremities were enrolled in this prospective study. 113 patients had DVT extending into the pelvis (Group A), 183 patients had a thrombus up to the thigh (Group B) and 74 patients isolated lower leg vein DVT excluding the popliteal vein (Group C). Table 1 shows clinical characteristics of the patients.

All patients were admitted to the ward, got firm bandages and were kept mobile. The legs were screened by venous occlusion plethysmography and Doppler and the diagnosis was made by Duplex scanning. In case of lower limb involvement 99mTc Plasmin test and- if inconclusive- phlebography was added. The suspicion of an iliofemoral DVT was confirmed by radionuclide venography in every case: 99mTc-labeled microspheres are injected into dorsal foot veins of both legs. A gamma camera placed over the proximal thighs and lower abdomen registers the tracer flow through the pelvic veins. The microspheres are trapped in the terminal pulmonary arterioles allowing perfusion scintigraphy of the lungs. In case of perfusion defects an inhalation scan using DTPA aerosol is added. In patients who are not investigated by radionuclide phlebography perfusion lung scans are performed by i.v.-injection of 99mTc-microspheres. Lung scans are repeated after 11 days in average in every patient.

All patients were screened for malignancy while staying on the ward.

Therapy

All 370 patients received LMWH (Fragmin). Patients suffering from iliofemoral DVT ,Group A (n=113), were randomized into two groups Group. A_1 (n=58) received Fragmin 200 IU / kg body weight once per day subcutaneously. Group A_2 (n=55) received 100 IU / kg body weight twice a day . Group B (n=183) and Group C (n=74) received Fragmin 200IU/kg once per day for 5-12 days and then oral anticoagulation (Marcoumar).
Anti- Fxa was checked 4 and 24 h after injection because of principal interest once during the treatment, platelet counts were performed once a week.

Results

The primary endpoint for the efficacy of our treatment was the incidence of new pulmonary emboli diagnosed by the control lung scan compared to the baseline scan. In the baseline scan pulmonary emboli (PE) were detected in 49/113 (45%) of group A , 95/183 (52%) in group B and 26/74 (35%) in group C. (Chi square-test: A and B vs. C $p<0.05$).The majority of these pulmonary emboli was clinically silent. New pulmonary emboli could be proved by the control scan after 11 days in group A_1 in 3/58 (5.2%) patients and in group A_2 in 3/55 (5,4%) . In group B 8/183 (4,4%) and in group C 3/74 (4%) developed new PE in the second lung scan (no statistically significant difference between the groups) (table 2).

The total incidence of malignant tumors was 53/370 (14.3%). (Group A: 23.9%, group B: 11.5%, group C: 6.8%. (Group A statistically significantly higher than B and C, $p>0.005$).
During the initial treatment period, minor bleeding occured in 5/370 (1,3%) patients.One patient of group A1 developed a major bleeding. A 73 y old man died of malignant disease five weeks after hospital discharge (table 2).

CONCLUSION

Regarding the incidence of new pulmonary emboli LMWH, which does not need special coagulation tests, seems to be effective and safe in a fixed dose once daily. ByTreating mobile patients suffering from DVT with firm compression bandages and LMWH, outpatient management of a large proportion of DVT-patients will be possible .

Acute DVT in 370 patients. Treatment by LMWH, compression, walking
(Feb 92-Dec 94)

	Group A[1] Iliofemoral (n=58)	Group A[2] Iliofemoral (n=55)	Group B Thigh n=183	Group C Lower leg n=74
LMWH (Fragmin)	1x200 U/kg	2x100 U/kg	1x200 U/kg	1x200 U/kg
Age	73 (23-92)	76 (27-92)	68 (24-92)	60 (23-87)
Sex m/f	25/33	27/28	105/78	28/46
l/r	32/26	43/12	88/95	42/32
Previous history DVT	31%	34,5%	26,2%	21,6%
Duration of symptoms(d)	3 (0-30)	3 (0-30)	6 (0-42)	5 (0-35)
Malignant disease (%)	24,1%	23,6%	11,5% (vs A p<0,05)	6,8% (vs A p<0,01)

Table 1: Characteristics

	Group A[1] Iliofemoral (n=58)	Group A[2] Iliofemoral (n=55)	Group B Thigh n=183	Group C Lower leg n=74
Primary PE	23 (40%)	26 (47%)	95 (52%)	26 (35%)
Symptomatic	8 (34%)	6 (23%)	34 (37%)	12 (46%)
New PE	3/58 (5,2%)	3/55 (5,4%)	8/183 (4,4%)	3/74 (4%)
New sympt.	-	-	1/8	-
Minor bleending	2 (3,4%)	-	2 (1,1%)	1 (1.4%)
Major bleeding	1 (1,7%)	-	-	-
Death	-	-	1*	-

*:5 wks after discharge
(bronchus-carcinoma)

Table 2:Results

REFERENCES

1. Albada J., Nieubenhuis HK., Sixma JJ.: Treatment of Acute Venous Thromboembolism with Low Molecular Weight Heparin (Fragmin). Circulation 1989;80: 935-940.

2. Prandoni P., Lensing AWA, Büller HR, Carta M, Cogo A, Vigo M, Casara D, Ruol A., Ten Cate J.: Comparison of subcutaneous low-molecular-weight   heparin with intravenous standard-heparin in proximal deep-vein thrombosis. Lancet 1992; 339:441-445.

3. Holmström M., Törnebohm E, Berglund M-C, Granqvist S, Lockner D. : Fragmin (Kabi) Subcutaneously once or twice daily in the Treatment of DVT. Jouroal of Internal Medicine 1990;228, suppl. 733.

4. Partsch H. Compression therapy of the legs. J. Dermatol. Surg. Oncol.1991;17:799-805.

5. Partsch H., Oburger K., Mostbeck A., König B., Köhn H.: Frequency of pulmonary embolism in ambulant patients with pelvic vein thrombosis: A prospective study. J. Vasc. Surg.1992; 5:715-722.

6. Harenberg J, Leber G, Raedsch R, Zimmermann R, Schwarz F, Kübler W.: Therapeutic application of subcutaneous LMW H in acute venous thrombosis. Haemostasis 1990; 20 (suppl.1), 205-219.

7. von Liebe S, Kissler M, Zumtobel V.: Zur Häufigkeit von Lungenembolien vor und nach Thrombektomie tiefer Bein-Beckenvenenthrombosen. Chirurg.l991; 62:482-485.

8. Cuppini S, Cattelan AM, Casara D, Prandoni P.: Occult pulmonary embolism in patients with proximal deep venous thrombosis. Ann Ital Med Int 1991; 6:1-5.

9. Plate G, Ohlin P, Eklöf B.: Pulmonary embolism in acute iliofemoral venous thrombosis. Br.J.Surg 1985; 72:912-915.

10.Hull RD, Raskob GE, Coates G, Panju AA.: Clinical validity of anormal perfusion lungscan in patients with suspected pulmonary embolism.Chest 1990; 97:23-26.

11.Pilger E, Obernosterer A, Lipp R, Decrinis M., et al:. Prävalenz und Inzidenz einer Pulmonalarterienembolie (PAE) bei Patienten mit tiefen venösen Thrombosen (TVT):VASA 1992; suppl 37:38-39.

12.Huismann MV, Büller HR, ten Cate JW, van Royen EA, Vreeken J, Kersten M-J, BakxR.::Unexpected High Prevalence of Silent Pulmonary Embolism in Patients with deep venous Thrombosis. Chest 1989; 95: 498-502.

Phlebology '95, D. Negus et al. (eds.). Phlebology (1995) Suppl. 1: 731-733

V/3.10

Surgical Treatment of Varicophlebitis

L. De Santis[1], F. Battocchio[1], M. Baldan[1], O. Terranova[1], G.P. Avruscio[2], G.P. Signorini[2] and A. Rugna[3]

[1] Cattedra di Chirurgia Generale e Divisione di Chirurgia Geriatrica, [2] Servizio di Angiologia, [3] Divisione Medica I', Università di Padova, Italy

INTRODUCTION

Superficial thrombophlebitis of the lower limbs represents a frequently observed pathology which complicates varicose disease in 15-20% of cases [1].

Usually blood stasis, coupled or not with a trauma, is the principal cause; more rarely it depends on coagulation pathologies, be they hereditary (C Protein, S Protein, Antithrombin III deficits) or acquired (malignant tumors, vasculitis, antiphospholipids antibody Syndrome).

If varicophlebitis was commonly considered as a favourable course illness, in the last years, due to the introduction of new diagnostic methodologies such as echo-doppler and echo-color-flow-doppler, the benignity of this disease has become matter of discussion. Recent studies, in fact, demonstrate a progression from superficial to deep venous thrombosis in a rate ranging from 10 to 32% [2]. This justify the carefullness and the radical therapeutic approach with which we treat the cases with proximal extention, when sapheno-femoral or sapheno-popliteal junctions are involved.

Aim of this study was to analize the characteristics of site and extention of varicophlebitic process in the proximal forms, the possible involvement of the deep venous system and the results of a radical surgical treatment.

METHODS

From January 1992 to December 1994, 105 patients (59 females and 46 males, with age ranging from 24 to 84 years), afflicted with proximal varicophlebitis underwent our observation.

The non invasive study with duplex scanning and color flow echo-doppler demonstrated a thrombosis of the greater saphenous vein in 75 cases , of the lesser saphenous vein in 21 cases and of a collateral varicose branch in 9 cases.

On making diagnosis the thrombosis involved the deep venous system in 19 cases, 14 of which represented a progression from the greater saphenous vein while 4 from the lesser saphenous vein and 1 from varicose collateral branch.

In 9 cases the thrombus involved the deep venous system and heparin treatment, at the usual dosage, was carried out.

In the other 10 cases the thrombus jutted into the deep venous system for a short span, so its exeresis was possible. These last patients, together with the others presenting only a superficial involvement, had been surgically treated.

The operation, sometimes under local anesthesia, consisted in a wide exposure and a careful isolation of the thrombosed vein to avoid embolization of thrombotic material. After tying and sectioning the collateral branches, a venotomy followed with removal of the thrombus and verification of patency of the deep venous system by means of Valsalva manouvre, prior to sectioning the superficial vein at its confluence with the deep system. The operation was then completed with exeresis of thrombosed and varicose collateral branches.

All the patients had a regular post-operative course, with no complication. The mean hospital stay was 2 days. Follow up of these patients revealed no recurrency of varicophlebitis and echo-doppler inspection confirmed the patency of deep venous system.

DISCUSSION

The incidence of deep venous thrombosis as complicating superficial varicophlebitis ranges from 2.8% of old series up to 20-30% of up to date studies [3,4,5,6].

Varicophlebitis affecting greater saphenous vein means a risk of deep venous thrombosis twice as much as that involving lesser saphenous vein or collateral branches, being otherwhile of 10% in these cases.

The rate is high even in our study, in which deep venous thrombosis complicated the 20.6 and 17% of cases respectively. If considering the frequency of varicose disease, these rates are not negligible.

A radical surgical treatment appears thus convenient in these cases to prevent extension of thrombosis to deep venous system and a possible pulmonary embolism.

The most important act of this operation is crossectomy with interruption of the superficial vein at its confluence with deep venous system. It can be performed under local anesthesia. To our opinion it's better, when possible, to complete the operation with saphenectomy as it permits a rapid relief from pain, a complete treatment of varicose disease and a prevention from varicophlebitic recurrency (occurring in 15% of cases). It further avoid the risks linked to anticoagulant therapy.

An early treatment of the disease means an easier surgical treatment as the thrombus is not jet organized. In this case the operation is similar to the saphenectomy for varicose veins. To these advantages we have to add a reduction of costs due to a single hospital stay.

In case of varicophlebitis at lesser risk, as in cases involving distal branches, we recommend a conservative treatment with non-steroid antiphlogistic drugs, compressive bandages and early deambulation. In the same way, in the cases with wide involvement of deep venous system, anticoagulant therapy and, in selected cases (phlegmasia coerulea dolens, hypersensitivity to heparin, serious pulmonary embolism), thrombolitic drugs remain the treatment of choice.

Echo-doppler evaluation has proven useful in the evaluation of this disease as it permits a clear morphologic definition of the involved venous system and allows a follow up showing an eventual progression to deep venous thrombosis, thus conditioning the therapeutic choice.

REFERENCES

1. Bergquist D, Jaroszeski H. Deep vein thrombosis in patients with superficial thrombophlebitis of the leg. Br Med J 1986; 292: 658-659.
2. Battocchio F, De Santis L, Signorini GP, Avruscio GP, Benedetti L, Terranova O. The role of noninvasive imaging in therapy for varicophlebitis of the saphenous system. Phlebologie 1992. Eds John Libbey Eurotext,Paris 1992; 648-650
3. Lofgren EP, Lofgren KA. The surgical treatment of superficial thrombophlebitis. Surgery 1981; 90:49-54.
4. Barrellier MT. Thromboses veineuses superficielles des membres inferieurs.Phlebologie 1993; 46: 633.
5. LutterKS, Kerr TM, Roedersheimer LE, Lohr JM, Sampson MG, Cranley JJ. Superficial thrombophlebitis diagnosed by duplex scanning. Surgery 1991; 110: 42-46.
6. Husni EA, Williams WA. Superficial thrombophlebitis of lower limbs. Surgery 1992; 91: 70.

Phlebology '95, D. Negus et al. (eds.). Phlebology (1995) Suppl. 1: 734-736

P259

Anticoagulant and Thrombolytic Treatment of the Deep Venous Thrombosis

J. Mazuch, P. Bruncak, K. Gec and L. Machan

The Department of Surgery, NsP Hospital Regional, Lucenenc, Slovakia

The venous thromboses are serious medicine problem. Especially the deep venous thromboses with complications like pulmonary embolia or post thrombotic syndrome.

Early diagnosis and effective treatment of the deep venous thrombosis can prevent these complications. The treatment is following: anticoagulant, thrombolytic or surgical. The aim of the treatment is to reach desobliteration of veins as soon as possible and to keep the vein valves undamaged /it is the prevention of post thrombotic syndrome./. The second aim of the treatment is to eliminate potential sources of the pulmonary embolia.

The indication for the surgical treatment is mostly ileofemoral thrombosis /2/. It is the fastest way how to do the desobstruction of the vein trunks by Fogarty. Disadvantages are quite often rethromboses and the necessity of A-V fistula and the second intervention to abolish the fistula. In early stages of DVT very good results could be obtained by anticoagulant and thrombolytic therapy. But the condition is early diagnosis and rational treatment /6/. The aim of the rational treatment is to find optimal therapeutic process and the way of application. Thrombolytic treatment by streptokinase is different than anticoagulant treatment by heparin. Streptokinase treatment is active, can solve the new thrombus and reach full desobstruction of vein river-bed. Heparin is polyvalent anticoagulant, that works in all 4 phases of the coagulation /especially like Antithrombin III/. Heparin's effect is slow and the time of the application is longer, 5-7 days.

The aim of our study was to objectify the results of anticoagulant and thrombolytic treatment and the way of application.

MATERIALS AND METHODS

At the Department of Surgery, NsP Lucenec we treated 354 patients from 1975 to 1992 for DVT. There were 202 males and 152 females, the mean age was 55.1 years. We treated 68.6% of the patients for DVT with history shorter than one week. To objectify our diagnosis, we used the phlebography in 64.4% of the patients, later on Doppler USG. After localisation we recognised 4 forms. The most frequent was crural form 232 /65.5%/ and ileofemoral form 74/20.9%/. We found signs of phlegmasia alba dolens in 21 patients and thrombolytic treatment was applied by 2 of them.

TREATMENT

We always started the anticoagulant therapy with Heparin in continual i.v. infusion. Dose was 5 mg/kg. That means 4 x 10,000 u/24 hours in 80kg patient. The treatment lasted 5-7 days and we controlled thrombin time, prothrombin time and Lee-White clotting time. After 5-7 days of treatment by Heparin we provided the phlebography again and changed Heparin for peroral anticoagulant Pelentan. Treatment was Pelentan lasted 3-6 months and prothrombin time was controlled regularly. We treated 331 patients for DVT with Heparin. General application of Heparin was done in 256/72.3%/patients. The topical application, that means perfusion of the limb with the thrombosis/Heparin applied into the periphery of great saphenous vein/ was done in 75/21.2%/ patients.

We used Streptokinase in 23 patients in 23 patients, all of them had ileofemoral thrombosis. The thrombolytic treatment we always started with titration dose 500,000 u. of Streptase and corticosteroids i.v. This initial dose was followed by continual 100,000 u of Streptase / hour in permanent i.v. application. The treatment lasted 48-72 hours, and we controlled fibrinogen, thrombin time and euglobin lysis time.

After Streptase we followed the treatment by Heparin and later on by Pelentan. The general application of Streptase we applied in 13 patients and the topical in 10 patients. The better results of the treatment/resolution of the thrombus/ we saw after the topical administration in 90% of the patients.

The complete lysis of the thrombus we found in 229 /64.7%/ cases and we call this excellent results. The partial lysis - an improvement of the status, we found in 114/32.2%/ of the patients. After topical administration of anticoagulant or thrombolytic treatment we achieved the higher numbers of the complete lyses.

To objectify the results of the treatment after general and topical administration /Heparin and Streptase/, we found out 120 patients. All these patients had phlebography before and after the treatment. The complete lysis of DVT before and after the treatment. The complete lysis of DVT we found in 73.3% of the patients after general application and in 92.18% after topical application.

The excellent result of the treatment / complete lysis of the thrombus in vein system/ was in 18.8% higher after the topical application than after the general application /p < 0.05/. But it is much better to prevent the thrombosis than to treat it. Physical and medicinal prevention and prophylaxis is overall accepted /4/.

After the administration of anticoagulant. and thrombolytic treatment the number of fatal pulmonary embolia decreased from 12.20% to 1-1.5% /3/. In our study of the patients treated for DVT we had 4 cases of fatal pulmonary embolia 1.12%. 3 cases were during the treatment by Heparin and 1 case during the thrombolysis. 2 elderly patients died for cardio-pulmonary decompensation. We had 8 hemorrhagic complications/2.25%/. In 2 cases it was serious bleeding, where we had to stop the therapy and we gave the blood transfusions. It was always by the Streptase application. The risk of the serious bleeding is from 1.3 to 15% /1.6/. We found 4 patients with post thrombotic syndrome. 1 patient was operated on, Palme's operation with good result.

REFERENCES

1.	Holm HA, Finnanger B, Hartmann A, Laerum F, Lohren O, Budd TE, Stray N, Woland T. Heparin treatment of deep venous thrombosis in 280 patients: symptoms related to dosage. Acta med. Scan., 215, 1984, 1:47-53.

2.	Kaspar S, Voboril Z, Jon B, Gneidy M. Surgical treatment of acute ileofemoral thrombosis. Prakt. flebol. 2, 1993, 2:38-41.

3.	Krcilek A, Thrombophlebitis and thromboses of limb veins. Praha, Avicenum 1970, 172.

4.	Mazuch J, Mihalovics T, Filo M. Prevention and prophylaxis of the thromboembolic complications by fractures of femur. Acta orthop. Traum. Czech, 53, 1986, 1:34-40

5.	Mazuch J, Filo M, Pelo J, Bruncak P, Mjsanik L, Mitacz K. Rational treatment of venous thromboses. Prakt. Lek 67, 1987, 12:466-470.

6.	Wilson J R, Lampman J, Heparin therapy: A randomised prospective study. Am. Heart J., 1979, 2:255-258.

Phlebology '95, D. Negus et al. (eds.). Phlebology (1995) Suppl. 1: 737-740

OP/19.5

Follow Up Study of 160 Iliofemoral Venous Thrombectomies

A. Hetenyi

Department of Vascular Surgery Magyar Imre Hospital, Ajka, Hungary

INTRODUCTION

The rational way of treating iliofemoral venous thrombosis is - in our opinion - thrombectomy. It is generally accepted in medical literature, that early surgical interventions have the best results (up to 7 davs from the development of the thrombus). However, we have only the approximate conceptions, that the really beginning of the thrombosis in the different parts of the venous system of the lower leg. The location, the type and the expansion of DVT is a very important factor in the surgical indication and in the judgement of the early and late results. We stove for interventions, for the surgical liberation of the "groin collector segment" (common femoral, deep femoral and long saphenous veins) and the iliac outflow tract. Therefore, for this reason, we have operated more aggressively the ascending thromboses, as others (14 - 21 days after the distal develops).

PATIENTS

From 1986 - 1992, we had operated on 160 patients: 52 women (average age 50.2 years) and 98 men (average age 54.8 years). In the women's group, there were 9 operations on the right, 52 on the left, and 1 on the both sides; in the men's group, there was 41 on the right, 50 on the left, and 7 on the both sides.

There was 83 ascending, 40 descending, 15 ascending-descending types (expanded from the thrombosed LSV) of the thrombosis, and in 22 cases we couldn't determine the starting-point of the thrombosis (most of these patients had concomitant malignant disease). There were generally two or more risk factors in the anamnesis of the patients. The most frequent were: immobilisation (45), different types of trauma and surgery (44), ascending varicophlebitis (19), gravidity and postpartum state (10), and malignant diseases (8).

DIAGNOSIS

Our routine was: clinical examination, CW-Doppler, Duplex-scan (venous and abdominal investigation), chest X-ray examination, ascending phlebography (expect in the phlegmasia coerulea cases).

SURGICAL MANAGEMENT

The "collector segment" is exposed, the veins are encircled. Transverse or longitudinal venotomy are made in the CVF just above the confluence. Fogarty-balloon is passed through the thrombus into the IVC and is than inflated. The thrombus is than extracted with another Fogarty-catether and suction. Since 1990 we have been able to control the iliac veins intraoperative with angioscopy, and we extract the remaining thrombi under visual control. If there were no other choices in exposing a large part of the CVF, we protected the vein from compression and collapse by an external PTFE-spiral.

We had created an arteriovenous fistula (AVF) in 90 cases (indications: poor inflow because of the partially or unsuccessful distal thrombectomy, stenosis of the outflow tract). Temporary AVF were created from the LSV trunk only in 24 cases - we protected the LSV if it has a good collateral function (adherent thrombus in the femoropopliteal veins).

Postoperative treatment were: continous Heparin (5 - 7 days), early mobilisation, compression therapy, long lasting anticoagulation (Warfarin).

We ligated the AVF-s 3 - 6 months after surgery.

Early complications

Postoperative death: 7 cases (pulmonary embolism 2 - 17 days after surgery in 4 cases). Early reocclusion: 12 cases (successful re-thrombectomy: 1; unsuccessful re-thrombectomy: 4; high PTFE-Palma bypass: 2; conservative treatment 5).

FOLLOW UP

We followed the the clinical status of patients from discharge to the latest control. In the first months we losted 7 patients (early postoperative death) and during the follow up period an additional 18 patients (late death complications: pulmonary embolism 2, cardiac arrest 3, malignant disease 7; insufficient cooperation 6). The average follow up time was 29.6 months (3 - 96 months).

We controlled all of our patients by clinical examination and CW-Doppler. At the suspicion of stenosis or reocclusion of the outflow tract (swelling, pain, CW-Doppler findings) we have made as ascending phlebography in 18 cases (negative results in 9, iliac or femoral occlusion in 5, iliac compression in 1, iliofemoral reflux in 3 cases) or at functioning AVF an aortophlebography in 31 cases (negative results in 11, iliac stenosis or occlusion in 17, femoropopliteal occlusion in 3 cases).

We indicated and performed, based on the phlebographic findings, 12 late iliofemoral reconstructions (PTFE-Palma bypass, iliac patch-plasty, decompression of the iliac arterial aneurysm).

Figure 1. illustrates the relation of the site and the extent of thrombosis and the early success of the surgical intervention. In some of the iliofemoral thrombosis, we could perform only a partial thrombectomy: the adherent femoropopliteal thrombus, we are unable to remove.

We classified the clinical status of the patients as:

1. -without complaints (with or without compression therapy)
2. -mild edema (1 - 2 cm difference in circumference)
3, -permanent edema (more than 2 cm difference in circumference), spontan Palma-veins, secondary varicosity
4. -lipodermatosclerosis, ulcus cruris postthromboticum.

Figure 2. illustrates the percentage of controlled patients, and the changing of their clinical status, connection with the follow-up time.

The clinical status of the thrombectomised patients are permanently successful in 60 - 70 % and obligate in 20 - 30 %, despite the relatively liberal surgical indication. In this result a significant role is played not only in the first operation, but the late surgical reconstructions, the compression therapy and the consistent care of the patients.

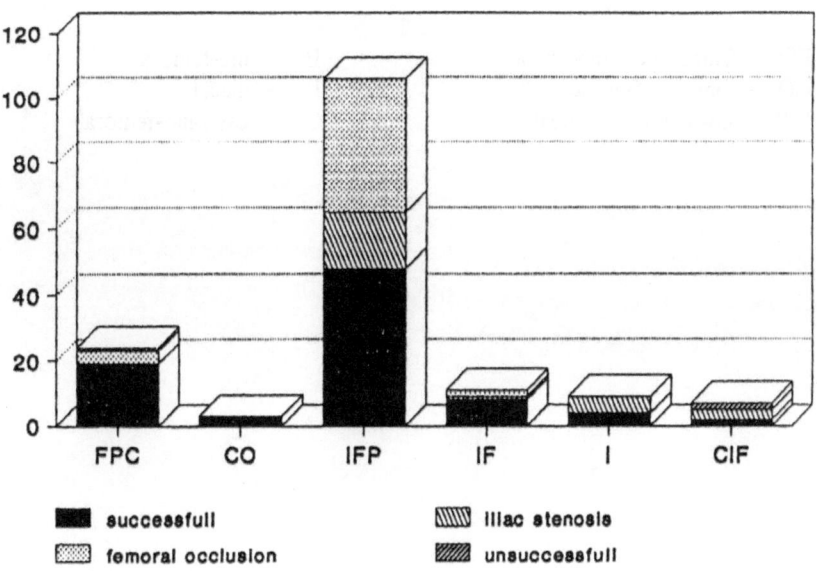

Fig. 1

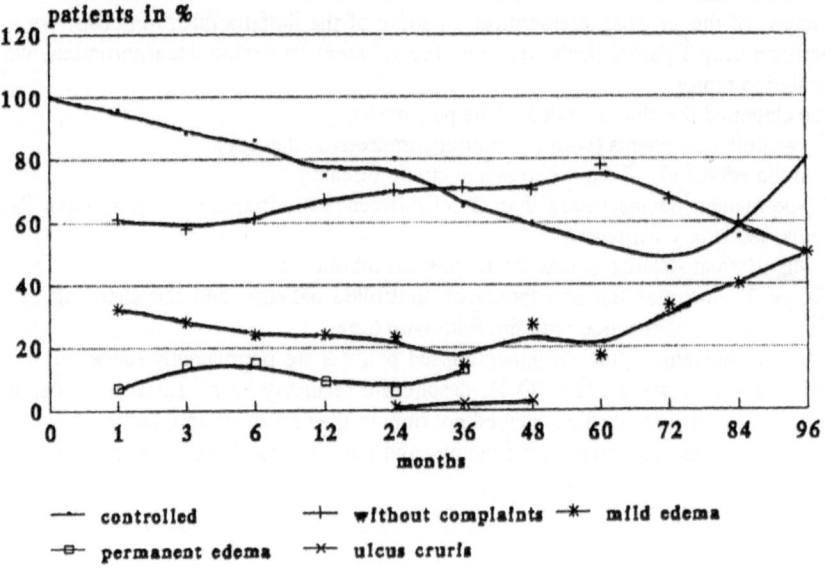

Fig 2.

FPC = femoro-popliteo-crural IF = ilio-femoral
CO = common femoral   I = iliacal
IFP = ilio-femoro-popliteal   CIF = cavo-ilio-femoral

Phlebology '95, D. Negus et al. (eds.). Phlebology (1995) Suppl. 1: 741-743

OP/19.4

The Evolution and Improvement of Treatment for Deep Venous Thrombosis and Pulmonary Thromboembolism

A. Lechter, C.A. Franco, G. Bayona, L.G. Cadavid and D.A. Rojas

Service of Vascular Surgery and Angiology, Hospital Militar Central, Bogota D.C., Columbia, South America

INTRODUCTION

Venous thrombosis and its sequelae are among the most challenging, least understood and neglected problems in medicine.

Diagnosis of this entity is difficult and the therapeutic modalities were ineffective in reducing its overall mortality and morbidity until the knowledge and succesful clinical use of thrombolytic agents.

These agents are Streptokinase and Urokinase, that were found to be effective in the management of both venous thrombosis and pulmonary embolism, provided faster and better resolution, restoration of physiologic function and greater clinical improvement in comparison with Heparin therapy alone.

METHODS

We used sistemic thrombolytic therapy with Streptokinase in 300 patients with clinical diagnosis of deep venous thrombosis of legs and/or pulmonary embolism during the years 1.985 to 1.994. In 285 cases these diagnosis were confirmed by at least one invasive or not invasive diagnostic method. The other 15 patients have no paraclinical study done, due to the very clear clinical findings and because it was not possible to realize the study in a very short time after the admission of the patient.

In 260 of the 300 patients, the thrombolytic therapy was done in the first week after the symptoms appeared. The other 40 cases were considered late thrombolysis, and this is a new concept to be kept in mind.

We have used only Streptokinase (*Streptase-HOESCHT*)

Our dosage scheme is initiated by a single dose of 100mg of Hydrocortisone I.V., followed by one dose of 250.000 international units of Streptokinase and doses of 100.000 units/hour for 12 hours. Then we apply other 6 doses of 250.000 units each 12 hours for 3 days. The total dose is near 3'000.000 international units.

RESULTS

The overall result was very good. 78% (234 patients) had a significant degree of benefit, 16% (48 patients) were clinically improved and only 6% (18 patients) were worst , including 1 fatal case.

Minor complications were observed in 10.66% (32 patients) and consisted of allergic reaction with rash (14 patients), myalgia (6 patients), vomit (5 patients) and gingival hemorrhage (3 patients). In these 28 patients the treatment was not interrupted.

Only 3 patients presented a mayor complication. In two cases we demonstrated a retroperitoneal hemorrhage with CT-Scan. The treatment was suspended and in one case it required transfusion of four units of fresh blood. Of special importance was a fatal case in a young woman, 32 years old, who presented a massive intracraneal hemorrhage at the second day of treatment, and finally death. The autopsy revealed an arterial malformation at the right PICA.

The most common affected sex were female with 64% (192 patients) .

The age limits were 16 and 82 years old with average of 46.

Late thrombolysis was used in 40 cases. Twenty six (65%) of these were treated one week to three months after the thrombotic episode. There were fourteen patients (35%) who had a very late thrombolysis, from three months to twenty four months after the initial episode. All of them had been treated with Heparin, Sodium Warfarin or Aspirin with very poor results. We decided to "activate" the fibrinolytic system and were surprised to find that most cases (90%=36 patients) had a response to thrombolysis. This response was moderate in 10 cases, good in 20 cases and excellent in 6 cases. We will demonstrate some of these spectacular cases.

CONCLUSION

Deep venous thrombosis is a common entity, the actual treatment must be based on thrombolytic therapy that has proven to be sure and effective.

The new indications were the cases not treated at the initial first week in which Streptokinase is more successful.

Late thrombolysis can be used with variable but promising results.

REFERENCES

1. Albrechtsson U, Anderson J, Einarsson E, et al: Streptokinase treatment of deep venous thrombosis and its postthrombotic syndrome. Follow-up evaluation of venous function. Arch Surg 116:33, 1.981

2. Altemeier WA, Hill EO, Fullen WD: Acute and recurrent thromboembolic disease: A new concept of etiology. Ann Surg 170:547, 1.969

3. Bell WR, Meek AG: Guidelines for the use of thrombolytic agents. N Engl J Med, 201: 1266, 1.979

4. Coon WW: Epidemiology of venous thromboembolism. Ann Surg 186:149, 1.977

5. Hirsh J, Genton E, Hull R: Venous thromboembolism. New York, Grune & Stratton, 1.981, pp 122-144.

6. Kakkar VV, Corrigan TP, Fossart DP, et al: Prevention of fatal postoperative pulmonary embolism by low doses of Heparin. An International multicentre trial. Lancet 2:45 1.975

7. Kakkar VV, Lawrence D, Bentley PG, et al: A comparativ study of low dose of Heparin and a Heparin analogue in the prevention of postoperative deep vein thrombosis. Thromb Res, 13: 111, 1.978.

8.   Sabiston   DC Jr: Pathophysiology, diagnosis and management of pulmonary embolism. Am J Surg 138:384, 1.979

P251

IN-HOSPITAL VERSUS OUTPATIENT TREATMENT OF ACUTE DEEP VEIN THROMBOSIS: THE PATIENTS' PREFERENCES

Werner Blättler and Eugen Frick
Clinic for Vascular Diseases, Zürich, Switzerland

Randomisation is an obligatory requirement for our ongoing trial of in-hospital versus outpatient treatment of acute deep vein thrombosis (DVT). Initial therapy in the hospital consists of immobilisation and heparin infusion, outpatient therapy of deliberate ambulation in compression stockings and Dalteparin subcutaneously. Eventual preferences of eligible patients are not taken into account. As a consequence, recruitment is slow. What could be worse, selection bias may occur, since both treatment forms are routinely available at our clinic and the indication of either therapy is at the discretion of the caring physician and his fully informed patient.

To assess eventual bias we surveyed the preferences of all patients referred to our clinic in the first semester of 1994. Of a total of 46 patients with confirmed acute DVT 25 were eligible but only 5 agreed to randomisation. Six requested in-hospital treatment and 14 prefered outpatient management. Opting for ward admission were mainly women (4 of 6) with symptoms of short duration (4.3d), presenting with risk factors such as cancer (5 of 6), but only rarely with triggering events (1 of 6). On the other hand, outpatient treatment was prefered by men (10 of 14) with a prior experience of DVT (6 of 14) but few severe risk factors (1 of 14), prevalence of triggering events (10 of 14) and longer duration of symptoms (8.2d). Age and extension of DVT (74% femoral) were no discriminating criteria.

We conclude that our randomised trial is biased because the majority of the opinionated patients refuse to accept the play of chance. Rather they deliberate the study objectives and develop strong preferences for either hospitalisation or outpatient treatment depending on their personal situation. Their preferences reflect reasonable judgement that has to be accepted although it jeopardizes the realisation of a controlled trial.

P252

A NEW CAVA-FILTER "SAND-GLASS".

Saveliev V., Yablokov E., Procubovsky V.

State Russian Medical University,
Department of Intervention Radiology,
Moscow, Russia.

OBJECTIVE: To review the preliminary experimental and clinical experience of a new device for the prevention of pulmonary embolism.
DESIGN: In vitro comparative study of some vena cava filters models and review of the first clinical experience with a new cava filter " Sand-Glass".
PATIENTS: 15 patients undergoing a new cava-filter placement.
MEASUREMENTS: Clinical outcome and results of the cavagraphy and ultrasound scanning documented at two weeks and six months follow-up after operation.
RESULTS: Experimental data: The "Sand-Glass" filter has better clottrapping features than " Basket " and " Bird's Nest" and minimally affects hydrodynamics in vena cava inferior model.
Clinical data: No history of recurrent embolism in patients undergone the "Sand-Glass" filter placement; vena cava inferior is patent in 14 of 15 patients.
CONCLUSION: Initial results with cava-filter "Sand-Glass" appear encouraging.

P284

FIBRINOLYTIC THERAPY IN PATIENTS WITH DEEP VEIN THROMBOSIS (DVT) IN SUBACUTE PHASE AFTER DELIVERY OR ABORTION

Batchvarova V, Lukanova D

National Centre of Cardiovascular Disease, Sofia, Bulgaria

Objective: The only indications for fibrinolytic therapy was considered the acute phase of DVT. The aim of our study is to evaluate the clinical effect of fibrinolytic therapy in patients with DVT in the subacute phase (1 to 4 weeks after the clinical beginning of the disease).

Design and patients: 19 patients after delivery or abortion with DVT of various localisation were subjected to fibrinolytic therapy. The mean age of the patients was 25 years. The standard initial and supporting dose of streptokinase were applied. The mean duration of fibrinolytic therapy was 34 A. To 1 month after delivery or abortion, for 2 weeks we perform minimal optimal heparin therapy and adequate treatment of the frequent pelvic infection (if available), until restoration of the uterus epithelium, following fibrinolytic therapy. The fibrinolytic therapy was followed by heparin, indirect anticoagulants and Gincor-fort for 6 months to 1 year.

Measurements: The stages of venous insufficiency of the extremities were assessed by oedema, cyanosis, secondary compensatory varicae, pigmentation, dermatosclerosis and venous ulcer.

Results and Conclusions: Fibrinolytic therapy in the subacute phase of DVT has shown a very good effect and should be applied in the first month of the disease.

P260

SURGICAL TREATMENT OF DEEP VEIN THROMBOSIS.

Pollice F., Salerno F.

Institute of Cardiovascular Surgery, University of Bari, Italy.

Objective: The aim of the study was to reevaluate the present role of indication for,and technique of surgery for acute deep vein thrombosis. The outcome of surgery is discussed,and the nonsurgical therapies are compared.

Patients: A series of 213 consecutive patients suffering from acute iliofemoral vein thrombosis who underwent venous thrombectomy is retrospectively analyzed.Surgery was performed from an inguinal approach with a Fogarty balloon catheter and by bimanual expriration from the femoral and popliteal veins.Angioscopy for control is recommended.Postoperative oral anticoagulation treatment was attempted whenever possible.

Measurements: Long-term results obtained in 130 patients after a median follow-up of 78 months(49% free of symptoms,35% PTS I,18% PTS II,8% PTS III)showed a significant correlation to the duration of preoperative anamnesis:<5 days:64% free of symptoms;>5 days:34% free of symptoms;the rate of PTS III was equally distributed in the group with long (<5 days)and short(>5 days)anamnesis(8% and 9% respectively).If the medication was canceled,aggravation of the clinical symptoms in one-third of patients was observed.

Conclusions: Venous thrombectomy is an important treatment option in patients with contraindications to thrombolytic therapy.With patients younger than 65 years and short anamnesis,functional results are acceptable. High risk patients(severe cardiac disease and previous pulmonary embolism)should be treated with medical therapy only.

OP/13.6

FOLLOW UP STUDY OF 160 ILIOFEMORAL VENOUS THROMBECTOMIES

Hetényi A. M.D.

Dept. of Vascular Surgery, Magyar Imre Hosp. Ajka, HUNGARY

Objective: To review the early and late results of the surgical management of deep venous thrombosis.
Design: To follow up our patients.
Patients: 160 were operated, 135 controled at least 3 months after surgery (mean 29.6).
Intervention: Iliofemoral venous thrombectomy with (70) and without (90) AV fistula. Our goal was the restoration of the venous flow in the iliac veins and in the subinguinal collector segment, therefore we made late interventions, too.
Measurements: We controled all of patients by clinical examination and CW-Doppler, 18 by late ascending phlebography, 31 by aortophlebography.
Results: We followed the clinical status of patients from discharge to the latest control. The patients having no complaints after the operation, remained permanent free from edema with or without compression therapy. The group of partially thrombectomised patients have some swelling and pain after the operation - the severe signs of postphlebitic syndrome broke out five years after surgery. The clinical and anatomical status wasn't the sam in all of the cases.
Conclusions: The resolution of the iliac veins and the subinguinal collector segment is an useful method for prevention of postphlebitic syndrome.

P262

RADICAL VARICECTOMY IN ASCENDING LSV VARICOPHLEBITIS

Hetényi A. M.D.

Dept. of Vascular Surgery, Magyar Imre Hosp., Ajka, HUNGARY

Objective: To compare the results of radical varicectomy (RV) with the less invasive methods in the surgical treatment of ascending LSV varicophlebitis.
Design: Retrospective open comparative study.
Patients: 148 patients were operated, 134 were controled 1 year after surgery. We report only the control patients.
Intervention: only crossectomy (C=10), crossectomy + stripping above the knee (CS=24), crossectomy + stripping + varicectomy (RV=100).
Measurements: Personal control. Residual varices, pain, edema, skin alterations observed.
Results: On the RV group far less residual varices and painful conglomerates (100/14) as in the C (10/6) and CS (24/10) groups. The mean hospitalisation time in the RV group was 5.8 days. There was no death, one bleeding, one infection occured. This patients return at their own daily activity and work earlier.
The details of the surgical procedure are discussed.
Conclusions: The RV results a definitive recovery of the patients, it isn't more dangerous but much more economic as the other surgical methods.

OP/8.3

SUBCUTANEOUS LOW-MOLECULAR-WEIGHT HEPARIN (LMWH) COMPARED WITH CONTINUOUS INTRAVENOUS HEPARIN (IVH) IN THE TREATMENT OF PULMONARY EMBOLISM.

Pineo G.E., Hull R.D., Brant R.F., Elliott C.G., Raskob G.E., Feldstein W. Canadian-American Thrombosis Group, University of Calgary, Calgary, Alberta, Canada.

Objective: To assess the efficacy and safety of LMWH compared with intravenous heparin (IVH) in the treatment of pulmonary embolism (PE).

Design: A multi-centre clinical trial comparing once daily, subcutaneous LMWH (Logiparin) with adjusted dose IVH given by continuous infusion for the inital treatment of patients with objective documented PE. Baseline ventilation-perfusion (V/Q) lung scans and chest x-rays were performed on all patients. The films were reviewed by two experts without knowledge of the patient's treatment group or clinical outcomes, and were interpreted as high probability (HP), nondiagnositc (ND) or normal (N) according to the PIOPED and Biello specifications. Patients from the four centres having the highest incidence of HP lung scan patterns were reviewed with respect to clinical outcomes (recurrent venous thromboembolism or death) and safety (major bleeding).

Results: None of the 51 patients who received LMWH and 1 of 46 patients who received IVH (2.2%) had new epidsodes of venous thromboembolism [p=0.47, 95% confidence interval (CI), for the difference, -2.0 to 6.4]. One patient (2.0%) receiving LMWH died, as compared to 4 patients receiving IVH (8.7%) (p=0.2), 95% CI for the difference, -2.2% to 15.7%. No patients in either group had major bleeding.

Conclusion: LMWH is at least as effectve as classical IVH therapy in patients with PE. Patients with uncomplicated PE could be treated as outpatients.

Deep Venous Reflux and Occlusion/Venous Ulcers

La gamme monodose
de
l'insuffisance veineuse

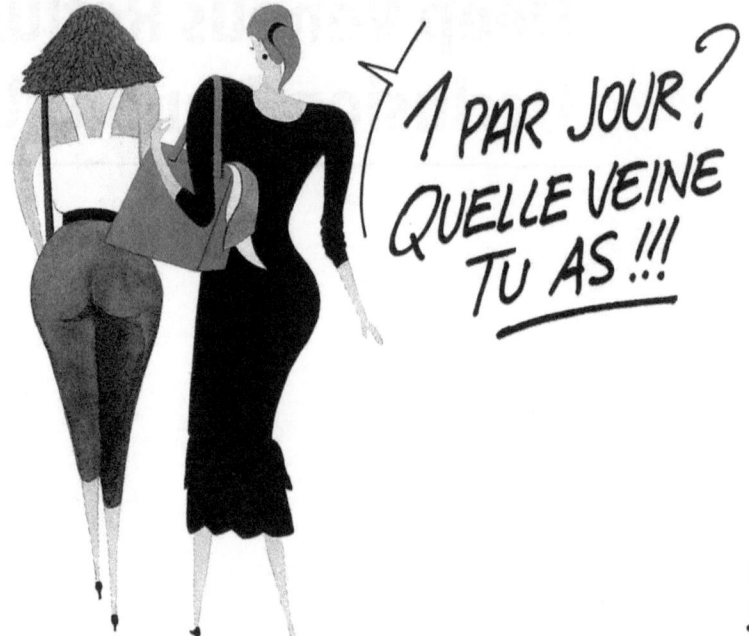

*1 PAR JOUR?
QUELLE VEINE
TU AS !!!*

Veinamitol® 3500mg

Troxérutine

Veinotonique et correcteur rhéologique

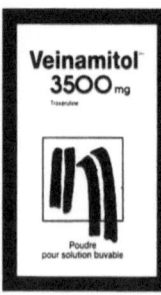
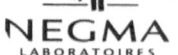
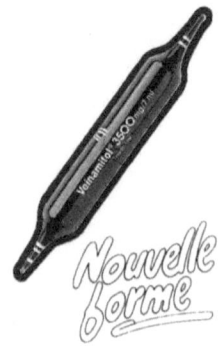

Deep Venous Reflux and Occlusion/Venous Ulcers

Natural History

Phlebology '95, D. Negus et al. (eds.). Phlebology (1995) Suppl. 1: 752-754

P002

The Natural Progression of Deep Venous Thrombosis (DVT) as Followed by Duplex Ultrasound over a One Year Period

A.M. O'Shaughnessy, D.E. FitzGerald

Department of Vascular Medicine, James Connolly Memorial Hospital, Blanchardstown, Dublin 15, Ireland

INTRODUCTION

It is still unknown why certain patients develop a post phlebitic limb following a deep venous thrombosis (DVT) while others appear to have no long term effects. (1) In the acute stage, the physician is primarily concerned with the risk of a pulmonary embolism and once this risk has passed the patient is very often forgotten until they present with venous ulcers a number of years later. Duplex scanning of the peripheral veins is a well established method to diagnose an acute thrombosis. This method allows visualization of the thrombus. (2) As the thrombus can be aged according to its ultrasonic appearance, Duplex scanning then becomes an excellent method to follow-up the ageing process of a DVT and to assess the long term effects on the patient. In this centre we are currently using Duplex scanning in an on-going study to assess patients over a one year period to try and establish what factors lead to the development of a post-phlebitic limb.

METHODS

One hundered patients (100) who presented with an acute DVT as diagnosed by Duplex Scanning were included in the study. Patients who were unavailable for follow-up or who had poor visualization of their veins were excluded. All patients were treated in the acute stage with intravenous Heparin followed by Warfarin for six months. (3,4) A Duplex Scan (Acuson) was performed at one week, one month, six months and one year following their initial presentation. At each examination the ultrasonic appearance of the thrombus and its anatomical site were noted. Extension, recanalization or resolution of the thrombus and the development of venous collateralization and valvular incompetence were assessed also. Patients were grouped according to the anatomical level of the DVT.

RESULTS

There was a 14% mortality rate, 4% of which were directly
related to the DVT (2 P.E.'s and 2 Phlegmasia Cerulea Dolens).
In the group of patients whose DVT was below the knee (N = 50),
the thrombus dissolves more quickly and they present with the
least long term effects. Thrombus above the knee (N = 52)
leads to the development of collaterals between one to six
months. Incompetence can take up to one year to develop and is
more frequent in the proximal DVT group. A small percentage of
the thrombi extend (N = 14) and a low percentage of recurrent
DVT's develop (N = 10) in both groups.

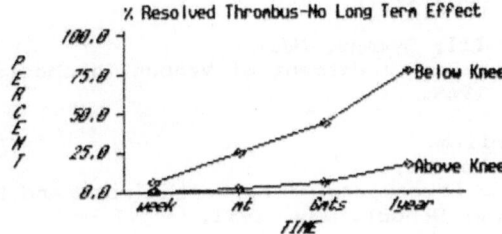

CONCLUSION

The long term effects of an acute DVT depend greatly on the
anatomical site of the DVT and on the speed at which it
resolves. The majority of patients whose thrombi are slow to
organise usually go on to develop an incompetent deep venous
system and therefore are at risk for a post-phlebitic limb.
Competent collateral channels are a better outcome than
recanalization within the lumen without directional control.
Duplex scanning is a safe and effective way to follow the
long term progress of an acute DVT and to assess the
development of a post phlebetic limb. It is hoped than this
method will lead to a better understanding of patients response
to treatment and eventually lead to a more succesful managment
of the acute deep venous thrombosis. (5)

REFERENCES

1. Incidence & Importance of Thromboembolism
    Venous Thrombosis & Pulmonary Embolism, Eds Hume, Sevitt &
    Thomas, Harvard University Press, Chapt. 1, 1970.

2. Talbot, S.R.
    Thrombus Identification and Characterization.
    Techniques of Venous Imaging, Eds. Talbot & Oliver, Appleton
    Davis, Inc., Chapt. 5, 1992.

3. Hull, R; Delmore, T; Genton, E. et al.
    Warfarin Sodium Versus Low Dose Heparin in the Long-Term
    Treatment of Venous Thrombosis.
    N. Eng. J. Med. 301: 855, 1979.

4. Coon, WW; Willis, PW III; Symons, MJ.
    Assessment of Anticoagulant Treatment of Venous Thrombolism.
    Ann. Surg. 170; 559, 1969.

5. Prevention of Thrombolism.
    European consenus Statement.
    Cardiovascular Disease Educational & Research Trust and St.
    Mary's Hospital Medical School, Nov. 1991.

Phlebology '95, D. Negus et al. (eds.). Phlebology (1995) Suppl. 1: 755-757

OP/7.6

What Factors are Associated with Leg Ulcer Recurrence

P.J. Franks[1], M.I. Oldroyd[2], D. Dickson[2], E.J. Sharp[2] and C.J. Moffatt[1]

[1] Centre for Research & Implementation of Clinical Practice, 5-7 Parsons Green, London
[2] Department of Surgery, Charing Cross & Westminster Medical School, London

INTRODUCTION

Compression stockings are considered to be the main line of defence against the recurrence of chronic leg ulceration, yet few studies have investigated the incidence of recurrence in patients with newly healed ulceration. The Lothian & Forth Valley study found that one third of all patients being treated for ulceration had experienced four or more previous episodes [1]. It has been estimated that there may be three times as many patients with healed ulceration at risk of recurrence than those with current ulcers, giving an 'at risk' population of 300,000 in the UK alone. The aim of this study was to determine the incidence of recurrence in patients with newly healed leg ulceration and to determine what factors are likely to be important in increasing the risk of recurrence.

METHODS

This observational study was set within a framework of a clinical trial comparing two class II below knee stocking types. In the trial the key interest was in the problems associated with stocking use such as ability of patients to put on and take them off, and reactions to the stocking material. The trial patients were a subset of the total group of patients with newly healed ulcers, the remainder being patients who did not fulfill the trial entry criteria of suitability for stockings or the requirement for 'made to measure' hosiery. All patients had newly healed leg ulceration. Those patients with venous disease were previously treated with the four layer bandage (4LB) a high compression system effective in healing venous ulceration in out-patient and community clinics [2,3]. Those patients with mild arterial disease were not excluded from this study, since these patients are often prescribed compression hosiery to prevent recurrence. However, the presence of arterial disease was examined as a potential risk factor for the leg ulcer recurrence.

All patients were treated in community clinics for their ulceration. Following healing, informed consent was given to take part in the study. Patients which the clinical nurse specialist considered to have skin too friable to attempt a stocking application were treated by alternative methods, most frequently the application of an elastocrepe bandage. Patients were followed up at three monthly intervals to a maximum of 18 months. In patients who experienced a stocking reaction a cotton sock was placed over the limb prior to the reapplication of the stocking.

Risk factor analysis was performed using a Cox proportional hazards model with results expressed as relative risk (RR) and 95% confidence intervals (95%CI).

RESULTS

Of the total of 188 patients entered into the study (mean age=72 years, 69% women), five patients required made to measure stockings and 17 could not tolerate them due to friable skin. The remaining 166 were considered suitable for the clinical trial and were randomised accordingly. The overall cumulative recurrence rate was 26% after one year and 31% after 18 months.

Table I. Comparison of selected risk factors for leg ulcer recurrence

Factor	n	events	RR (95%CI)	p
History of hypertension				
No	151	60	1.0	
Yes	37	9	0.50 (0.24, 1.00)	0.036
History of deep vein thrombosis				
No	168	58	1.0	
Yes	20	11	1.97 (1.02, 3.81)	0.057
Original ulcer size				
<10cm^2	149	49	1.0	
$\geq$10cm^2	37	20	2.11 (1.23, 3.60)	0.009
Weeks to heal				
<12	137	46	1.0	
$\geq$12	50	23	1.59 (0.95, 2.63)	0.079
Suitability for stockings				
yes	171	58	1.0	
no	17	11	2.58 (1.33, 5.01)	0.010

Other potential risk factors for ulcer recurrence which were examined but which failed to approach statistical significance included poor mobility (RR=0.82, 95%CI 0.48,1.37), ankle ABPI >0.9 (RR=2.17, 95%CI 0.78, 6.10), and never wearing stockings (in patients randomised to them), RR=1.44, 95%CI 0.52,3.99.

Stepwise analysis indicated that the independent factors for leg ulcer recurrence were previous ulcer size $\geq 10cm^2$ (RR=2.13, 95%CI 1.25, 3.72), history of deep vein thrombosis (RR=2.34, 95%CI 1.19, 4.57) and unsuitability for compression stockings (RR=2.52, 95%CI 1.28, 4.94).

DISCUSSION

This study has indicated the risk of recurrence in patients with newly healed leg ulceration was 26% after one year. This compares with a study in north London which found a recurrence rate of 69% after one year in out-patients [4]. More recent studies have produced much lower results, though these studies may be in selected groups, whereas the current study was an examination of consecutively healed patients. The current study has indicated that factors associated with the severity of venous disease in the patients, namely large ulcer size and history of deep vein thrombosis appear to be important in recurrence, whilst the skin structure as given by the unsuitability of patients for compression hosiery is also indicative of a poor outcome. Both skin and venous factors appear to play important roles in the recurrence of previously healed leg ulceration.

REFERENCES

1. Callam MJ Harper DR Dale JJ Ruckley CV: Chronic ulcers of the leg: clinical history. Br Med J 1987; 294: 1389-91

2. Blair SD Wright DDI Backhouse CM Riddle E McCollum CN:
Sustained compression and healing of chronic venous ulcers
Br Med J 1988; 297: 159-61

3. Moffatt CJ Franks PJ Oldroyd M Bosanquet N Brown P Greenhalgh RM McCollum CN: Community leg ulcer clinics and impact on ulcer healing.
Br Med J 1992; 305: 1389-92

4. Monk BE Sarkaney I: Outcome of treatment of venous stasis ulcers.
Clin Exp Dermatol 1982; 7: 397-400

Phlebology '95, D. Negus et al. (eds.). Phlebology (1995) Suppl. 1: 758-760

OP/3.7

Malignancy in Patients Presenting With Chronic Leg Ulcers

D. Yang, M.C. Stacey, B. Morrison and S. Hoskin

University Department of Surgery, Fremantle Hospital, Fremantle, Western Australia

INTRODUCTION

Malignancy is one of the differential diagnoses for ulcerated lesions on the leg. This may arise either as an ulcerating skin cancer or alternatively as malignant change in an existing ulcer. The frequency of skin cancer in patients presenting with a leg ulcer is difficult to determine because reports are generally of only a few cases[1-3].

The lower limbs are not a common site for skin cancer, representing only 2.8% of skin cancers in one reported study in the USA[4]. In Australia however, lower limb amelanocytic skin cancers have been demonstrated to comprise 11% of all skin cancers[5]. The highest incidence of such skin cancers was in patients over 70 years of age. Patients of this age also have a higher prevalence of chronic venous ulcers[6]. A relatively high frequency of skin cancer in patients presenting to the leg ulcer clinic at Fremantle, might therefore be expected.

In this study we have evaluated the frequency of skin cancer in patients presenting to the Leg Ulcer Clinic at Fremantle, and have attempted to identify some of the clinical features which may help to achieve earlier diagnosis.

METHODS

Patients considered in this study have all been referred to the Leg Ulcer Clinic with a chronic leg ulcer. Patients reported here presented during a period of six and a half years.

On referral to the clinic patients have a number of investigations performed to assess the aetiology of their ulcer. The investigations used to establish the cause of ulceration are - arterial Doppler pressures, photoplethysmography, haemoglobin, urea and electrolytes, blood glucose, rheumatoid serology, and autoantibody screen.

A biopsy is taken if there are any features that might suggest malignancy. Biopsies may also be performed at a later date if treatment has been initiated for a different diagnosis, and the ulcer either fails to respond to treatment or develops features that might suggest a neoplastic lesion. When biopsies are performed, these are taken under local anaesthetic using 1% lignocaine with adrenaline. An ellipse of tissue 1 cm in length, including intact skin and ulcer base, is excised from the edge of the ulcer.

RESULTS

During a six and a half year period, 890 patients were referred to the leg ulcer clinic at Fremantle Hospital for treatment of their chronic leg ulcer. During this time 41 patients were found to have histological evidence of skin cancer in ulcers on 46 limbs. Basal cell carcinoma was identified in 35 limbs and squamous cell carcinoma in 11 limbs. In addition 7 patients had evidence of a premalignant condition in 7 limbs. These consisted of solar keratosis in 3 limbs, squamous cell carcinoma in situ in 2 limbs, squamous keratosis in 1 limb and basal cell papilloma in 2 limbs.

There were 28 female and 20 male patients with a median age of 76.5 years. Only one ulcer could really be considered to be a Marjolin's ulcer, since this had been biopsied on several previous occasions without evidence of skin cancer. This ulcer had been present for 36 months. An estimate of the ulcer size, number of previous ulcers and the duration of the ulcers was present in 35 of the remaining limbs. The size of the ulcers ranged from 0.59 to 57.5 square centimetres, with a median area of 3.85 square centimetres. These ulcers had been present for between 2 weeks and 7.2 years with a median of 20 weeks. In 18 limbs (51.4%) this was the first episode of ulceration, and in 177 limbs (48.6%) there had been previous ulceration.

Assessment for other causes of ulceration were performed in 45 of these limbs. In the other 8 limbs these investigations were not performed as the appearance of the ulcer at the time of presentation was strongly suggestive of skin cancer only and a biopsy was the first investigation performed. Thirty one limbs had evidence of venous disease based on photoplethysmography, 11 limbs had evidence of both venous disease and arterial disease, and in 3 limbs there was no evidence of venous or arterial disease. The ulcerating skin cancers were found in the gaiter region of 30 of the 43 limbs with evidence of venous disease.

The diagnosis of skin cancer or premalignant condition was made on a biopsy taken during the initial assessmentor at the time of presentation with a new ulcer in 34 limbs (64.2%). In 19 limbs the diagnosis was made during the course of treatment of their leg ulcer which had been presumed to be due to another cause. The biopsy was taken in these patients because their ulcer was not responding as would have been expected. In these cases there was little change in the ulcer to suggest that it was in fact a skin cancer.

Discussion

This study has indicated that skin cancer was present in 4.5 % of patients referred to a specialist clinic for the treatment of leg ulcers. In addition premalignant skin conditions were identified in a further 0.8% of patients.

In the majority of these patients (64%) the diagnosis was suspected at the initial evaluation at the clinic, even though it had not been suspected by the referring practitioner. However, in 36% of these patients the diagnosis was not suspected on initial assessment in the clinic, and patients were commenced on treatment for other identified causses for chronic leg ulcers. The diagnosis was eventually made after the patients had failed to respond to treatment and a biopsy was performed. This highlights the fact that ulcerating skin cancers on the lower leg can be very difficult to differentiate from chronic leg ulcer due to other causes. They do not necessarily have all of the clinical features that one would normally associate with a skin cancer.

One of the features highlighted in this study that might help clinicians to suspect an ulcerating skin cancer are the failure of the ulcer to respond to appropriate treatment, especially in patients with evidence of venous disease. In addition, in patients with venous disease, the ulcerated skin cancer was not present in the gaiter region in 35% of patients. The absence of any other cause of a leg ulcer on initial evaluation may also suggest that the lesion could be a skin cancer.

In the patients identified in this study, only one could be considered to have a Marjolin's ulcer. The remaining lesions most likely arose as malignancies de novo. Traditionally, the incidence of basal cell carcinoma in the lower limb was thought to be low. More recently it has been suggested that basal cell carcinoma arises more frequently on the lower limb. One recent study has indicated that as many as 8% of all basal cell carcinoma may occur on the lower limb, and that this was the predominant skin cancer at that site with a frequency 1.5 times that of squamous cell carcinoma[5]. It has also been postulated that the changes in dermal connective tissue which occur in chronic venous disease may predispose to the development of basal cell carcinoma[7,8]. The findings of this study would tend to support such an assertion.

Biopsy of ulcerating lesions on the leg is a simple investigation and should be employed if there are any features to suggest that the lesion is actually a skin cancer. However, the lack of features of skin cancer should not delay the clinician from taking a biopsy in an ulcer that is not responding to appropriate treatment.

REFERENCES

1. Browse NL, Burnand KG, Lea Thomas M. Venous ulceration - diagnosis. In: Diseases of the veins: pathology, diagnosis, treatment. London: Edward Arnold, 1989: 371-409.
2. Lagattolla NRF, Burnand KG. Chronic venous disease may delay the diagnosis of malignant ulceration of the leg. Phlebology, 1994; 9: 167-9.
3. Ryan TJ, Wilkinson DS. Diseases of the veins and arteries - leg ulcers. In: Rook A, Wwilkinson DS, Ebling FJG, editors. Textbook of dermatology, 4th edn. Oxford: Blackwell Scientific, 19886; 7: 219-27.
4. Scotto J et al. Incidence of non melanoma skin cancer in the United States. Publication no. (NIH) 82-2433. US Department of Health and Human Services. December, 1981.
5. Giles G, Marks R, Foley P. Incidence of non-melanocytic skin cancer treated in Australia. BMJ 1988; 296: 13-7.
6. Baker S, Stacey M, Singh G, Hoskin S, Thompson P. Aetiology of chronic leg ulcers. Eur J Vasc Surg 1992; 6: 245-51.
7. Black MM, Walkden V. Basal cell carcinomatous changes on the lower leg: a possible association with chronoc venous stasis. Histopathology 1983; 77: 219-27.
8. Mitrani E. Possible role of connective tissue in epidermal neoplasia. B J Dermatol 1978; 99: 233-44.

Phlebology '95, D. Negus et al. (eds.). Phlebology (1995) Suppl. 1: 761-763

P164

Leg Ulcers. Casuistry From January 1985 to December 1994

S. Massi, C. Ruggieri, G. Botta, A.M. Peccatori and S. Mancini

III Department of General Surgery and Center of Phlebology "W. Pabisch" Faculty of Medicine and Surgery, University of Sinea, Italy

INTRODUCTION

The lower limbs ulcers are the expression of a local or a systemic disease, able to produce some necrotic phenomenous to which a loss of substance concerning epidermis, derma, subcutateous tissue and more rarely fascia is united.

The lower limbs ulcers treatment represents a difficult problem. The expensive costs of the therapy and the invalidness of the same disease have a negative influence on public sanitary expense and on the way of life of the patient, whose working ability may result compromised for ever.

Though the old are hit more, it has been possible to evict, thanks to new epidemiological studies, that in 22% of the cases the ulcerations arise about 40 years.

In accordance with the international literature data, we can affirm that about the 1% of the people is suffering from ulcerative lesions to lower limbs and that, in 75% of the cases, these may result bound to a peripheral venous insufficiency.

Therefore a careful diagnostic study is necessary to be able to carry out a patient's right management.

Our experience agrees with the literature data, asserting that the most frequent reasons of the ulcerative lesions in lower limbs are, in order of incidence: venous insufficiency, arterial insufficiency, neuropathies and others factors

CASUISTRY

From january 1985 to december 1994, 820 patients (females 590 and males 230), affected with ulcers in lower limbs, have been treated. 82 of them had bilateral lesions:

we have reached a total of 1014 ulcers. The data extracted and the relative percentage to the age, to the ethiopathogenesis, to the exetnsion, to the localization and to the time of healing are resumed in the following list:

Females=590 (72%)   Males=230 (28%)

Age: min.19 years - middle 55 years - max 92 years

Ethyology:

Varicose	524 (51.7%)
P:T:F.S.	147 (14.5%)
Mixed	131 (12.9%)
Arterial	74 (7.3%)
Traumatic	59 (5.8%)
Diabetic	52 (5.1%)
Neurologic	9 (0.9%)
Other	18 (1.8%)

Extension:

0 - 4 cm	569 (56.1%)
4 -10 cm	290 (28.6%)
10 -20 cm	106 (10.6%)
>20 cm	48 (4.7%)

Localization:

leg medial	402 (39.6%)
" lateral	160 (15.8%)
" anterior	177 (17.5%)
" posterior	43 (4.2%)
malleolus	148 (14.6%)
foot:dorsum	54 (5.3%)
" toes	18 (1.8%)
" plant	12 (1.2%)

RESULTS

The healing of the ulcers is obtained in 91% of the cases. Total recurrence rates of ulcers was in 11% of the cases. All patients are subjected to a complete clinical test and to a non-invasive or invasive study for a perfect ethyopathogenetic framing, to a photografic and morphometric relief of the ulcer combined with a taking of local material for the cultural test and biopsy for histological test added to a complete haematologic study of the patient.

Our treatment includes, for all types of ulcers: the ozonized hydromassage, the curettage, the application of one or more topical dressings and inelastic bandage.

The treatment, in 98% of the patients, was ambulatorial.

REFERENCES

1.   Mancini S. La terapia delle ulcere degli arti inferiori. Casa Ed Grafica Sturli, sett 1990.
2.   Massi S., Ruggieri C., Mancini S. Traitement des ulcères des membres inférieus. Intensive Practical Course in Phlebology,Montreal,1992,283-290.

Phlebology '95, D. Negus et al. (eds.). Phlebology (1995) Suppl. 1: 764-766

PI/1.3

Results From the Study of the French Epidemiological Observatory of Leg Ulcer: Study Conducted by 265 MDs on 1300 Patients

S. Sadoun, L. Marzin, J. Seror and F.A. Allaert

10 Rue Benjamin Moloise 9400 Créteil, 5 Rue Jacques Duclaux 75015 Paris, 24 Boulevard de la Libération 94300 Vincenes, CHRU du Bocage 21000 Dijon

INTRODUCTION:

Recently better knowledge of the post thrombotic syndrome and of arterial diseases of the lower limbs have lead to improved treatment of leg ulcers.

There is a general feeling that the incidence of the disease is decreasing. Epidemiological studies show variable prevalences of leg ulcers in general or selected populations : 0.1 to 0.2% for Callam (3); 6.2/10 000 inhabitants for Baker (2) in Australia, with 90% older than 60 years old (prevalence: 3.3%); 0.18% and 1.3% for the Alexander House Group consensus conference (1); between 0.11 and 0.3% for Nelzen (4) in Sweden. In France, the prevalence is approxiamtely 1.45%, and less than 2% of first consultations are motivated by an ulcer (5).

OBJECTIVE:

To study the evolution of the epidemiological parameters of leg ulcers from an annual-sequential analysis of the incidence and the prevalence, with the help of investigators throughout France.

MATERIAL AND METHODS:

Each investigator had to examine each consecutive patient seen at the clinic for a leg ulcer.

The record form consisted of 8 questions with potentially 25 answers, and the following information was collected:

    - Number of leg ulcer patients

- Number of new patients
- Gender
- Age scale (<40, from 41 to 50, 51 to 60, 61 to 70, >70).
- General evolution (first time, recurrence, evolution >3 months).
- Number of ulcers per patients (one, two, >3 ulcers).
- Ulcer localisation (right leg, left leg, inferior half of the leg, lateral, medial malleolus, bilateral, other).
- Ulcer cuases (Venous, arterial, other)

RESULTS:

The study was conducted from March till October 1993.

265 Doctors in France comprising of 30% GPs, 40% dermato-Phlebologists and 30% Phlebologists-angiologists participated in the study.

1300 patients were examined i.e. 5 per investigator.

1012 new patients have been examined i.e. 3.8 per investigator.

The sex ratio is 70% women and 30% men.

50% of the paients are older than 70 years, 33% are between 61 an d70 years and 17% are younger.

61% of the patients have 1 ulcer, 22% have 2, and 17% have 3 or more.

20% of the ulcers are less than 3 months old, 45% are 3 months old or more, 35% are recurrent ulcers.

75% of the ulcers are from venous origin, 15% are arterial and 10% are of mixed origin.

The relative incidence is 0.3 new ulcers per month per investigator, the incidence is constant over the period.

CONCLUSION:

This study is sponsored by eminent French specialists (Pr Fiesinger, Drs Marzin, Megret, Perrin, Stemmer) and the authors have calculated the epidemiological parameters of leg ulcer for the first time in France.

Repetition of the study every year will give the evolution of the disease by the calculation of the incidence and the prevalence of the disease for each investigator, thus indirectly studying the general efficacy of treatment.

BIBLIOGRAPHY:

1. The Alexander House Group : consensus paper on venous leg ulcer, J Dermatol Surg Oncol 1992; 18(7): 592-602.

2. Baker SR, Stacey MC, Jopp-MacKay AG, Hoskin SE, Thompson PJ : Epidemiology of chronic venous ulcers, Br L Surg 1991 Jul; 78(7): 864-867.

3. Callam M : prevalence of chronic leg ulceration and severe chronic venous disease in western countries? Phlebology 1992, Suppl 1: 6-12.

4. Nelzén O, Berqvist D, Lindhagen A : leg ulcers : a hidden problem in the community, Phlébologie 92, Eds Raymond-Martimbeau, R Prescott, M Zummo. John Libbey Eurotext 1992, pp. 247-249.

5. Sadoun S, Vin F, Garde C, Henriet JP, Allaert FA : Approche Clinique et Thérapeutique de l'Insuffisance Veineuse (ACTIVE), Artères et Veines 1993; vol XII, n°1: 44-51.

Phlebology '95, D. Negus et al. (eds.). Phlebology (1995) Suppl. 1: 767-773

OP/3.2

La Prevalence de la Maladie Veineuse Evalueé Chez Pres de 40,000 Patients

C. Janbon, I. Quéré and J.C. Laborde

Service de médecine interne B, Hôpital St-Eloi, 34295 - Montpellier Cedex 5, France

The Prevelence of Venous Disorders Evaluated in Nearly 40,000 Patients

SUMMARY

The DEFI Programme, by its methodology and the size of the population studied, nearly 40,000 patients, is an essential contribution to knowledge of venous pathology in France.

The most important finding is the significant prevalence of venous pathology (52.6%) but above all, the hidden venous pathology which can only be found by questioning or by clinical examination.

This information should encourage further research into venous disorders, because very efficient methods of treatment are available and adaptable to each stage of varicose disorders.

D.E.F.I.

LA PREVALENCE DE LA MALADIE VEINEUSE EVALUEE CHEZ PRES DE 40 000 PATIENTS

C. Janbon, I. Quéré, JC Laborde
Service de médecine interne B, Hôpital St-Eloi, 34295 - Montpellier Cedex 5, France

INTRODUCTION

La prévalence de la pathologie veineuse est extrêmement variable d'un continent à l'autre et même d'un pays à l'autre. On connaît sa **forte prévalence dans les pays développés** : il y a, par exemple, cinquante fois plus d'insuffisants veineux au Pays de Galles qu'en Nouvelle-Guinée.

Parmi les pays occidentaux, le Japon fait exception, la fréquence de cette pathologie y étant particulièrement faible. Il semblerait donc que ce ne soient ni l'urbanisation, ni l'industrialisation qui soient en cause dans la genèse de la pathologie veineuse mais d'autres facteurs environnementaux dont les principaux sont **l'alimentation et la sédentarité**. Parallèlement, **l'hérédité** joue bien entendu aussi un rôle essentiel.

En France, on le sait, la pathologie veineuse est très fréquente comme en témoignent le nombre de traitements chirurgicaux réalisés chaque année : entre 100 et 200 000, ainsi que le nombre de séances de sclérothérapie pratiquées chaque jour : environ 2 à 3 000 (1)

Malgré cette forte prévalence supposée, aucune étude n'a permis de déterminer la fréquence de l'insuffisance veineuse dans la population française. C'est précisément l'objectif du programme D.E.F.I. qui pour la première fois a permis d'obtenir des **données épidémiologiques précises sur la pathologie veineuse en France.**

PATIENTS ET METHODES

Ce programme a été conduit en **médecine générale** entre le mois d'octobre 1993 et le mois de février 1994. Deux mille six cent neuf médecins généralistes y ont participé ; ils ont recherché une insuffisance veineuse, quel que soit son type : fonctionnel ou organique, chez 15 patients consécutifs et cela quel que soit leur motif de consultation. Au total, la recherche d'une insuffisance veineuse a été effectuée chez 39 135 patients.

La présence d'une insuffisance veineuse chez ces patients était déterminée grâce à un questionnaire réalisé en collaboration avec la SOFRES et comportant un arbre décisionnel (fig. 1).

Dans le premier cas de figure, l'insuffisance veineuse était le motif principal de la consultation, dans ce cas le patient était identifié, d'emblée, en tant qu'insuffisant veineux.

Si le patient venait consulter pour une autre raison, l'insuffisance veineuse était recherchée par l'interrogatoire.

Enfin, en cas d'absence de signes d'insuffisance veineuse à l'interrogatoire, un examen clinique était réalisé à la recherche de télangiectasies, variscosités, varices, signant l'existence d'une maladie veineuse.

RESULTATS

Au total, une **insuffisance veineuse** a été retrouvée **chez 52,6 % des patients** consultant en médecine générale (Fig.2).

Les circonstances de découverte se sont réparties (Fig. 3) de la façon suivante :

* pour **11 %** des patients consultants, l'insuffisance veineuse était le **motif principal de la consultation.**

* pour **33,3 %** des patients, celle-ci a été retrouvée à l'interrogatoire,

* enfin, pour **8,3 %** des patients, c'est **l'examen clinique** qui a permis de déterminer la présence d'une insuffisance veineuse.

D'autres éléments intéressants ressortent de cette enquête, en particulier **la prépondérance féminine** de la maladie veineuse, qui est une donnée classique de cette pathologie, a été ici clairement mise en évidence et quantifiée : 64,1 % des femmes avaient une insuffisance veineuse contre 35 % des hommes seulement (Fig. 4).

Par ailleurs, la prévalence de la pathologie veineuse a été étudiée par classe d'âge de 10 ans et il apparaît, là aussi clairement, que **la prévalence augmente avec l'âge** et que, à partir de la tranche d'âge 40-49 ans, les patients insuffisants veineux deviennent majoritaires (Fig. 5).

DISCUSSION

L'objectif et l'intérêt de ce programme étaient de déterminer la prévalence de l'insuffisance veineuse dans la population française. Il a été réalisé en médecine générale ce qui nous a permis d'obtenir les données les plus fiables possibles sur une population "*tout venant*".

Le programme D.E.F.I. confirme la forte prévalence de l'insuffisance veineuse dans la population française : 52,6 % de la population étudiée présentait une insuffisance veineuse. Mais dans la majorité des cas, cette insuffisance veineuse n'était pas spontanément mentionnée, et n'a été découverte qu'à l'interrogatoire ou à l'examen clinique.

Par ailleurs, la prépondérance féminine de l'insuffisance veineuse a été pour la première fois quantifiée : 64,1 % des femmes ayant participé à ce programme avaient une insuffisance veineuse contre 35 % des hommes. Enfin, l'augmentation de la prévalence avec l'âge a, elle aussi, été confirmée : elle atteint 72 % après 70 ans.

CONCLUSION

Le programme D.E.F.I. par sa méthodologie et l'importance de la population étudiée, près de 40 000 patients, apporte une contribution essentielle à la connaissance de la pathologie veineuse en France.

Son plus important enseignement est la forte prévalence de la pathologie veineuse (52,6 %) mais surtout de la pathologie veineuse méconnue qui n'est retrouvée qu'à l'interrogatoire ou à l'examen clinique. Cette information doit nous inciter à rechercher activement une insuffisance veineuse chez nos patients, car nous disposons actuellement de thérapeutiques très efficaces permettant une prise en charge adaptée à chaque stade de la maladie variqueuse.

REFERENCE

1.   Chantereau JP, Davinroy M
      Les varices des membres inférieurs : données épidémiologiques
      Actu. Vasc. Int. n° Hors Série, *oct. 93*

Ce programme a été réalisé grâce au soutien des Laboratoires SERVIER

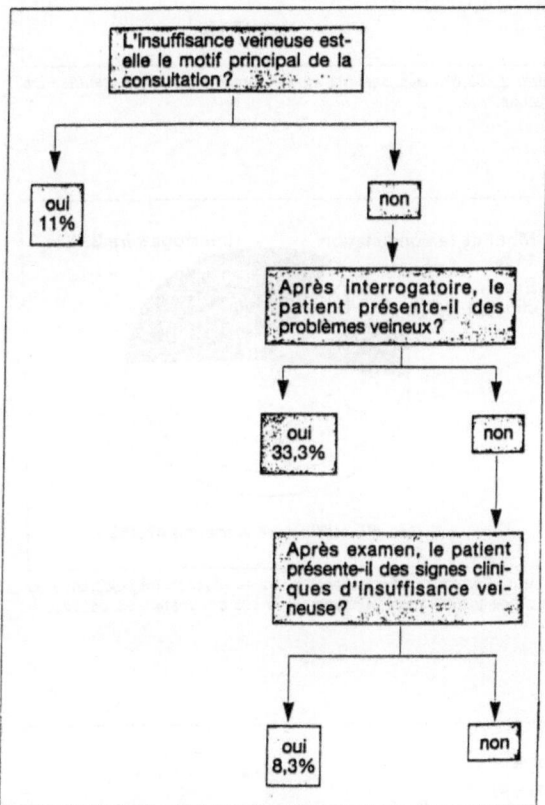

Figure 1: La prévalence de l'insuffisance veineuse a été déterminée pa
les médecins grâce à un questionnaire comportant un arbre décisionnel.

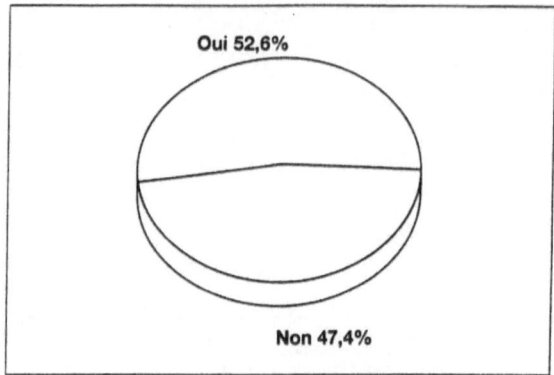

Figure 2: 52,6% des patients étudiés présentaient une insuffisance veineuse.

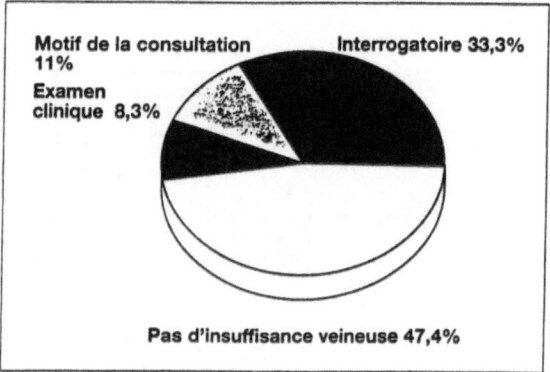

Figure 3: Répartition des patients inclus en fonction de l'existence ou non d'une insuffisance veineuse et de ses circonstances de découverte.

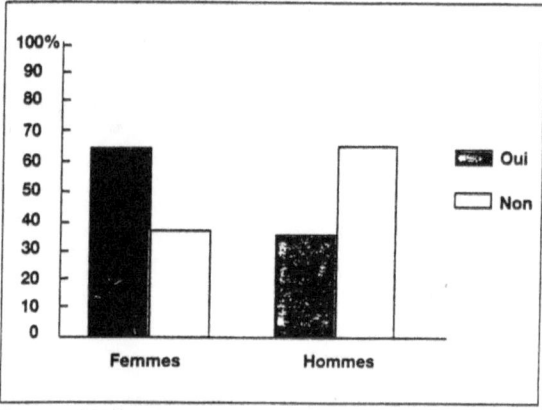

Figure 4: 64,1% des femmes et 35% des hommes présentaient une insuffisance veineuse.

773

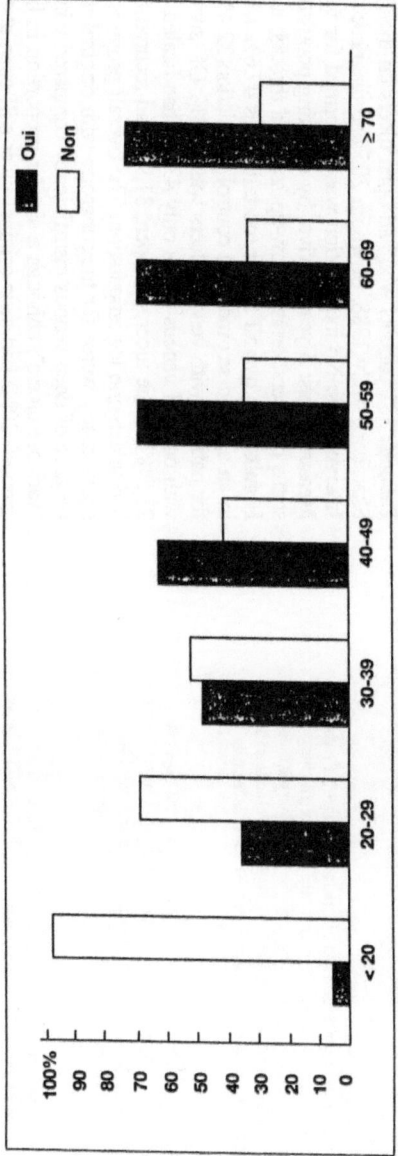

Figure 5: La prévalence de l'insuffisance veineuse augmente avec l'âge. Les patients insuffisants veineux deviennent même majoritaires à partir de la classe d'âge 40-49 ans.

OP/3.1
THE NATURAL HISTORY OF VENOUS LEG ULCERS

Nelzén Q, Bergqvist D*, Lindhagen A.

Depts of Surgery, Kärnsjukhuset Skövde and *University Hospital
Uppsala, Sweden

Objective: To assess the long term outcome for patients with diagnosed venous ulcers treated in the community.
Design: A prospective 5 year follow-up of unselected patients with leg ulcers.
Patients: 382 patients who had open ulcers on inclusion in the Skaraborg study 1988, of whom 205 had diagnosed venous ulcers.
Interventions: No intervention was performed for venous ulcers.
Measurements: 5 year survival by checking population registers and status of ulceration at follow-up assessed through a questionnaire.
Results: The overall 5 year mortality was 47,6% which is higher than in an age and sex matched control population(32,4%). The mortality for patients with venous ulcers was 37,4%. Of surviving patients with original venous ulcers only 43,7% had healed their ulcers, 21,5% had the ulcer still open, 31,9% had recurrent ulcers and 3% had undergone leg amputation. The overall prognosis was significantly worse for the subgroup with original venous ulcers because of deep venous insufficiency compared with those with "varicose ulcers", although a similar proportion in both groups(~20%) had their original ulcer still open at follow-up. The overall healing was worst among patients with venous ulcers if compared with the outcome in patients with ulcers of arterial or other cause.
Conclusions: The long term prognosis for patients with venous ulcers treated in the community is poor. Less than half being healed after 5 years. About 20% never heal and 30% recur. These results are not acceptable and indicate present treatment regimes to be insufficient. Improvement of the care of patients with venous ulcers is nesessary.

P151
COMPLICATIONS CARCINOMA OF ULCERS VENOUS

IGARZABAL CARLOS, FEINSILBERG DANIEL.

DEPT.SURGERY, DIV. DERMATOLOGY
HOSPITAL GRAL AGUDOS "DR.J.M.RAMOS MEJIA", BUENOS AIRES, ARGENTINA.

OBJETIVE: revision retrospective of our series of cases.

DESIGN: fact little frequent that occurs among 0.5 to the 2% of the C.A. EPIDER-MOIDES.

PATIENT: 3 female and 1 male.The age range was among 58 and 61 years old with an average of 69 years. the free time of the tumor was of 29 years. were all located in 1/3 inf.leg, 3 to left and 1 to right leg. Clinic 2 were ulcerosivos, 1 case vegetate you and the remainder ulcerovegetate. The histopatology in 4 cases was carcinomaepidermoi semimadure. The time of evolution was of 5-10-12 and 36 months to the moment.

MEASUREMENTS: the treatment erfected in two cases was that of the amputation infrascondilea, being found 3 and 5 years free of tumor. One case se to received cobaltoterapy for be denieo to the amputation the varon this series development M.T.I. ganglinic and cervical ex-piring after to 3 months.

RESULTS: in our experience on a total of 431 C.A. EPIDERMOIDES skin excluding the mucous and semimucous, 4 were developed on U.V. CHRONICLE, what represent 0.92% and of a total of 2880 alone U.V.C. developed C.A. 0.14%.

CONCLUSIONS: the controlof the patients with U.V. must be continued to detect the possibles changes C.A. of evil predict, by the invasio conti-quous oseous and the posibility of M.T.I. ganglionic and to distance.

V/3.5

VENOUS LEG ULCER : PHYSIOPATHOLOGY AND PRATICAL DATA FOR ITS TREATMENT

RETTORI René M.D., PARPEX Patrick and NGO Patrick

Hôpital Corentin Celton (Paris VI), Policlinique, 37 boulevard Gambetta, 92133 Issy-les-Moulineaux

Objective : Review of physiopathological and pratical data for the choice of the treatment.

Design : Study of macro and microvascular changes caused by high ambulatory venous pressure in the valvular insufficiency of varicose veins, thrombophlebitis and congenital anomalies. This insufficiency is demonstrated clinicaly, by ultrasounds (dupplex scanning), dynamic phlebography and venous angioscopy.

Results : Greater is venous insufficiency, greater is the risk of a ulcer developing. If compression therapy is applied in correct way, ulcer cicatrisation obtained in majority of cases. To prevent ulcer recurrence it is necessary to treat the causal venous disease. When ulcer fails to heal or recours despite the usual treatment, two possibilities are stressed :
- progressive aggravation of the causal venous insufficiency ;
- combination of venous insufficiency with a loco-regional or general factor. It is thus at a loco-regional level that ankle stiffness, major subulcer sclerosis with possibility of calcified plaques, lymphatic stasis and exceptionally malignant degeneration. Howewer the most important occurence in the event of resistant ulceration is due to a combination of arterial and venous insufficiencies. In these "mixed ulcers" arterial lesions are most frequently peripheral and epidural spinal cord electrical stimulation is specially indicated.

Conclusions : The local leg ulcer treatment appears of minor importance ; the most important is the etiologic treatment wich is alone able to prevent the recurrence .

P174

LEG ULCER AND MALIGNANT MELANOMA

Titon J-P

Dept of Angiology, Centre Médical Montréal, La Fleche, France

Objective: To present a patient with a leg ulcer associated with a malignant melanoma

Design: A study of a particular association of phlebologic and dermatologic disease. Skin ulceration and cancer with the necessity to think about, in front of special clinical symptoms of an ulcer.

Results: A patient, already followed by several physicians since two years for a leg ulcer with an important varicosis of his legs, was seen for this ulcer which became localised on the sole of his left foot. The evolution of this special ulcer was better with the classical treatment of a leg ulcer and of the varicosis of his leg. But it was very red, fleshy, bleeding and after a good detersion, some little black points became visible just beside. The biopsy revealed that this ulcer was associated with a malignant melanoma.

Conclusion: This patient is very interesting for two reasons: first, it is an association leg-ulcer and malignant melanoma or an ulcerated melanoma (but two years of evolution without adenopathy) ? Secondly the pathology that he presents allowed to put the phlebologists on their guard against the melanoma in front of a leg ulcer, bleeding, with granulation, with sometimes, little black points beside. This pathology seems to be rare, therefore.

THE NECROTIC ULCER FOLLOWING A TRAUMATISM AMONG OLDER PATIENTS : A PARTICULAR ENTITY.

Coget J.M., Millien J.P.

61 Rue de Turenne 59000 LILLE - FRANCE

Objective : Clinical and nosological analysis of the necrotic ulcer of the lower limb among older patients, secondarily following a traumatism.

Project : To study the mechanisms by which this type of ulcer appears, which does not respond to the classical aetiologies.

Patients : 10 patients : 10 women (older than 50 years).

Measurements : Clinical analysis : general criteria - characteristics of the ulcer and surrounding tissues. General examination. Arterial and venous duplex scanning. Standard biological checking. Identical therapeutic protocol.

Results : Similar clinical aspect : association of a cutaneous necrosis and widespread diffuse periulcerous hematoma. Absence of associated vascular pathologies at the origin of those ulcers. Clinical evolution always favourable. Physiopatholgy linked to a topographical ischaemia and vessel rupture.

Conclusion : By its specific clinical aspects, the necrotic ulcer following a traumatism among older patients, constitutes a real entity. Its aetio-pathogeny seems to be linked to the aging process of the cutaneous tissue and to the physiological arteriolosclerosis.

Deep Venous Reflux and Occlusion/Venous Ulcers

Clinical Research

Phlebology '95, D. Negus et al. (eds.). Phlebology (1995) Suppl. 1: 778-780

P274

Chronic Venous Ulcers are Associated with Elevated Systemic Markers of Coagulation and Increased Systemic Fibrinolytic Activity

L.J. Fligelstone, R.A. Salaman[1], S.V. Davies[2], I.F. Lane and K.G. Harding[1]

Cardiff Vascular Unit, [1] Wound Healing Research Unit, [2] Department of Haematology University Hospital of Wales, Heath Park, Cardiff CF4 4XW, UK

INTRODUCTION AND HYPOTHESIS

Venous ulceration is a common condition associated with significant disability and consumption of resources. The prevalence in the United Kingdom for all ages is 1.5-1.8/1000 total population. In the elderly this increases to 3/1000 in the 61-70 year age group, and 20/1000 in those over 80 years. The common denominator in venous ulceration is defective venous return, this may be secondary to calf pump failure, incompetent perforating or deep veins. This leads to excessive post-capillary venous pressure that is found in patients with venous ulceration and lipodermatosclerosis.

The *current theories* of the pathogenesis of venous ulceration are:

1 White Blood Cell Entrapment

White blood cells have been shown to be trapped within the capillary microcirculation and lead to plugging of capillaries, leading to decreased perfusion and supply of oxygen and nutrients (1).

2 White Cell Activation Associated With Ischaemia And Reperfusion

White cells that become trapped in the capillary microcirculation have been shown to be released on reduction of the venous pressure but show marked respiratory burst activity. These activated neutrophils release free radicals that may cause tissue damage leading to venous ulceration (2, 3).

3 Fibrin Cuff Theory

The excessive back pressure leads to capillary leakage of fibrin, leaving a cuff of fibrin that may impede oxygen and nutrient diffusion and the changes of skin necrosis and ulceration. The fibrin cuffs were thought to be due to defective fibrinolysis (4).

4 Hypercoagulability

There have been several case reports of venous ulceration secondary to hypercoagulable states. Antiphospholipid antibodies, and a defective protein C pathway have been implicated in the pathogenesis of venous ulceration (5, 6).

It is very likely that the cause of venous ulceration is multifactorial and that all the theories to date may each contribute to the formation of the venous ulcer.

AIMS

To determine the presence of hypercoagulable states in patients with non-healing venous ulcers. Secondly to re-evaluate the function of the coagulation and fibrinolytic pathways in patients with non-healing venous ulcers.

EXPERIMENTAL DESIGN AND METHODS

Twenty patients with non-healing venous ulcers and twenty control subjects were assessed. All control subjects were fit, non-smokers, without history or clinical evidence of peripheral vascular disease. A non-healing venous ulcer was defined as "a venous ulcer that had failed to heal despite three months therapy with the four layer Charing Cross bandage technique within the dedicated Wound Healing Research Unit". Significant arterial disease was excluded by examination, ankle brachial index pressure and arterial duplex where appropriate. Venous disease was assessed by hand held bi-directional Doppler and colour duplex scanning, using a Toshiba SP270A scanner and 5 MHz and 8 MHz linear array probes. The coagulation and fibrinolytic pathways were assessed on a 20 ml blood sample obtained without the use of a tourniquet. The following assays were performed:– One stage prothrombin time, activated partial thromboplastin time, fibrinogen concentration (Coagulation diagnostics, Boehringer, Mannheim, following the method of Clauss), prothrombin fragments 1&2 (sandwich enzyme-immunoassay, Behringwerke, Marburg, Germany), dilute Russell's viper venom time with platelet neutralisation procedure (7), anticardiolipin antibodies by ELISA for IgG and IgM (solid phase ELISA), thrombin antithrombin III complex (sandwich enzyme-immunoassay, Behringwerke, Marburg, Germany), D-dimer (Sigma Diagnostics, Poole, UK, semi-quantitative latex agglutination assay), and plasmin – alpha 2 antiplasmin complex (sandwich enzyme-immunoassay, Behringwerke, Marburg, Germany).

RESULTS

All patients and controls had ankle brachial indices ≥ 0.8. The median (range) age was 75(61-90) for patients and 49(40-65) for controls. There were 8 male and 12 female patients and 7 male and 13 female controls. The median (range) ulcer area was 55 (4 – 150) cm^2. The duration of ulcer and duration of therapy are given below:

	Duration of Ulcer (months)	Duration of Therapy (months)
Median	90	18
Range	8 – 480	6 – 72

The full blood count, urea and electrolytes and liver function tests were all within normal limits. Standard coagulation assays, i.e. OSPT, APTT, KCT were all normal.
There were no abnormalities of antiphospholipid antibody activity, neither lupus anticoagulant or anticardiolipin antibody activity. Fisher's exact test was used to analyse the data below.

Thrombin antithrombin III complex

TAT complex	Controls	Subjects	
Elevated	0	12	
Normal	20	8	p <0.0001

Fibrinogen

Fibrinogen	Controls	Subjects	
Elevated	0	5	
Normal	20	15	p = 0.0471

Prothrombin fragments 1&2	Controls	Subjects	
Elevated	1	17	
Normal	19	3	p = 0.0471
Plasmin antiplasmin complex	Controls	Subjects	
Elevated	0	7	
Normal	20	13	p = 0.0042

DISCUSSION

Fibrinogen elevation is seen in patients with advanced atherosclerosis, however those studied did not have overt evidence of atherosclerosis. Fibrinogen is a positive risk factor for myocardial infarction and is becoming recognised as a prognostic indicator for vein graft stenosis. However fibrinogen is often elevated as part of the acute phase response of inflammation, therefore in the presence of an open healing wound this finding must be considered with caution.

The assays used show that there is evidence of fibrin formation, within the systemic circulation. The site of this activity can not be demonstrated by these assays but it is likely to be in the region of the venous ulcer. There is also evidence of increased fibrinolytic activity in the systemic circulation. Previous work has reported defective fibrinolysis in the lower limbs of patients with venous ulcers. The former studies were performed using the euglobulin clot lysis time, a relatively insensitive non-specific assay. The assays used in this study, specifically assess certain steps of the coagulation and fibrinolytic pathways and show activation of these pathways unlikely to be otherwise detected.

The activity of the coagulation and fibrinolytic pathways are complementary and an imbalance favouring the formation of fibrin may explain the formation of fibrin cuffs. The findings of our study must be interpreted with care, as the patients are a subgroup with non-healing ulcers. We are currently assessing two further groups of patients one with lipodermatosclerosis and the other with newly diagnosed venous ulcers. These studies are necessary to determine whether the changes observed are part of the pathogenesis of the ulceration or a systemic reflection of a chronic granulating wound. Studies also need to be carried out to assess if there is a local defect in the affected limbs and therefore we plan to assess coagulation and fibrinolytic activity in arm and leg samples from subjects.

REFERENCES
1. Coleridge-Smith P, Thomas P, Scurr J, Dormandy J. Causes of venous ulceration: a new hypothesis. British Medical Journal 1988;296(6638):1726-7.
2. Cheatle T. Venous ulceration and free radicals [letter]. British Journal of Dermatology 1991;124(5):508.
3. Falanga V, Kruskal J, Franks J. Fibrin- and fibrinogen-related antigens in patients with venous disease and venous ulceration. Archives of Dermatology 1991;127(1):75-78.
4. Browse N, Burnand K. The cause of venous ulceration. Lancet 1982;(ii):243-245.
5. Blanchemaison P, Griton P, Cloarec M. Les Ulcères hypercoagulables. A propos d'un cas récent. Phlébologie 1987;40(4):949-954.
6. Blanchard B, Lazareth I, Brossel C, Saporta L, Letanoux M, Priollet P. Lupus anticoagulant and leg ulcers associated with ankylosing spondylitis. Journal of Rheumatology 1991;18:1922-1923.
7. Exner T, Triplett DA, Taberner D, Machin SJ. Guidelines for testing and revised criteria for lupus anticoagulants. Thrombosis and Haemostasis 1991;65(3):320-322.

Phlebology '95, D. Negus et al. (eds.). Phlebology (1995) Suppl. 1: 781-783

PI/7.5

Influence of Erythema and Sclerosis on Skin Oxygenation and Microcirculation around Venous Ulcers

S. Roszinski and W. Schmeller

Department of Dermatology and Venereology, Medical University of Lübeck, Germany

INTRODUCTION

It is known that in lipodermatosclerosis (LDS) laser Doppler flux (LDF) values are higher and transcutaneous PO_2 ($tcPO_2$) values are lower than in healthy skin [1,2]. Previously we introduced the method of *intracutaneous* PO_2 ($icPO_2$) measurement in patients with chronic venous insufficiency (CVI) [3]. The tissue oxygenation of dermis and subcutis was directly measured with needle probes. The mean $icPO_2$ values obtained from the ulcer border showed a large variation from patient to patient (from 6 mmHg up to 42 mmHg) [4]. This finding could be explained by a different intensity of sclerotic alterations and a variable vessel density and/or inflammation ("hypodermitis") in these areas.

The objective of this open, prospective study was to evaluate the influence of trophic skin changes ("hypodermitis", LDS) on $icPO_2$ in contrast to well established non-invasive methods of microcirculation around venous ulcers.

METHODS

On a group of 21 patients (27 legs) with venous ulcers caused by deep venous insufficiency measurements were performed in healthy appearing skin at the proximal part of the lower leg and at the distal part of the lower leg within 1 cm of the ulcer border.

According to the degree of erythema (mean a-value by skin colorimetry; Chroma-Meter CR-200, Minolta, Japan) and the amount of sclerosis (graded by palpation) at the ulcer edge parameters were divided into two groups: a.) 1. mild erythema - 2. extensive erythema and b.) 1. moderate sclerosis - 2. extensive sclerosis.

$IcPO_2$ values were measured as described earlier by our group [3]. For the determination of the $icPO_2$ steel shafted PO_2 needle probes were used (tip diameter 250 μm, response time $T_{90} < 500$ ms; GMS, Kiel, Germany). The electrode signals were processed by a LICOX-PO_2-channel; GMS, Kiel, Germany) and displayed on line. PO_2 readings were corrected for actual skin temperature. The PO_2 probes were inserted into the skin at an insertion angle of 10° (perspax angle fixed on the skin) and then pushed forward in steps of about 1 mm by hand in short intervals. At the end of each step a single local PO_2 value was registrated during the standstill of the probe. In each puncturing channel 6 local PO_2 values were measured. PO_2 values up to a penetration depth of about 3 mm at the ulcer border (2 mm in healthy skin) were designated as intracutaneous PO_2 values.

$TcPO_2$ was measured using an Oxymonitor (Oxymonitor SMK 363, Hellige, Freiburg, Germany) at electrode temperatures of 37°C and afterwards at 44°C at the same site. LDF was measured with an MBF3D equipment by Moor Instruments (Devon, England).

All measurements were performed with subjects resting supine. The room temperature was between 21 - 24°C.

Statistical evaluation: Statistical analysis were performed with the Mann-Whitney Rank Sum Test. The correlation between two parameters was calculated by Pearson correlation coefficient.

RESULTS

All results are presented in Table 1.

Table 1.

	$tcPO_2 37$ (mmHg)	$tcPO_2 44$ (mmHg)	$icPO_2$ (mmHg)	LDF (AU)	a	Temp. (°C)
I. Healthy skin						
n=27	9	60	46	15	4.8	31.2
II.a.) LDS moderate sclerosis	0	5	29	178	14.4	32.9
n=15						
	n.s.	n.s.	p<0.05	n.s.	n.s.	n.s.
extensive sclerosis	0	1	14	187	13.0	32.9
n=12						
II.b.) LDS mild erythema						
a < 13.3	1	6	19	116		33.0
n=12						
	p<0.05	p<0.005	n.s.	p<0.01		p<0.05
extens. erythema						
a > 13.3	0	0	16	235		34.2
n=15						

(Median values shown for $tcPO_2$ 37°C, $tcPO_2$ 44°C and $icPO_2$; mean values for LDF, a-value and skin temperature)

At the ulcer border (LDS) Median $icPO_2$ was 29 mmHg in moderate sclerosis and 14 mmHg in extensive sclerosis (difference significant, $P < 0.05$). Other parameters ($tcPO_2$, LDF, a-value, skin temp.) showed no significant difference if measuring sites were divided into moderate and extensive sclerosis.

On the other hand icPO$_2$ was not influenced by skin erythema whereas all other parameters were dependent on the degree of "inflammation".

In healthy appearing skin there was no positive correlation between icPO$_2$ and the parameters tcPO$_2$ 37°C, tcPO$_2$ 44°C and LDF. There was no correlation between icPO$_2$ and LDF in LDS too, but a moderate correlation between icPO$_2$ and tcPO$_2$ 37°C ($r=0.41$, $P<0.03$) and between icPO$_2$ and tcPO$_2$ 44°C ($r=0.47$, $P<0.014$) at the ulcer border was found.

The best correlation between two of the parameters was found between LDF and a-value ($r=0.58$, $P<0.002$) in lipodermatosclerosis.

CONCLUSIONS

In preliminary studies a great heterogeneity of icPO$_2$ values around venous ulcers has been observed. Our new results show, that skin oxygenation at the ulcer border is mainly dependent on the amount of sclerotic tissue changes (LDS) and not by the degree of skin erythema. The poor correlation between icPO$_2$ and tcPO$_2$ values indicates that O$_2$ molecules in different parts of the dermis are registrated by these methods. TcPO$_2$ values represent morphological and/or functional changes mainly in the *papillar* dermis while icPO$_2$ values obtained by our method represent the ratio of oxygen supply to oxygen consumption in *deeper* parts of the dermis.

Skin erythema ("hypodermitis") is characterized by maximal dilatation of papillary and subpapillary vessels, indicated by high LDF values and a lacking increase of tcPO$_2$ during heating of the tcPO$_2$ electrode from 37°C up to 44°C. LDF values reflect dilatation of dermal vessels (hyperemia) which are obviously not involved in the oxygen supply to the skin.

REFERENCES

1. Franzeck UK, Bollinger A, Huch R, Huch A. Transcutaneous oxygen tension and capillary morphologic characteristics and density in patients with chronic venous incompetence. Circulation 1984; 70: 806-811.
2. Jochmann W, Mostbeck A, Partsch H. Postocclusive reactive hyperemia and postural vasoconstriction in different kind of leg ulcers - Investigations with laser Doppler. VASA 1993; 22: 306-315.
3. Roszinski S, Köser T, Wilhelm KP, Schmeller W. Untersuchungen der Oxygenierung von Dermis und Subkutis bei Dermatoliposklerose. VASA 1993; 22: 297-305.
4. Roszinski S, Schmeller W. Differences between intracutaneous and transcutaneous skin oxygen tension in chronic venous insufficiency. J Cardiovasc Surg 1995; in press.

Phlebology '95, D. Negus et al. (eds.). Phlebology (1995) Suppl. 1: 784-786

PI/2.1

Clinical Trials in the Treatment of Chronic Venous Ulceration

M.C. Stacey

University Department of Surgery, Fremantle Hospital, Western Australia

INTRODUCTION

Clinical trials in the treatment of venous ulcers have been used to evaluate a wide range of materials, methods and substances. These can be considered as evaluations of either methods of dressing the ulcerated leg or evaluations of active agents. The discussion in this paper is limited to randomised controlled trials and does not touch on single arm evaluations which can serve only as a guide to what treatments should be more thoroughly investigated.

STUDY DESIGN

The design of the study is crucial to producing a meaningful evaluation. The aim of the study will influence the treatment to be used in both the study and control groups, as well as the specific methods used to evaluate the treatment. The object of the study may be a) to evaluate the influence of a specific type of treatment on the biological healing process, either during a certain phase of the healing process or the whole of the process, or b) to evaluate the treatment as an overall method of treating chronic venous ulcers in clinical management. Which of these types of studies is undertaken will determine whether the design is intention to treat or whether withdrawals are excluded from the study. It will also determine the measurement used to assess healing, in particular whether time to total healing of the limb or ulcer or simply a reduction in size over a given time interval is to be used.

If the treatment is to be evaluated for use in the clinical management of leg ulcers, it is important to use a control group that has optimal conservative treatment and not a form of treatment that may be regarded as sub-optimal. If the study is being undertaken to determine whether a particular treatment has a physiological effect, this may be done in comparison with treatment that is perhaps sub-optimal. In a number of published studies this aspect of the evaluation has not been well planned or well thought out, and as a result incorrect conclusions have been made from these studies.

A number of reported studies are simply phase 1 or phase 2 clinical trials of new agents and have been over interpreted. Clearly if these new agents are to be adequately and accurately assessed, proper phase 3 trials are necessary.

A further aspect of study design that can lead to inconclusive results is the determination of the sample size to be used in the studies. The size of the sample required to provide a meaningful result statistically will determine whether particular studies should be done over one or multiple sites. This may therefore determine whether it is in fact feasible to undertake a specific study at all.

TREATMENTS ASSESSED IN CONTROLLED TRIALS

The treatments that have been assessed in controlled clinical trials include the following :

1. Method of dressing - These include dressings, different types of bandages, the sequential compression device, elastic stockings and the use of the non-stretch device "Circaid".
2. Active agents
   (a) Topical agents. These include topical antibiotics, antiseptics, growth hormone, Prostaglandin E1, a number of different cytokines, the use of magnetism and skin substitutes.
   (b) Systemic pharmaceuticals. These includes vasodilators, vasoconstrictors, agents to increase capillary permeability, agents to alter cell deformability, fibrinolytic enhancing agents, and antibiotics.

Several treatments have been shown to improve the healing of chronic venous ulceration when compared with less than optimal treatment. These include

a) The addition of oxypentifylline[1]
b) The use of skin substitute[2]
c) Sequential compression device[3]
d) Optimal compression therapy[4]

The studies reported above have been performed by single investigators only and have not been repeated to date. The central groups in all of these studies have had treatments that have either not been well controlled or that have not received optimal compression therapy.

There has been no treatment method that has been demonstrated to improve the healing obtained with optimal compression therapy. In addition, to date there is no good evidence to suggest that any specific dressing has a direct influence on the healing process.

Some agents have been shown to reduce the size of wounds without an indication as to whether they reduce the time to total healing. This may in fact be of particular benefit for use during part of the healing process. However, frequently excessive claims are made about the benefit of using these agents. Many of the agents tested are not specifically directed towards a known abnormality in the healing process in the chronic wounds. It is extremely important to understand more about the pathophysiology of the wound healing process in order to help direct the types of treatment that may be evaluated in well controlled and well designed clinical trials.

REFERENCES

1. Colgan MP, Dormandy JA, Jones PW, Schraibman IG, Shanik DG, Young RAL. Oxpentifylline treatment of venous ulcers of the leg. Br Med J 1990; 300 : 972-5.
2. Sabolinski M, Rovee D, Parenteau N, Mulder G, Jensen J. The efficacy and safety of Graftskin;tm for the treatment of chronic venous ulcers. Presented at Wound Healing Society Meeting, Minneapolis, 27-30 April 1995.
3. Coleridge Smith PD, Sarin SA, Wilson LAA, Scurr JH. Intermittent pneumatic compression improves venous ulcer healing. Proceedings of International Union of Phlebology Meeting, Strasbourg; 25-29 September 1989, Vol 2 : 1146-48.
4. Stacey MC, Vandongen Y, Trengove N, Hoskin S, Thompson P, Pearce C. The effectiveness of compression in healing chronic venous ulcers. Presented at the International Union of Phlebology Meeting, London, September 1995 (Proceedings In Press)

Phlebology '95, D. Negus et al. (eds.). Phlebology (1995) Suppl. 1: 787-789

OP/15.2

The Influence of Graduated Compression Elastic Stockings on Venous Refilling Time

Y.K. Vandongen, P. Rashid and M.C. Stacey

Department of Surgery, University of Western Australia, Fremantle Hospital, Fremantle, Western Australia

INTRODUCTION

Compression stockings have long been used in the treatment of venous insufficiency and venous ulceration. Their action is thought to result in an improvement in venous return from the leg. For optimal effect it is suggested that the stockings should provide graduated compression Highest pressures should be at the ankle and these should reduce towards the knee[1,2].

Studies have shown that venous refilling time can be improved with the use of elastic compression stockings[2,3]. These studies however have focused predominantly on patients with venous insufficiency and not patients with previous ulceration.

The aim of this study was to determine whether below knee graduated compression elastic stockings would improve venous refilling time in patients with a history of venous ulceration. The aim was also to investigate whether there was any relationship between graduated compression and venous refilling time.

METHOD

Patients in this study were participating in a larger trial assessing the role of graduated compression stockings in the prevention of ulcer recurrence. All had venous ulcers which had healed two weeks before entering the study.

Patients were randomized to receive either stockings (Venosan[R] 2003, Salzman AG. St Gallen, Switzerland) or no stockings. Patients were instructed to wear the stockings at all times, removing them to go to bed.

Venous refilling time was measured using a photoplethysmograph (Parks Vascular Mini-Lab III). The transducer was placed 7.5 cms above the medial malleolus with patients in a sitting position.

Stocking pressures were measured using a Borgnis Medical Stocking Tester. Pressure readings were recorded at four points between the ankle and the knee on the medial side of the leg.

All measurements were performed on entry into the study and repeated at two weeks, three months and six months.

RESULTS

Over a two year period 118 patients with 128 healed limbs were recruited into the study. Twenty seven females and 30 males were recruited into the stocking group (62 limbs). Mean age of the females was 70.2 years (range 47-83 years) and males 64.1 years (range 37-93). The no stocking group comprised 34 females and 27 males (66 limbs). Mean age of the females was 69.5 years (range 39-84 years) and of males, 66.8 years (range 33-84).

Venous refilling time was not altered when stockings were applied (paired t-test, $p > 0.05$). Nor was there an improvement in refilling time in patients who regularly wore the stockings for six months (repeated measures ANOVA, $p = 0.56$).

A comparison between patients wearing stockings and those who did not wear them also failed to show a difference in refilling time (repeated measures ANOVA, $p = 0.32$, Fig 1).

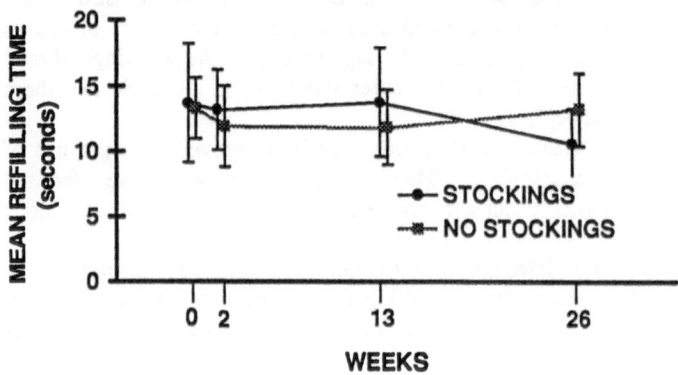

Fig 1. Comparison of venous refilling time between the stocking group and the no stocking group.

In patients wearing stockings, the mean pressure under the stockings when first applied was greater at the ankle (27mmHg) and reduced at consecutive points to the knee (13mmHg). Mean pressures remained graduated although they were reduced at the end of six months (Fig 2). Observed on an individual basis however, graduated pressure was achieved in only 55% of limbs.

Venous refilling time in patients whose stockings provided graduated compression was not significantly different from those in whom graduated pressure was not present. In fact there appeared to be a trend for those with graduated compression to have a lower refilling time (t-test, $p > 0.05$).

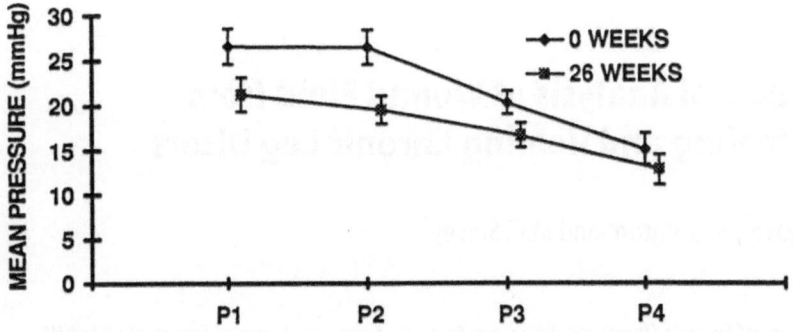

Fig 2. Mean pressure under the stockings at the beginning of the study and after six months.

DISCUSSION

The findings from this study indicate that venous function in patients with recently healed venous ulcers is not improved with the application of compression stockings. This contrasts with reports from others[2]. However this may be explained by the fact that all patients in this study had experienced past venous ulceration whereas this was not the case in previously reported work.

As a result of laboratory testing of the stockings, it is currently thought that to improve venous function the stockings must provide a pressure of approximately 40-50mmHg at the ankle. In this study mean pressures were found to be somewhat less than this. The observed pressure range however was similar to that reported in other studies in which pressure beneath the stockings was measured on the patient's leg[2].

Much emphasis has also been placed on the need to provide graduated compression to the limbs for proper effect[1,2]. Mean pressure between ankle and knee was found to be graduated in this group of patients even over an extended period. However on an individual basis compression was graduated in only approximately half of the patients, a finding which has not been previously reported. Clearly this must be a problem associated with all types of custom made stockings and does raise the question as to whether graduated compression is really necessary.

REFERENCES

1. Horner J, Fernandes J, Fernandes É, Nicolaides AN. Value of graduated compression stockings in deep venous insufficiency. Br Med J 1980; 280:820-821.

2. Cornwall JV, Doré CJ, Lewis, JD. Graduated compression and its relation to venous refilling time. Br Med J 1987; 295:1087-1090.

3. Evander E, Scigala EM, McDonnell AE, Evander A, Gewertz BL, Zarins CK. Influence of support stockings on photoplethysmography (PPG) recovery time in venous insufficiency. Bruit 1984; VIII:287-289.

Phlebology '95, D. Negus et al. (eds.). Phlebology (1995) Suppl. 1: 790-792

PI/2.4

Biochemical Analysis of Wound Fluid from Non-Healing and Healing Chronic Leg Ulcers

N. Trengove[1], S. Langton[2] and M.C. Stacey[1]

[1] Department of Surgery, University of Western Australia, Fremantle Hospital, Fremantle, 6160 WA.
[2] Department of Clinical Biochemistry, Fremantle Hospital, Fremantle, 6160 WA

INTRODUCTION

Currently, there is considerable clinical research into the treatment of chronic venous leg ulcers, however the underlying pathophysiology of the disease process is largely unknown.[1,2] The majority of patients with chronic leg ulcers are managed successfully in the community, however a small percentage of patients do not respond to outpatient treatment and require hospitalisation for skin grafting. It has been observed that after 2 weeks bed rest in preparation for skin grafting the leg ulcers show obvious signs of healing with the formation of granulation tissue and epithelialization. Therefore it is possible to study these wounds in both a non-healing and healing phase.

Recently the analysis of wound fluid has been used to gain an insight into the wound environment.[3,4] This research is based on the assumption that wound fluid reflects the extra cellular fluid of the tissue. If this is the case then analysis of wound fluid can give valuable information about the growth conditions of cells within the wound.

It was therefore the purpose of this study to compare wound fluid and serum in order to understand more completely what wound fluid is and then by comparing the non-healing and healing wound fluid gain an understanding of chronic wound healing.

MATERIAL AND METHODS

This is a comparative study of paired wound fluid and serum samples from 8 patients admitted to hospital for skin grafting. Wound fluid and blood samples were collected when patients were first admitted to hospital (non-healing phase) and after 2 weeks bed rest in preparation for skin grafting (healing phase).

Wound fluid and serum samples were screened for a range of general biochemical parameters, eg: electrolytes, creatinine, urea, lactate, lactate dehydrogenase (LDH), glucose, & protein levels.

Median values were calculated and samples compared statistically using Wilcoxon Sign Rank Test.

RESULTS

A summary of results comparing wound fluid and serum are listed in table 1.

When comparing wound fluid to serum it was noted that electrolyte, urea and creatinine levels were similar in wound fluid and serum samples. However, lactate levels were significantly increased in wound fluid (10.9 mmol/L) relative to serum (2.7 mmol/L) (p< 0.01)and glucose levels were significantly lower in wound fluid (1.8 mmol/L) when compared to paired serum samples (6.4 mmol/L) (p< 0.01). Also the levels of bicarbonate were significantly lower in wound fluid (19 mmol/L) when compared to serum (26 mmol/L) (p=0.0004) and most notably the levels of lactate dehydrogenase (LDH) in wound fluid (5949 u/L) were almost 20 x that of serum (381 u/L). Other results show that both albumin and total protein levels in wound fluid (21 & 38.5 g/L) were approximately half that of serum levels (40 & 72 g/L). The levels of C-reactive protein were similar in wound fluid (8.5 mg/L) and serum (6.4 mg/L) (p=0.2).

Table 1. Comparison of Serum and Wound Fluid

	SERUM		WOUND	FLUID
	median	range	median	range
Sodium (mmol/l)	142	138-145	141	133-146
Potassium (mmol/l)	4.9	3.4-6.6	4.4	3.2-5.7
Chloride (mmol/l)	100.5	95-106	104	96-109
Bicarbonate (mmol/l)	26	19-31	19	14-22
Urea (mmol/l)	8.7	2.7-23.1	8.9	2.5-22.6
Creatinine (μmol/l)	111.5	59-342	116.5	46-335
Glucose (mmol/l)	6.4	4.6-9.9	1.8	0.6-5.9
LDH (u/l)	381.5	275-567	5949	789-9901
Lactate (mmol/l)	2.7	1.3-6.5	10.9	5.4-16.7
Albumin (g/l)	40	35-48	21	14-28
Total Protein (mg/l)	72.5	65-83	38.5	26-51
C-Reactive Protein (mg/l)	6.4	2.9-115	8.5	2.5-25

Table 2. Comparison of non-healing and healing wound fluid.

	NON-	HEALING		HEALING
	median	range	median	range
Sodium (mmol/l)	140	135-146	141	133-143
Potassium (mmol/l)	4.3	3.2-5.7	4.3	3.6-5.4
Chloride (mmol/l)	104.5	96-109	103.5	95-108
Bicarbonate (mmol/l)	17.5	14-20	19	16-22
Urea (mmol/l)	9.3	2.5-21.3	8.9	2.1-28.8
Creatinine (μmol/l)	105	46-335	120	70-288
Glucose (mmol/l)	1.2	0.6-3.7	2	1.1-5.9
LDH (u/l)	6005.5	789-7795	5728	1308-9901
Lactate (mmol/l)	12	6.2-13.8	10.4	5.4-16.7
Albumin (g/l)	18.5	14-24	23	18-28
Total Protein (mg/l)	34	26-46	41	36-51
C-Reactive Protein (mg/l)	12.5	5-25	5.8	2.5-21

A summary of results comparing non-healing and healing wound fluid are listed in table 2. When analysing changes from the non-healing to the healing phase it was noted that there was a significant increase in the levels of bicarbonate ($p=0.018$), albumin ($p=0.011$.), and total protein ($p=0.011$) and a significant decrease in the levels of C-reactive protein ($p=0.018$).

DISCUSSION

Based on this analysis it can be said that wound fluid collected from chronic leg ulcers is an exudate that represents the components of the extra-cellular fluid and hence reflects the cellular environment of the wound. The altered levels of lactate, bicarbonate, and glucose in wound fluid when compared to serum suggest an anaerobic environment while the high levels of LDH indicate a state of tissue destruction. The decrease in the levels of C-reactive protein from the non-healing to the healing phase suggest a decreased inflammatory state in the healing wound.

In summary these results demonstrate that wound fluid is a useful tool for analysing the wound environment. Biochemical analysis of wound fluid has not been previously reported and as shown here can give information about the metabolic state of the wound. By extending this analysis to examine both non-healing and healing chronic wounds valuable information can be gained about changes occurring in the wound during healing.

REFERENCES

1. Robson M, Phillips L, Thomason A, Robson L, Pierce G.
    Platelet-derived growth factor BB for the treatment of chronic pressure
    ulcers. The Lancet, 1992 ;339: 23-25

2. Finetti G, Farina M. Recombinant human basic fibroblast growth factor :
    different clinical dressings for clinical application in wound healing.
    Il Farmico, 1992; 47: 967-978

3. Dvonch MD, Murphey RJ, Matsuoka J, Grotendorst GR. Changes in growth
    factor levels in human wound fluid. Surgery, 1992; 112: 18-23

4. Hunt TK. Wound fluid : The growth environment. Clinical and experimental
    approaches to dermal and epidermal repair: normal and chronic wounds. Wiley-
    Liss, Inc. 1991; p223-230

Phlebology '95, D. Negus et al. (eds.). Phlebology (1995) Suppl. 1: 793-795

OP/9.1

Alterations in Immune Cells in Human Chronic Leg Ulcers

M.C. Stacey, S. Lainez, T. Skender-Kalnenas and B. Morrison

University Department of Surgery, Fremantle Hospital, Fremantle, Western Australia

INTRODUCTION

The complex of immune response associated cells and humoral factors present in the skin has been referred to as the skin immune system[1]. The various cellular components of this system include tissue macrophages, monocytes, granulocytes, mast cells, Langerhans cells, dendritic cells, T cells, endothelial cells and keratinocytes[2]. The humoral factors involved in this system include fibrinolysins, antimicrobial peptides, complement peptides, eicosanoids, neuropeptides, cytokines, secretory immunoglobulins, interleukins, interferons and colony stimulating factors[2]. This system plays a significant role in the response of the skin to injury and the repair process that follows.

Previous work in our department has demonstrated increased levels of the proinflammatory cytokines interleukin-1, interleukin-6, and tumour necrosis factor-α in non-healing chronic leg ulcers. However, the precise role of the cells of the skin immune system in the healing of chronic wounds, and in particular chronic venous ulcers, remains uncertain. Changes in the populations or functions of these cells during healing of chronic ulcers have not been established.

The aim of this study was to assess changes that occur in the populations of these cells in chronic leg ulcers when they enter a healing phase.

METHOD

This study has examined biopsies taken from the leg ulcers of 13 patients. All patients had evidence of chronic venous disease as confirmed by an abnormal venous refilling time on photoplethysmography. In addition, 6 patients also had evidence of arterial disease proven by arterial Doppler ratios of less than 0.90. The ulcers were present in the legs and not the feet of all patients examined.

In all patients in this study their ulcers had either failed to reduce in size with appropriate compression therapy, or had shown a gradual increase in size. These patients were admitted to hospital for bed rest, regular dressings, and subsequent skin grafting. Biopsies and tracings of the ulcer were taken on admission to hospital, and again after two weeks of dressings, and just prior to skin grafting. In all cases there was a reduction in the area of the ulcer.

The biopsies consisted of two adjacent pieces of tissue that were one centimetre in length, 3 mm wide, and 5 mm deep. One segment was placed in formalin for routine paraffin embedding and the other piece was stored at -70°C until processed.

The formalin fixed tissues were stained with haematoxylin and eosin to assess the number of neutrophils present, and with toluidine blue to assess the number of mast cells. The frozen sections were incubated with immunohistochemical markers for different cellular components of the immune system, and the streptavidn-biotin system was used in combination with alkaline phosphatase as the reporter molecule. The markers used were - CD20 (B lymphocytes), CD2 (T lymphocytes), CD4 (Inducer T lymphocytes), CD8 (Suppressor T lymphocytes), MAC 387 (macrophages), Factor XIIIa (Dermal dendritic cells) and CD1a (Langerhans cells).

Sections were examined at a magnification of 40x, at the ulcer base, beneath the ulcer edge, and beneath the intact skin at a distance of 5 high power fields (HPFs) from the ulcer edge. Ten fields were examined consisting of two adjacent fields for a depth of 5 HPFs. Intact cells staining positive for the particular marker, or in the case of neutrophils - those with typical appearances of neutrophils, were counted in each field, and the total number for each 10 HPFs was calculated. All tissue sections were assessed in duplicate on two separate occasions, and without knowledge of the phase of healing. Healing and non-healing biopsies for the same patient were stained at the same time.

RESULTS

There were a total of 13 patients who had their biopsies assessed in this study. There were 8 males and 5 females. The median age was 80 years (range 68 - 87). The number of paired biopsies for each analysis varied slightly due to technical difficulties with sections.

The major changes identified with healing occurred with CD4 positive lymphocytes and mast cells. There was a significant increase in the number of CD4 positive lymphocytes in the healing phase in the biopsies taken from the base of the ulcer (Table 1, $p<0.01$, Wilcoxon signed rank test). This trend was not observed in the biopsies from the ulcer edge or the intact skin.

		Base			Edge			Skin	
	n	NH	H	n	NH	H	n	NH	H
T lympho (CD2)	9	58	62	11	92	40	11	44	46
T lympho (CD8)	6	18	26	9	38	12	9	19	5
T lympho (CD4)	9	24	60	10	52	37	10	40	39
Mast cells (Tol blue)	8	5	0	11	19	2	11	26	11
PMN (H&E)	11	20	12	12	13	19	12	0	1
Macro (MAC387)	8	58	59	10	14	16	9	20	9
B lympho (CD20)	6	26	19	6	10	2	5	7	2
DDC	7	0	0	7	0	0	7	3	1
Langerhans (FXIIIa)	9	0	0	9	3	1	9	3	3

Table 1. Numbers of cells staining in 10 HPFs for each cells type at each site of the biopsy in the non-healing (NH) and healing phases (H). The numbers of paired comparisons for each site are shown (n).

There was a significant reduction in the number of mast cells in the healing phase in the biopsies taken from the edge of the ulcer (Table 1, p = 0.02). There were very few mast cells in the base of the ulcer in either the non-healing or the healing phase. A similar trend to reduction of the number of mast cells in the healing phase in the intact skin was observed but this was not statistically significant.

Neutrophils were abundant in the ulcer base and ulcer edge, and few were seen in the intact skin, however, there was no alteration between healing and non-healing. Macrophages were most abundant in the ulcer base, but were also evident in other areas of the biopsies, without any change with healing. Total T lymphocytes and CD8 positive T lymphocytes were present in all parts of the biopsies without any trend with healing. B lymphocytes were most abundant in the ulcer base without any significant trend in the healing phase. Very few dermal dendritic cells or Langerhans cells were seen in any of the biopsy sites, with no evidence of alteration with healing.

DISCUSSION

These studies were limited by the technical difficulties with some of the sections, and as a consequence the numbers of paired sections available for comparing healing and non-healing phases were possibly too few to make firm conclusions. However, a number of clear observations can be made from this data. Neutrophils, macrophages, T lymphocytes, B lymphocytes and mast cells were all present in these chronic ulcers in both the healing and non-healing phases. These were present in all areas examined with the exception of neutrophils that were present in very low numbers beneath the intact skin, and mast cells that were present in very low numbers in the ulcer base. There were few dermal dendritic cells or Langerhans cells present in any areas of these sections, with none of these being present in the base of the ulcers.

CD4 positive T lymphocytes were present in increased numbers in the base of the ulcers when they were healing. This could be either a causative factor in the healing of the wound or could be a result of the wound entering a healing phase. Previous studies have demonstrated an enhancement of wound healing parameters in animals with depletion of CD8 positive T lymphocytes[3], and it might follow that an increase in CD4 positive T lymphocytes could be associated with improved wound healing.

The release of granules from mast cells is associated with activation of phospholipase A2. This and its immediate metabolite lysolecithin are cytotoxic agents that have been associated with inflammatory and necrotising disorders[4]. These have previously been found to be elevated in wound fluid from chronic leg ulcers in a non-healing phase, in work from our department.

The function of the cellular immune system does need to be further examined in order to adequately understand the mechanism of the impaired healing in chronic leg ulcers.

REFERENCES

1. Bos JD, Kapsenberg ML. Immunol Today 1986; 7: 235-240.
2. Bos JD, Kapsenberg ML. The skin immune system: progress in cutaneous biology. Immunol Today. 1993; 14: 75-8.
3. Barbul A, Breslin RJ, Woodyard JP, et al. The effect of in vivo T Helper and T Suppressor lymphocye depletion on wound healing. Ann Surg 1989; 209: 479-485.
4. Langton SR. Phospolipase A2: its measurement and indications in disease. Aust J Medical and Laboratory Science 1990; 11: 78-86.

Phlebology '95, D. Negus et al. (eds.). Phlebology (1995) Suppl. 1: 796-798

OP/6.1

Popliteal Vein Reflux Demonstrated by Duplex Ultrasonography is Associated with Delayed and Non-Healing of Chronic Venous Ulceration

J. Brittenden, A.W. Bradbury, A.A. Milne, P.L. Allan[1] and C.V. Ruckley

Vascular Surgery Unit, University Department of Surgery and [1] Department of Medical Radiology, Royal Infirmary, Edinburgh EH3 9YW, Scotland

INTRODUCTION

Venous reflux, with or without obstruction, is generally accepted as the primary cause of chronic venous ulceration. However, the relative importance of reflux at different sites within the deep and superficial venous systems remains unclear [1]. The aim of the present study was to determine the relationship between deep and superficial venous reflux at different anatomical sites and healing of chronic venous ulceration.

PATIENTS AND METHODS

The study population consisted of 155 patients with chronic venous leg ulceration who presented to a hospital based venous clinic. All patients were treated with compression therapy for a period of 6 months and healing was assessed at monthly intervals. Patients with evidence of arterial disease (ankle:brachial pressure index <0.8), diabetes or connective tissue disease were excluded. Prior to treatment all patients underwent duplex ultrasonography which was performed by one consultant radiologist at pre-designated sites using an Auroscan 125 colour flow duplex scanner (Mountain View, California,USA). Patients were examined standing and in a 30^0 head up tilt. using manual calf compression and the Valsalva manoeuvre. Venous reflux was defined as the presence of reverse flow lasting greater than 0.5 seconds (2).

The male to female ratio was 1.8:1, with a median age of 69 years. The median (range) of the maximum ulcer diameter was 29mm (10-140mm). The median (range) duration of the current ulcer was 5 months (2-144), and the median number of previous episodes of ulceration was 2 (1-20).

RESULTS

At 24 weeks, 104 (67%) ulcers had healed. There was no significant difference in the pattern of deep or superficial venous reflux between the healed and non-healed group at the following sites: common femoral, superficial femoral, peroneal, anterior and posterior tibial, long saphenous (origin and mid-thigh segments) and short saphenous .

However, there was a significant correlation between the presence of popliteal vein (PV) reflux and healing (Table 1). In healed legs, 39 (38%) scans indicated competence of the above-knee PV compared with 5 (10%) scans in the non-healing group (p < 0.001 by X^2-test). Similarly, 44 (43%) scans showed below-knee PV competence in the healed legs compared with only 5 (10%) scans performed in legs remaining ulcerated (p < 0.001 by X^2-test). Combining above and below knee popliteal segments resulted in an even stronger correlation with rates of non-healing. Four of 42 (10%) patients with competent, and 45 of 103 (44%) patients with incompetent, above and

Table 1. Relationship between venous reflux and healing

VENOUS SEGMENT	NO REFLUX	NO RELUX HEALED	REFLUX	REFLUX HEALED	P value
Long saphenous (origin)	24	18	108	70	0.47
Long saphenous (mid-thigh)	21	17	116	75	0.23
Short saphenous	35	28	110	69	0.09
Common femoral	25	21	127	80	0.072
Superficial femoral	53	35	98	65	0.89
Proximal popliteal	44	39	110	64	**0.0006**
Distal Popliteal	49	44	105	59	**0.0008**
Posterior tibial	52	36	79	51	0.72
Peroneal	54	37	53	34	0.78

below knee PV failed to heal (p < 0.001 by X^2-test, sensitivity 40%, specificity 90%, positive predictive value 44%, negative predictive value 90%).

CONCLUSIONS

This prospective study has demonstrated that popliteal vein incompetence is strongly associated with delayed and non-healing of venous ulcers. Although there was considerable incompetence at other sites, including the superficial venous system, this had no effect on ulcer healing. In addition, the presence of both short saphenous and popliteal incompetence did not significantly affect healing.

At present most surgical treatment is aimed at the superficial venous system. Whereas some studies have shown excellant results from long saphenous stripping (3), others have shown that perforator and saphenous ligations alone are ineffective in promoting long term ulcer healing in the presence of deep venous incompetence (4). Venous valve surgery remains complex, and single valve replacement or repair is currently recommended (3). This study supports previous publications which have emphasised the importance of the popliteal segment in venous ulceration (5,6,7). In conclusion, popliteal vein incompetence in patients with venous ulceration is an indicator of poor prognosis and future developments in deep venous reconstruction should be aimed at addressing this problem.

REFERENCES

1. Milne AA, Stonebridge PA, Bradbury AW, Ruckley CV. Venous function and clinical outcome following deep venous thrombosis. Br J Surg 1994; 81:847-9.

2. Sarin S, Sommerville K, Farrah J, Scur JH, Coleridge Smith PD. Duplex ultrasonography for assessment of venous valvular function of the lower limb. Br J Surg 1994;81:1591-1595

3. Seitha K, Darke S. Long saphenous incompetence as a cause of venous ulceration. Br J Surg 1984;71:754-5.
4. Bradbury AW, Ruckley CV. Foot volumetry can predict recurrent ulceration after subfascial ligation of perforators and saphenous ligation. J Vasc Surg 1993; 18:789-95.

5. Wilson NM, Rutt DL, Browse NL. Repair and replacement of deep vein valves in the treatment of venous insufficiency. Br J Surg 1991;78:388-94.

6 Gooley NA, Sumner DS. Relationship of venous reflux to the site of venous valvular incompetence: Implications for venous reconstructive surgery. J Vasc Surg 1988;7:50-9.

7. Payne SPK, London NJM, Jagger C, Newland CJ, Barrie WW, Bell PRF. Clinical significance of venous reflux detected by duplex scanning. Br J Surg 1994;81:39-41.

Phlebology '95, D. Negus et al. (eds.). Phlebology (1995) Suppl. 1: 799-801

OP/3.6

Chronic Venous Ulceration: Comparison of Duplex Assessment of Venous Reflux in the Affected and Non-Affected Legs

A.W. Bradbury, J. Brittenden, P.L. Allan[1] and C.V. Ruckley

Vascular Surgery Unit, University Department of Surgery and [1] Department of Medical Radiology, Royal Infirmary, Edinburgh EH3 9YW, Scotland

INTRODUCTION

It is generally accepted that venous ulceration is most commonly a consequence of venous reflux with or without obstruction. However, the relative importance of reflux at different sites in the deep and superficial venous systems remains unclear [1]. The aim of the present study was to determine the pattern of venous reflux in the legs of patients affected by chronic venous ulceration and to compare this with the pattern of reflux in the contralateral unaffected leg.

PATIENTS AND METHODS

Fifty-four patients who had venous ulceration in one leg but who had never developed ulceration in the other. There were 26 males and 28 females. The median age was 69 (range 45-92) years. There were 26 ulcers on right legs and 28 on left legs. All patients had an ankle:brachial pressure index in excess of 0.8 in both legs. No patient was diabetic or had clinical or serological evidence of connective tissue disease or rheumatoid arthritis.

The median duration of the current episode of ulceration was 7 (range 2-120) months; the median number of episodes of ulceration was 2 (range 1-20); and the median time since onset of first ulcer was 14 (range 1-43) years.

Colour flow duplex ultrasonography of the deep and superficial venous systems of both legs was performed by a single Consultant Radiologist (PLA) using an Acuson 128 machine (Acuson, Mountain View, California, USA) and either a 5-MHz or 7.5-MHz transducer. Patients were examined standing and in a 30° head up tilt. Venous reflux was elicited using manual calf compression and Valsalva manoeuvre and was considered pathological if reverse flow exceeded 0.5 secs [2].

RESULTS

There was no significant difference between ulcerated and non-ulcerated legs in the pattern of venous reflux in the common femoral, proximal and distal superficial femoral, peroneal, long saphenous (origin and mid-thigh segments), and short saphenous (origin) veins.

By contrast, 42 ulcerated legs had proximal (above knee) popliteal vein reflux compared with 31 non-ulcerated legs (p = 0.034, $\chi2$ = 4.53, with Yates correction). Similarly, 39 ulcerated legs had distal (below knee) popliteal vein reflux compared with 26 non-ulcerated legs (p = 0.024, $\chi2$ = 5.09, with Yates correction). The above knee popliteal vein was visualised in all patients and the below knee popliteal vein in all but one patient.

The proportion of uninformative scans was much higher when examining the crural veins. Nevertheless, ulcerated legs were also significantly more likely to exhibit venous reflux in the posterior tibial (27/44 vs. 16/47 informative scans, p = 0.016, $\chi2$ = 5.75, with Yates correction) and anterior tibial (9/42 vs. 2/44 informative scans, p = 0.044, $\chi2$ = 4.08, with Yates correction) veins than legs that had never developed ulceration.

CONCLUSIONS

The present study demonstrates that deep and superficial venous reflux is common in legs clinically unaffected by the skin changes typical of chronic venous insufficiency. Thus the only significant difference between legs affected by chronic venous ulceration and the contra-lateral unaffected leg (without any history of ulceration) was the degree of popliteal, anterior and posterior tibial vein reflux. There was no difference in the presence of reflux at other sites within the deep system or with respect to long and short saphenous incompetence.

These observations suggest that the clinical significance of a particular pattern of venous reflux within a leg affected by chronic venous ulceration cannot be determined without reference to the contralateral non-ulcerated limb. This may explain why studies attempting to correlate the pattern of deep and superficial venous reflux with the severity of clinical disease have reported such disparate results. In addition, the present data may explain why some authorities obtain excellent results from superficial venous surgery alone [3] and others do not [4,5]. For the individual patient there must be additional factors, perhaps at a microvascular level [6], that determine whether a particular pattern and severity of reflux leads to skin changes and ulceration. For example, it is common in clinical practice to see patients with gross superficial varicosities but without any skin changes. Similarly, in patients with the post-thrombotic syndrome there is a poor correlation between the pattern and severity of reflux and symptoms [1]

In absence of a clear understanding of what these additional factors might be, and so how to influence them, the surgeon must adopt a somewhat pragmatic approach. When contemplating surgery it would seem reasonable to advocate correction of that reflux which is present in the ulcerated, but not in the unaffected, limb. In a minority of patients this is straightforward as it entails superficial venous surgery alone. However, the present study confirms the results of earlier work, from both our own department [5,7] and from others [8], that clearly demonstrates the importance of the popliteal vein in maintaining clinical and haemodynamic normality of the calf. Novel surgical methods of correcting reflux within the popliteal segment are urgently required.

REFERENCES

1. Milne AA, Stonebridge PA, Bradbury AW, Ruckley CV. Venous function and clinical outcome following deep venous thrombosis. Br J Surg 1994; 81:847-9.

2. Sarin S, Sommerville K, Farrah J, Scurr JH, Coleridge Smith PD. Duplex ultrasonography for assessment of venous valvular function of the lower limb. Br J Surg 1994; 81:1591-1595.

3. Darke SG, Penfold C. Venous ulceration and saphenous ligation. Eur J Vasc Surg 1992; 6:4-9.

4. Burnand K, Lea Thomas M, O'Donnell T, Browse NL. Relation between post-phlebitic changes in the deep veins and results of surgical treatment of venous ulcers. Lancet 1976;

5. Bradbury AW, Ruckley CV. Foot volumetry can predict recurrent ulceration after subfascial ligation of perforators and saphenous ligation. J Vasc Surg 1993; 18:789-95.

6. Bradbury AW, Murie JA, Ruckley CV. The role of the leucocyte in the patho-genesis of vascular disease. Br J Surg 193; 80:1503-12.

7. Bradbury AW, Stonebridge PA, Callam MJ, Ruckley CV, Allan PL. Foot volumetry and duplex ultrasonography after saphenous and subfascial perforating vein ligation for recurrent venous ulceration. Br J Surg 1993; 80:845-48.

8. Payne SP, London NJ, Newland CJ, Bell PR, Barrie WW. Investigation and significance of short saphenous incompetence. Ann R Coll Surg Eng 1993; 75:354-7.

Phlebology '95, D. Negus et al. (eds.). Phlebology (1995) Suppl. 1: 802-804

PI/3.5

Growth Factors in Venous Ulcers

N.R.F. Lagattolla, D. Gill and K.G. Burnand

Department of Surgery, St Thomas' Hospital, London, England

INTRODUCTION

Growth factors are implicated in acute and chronic wound healing [1,2]. As part of a project to determine why some venous ulcers heal rapidly and some remain unhealed for years, we investigated transforming growth factor-β_1 (TGF-β_1), basic fibroblast growth factor (bFGF) and platelet-derived growth factor (PDGF) by enzyme-linked immunoassay (ELISA) and immunohistochemistry, and epidermal growth factor (EGF), insulin-like growth factor (IGF-1), tumor necrosis factor (TNFα), and receptors to bFGF and PDGF by immunohistochemistry, in venous ulcer and normal skin biopsies.

METHODS

Biopsies were taken from 19 venous ulcers and 7 specimens of normal skin under local anaesthetic from patients attending the St Thomas' Ulcer clinic. A reprasentative block was taken from every sample and this was fixed in neutral buffered formalin for immunohistochemical localisation of the above growth factors, and EGF, IGF-1, TNFα, receptors to bFGF and PDGF, α-smooth muscle actin, vascular endothelium (factor VIII), and macrophages (CD68). The residual parts of the ulcer biopsies were divided into two portions consisting of the base and the edge of the ulcer. All samples were immediately frozen in liquid nitrogen for TGFβ_1, bFGF and PDGF ELISA.

The immunohistochemistry was performed on paraffin wax embedded 4μ sections. The optimal dilutions for the primary antibodies had been previously established. Each antibody-treated section had a negative control treated with murine IgG or buffered saline as appropriate in place of the primary antibody. The technique involved an overnight incubation with the primary antibody at 4°C, followed by biotinylated secondary antibody, streptavidin and diaminobenzidine. Commercially available ELISA kits were used for bFGF and PDGF-AB (Quantikine), and we used a modified assay based on that of Danielpour for TGF-β_1[3].

Details of the duration of current ulceration, ulcer size, and the length of time taken to complete ulcer healing from the time of the biopsy were obtained from each patient.

RESULTS

Immunohistochemistry

The distribution of PDGF, PDGF-receptor, bFGF, bFGF-receptor, and EGF was similar, both in normal skin and venous ulcer biopsies. These were present in the epidermis, vascular smooth muscle, eccrine gland acini and ducts, and in dermal fibroblasts. EGF and bFGF was identified in the basal layer of the epidermis only at the very edge of the ulcer. TGF-β_1 was prominent in the dermis of ulcer specimens, but was rarely observed in normal skin. Nests of TGF-β_1 staining cells were occasionally seen in mid epidermis of normal and ulcerated skin. IGF-1 and TNFα stained heavily in both dermis and epidermis of normal and ulcerated skin. Macrophages and myofibroblasts were prominent in the bases of ulcer biopsies. Factor VIII was observed in endothelium and in perivascular cuffs in ulcer biopsies.

Table 1. Growth factor levels (pg/mg tissue, median value and range) in normal skin, and venous ulcer edge and base specimens

| | Normal skin (n=7) | Venous ulcer (n=19) | |
		Edge	Base
TGF-β_1	5*	5* (5-26.3)	16.6 (5-42.7)
bFGF	21.2 (8.4-56.4)	32.4 (11.5-52.1)	48.6 (10.4-89.4)
PDGF	0.7* (0.7-14.1)	0.7* (0.7-2.2)	1.4 (0.7-4.6)

*lower limit of assay

Normal Skin and Venous Ulcer Growth Factors

There was no demonstrable TGF-β_1 in any normal skin specimen, but this was detected in 9/19 edge samples, and 13/19 base samples. Assuming the lowest detectable TGF-β_1 level in normal skin, there is significantly more TGF-β_1 in both ulcer edge (p=0.03) and base (p=0.004) than in normal skin. The median value of bFGF in ulcer edge is greater than in normal skin, but the difference is not significant (p=0.31). There is, however, significantly more bFGF in ulcer base than in normal skin (p=0.013). PDGF levels are not significantly different in normal skin and edge (p=0.46) and base (p=0.1) samples (all Mann-Whitney U-Test).

Growth Factors in Ulcer Edges and Bases

For all the growth factors assayed, there was significantly greater amount in the ulcer base compared to the edge (TGF-β_1 p=0.004; bFGF p=0.007; PDGF p=0.026; Wilcoxon Rank Sum Test)

Growth Factors Related to Ulcer Size, Duration and Time to Ulcer Healing

There was no relation between ulcer edge or base bFGF, PDGF and TGF-ß$_1$ and duration prior to biopsy or ulcer size. Within six months of biopsy, 10 ulcers had healed. Ulcer edge TGF-ß$_1$ exhibited a negative correlation with time to healing ($r = -0.6$) which approached significance ($p=0.065$). There was no significant correlation between either edge or base bFGF and time to healing. However, bFGF was greater in ulcers that healed within six months compared to those remaining unhealed (median bFGF pg/mg [range]: edge 34.2[21.2-52.1] vs 17.1[11.5-38.3] p=0.036; base 56.2[22.3-89.4] vs 42.2[10.4-58.9] p=0.069; Mann-Whitney U-Test). There was no relation between PDGF to time to healing.

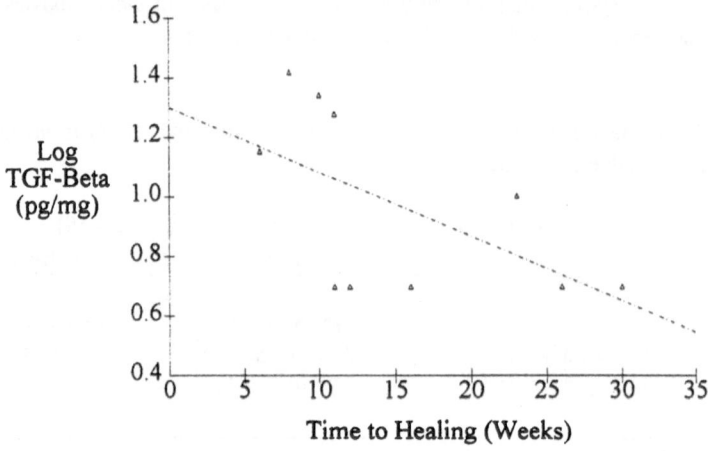

Figure 1. Correlation of ulcer edge TGF-ß$_1$ (pg/mg) and time-to-ulcer healing in weeks

SUMMARY

Growth factors appear to have a role in venous ulceration. Increased levels of TGF-ß$_1$ and bFGF may be associated with ulcer healing. Growth factors are present in greater amounts in the bases of venous ulcers compared to their edges, but activity at the ulcer edge may bear more relation to ulcer healing.

REFERENCES

1. McKay IA, Leigh IM. Epidermal cytokines and their roles in cutaneous wound healing. Br J Dermatol 1991; 124:513-8

2. Appleton I. Wound repair: the role of cytokines and vasoactive mediators. J R Soc Med 1994; 87:500-2

3. Danielpour D. Improved sandwich enzyme-linked immunosorbent assays for transforming growth factor-ß$_1$. J Immunol Methods 1993;158:17-25

Phlebology '95, D. Negus et al. (eds.). Phlebology (1995) Suppl. 1: 805-807

OP/9.4

A Comparison of Sources of Keratinocytes for Culture

N.R.F. Lagattolla, D. Gill and K.G. Burnand

Department of Surgery, St Thomas' Hospital, London, England

INTRODUCTION

Cultured keratinocytes have been used to treat chronic leg ulcers [1], burns [2] and surgical defects [3]. As part of a project to investigate cultured keratinocytes in venous ulceration, we assessed the potential of skin from different sources to produce viable keratinocyte cultures under different culture methods. The aim was to culture keratinocytes from adult skin samples to confluence as efficiently as possible.

METHODS

Skin was obtained from 45 surgical specimens. These were 27 adult surgical biopsies (mean age 65, range 20-86), 12 neonatal foreskins, and 6 lower limb lymphoedema reduction operations (mean age 34, range 26-41). The skin was washed in Dulbecco's Minimal Essential Medium (DMEM) with 5% foetal calf serum (FCS), and stored overnight at 4°C in DMEM with 5% FCS containing amphotericin, penicillin and streptomycin. The samples were cut into 5mm strips and placed in dispase (2.4 iu/ml) for 2 hours at 37°C. After the dispase was pipetted away, the epidermis was removed with fine forceps, and placed in 10ml 0.25% trypsin in a 50ml centrifuge tude and skaken for 5 minutes before neutralisation with 3:1 DMEM with 10% FCS. The suspension was passed through a sieve, and centrifuged at 1000rpm for five minutes. The pellet was suspended in 4ml of medium, the cells were counted, and plated at a mean density of $3.0 \times 10^4/cm^2$ in $25cm^2$ culture dishes.

Primary cultures were initiated on bovine type IV collagen, recombinant fibronectin (Pronectin), gelatin, mitomycin treated 3T3 feeder cells, and on uncoated culture dishes in both serum-free medium (Sigma, containing bovine insulin and pituitary extract, EGF, hydrocortisone, gentamicin and amphotericin) and in 3:1 DMEM:F12 (containing 10% FCS, transferrin, cholera toxin, tri-iodothyronine, adenine, EGF, hydrocortisone, tetracycline, penicillin, streptomycin and amphotericin). Ten primary cultures were initiated using each method. 29 successful primary cultures were passaged onto uncoated dishes in serum-free medium.

The outcomes were determined microscopically. A successful outcome comprised the presence of confluent cells or multiple colonies. An unsuccessful outcome comprised failure of the culture to grow, or overgrowth of the culture by fibroblasts.

RESULTS

Plating Substrate

Primary cultures failed to grow on 11 occasions in serum-free medium and 7 times with serum. 10 of 17 fibroblast overgrown cultures had been plated on fibronectin. Though uncoated dishes produced less keratinocyte cultures, this was not significantly less than pre-treatment of dishes with 3T3s, collagen or gelatin ($p>0.3$, $\chi^2 =0.52$, 1df).

Table 1. Numbers of successful cultures out of ten initiated using each method

Plating substrate	Serum-free	Serum-supplemented
3T3 cells	9	8
Collagen	9	7
Gelatin	9	7
Fibronectin	4	2
Uncoated dish	8	4

Serum Supplementation

Successful keratinocyte cultures were usually confluent in serum-free and colonial in serum-supplemented medium. 7/50 cultures (14%) failed in serum-supplemented, and 9/50 (18%) in serum-free medium. There was fibroblast overgrowth in 15 cultures (30%) in serum-supplemented, and in two cultures (4%) in serum-free medium ($p<0.001$, $\chi^2=11.71$, 1df). Successful keratinocyte cultures were obtained significantly more often in serum-free medium than serum-supplemented medium (39/50 vs 28/50, $p<0.05$, $\chi^2=4.95$, 1df).

Keratinocyte Source

The mean time-to-confluence for primary cultures was 7 days for neonatal foreskin (range 5-11, SE 2.0), 15 days for adult surgical biopsies (range 11-27, SE 1.2), and 26 days for lymphoedematous skin (range 17-35, SE 4.9). The differences are significant ($p=0.0001$ H=19.95, Kruskal Wallis; adult vs lymphoedema $p=0.024$, adult vs neonatal $p=0.0002$, neonatal vs lymphoedema $p<0.0007$ Mann-Whitney U-test). Keratinocytes obtained from lymphoedema reduction operations can be cultured, though primary cultures take longer to reach confluence than normal skin.

Effect of Passage

All passaged cultures reached confluence, irrespective of keratinocyte source, in a mean of 5 days (n=29; range 3-18).

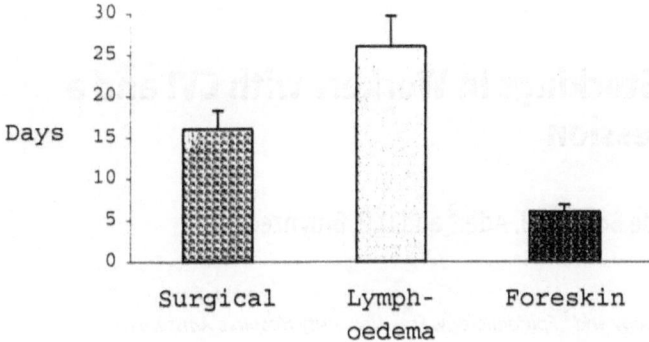

Figure 1. Mean time to confluence in days for different keratinocyte sources (standard error; p=0.001, Kruskal Wallis).

SUMMARY

Keratinocytes derived from lymphoedematous skin can be cultured, though the primary cultures take significantly longer to reach confluence than keratinocytes from normal skin. Neonatal foreskin keratinocytes reach confluence faster than adult skin keratinocytes. The passage of confluent primary cultures results in confluence most rapidly of all and is appears not to reflect the origin of the keratinocytes.

The use of recombinant fibronectin as a plating substrate and culture medium containing supplements including foetal calf serum both promote fibroblast overgrowth. The culture of human cells in serum-free medium is equally successful on 3T3 feeder cells, bovine type-IV collagen, gelatin or on uncoated tissue culture dishes, and results in confluent keratinocyte sheets rather than keratinocyte colonies.

REFERENCES

1. Hefton JM, Caldwell D, Biozes DG, Balin JK, Carter DM.
    Grafting of skin ulcers with cultured autologous epidermal cells.
    J Am Acad Dermatol 1986; 14:399-405

2. O'Connor NE, Mulliken JB, Banks-Schlegel S, Kehinde O, Green H.
    Grafting of burns with cultured epithelium prepared from autologous
    epidermal cells. Lancet 1981;1:75-8

3. Gallico GG, O'Connor NE, Compton CC, Remensnyder JP, Kehinde O, Green H.
    Cultured epithelial autografts for giant congenital naevi.
    Plast Recon Surg 1989; 84:1-9

Phlebology '95, D. Negus et al. (eds.). Phlebology (1995) Suppl. 1: 808-810

OP/15.4

Compression Stockings in Workers with CVI and a Standing Profession

R.M.A. Krijnen[1], E.M. de Boer[1], H.J. Adèr[2] and D.P. Bruynzeel[1]

Departments of [1] Dermatology and [2] Epidemiology, Free University Hospital, Amsterdam, The Netherlands

INTRODUCTION

Chronic venous disorders occur frequently in the occupational population [1]. Literature shows evidence that venous disorders lead to incapacity to work in approximately 2% of the occupational population [2]. Many workers with venous disorders never consult a doctor and are not treated for this reason [2].

In this study medical compression stockings were distributed to workers with chronic venous insufficiency (CVI) who have a standing profession. The aim of the study was to investigate the practical implications of wearing stockings on the work floor, the acceptance by the workers and the effects on subjective complaints of the legs.

MATERIALS AND METHODS

A randomized trial was performed in 9 factories, mainly in the meat industry. 308 male workers were examined for the presence of CVI by physical examination, Doppler ultrasound investigation and light reflection rheography. Out of these 308 subjects, in 90 subjects CVI was diagnosed. One third of these subjects had progressed CVI with skin disorders such as hyperpigmentation (Widmer II) or trunk varicosis. The others had less severe disorders such as side branch varicosis and ankle flare (Widmer I). None had active ulceration. Individuals with only intracutaneous varices were considered not to have CVI.

Subjects having CVI were randomized into an intervention group and a control group. Subjects in the intervention group received below-knee compression stockings (30-32 mmHG). All stockings were measured by a qualified bandager (orthotist) and made-to-measure. After three months of intervention, all subjects having CVI were examined again.

Subjects were asked for the presence of complaints of the legs, such as a tired or heavy feeling and pain in the legs. The severity of these complaints was scored on an ordinal scale (never/ sometimes/often). The rates scored before and after the follow-up were compared.

RESULTS

Out of the 50 workers randomized into the intervention group, in 45 the use of the stockings could be evaluated (5 subjects were lost for follow-up because of unrelated reasons).

Thirty out of 45 workers had used their stockings (almost) every day. In the 30 subjects that had worn their stockings every day, significantly less complaints were present after three months of intervention compared to themselves and to the controlgroup (p < 0.005). Figure 1 shows the percentage of subjects with complaints of the legs. Before the intervention, 21 out of the 30 persons complained of a tired feeling in the legs. After three months of interventions, only 8 persons reported such complaints. Pain in the legs was reported by 10 out of 30 subjects before, and by 2 out of 30 subjects after the interventions. In the subjects randomized into the control group no mean difference in complaints before and after intervention was found.

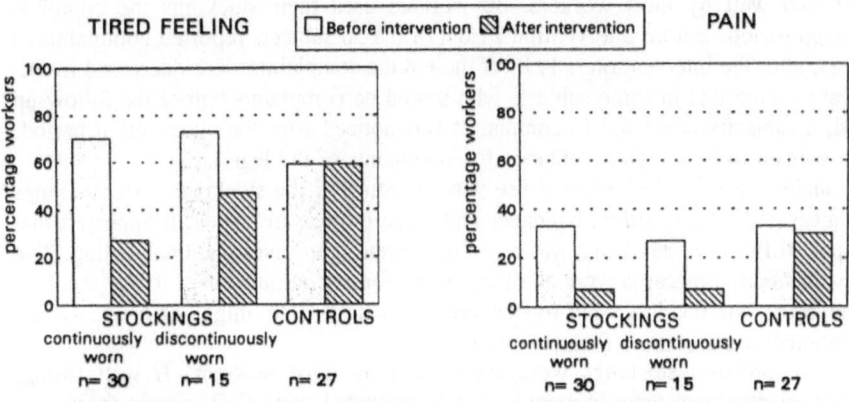

Fig. 1. Percentage of workers with complaints of the legs before and after intervention. Subjects that did not use the stockings during the whole period were listed separately.

After intervention all subjects were asked if the complaints of the legs were changed compared with before the intervention (table 1). A decrease of complaints was reported by 57% of the subjects wearing stockings and by no subjects in the control group. In case of discontinued use of the stockings, a decrease of complaints was reported by 27% of the subjects. The results were approximately the same for persons with minor venous disorders as for persons with progressed CVI.

Table 1. Changes in complaints of the legs after intervention, as reported by the subjects.

| | STOCKINGS | | | | CONTROLS | |
| | continuously worn | | discontinuously worn | | | |
	n=30	%	n=15	%	n=27	%
decrease complaints	17	57%	4	27%	0	0%
unchanged	13	43%	11	73%	25	93%
increase complaints	0	0%	0	0%	2	7%

All persons who had infrequently used the stockings were asked for the reason. Discontinued use of the stockings was in 7 cases attributed to stocking related factors (pinching: 5, sliding down: 2), in 4 cases attributed to skin related factors (itch: 2, red and swollen skin:2), in 1 case attributed to workplace related factors (wet work), in 1 case attributed to a sporting injury and in two cases the subjects could not explain the reason for discontinued use.

DISCUSSION

A standing profession is associated with an increased risk for venous disorders. And during standing, complaints of the legs associated with the disease might aggravate. Compression stockings can be useful in slowing down the development of CVI and in reducing the subjective complaints of the legs associated with CVI. No information was available about the use of elastic stockings in an industrial population.

In 45 workers with CVI who received elastic stockings, the stockings were appreciated well by most workers. 30 workers used their stockings the complete follow-up period. Before intervention 21 out of the 30 subjects reported complaints of the legs, after the intervention only 8 (of these 8 the complaints were decreased in 5).

It was striking that in some subjects who scored no complaints before the follow-up period, a subjective decrease in complaints was noticed after the intervention period. There seemed to be a high acceptance for complaints of the legs.

The main cause for discontinued use was ill fitting of the stockings. All stockings were measured by a qualified bandager and made-to-measure. Thus, it appeared that sub-optimal fitting of stockings was a problem even in an investigational setting. The occupational circumstances were an other reason for discontinued use. It was reported in one case, but possibly skin-related factors such as itch might also depend on occupational circumstances (heat, moist.)

Elastic compression stockings were appreciated by most workers. If well fitting, compression stockings were of great benefit to workers having CVI, also in those with minor disorders.

ACKNOWLEDGMENTS

We thank Bauerfeind for kindly supplying the compression stockings.
This study was made possible by a grant of the Praeventiefonds, The Netherlands

REFERENCES

1. Widmer LK, Plechl S-Ch, Leu HJ, Boner H. Venenerkrankungen bei 1800 Berufstätigen. Basler Studie II. Schweiz. med. Wschr. 1967;97:107-10.

2. Fischer H, Widmer LK, Biland K. Sozioepidemiologische Studie über die Venenleiden bei einer erwachsenen Wohnbevölkerung in der Bundesrepublik Deutschland. Phlebol. u. Proktol. 1980;9:147-52.

Phlebology '95, D. Negus et al. (eds.). Phlebology (1995) Suppl. 1: 811-813

OP/21.1

Comparison of Duplex Valve Closure Time and Air Plethysmography in Assessing Venous Reflux

H.J. Welch, M.D. Iafrati, A.A. Rodriguez and T.F. O'Donnell

Division of Vascular Surgery, New England Medical Center and Tufts University School of Medicine, Boston, Massachusetts, USA

INTRODUCTION

Venous reflux is a significant cause of chronic venous insufficiency (CVI), whether it be in the superficial and/or deep venous system. Identification of the system(s) involved and quantification of the degree of reflux has significant therapeutic implications. Non-invasive testing is now indispensable in the evaluation of the CVI patient, however, selecting the best test to measure reflux is a matter of considerable investigation and debate. We compared Duplex derived valve closure time (VCT) and air plethysmography derived venous filling index (VFI) with and without tourniquet to determine the correlation between the tests in measuring reflux.

METHODS

Using a retrospective review of non-invasive data from a vascular registry at a university teaching hospital, we examined 33 limbs in 26 patients (13 male, 13 female). Duplex VCT, using the cuff deflation technique as described by van Bemmelen et al[1], was measured at the saphenofemoral junction (SFJ), mid-portion of the greater saphenous vein (GSV), superficial femoral vein (SFV), and popliteal vein (PV). Superficial venous reflux by duplex was calculated as SFJ + GSV, and total limb reflux as SFJ+GSV+SFV+PV. An abnormal total VCT was defined as ≥ 4 seconds. Abnormal superficial reflux was defined as $\geq 50\%$ of total VCT when the total VCT was ≥ 4 seconds. VFI was measured in standard fashion and repeated with an above knee tourniquet (penrose drain) if initially abnormal.

RESULTS

Of the 33 limbs, 12 were clinical class 1, 9 were class 2, and 12 were class 3. The average age of the patients was 47.4 years (range 25 - 79). Previous surgery had been performed in 3 patients including 2 limbs with vein valvuloplasty and ligation of varicose veins or incompetent perforators, and 2 limbs with ligation and stripping of varicose veins. Twenty-one limbs had abnormal TVCT and 18 limbs had an abnormal VFI. Two limbs had an abnormal VFI and normal TVCT, while conversely 5 limbs had abnormal TVCT and normal VFI. Of the thirty-three limbs, there was agreement between TVCT and VFI in 26 and disagreement in 7 limbs. Twenty-three limbs had an abnormal superficial reflux of $\geq$50% of total reflux by duplex VCT.

With the above selected values, VFI was found to discriminate normal from abnormal TVCT with a sensitivity of 76% and specificity of 83%. The positive predictive value for VFI with TVCT as the "gold standard" was 89% and the negative predictive value was 67%. When comparing the absolute values for VFI and TVCT, the correlation coefficient was $r = 0.34$. Thus, the magnitude of reflux as measured by these two tests does not follow a linear relationship.

When an abnormal VFI was initially obtained, a tourniquet consisting of a penrose drain was placed around the mid thigh in an attempt to eliminate superficial reflux in the greater saphenous vein as measured by the APG calf cuff. In 13 limbs with an abnormal VFI and superficial reflux documented by duplex, the addition of a tourniquet caused the repeat VFI to decrease in four limbs, increase in 5 limbs and had no change in 4 limbs. In 5 limbs with an abnormal VFI but no evidence of superficial reflux by duplex, addition of a tourniquet decreased the repeat VFI in 2 limbs, increased it in 1 limb, and had no effect in 2 limbs. Analysis of the change in VFI with tourniquet using a two-tailed t-test failed to discriminate ($p = 0.46$) limbs in which venous insufficiency was primarily superficial ($\geq$50% of TVCT) from those in whom insufficiency was primarily deep.

DISCUSSION

Non-invasive testing of venous reflux is performed to quantify the severity of the reflux and select those patients who may require a descending phlebogram and possible deep venous reconstruction, or a more simple superficial procedure. Several non-invasive tests are available, including duplex, air plethsymography, and photoplethysmography. Duplex valve closure times have been shown both by van Bemmelen et al[1], and our own vascular laboratory[2] to be an accurate method of quantify venous reflux. We currently use duplex VCT's to assess both the superficial (saphenofemoral junction, mid greater saphenous vein, and lesser saphenous vein if applicable) and the deep system (superficial femoral vein, popliteal vein, and profunda femoris vein). Additionally, we perform air plethysmography to obtain a global assessment of the limb in question.

While we have shown good agreement between VFI and VCT as tests that assess reflux, the lack of absolute correlation is not surprising. Valve closure times measure length of reflux at the imaged site, and as we have shown, do not correlate with reflux volume[3]. Venous filling index measures venous volume of the calf and will be influenced by the degree of reflux at individual proximal levels. However, both tests show increases as the severity of reflux increases by descending phlebography[3], and worsening clinical stage[4], as one would expect.

Others have presented VFI as a singular test to assess reflux and plan invasive procedures[5]. While changes were seen in the VFI with the addition of a tourniquet, it is unclear whether the changes corresponded to descending phlebography. From the present study, when comparing VFI to duplex VCT, the addition of a superficial thigh tourniquet does not aid in defining the contribution of superficial reflux to overall reflux. It is acknowledged that these results may be related to the potential variability of the penrose drain tourniquet technique and thus demand that a more standard superficial occlusion be performed, ie an inflatable cuff. This area will require further evaluation. Currently, we cannot rely on VFI changes with tourniquet to define the degree of superficial reflux.

Because no test is infallible, including physical examination, we and many others believe that the best evaluation for venous reflux requires a combination of noninvasive tests, primarily duplex valve closure times and air plethysmography. With the present study there is reassuring agreement between VCT and VFI identifying reflux in most cases. However, when we have discordance between tests, we generally rely on the duplex VCT.

REFERENCES

1. van Bemmelen PS, Bedford G, Beach K, Strandness DE. Quantitative segmental evaluation of venous valvular reflux with duplex ultrasound scanning. J Vasc Surg 1989;10:425-31

2. Welch HJ, Faliakou EC, McLaughlin RL, Umphrey SE, Belkin M, O'Donnell TF. Comparison of descending phlebography with quantitative photoplethysmography, air plethysmography, and duplex quantitative valve closure time in assessing deep venous reflux. J Vasc Surg 1992;16:913-20

3. Rodriguez AA, Whitehead CM, McLaughlin RL, Welch HJ, O'Donnell TF. Duplex-derived valve closure times fail to correlate with flow velocities and flow volumes in patients with chronic venous insufficiency. Presented at the American Venous Forum, Seventh Annual Meeting, Ft. Lauderdale, FL. February 23, 1995

4. Iafrati MD, Welch HJ, O'Donnell TF, Belkin M, Umphrey SE, McLaughlin RL. Correlation of venous noninvasive tests with the Society for Vascular Surgery /International Society for Cardiovascular Surgery clinical classification of chronic venous insufficiency. J Vasc Surg 1994;19:1001-7.

5. Harada RN, Comerota AJ, Katz ML. A noninvasive screening test to detect "critical" deep venous reflux. Presented at the American Venous Forum, Seventh Annual Meeting, Ft. Lauderdale, FL. February 23, 1995

Phlebology '95, D. Negus et al. (eds.). Phlebology (1995) Suppl. 1: 814-816

P176

Therapeutical Indications in View of the Phases of Healing Cycle of the Leg Ulcers

C. Ruggieri, S. Massi, A.M. Peccatori, G. Botta and S. Mancini

III Department of General Surgery and Pabisch Center of Phlebology, Faculty of Medicine and Surgery, University of Siena, Italy

INTRODUCTION

The ulcer's therapy avails itself now of a wide range of products with peculiarities and properties partly laid upon, partly peculiar of everyone of them. No type of treatment assures either the whole management of every single ulcer or the management of all types of ulcera. We have keep in mind that the ulcer healing depends on a process extremely dynamical and the treatment has to adapt itself constantly to the ulcer peculiarities that are: the depth (superficial, at full thickness, of the hollow); the condition (necrotic, fibrinous, granular, reepithelial); the secretions (dry, wet, very much exuding, bleeding, ill-smelling); the pain modalities and the bacteriological sketch (sterile, colonized, infected, overinfected). One ideal treatment should therefore possess the following requisites: conformation, absorption ability, no toxie contaminators possession, antibacterial activity, haemostatic property, application aptitude, pain control, thermie insulation, cheap costs and long intervals of substitution, atraumatic to the rimoval. In spite of the improvements in this field, it doesn't exist any product with all the requested qualifications, therefore no treatment may be exploited for the management of all kinds of ulcers and few may be exploited for one single ulcer treatment during all the phases of the treatment cycle.

PATHOGENESIS

While the arterial and neuropathic ulcer pathogenesis is well determined, the venous ulcer pathogenesis is much more debated. Recent observations show a very close correlation between the origin of hypodermities, ulcerative lesions and local impairments of the cutaneous capillary microcirculation The capillaries pathological alterations in the venous chronic stasis of the lower limbs show themselves from the first moments with abnormal capillary permeability, with macromolecules filtration and particularly with the fibrinogen filtration that goes by into the pericapillay liquid where it creates fibrin complexes. The fibrin stratum creates a barrier to the scattering of oxygen and nourishing factors, indispensable to the cutaneous trophism. A newer hypothesis proposes the alterated rheology of the leucocytes like the venous ulcerations reason. It has been observed with regard to the leucocytes that they remain entrapped in the capillaries becouse of a precapillary vessel constriction, creating so a stoppage with a following increase of the permeability of the vessels. The reduced pression of perfusion secondary to the venous hyperpression causes one entrapment of leucocytes in the microcirculation with a capillary stoppage and a release of substances like ozone, free radicals and proteolytical enzymes, that contribute to increase the permeability with a further fibrin deposition in the pericapillary space. The arteriosclerosis is the principal reason of the ulcerative arterial lesions. It determines, through a lipids, cells, fibrous matrix accumulation in the vessel deep, the reduction of the vessel lumen with a stoppage of the bloody flux, with a following anoxia of tissue and cellular necrosis. The neuropathic ulcera arise in the tissues with adulterated sensitivity owing to repeated traumas. Particularly in the diabetic ulcera pathogenesis a microangiopathy joins with the neuropathy.

THERAPY

The treatment can't be disregarder from the diagnosis that at present can benefit by clinical- instrumental structures extremely transtworthy. After having established and discussed the reason of the ulcerative lesion, the topical treatment of ulcer begins. Our therapeutical protocol foresees to leave out of aetoiology of the ulcers, photographic and morphometric observations, tampons of the secretions for the examination of the culture, bioptics drawings of the bottom and of the borders for the histological examination and the ozonized hydromassage of the limb. The treatment success is influenced by the extreme variability of the individual answer binding to idiopathical primitive factors (immunologics...) and to acquired factors (allergies, intollerances...) that may annul our results. We try to suggest the use of a products series for all four phases of the recovery cycle of the ulcer:

1) Necrotic ulcer: when we face a necrotic tissue it is advisable the use of products able to be opposed to the dehydration and to make easier the same necrosis removal, praticable by the hydrocolloides application, by hydrocellular plaques. They create a physical barrier that prevents the substance and water loss, limiting the loss of heat, maintaining the ideal microenvironnement to which we can bring a further hydration by the use of a gel with an high watery contents to place under the occluded and semioccluded palques. The microenvironnement wetness, promoting the autolysis, causes the necrotic tissue removal.

2) Fibrinous ulcer: when the ulcer presents itself covered with a fibrinous stratum with a cellular infiltrations high contents, it results predisposed to the contagious and to the overinfections. The surgical cleanliness is in this phase fitter for a good detergency; if it isn't praticable we can apply products with polysaccharides and equine catalase, useful hydrocolloides, the hydrocellular plaques and the alginates that create the ideal microenvironment and have the high absorption ability of the secretions that in this phase are particularly abundant.

3) Granular ulcer: The ulcer in this phase is accompanied by granulation checks easily bleeding, and the secretions may be still abundant. As well as in the previous phase we have to resort to some highly absorbing treatments, with haemostatic properties and as

much possible atraumatic for the removal becouse of the presence of little reepithelial isles. Therefore in this phase the hydrocellular treatments are indicated aspecially those with alginate and with lyophilized heterologous collagen. From the surgical point of view, this phase represents the elective information for the dermepidermic autologous inoculations (Davis grafts, limb grafts) that may be consolidated by human fibrin glue and covered with polyuretane or biosynthetical pellicles to be applied also in the drawing zone.

4) <u>Reepithelial ulcer</u>: It is a superficial ulcer that, in most cases, doesn't produce high quantities of exudate. In this phase it is useful the employement of heterologous cutis of swuine, polyuretano or biosynthetical pellicles, hydrocellular treatments, but also simply paraffined or pretreated, but not adhesive, gauzes. The mesh-graft autologous inoculations are the most selected. We should pay much attention to the removal moment of the treatment to avoid the damage of the new epidermie cells.

In every phase the treatment changes are executed on the ground of the secreting power of the ulcer with intervals that may vary from 1 to 7 day; it's very important to try to avoid the periulcerous tissue soaking, that has to be cleansed and protected carefully. We have to remove crustes, hyperkeratosis scales, previous treatments residues, using physiological solution, ether, paraffin oil, zine oxide paste. It is necessary to proscribe the topical use of antibiotics and corticosteroids for their verified contrast and dilay action of the recovery, for the overinfections origin and frequent phenomena origin of bacterial and mycotic sensitizations. Particularly it is effective the use of vital dyestuffes (eosin, basic fuxin) for their antimycotic and bactericidal action on the GRAM+.

To complete every treatment and excepted rare exceptions, we use to apply a compressive inelastic bandage united to eccentric compressions. The compressive therapy represents really a fundamental moment in the ulcers therapy. This because of the action it carries out at macro and microcirculatory level, aimed at promoting the healing process. Generally we don't reserve the bandage to the venous ulcers, for whose healing it is indispensable, but we extend the use also to the other aetiology ulcers, modifying in case the application modalities.

CONCLUSIONS

The lower limbs ulcers treatment respresents still a problem to be solved. In spite of during tha last years notable progresses have been made, it is not possible yet to standardize one therapeutical protocol. The therapeutic strategy has to be, according to our experience, subtended to individualize and to treat precociously the reasons that have fixed the lesion, becouse only their removal will be able to shorten the healing time of the ulcer and to avoid the origin of probable relapsings

REFERENCES

1.   Mancini S. La terapia delle ulcere venose degli arti inferiori. Casa Ed Grafica Sturli, Sett 1990.
2.   Coleridge Smith P.D. et al. Causes of venous ulceration: A new hypothesis. Br Med J 1988; 296:1726-1727.

Phlebology '95, D. Negus et al. (eds.). Phlebology (1995) Suppl. 1: 817-819

PI/2.3

Is Reperfusion Injury a Cause of Venous Ulcers?

C.F. He[1], J. O'Brien, G.W. Cherry and F. Arnold

Wound Healing Institute, Department of Dermatology, Oxford Radcliffe Hospital, Oxford, UK
1 Visiting doctor from Tongji Medical University, Wuhan, CHINA

INTRODUCTION

The pathophysiology of venous leg ulcers is still not well understood. According to the "white cell" theory, trapped leukocytes occlude capillaries, and cause cutaneous ischaema and capillary damage [1]. Recurrent ischaemia and reperfusion may be a significant feature in venous ulceration [2]. A change from the horizontal position to dependency results in reflex vasoconstriction. It is proposed that while this phenomenon is not pathogenic in normal individuals, it may cause tissue damage or impair healing in patients with venous hypertension. When the leg is re-elevated, or calf pumping is rendered effective by bandaging the reperfusion occurs leading to generation of mediators of tissue damage [3].

The skin microcirculation disturbances in these patients are also incompletely understood. Superficial blood flow has been examined with laser Doppler flowmeters (LDF) [4]. Tissue blood flow is heterogeneous, and spatial variations cannot readily be assessed by LDF [5]. A newly developed laser Doppler perfusion imaging(LDI) device, which sequentially scans up to 4,096 measurement points over the tissue under study, and produces a perfusion image of a large area (approximately 12 x 12 cm²) almost in real time [6], may offer a solution to this problem.

The present study was designed: 1) to explore a possible link between limb posture and concentrations of cytokines and other mediators of reperfusion injury in patients with venous ulceration. Concentrations of platelet-activating factor (PAF), TNF-α, IL-1β, IL-1RA, IL-6, thromboxane(Tx) B2, leukotriene(LKTN) B4, and P-selectin were measured in venous blood draining ulcers before and after dependency, and re-elevation; 2) to examine the microcirculation of the ulcers and surrounding skin following ischaemia and reperfusion with LDI; 3) to examine possible correlations between mediators, blood flow, and clinical outcome of leg ulcers in a small number of patients.

MATERIALS AND METHODS

With ethical committee approval and informed consent, 10 leg ulcer patients (aged 56-80 years, 6 female) without significant arterial impairment, diabetes, or rheumatoid arthritis, were entered into this study. Light Reflective Rheography showed abnormal capillary refilling in all cases, which was due to deep venous disease in 9/10. All patients were under treatment at the Wound Healing Institute, Department of Dermatology, Oxford. Ulcers were treated with maximum tolerated below-knee compression bandaging. Patients were followed up for 6-12 months (average 8.2 months) after this study.

Blood sampling and measurements of cytokines and mediators: A 16 gauge siliconised cannula (Vygon) was inserted in the long saphenous vein (or a tributary) below the knee as near the ulcer as possible. Blood flow was allowed to stabilise with the leg horizontal for 20 mins, after which time, systemic (arm) and (leg) blood samples were obtained without occlusion. The leg was then lowered to dependency for 1 hour. At the end of 1 hour, the leg was re-elevated to the horizontal, and sequential blood samples were taken immediately, and at 10, 30, 60, and 120 mins.

PAF in plasma was detected using radioimmunoassay. TNF-α, IL-1β, IL-1RA, IL-6, P-selectin in serum were determined using the Quantikine immunoassay kits. TxB2 and LKTN B4 in plasma were measured using enzyme-linked immunosorbent assay.

Blood flow measurement by LDI: At each of a sequence of measurement points, laser light penetrates the tissue, becomes Doppler-shifted on moving red blood cells, and is partially backscattered by them. A fraction of the Doppler-shifted and returned light is received by a photodetector in the scanner head and converted to an electrical output signal, which is proportional to the concentration and velocity of moving blood cells in the sampling volume, and is defined as tissue perfusion.

During the study period, the laser beam was orientated perpendicular to the skin surface, with the scanning head at a distance of 14 cm. Small black paper markers were applied to the margins of ulcers for identification of regions of interest within scans. Laser Doppler scans of the ulcer proper and surrounding skin were performed with the leg horizontal for 20 mins, and repeated immediately before re-elevation, and at 20, 60, and 120 mins thereafter. Scans were analysed as follows: the perfusion value for the ulcer centre was determined from 25 contiguous measuring sites (2.5x2.5 mm), and the value for the surrounding intact skin a minimum of 25 equivalent sites.

Statistical Analysis: Because data could not be assumed to be normally distributed, Wilcoxon's signed rank test was used to analize the data on superficial blood flow and blood borne mediators. A p value of 0.05 or less was considered significant.

RESULTS

Blood flow: The mean perfusion values in ulcer proper at all time points were greater than those in intact skin surrounding ulcers. These differences are statistically significant ($p<0.05$). Postural change has an effect on blood flow both in ulcer proper and in intact skin. When leg position was changed from supine to dependency, the LDI perfusion values decrease significantly ($p<0.05$). After leg re-elevation to the supine position, blood flow returned slowly to, and often eventually exceeded baseline levels. In 4/10 cases, ulcer perfusion was still below initial values at 20 minutes. The same was true of adjacent normal skin in 5/10. At the 1 or 2 hour time points, both ulcer and normal skin blood flow exceeded resting values in 7/10 cases.

Cytokines and mediators:

PAF: In the supine position, PAF values in venous blood obtained from the leg were significantly higher than those from arms ($p<0.05$).

IL-1RA: Ten out of 10 samples showed greater IL-1RA values in the leg in the supine position than in the arm ($p<0.01$). Compared with the supine position, all IL-1RA values were decreased at 2 hour re-elevation ($p<0.01$).

IL-6: Supine leg values were higher than those for supine arm ($p<0.05$). Although 8/10 cases had greater IL-6 values after re-elevation, the differences between the supine leg values and the post-elevation values (10 mins and 30 mins) were not significant.

P-selectin: The supine P-selectin values for arms were greater than those for legs in all cases ($p<0.01$). The differences between the supine leg values and the re-elevation values were not significant.

TNF-α, IL-1β, TxB2, and LKTN B4: Only 2 patients had detectable levels of TNF-α. There was no detectable IL-1ß levels in any case. The differences in TxB2 values and LKTN B4 between different sampling time points were not significant.

Correlation of mediators, blood flow, and clinical outcome: We found no statistically significant association between baseline levels of mediator or changes in their concentration in venous blood with either blood flow, ulcer size or outcome of treatment. Only IL-1RA concentration was significantly correlated with postural change. However, basal PAF levels were >580 pg/ml in 4 of 5 patients whose ulcers healed within the treatment period, while in all non-healing patients, PAF was < 400 pg/ml. After dependency and 2 hours' re-elevation, PAF levels in all 5 healing patients were lower than at baseline, while in 3/5 with persistent ulceration, levels were elevated as compared with initial values.

Correlations were sought between changes in perfusion, and clinical outcome. While study numbers were too small for statistical significance, we noted that resting ulcer LDI values were > 2.2 V in 4/5 patients who went on to heal, while they were less than this value in 4/5 who did not.

DISCUSSION

The change of limb position from the horizontal to dependency is known to reduce blood flow in normal skin and venous ulcers [7], via the veni-arteriolar reflex. However, few studies have been performed to evaluate the events which follow re-elevation. We found that reperfusion was slow, and commonly resulted in an "overshoot" above initial values, often an hour or more after re-elevation.

PAF, IL1-RA and IL-6 values in venous blood draining ulcers at rest were significantly greater than those found in the arm, while the reverse was true for P-selectin. We can not say whether these findings relate to differences between arms and legs, or whether they are due to the presence of leg ulcer. A comparison between age matched patients with and without ulcers will be required to resolve this question.

The trend toward an association between higher levels of PAF in draining venous blood and healing also warrants further study. Exogenous PAF has been shown to accelerate gain in tensile strength in experimental incisional skin wounds; however, PAF antagonists had no effect on repair [8].

Changes in posture, and hence in blood flow, caused no consistent changes in any of the mediators studied here, except IL-1RA. Thus, although ischaemia and reperfusion clearly occurred, we are left with the conundrum that this was not associated with the biochemical events commonly found during reperfusion injury. However, unlike the situation of arterial occlusion and release, ischaemia due to venous hypertension is relatively mild, and reperfusion occurs far more slowly. We suggest that the rate of reperfusion is a critical determinant of damage and of the generation of these mediators. Thus if O_2^- radicals are generated sufficiently slowly, the buffering capacity of adjacent tissue may be adequate to prevent injury.

ACKNOWLEDGEMENTS. We are grateful for financial support and mediator assays, which were provided by British Biotechnology Ltd.

REFERENCES

1. Coleridge-Smith PD, Thomas P, Scurr JH, Dormandy A. Causes of venous ulceration: a new hypothesis. Br Med J 1988;296:1726-7.
2. Wilkinson LS, Bunker C, Edwards JCW, Scurr JH, Coleridge-Smith PD. Leukocytes: Their role in the etiopathogenesis of skin damage in venous disease. J Vasc surg 1993;17:669-75.
3. Welbourne CR, Goldman G, Paterson IS. Pathophysiology of ischaemia reperfusion injury: central role of the neutrophil. Br J Surg 1991;78:651-5.
4. Nilsson GE, Tenland T, Oberg PA. Evaluation of a laser Doppler flowmeter for tissue measurement of blood blow. IEEE Trans BME 1980;27:597-604.
5. Bircher A, Boer EMD, Agner T, Wahlberg JE, Serup J. Guidelines for measurement of cutaneous blood flow by laser Doppler flowmetry. Contact Dermatitis 1994;30:65-72.
6. Wardell K, Jakobsson A, Nilsson GE. Laser Doppler perfusion imaging by dynamic light scattering. IEEE Trans Biomed Eng 1993;40:309-16.
7. Svedman C, Cherry GW, Ryan TJ. Postural changes in the circulation of venous leg ulcer patients studied by laser Doppler imager. J Invest Dermatol 1991;98:604a.
8. Porras-Reyes BH, Mustoe TA. Platelet-activating factor: Improvement in wound healing by a chemotactic factor. Surgery 1992;111:416-23.

Phlebology '95, D. Negus et al. (eds.). Phlebology (1995) Suppl. 1: 820-822

P164

Leg Ulcers, Casuistry from January 1985 to December 1994

S. Massi, C. Ruggieri, G. Botta, A.M. Peccatori and S. Mancini

III Department of General Surgery and Center of Phlebology "W Pabisch", Faculty of Medicine and Surgery, University of Siena, Italy

INTRODUCTION

Lower limbs ulcers are the result of local or systemic disease, producing loss of epidermis, dermis, subcutaneous tissue and more rarely fascia.

Lower limb ulcer treatment is a difficult problem. The high cost of treatment and the morbidity of the disease have a substantial impact on healthcare expenditure and on the way of life of the patient, whose working ability may be permanently compromised.

Though the old are more often affected, it has been possible to discover, thanks to new epidemiological studies, that in 22% of the cases ulceration commences at about the age of 40 years.

In accordance with the international literature data, we can confirm that about the 1% of the population suffers from ulcerative lesions of the lower limbs and that, in 75% of the cases, these may result from peripheral venous insufficiency.

Therefore careful diagnostic investigation is necessary to establish the correct patient management.

Our experience agrees with the literature in that the most frequent reasons for ulcerative lesions in the lower limbs are, in order to incidence: venous insufficiency, arterial insufficiency, neuropathies and other factors.

REGISTRY

From January 1985 to December 1994, 820 patients (females 590 and males 230), with lower limb ulcers have been treated. 82 of them had bilateral lesions. The data extracted and the distribution according to age, the aetiopathenogenesis, the extent, the location and the time of healing are summarised in the following list:

Females = 590 (72%)   Males = 230 (28%)
Age: min. 19 years - middle 55 years - max 92 years

Aetiology

Varicose	524 (51.7%)
P:T:F:S	147 (14.5%)
Mixed	131 (12.9%)
Arterial	74 (7.3%)
Traumatic	59 (5.8%)
Diabetic	52 (5.1%)
Neurologic	9 (0.9%)
Other	18 (1.8%)

Size

0 - 4 cm	569 (56.1%)
4 - 10 cm	290 (28.6%)
10 - 20 cm	106 (10.6%)
>20 cm	48 (4.7%)

Location

leg medial	402 (39.6%)
leg lateral	160 (15.8%)
leg anterior	177 (17.5%)
leg posterior	43 (4.2%)
malleolus	148 (14.6%)
foot: dorsum	54 (5.3%)
foot: toes	18 (1.8%)
foot: plant	12 (1.2%)

RESULTS

Healing of the ulcers was obtained in 91% of the cases. Recurrence of ulceration occurred in 11% of the cases. All patients are subjected to a complete clinical test and to a non-invasive or invasive study to determine aetiology, to a photographic and morphometric examination of the ulcer combined with a taking of material for microbiology and a biopsy for histological examination and a complete haematologic study of the patient.

For all types of ulcers our treatment includes ozonized hydromassage, curettage, application of one or more topical dressings and inelastic bandage.

98% of the patients were treated.

REFERENCES

1. Mancini S. La terapia delle ulcere degli arti inferiori. Casa Ed Grafica Sturli, sett 1990.
2. Massi S, Ruggieri C, Mancini S. Traitement des ulcères des membres inférieus. Intensive Practical Course in Phlebology, Montreal, 1992, 283-290.

Phlebology '95, D. Negus et al. (eds.). Phlebology (1995) Suppl. 1: 823-825

P043

A New Tripod Laser Doppler Probe Holder for the Evaluation of Skin Blood Flow in Chronic Venous Insufficiency and Venous Ulceration

Th. Klyscz, M. Hahn, A. Steins and M Jünger

*Department of Dermatology, University of Tübingen, Liebermeisterstr. 25,
D-72076 Tübingen, Germany*

INTRODUCTION

The supply of blood to the upper 1.5 mm of the cutaneous vascular plexus is closely correlated with the Laser Doppler Flux (LDF). Because LDF is easy to calculate in many skin areas, it was quickly accepted in clinical medicine.

Laser Doppler Flux measurements are used today in a number of different medical fields, especially in the diagnosis of microangiopathy, for example as a result of peripheral arterial occlusive disease (3,5) or chronic venous insufficiency (1,2). Other areas of application include venous ulcus cruris (2) and monitoring the blood supply to skin grafts (7). In day-to-day practice, it is often difficult to carry out measurements in the last two areas because, for example, a probe cannot be set up on a sterile wound or because there is simply no good place to attach the probe in an ulcer. The inadequacy of the peripheral equipment presently available for such potentially significant areas of application contrasts starkly with the high technological standard of LDF-technology touted by the manufacturers. The solutions devised by industry to these specific problems are limited to special probe models, usually offset probes which are supposed to be mounted outside the area to be examined. The head of the probe itself is supposed to reach the cutaneous area to be examined without touching it. When this site exceeds a certain size the static problems involved in mounting the arm of the probe become immense. If a probe holder is to perform well in the applications cited above, intentional and unintentional movement of the area being examined should not cause position shifts of the probe head or artefacts while the measurements are being carried out.

We have developed a completely new tripod probe holder for both standard and special probes to make LDF measurements possible under the conditions above. The construction and possible applications of this novel peripheral device are explained below.

CONSTRUCTION

In designing this new probe holder our goal was to make it possible to reproducibly carry out LDF measurements with standard probes of all kinds and a number of different examination site sizes up to 15cm in length without touching the site itself. We wanted to be able to attach the holder to the surrounding skin and adjust for the sloping and curved surfaces found in actual clinical practice. Materials were selected which combined good stability and low weight. We wanted the tripod to be compatible with LDF equipment aready on the market in order to keep running material costs as low as possible. It should also be easy for nursing staff to operate.

We chose to base our design on a tripod with a central platform. The Y-shaped platform is made of 4 mm-thick clear Plexiglas with several holes drilled in it. The three legs of the tripod are positioned at each of the three ends of the Y. The tripod legs are made of aluminium rods or laminated plastic and end in the proven LDF cup feet which can be stuck to the skin with double adhesive rings. In order to make the construction flexible enough to fit all possible skin surfaces, the cup feet were mounted on the tripod legs with universal joints. The tripod legs themselves are fastened in the platform with chucks so their height is continuously adjustable. In addition, the elongated holes in the three ends of the Y-shaped platform make it possible to slide the legs back and forth to match the size of the measuring site. In the middle of the platform several holes have been drilled to accommodate mounting arms so that the LDF probe can be fastened underneath the platform. All of the tripod legs and mounting arms have the same outer diameter so that the probe could even be mounted at one of the outer ends of the Y-shaped platform for special applications. An engraved scale makes it possible to accurately document the configuration of the holder. The combination of these measuring coordinates with the positioning of the entire construction makes reproducibly exact measurements possible.

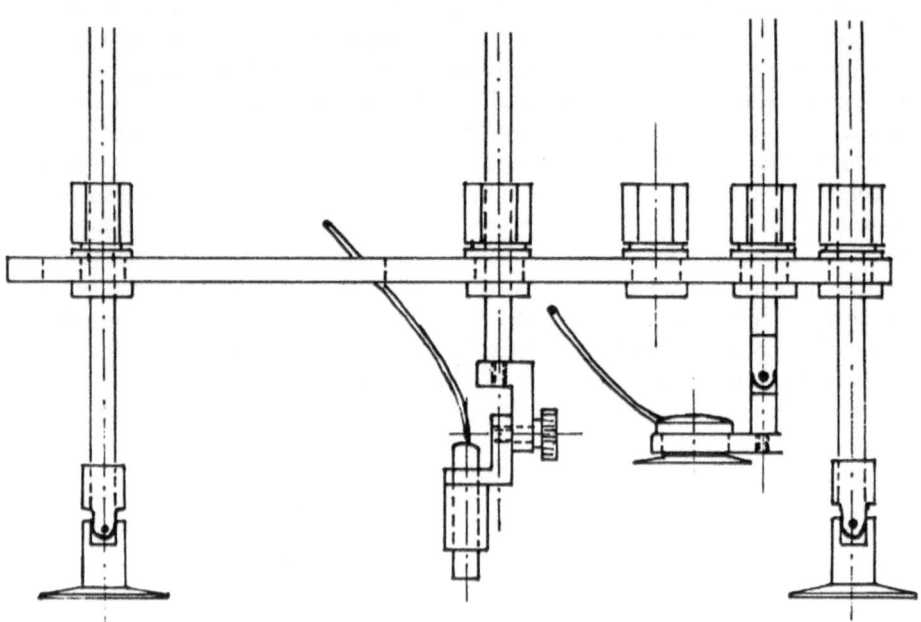

Fig. 1: Side view of the LDF tripod probe holder (schematic drawing).

DISCUSSION

Laser Doppler fluxmetry makes it possible to non-invasively quantify the average flow velocity of moving cells in a skin segment. Most equipment, like the 2mW helium-neon laser we used (Periflux PF2, Perimed, Stockholm), emits monochromatic light with a wavelength of 632.8 nm. The laser light is conducted to the skin through a glas fibre which is mounted in a probe above the side to be examined. It is emitted out of the end of the fibre and penetrates a semispherical area of skin about 1.5 mm in radius, where the blood flow in the subpapillary vascular plexus is measured. The frequency of the laser light is shifted when it is reflected from the moving blood cells (the Doppler effect) by an amount in linear correlation with the velocity of the reflecting cells. The reflected part of the emitted light returns to the measuring device through separate glass fibres to be analysed. The output produced - the Laser Doppler Flux (LDF) - corresponds to the product of the average frequency shift and the concentration of the moving blood cells. Since the LDF cannot be calibrated for different tissues, the absolute flux values should always be determined in relationship to a comparative or initial value (1,6,8). Continuous, non-invasive flux recordings in real time are thus made possible at any area of the body desired. The extremely short response time of about 0.2 sec gives the Laser Doppler Fluxmeter the advantage that it is able to detect even rapid changes in tissue perfusion.

Since this method was introduced, a number of attempts have been made to modify the LDF measuring system with peripheral equipment which would widen its range of applications. The construction presented here takes this aspect into consideration, too. It now makes the atraumatic placement of a probe possible in tissue areas which have not been accessible to LDF exploration until now. At the same time, function studies such as postural changes at the extremities and the examination of the venulo-arterial reflex in ulcus cruris can also be carried out.

REFERENCES

1. Holloway GA, Watkins DW. Laser Doppler measurement of cutaneous blood flow. J Invest Dermatol 1977;69:306-9.
2. Jünger M, Rahmel B, Rassner G. Laser-Doppler-Flux in venous ulcers. Int J Microcirc Exp 1988;7:88.
3. Moneta G, Schneider E, Jäger K, Brülisauer M, Thüring-Vollenweider U, Bollinger A. Laser Doppler flux and vasomotion in patients before and after transluminal angioplasty for limp salvage. Vasa 1988;17:26-31.
4. Nilsson GE, Tenland T, Öberg PA. Evaluation of Laser Doppler Flowmeter for measurement of tissue blood flow. IEEE Trans. Biomed Eng 1980;27:597-604.
5. Seifert H, Jäger K, Bollinger A. Analysis of flow motion by the Laser Doppler technique in patients with peripheral arterial occlusive disease. Int J Microcirc: Clin Exp 1988;7:223-36.
6. Stern MD. In vivo evaluation of microcirculation by coherent light scattering. Nature 1975;254:56-8.
7. Svensson H, Svedman P, Holmberg J, Wieslander B. Detecting changes of arterial and venous blood flow in flaps. Annals Plast Surg 1985;15:35-40.
8. Tenland T, Salerud EG, Nilsson GE, Öberg PA. Spatial and temporal variations in human skin blood flow. Int J Microcirc: Clin Exp 1983;2:81-90.

Phlebology '95, D. Negus et al. (eds.). Phlebology (1995) Suppl. 1: 826-828

P044

Transcutaneous Oxygen and Carbon Dioxide Measurements and Laser-Doppler Flowmetry in the Assessment of Periulcerous Leg Skin Microcirculation

E. Melillo, M.L. Iabichella, R. Berchiolli, M. Ferrari and R. Pedrinelli

Medinica Interna, Istituto di Chirurgia Generale e Sperimentale, Clinica Medica I, Azienda Ospedaliera Pisana, Università di Pisa, Pisa, ITALY

INTRODUCTION

Estimated prevalence of chronic venous ulceration ranges from 0.06 to 1.3%, some degree of venous disease is present in about 57 to 80% of patients with leg ulcers (1).

The sequence of events which leads to leg skin ulceration is not yet clearly understood. Venous hypertension may set the stage for subsequent ulcer development due to observed changes in skin microvessels and the interstitium.

In recent years, an increasing number of non invasive vascular techniques has become available for the evaluation of skin microcirculation (2-4).

Among those, Transcutaneous oxygen ($TCpO_2$) and Carbon Dioxide ($TCpCO_2$) tension can provide information on gas exchanges in the skin, and the Laser-Doppler Flowmetry (LDF) allows a reliable measurement of the skin blood-flow.

Aim of this work is the assessment of periulcerous skin microcirculation by $TCpO_2$, $TCpCO_2$ and LDF in patients affected leg ulcers.

PATIENTS AND METHODS

We have studied six consecutive patients (mean age 68.3, range 61-81 years, 4 females), presenting unilateral (n=3) or bilateral (n=3) leg ulcers, aged 2 to 24 months.

Three patients suffered from venous ulcers (VU) and the remaining complained of mixed arterial-venous ulcers (MU).

Demographics of all patients were represented in Table I.

DEMOGRAPHICS OF 6 PATIENTS WITH LEG ULCERS									
Pts n.	Sex	Age	BMI	Smoke	Chol.	Diabetes	Hypertension	**LEG ULCER**		
								Type	Site	Duration
1	M	61	27	Y	Y	N	Y	VU	B	4
2	F	69	24	N	N	N	N	VU	M	2
3	F	65	33	N	N	N	N	VU	M	2
4	F	81	26	N	N	N	Y	MU	M	24
5	F	62	38	Y	N	N	Y	MU	B	24
6	M	72	39	N	Y	Y	Y	MU	B	24

BMI=Body Mass Index   Y=Yes   N=N0   VU=Venous Ulcer   MU=Mixed Ulcer   B=Bilateral
M=Monolateral   Duration in Months

The diagnosis of vascular disease was performed by Plethysmography, Doppler C.W. and Duplex Imaging.
We evaluate the microcirculation of the skin in 2 sites just around the ulcer and 5 cm from it, using a combined measurements of $TCpO_2$ and $TCpCO_2$, after preheating at 44°C (Kontron Microgas 7640, mmHg) and LDF (Perimed 4001, Perfusion Unit, -PU-), at body temperature, 36° C and 44°C.

RESULTS

In Table II instrumental and non-invasive measurements with $TCpO_2$, $TCpCO_2$ and LDF in our cases were represented:

SKIN INSTRUMENTAL MEASUREMENTS IN 6 PATIENTS WITH LEG ULCERS									
PERIULCEROUS					**DISTAL (5cm)**				
Pts n.	TENSIOMETRY mmHg		LASER DOPPLER pu			TENSIOMETRY mmHg		LASER DOPPLER pu		
	pO_2	pCO_2	b	36°C	44°C	pO_2	pCO_2	b	36°C	44°C
1	0	62	209	247	195	2	52	76	81	88
2	9	43	111	127	140	34	38	46	47	108
3	21	37	7	17	268	30	37	7	90	151
4	0	48	42	58	77	10	41	46	50	58
5	1	48	45	45	138	10	42	26	30	48
6	2	72	40	42	45	3	49	19	21	24

Laser Doppler determinations were made at body temperature (b) and at probe heated at 36° and 44° C.

Periulcerous skin measurements showed decreased transcutaneous oxygen tension values ($TCpO_2$ was lower than 10 mmHg in 5 cases) and increased carbon dioxide tension values (higher than 43 mmHg in 5 patients): $TCpO_2$ and $TCpCO_2$ values were inversely correlated, revealing severe regional tissue impairment.
Distal evaluations, 5 cm far from the ulcer, confirmed a persistent tissue microvascular damage in four patients ($TCpO_2 \leq 10$ mmHg, $TCpCO_2 \geq 40$ mmHg), while in two

remaining cases we observed a significant increase in $TCpO_2$ (from 9 to 34 mmHg and from 21 to 30 mmHg, respectively) and a physiological decrease in $TCpCO_2$.

Periulcerous LDF measurements, performed at body temperature, showed high Perfusion Units values, probably indicating a desaturated blood stasis of capillaries.

LDF values in the same site with a heated probe, at 36° and 44°C, showed, generally, only a poor increase in microvascular perfusion, perhaps due to a reduced functional microcirculatory reserve or to the occurrence of neoangiogenesis or both.

Other Author's results in microcirculatory evaluations of patients with moderately severe venous insufficiency by dynamic capillaroscopy, before and after Na-fluorescein, demonstrated greatly dilated, elongated and winding capillaries and an increased in the pericapillary space (4).

Distal LDF evaluations showed lower mean PU values than those performed in periulcerous skin site and, at body temperature, an increased mean response to heated probe at 36°C and 44°C, compared to the values performed in periulcerous area.

On the contrary, a VU female patient (n.3) showed nearly physiological LDF values at body temperature and after heating both in the periulcerous skin site (from 7 PU to 17 PU at 36°C to 268 PU at 44°C) and in the distal area (from 7 to 90 PU at 36°C to 151 PU at 44°C).

All the patients underwent a conventional therapy (antibiotic, wound cleaning and elastic compression).

After a three months follow-up, only the patient (n.3) (VU, with both higher $TCpO_2$ and a better LDF heating response) recovered. Another VU patient (n.2), presenting a significant distal increase of $TCpO_2$, associated with a good LDF heating response, improved.

The remaining patients showed no relevant changes.

CONCLUSIONS

On the basis of our data we can suggest:

1) a decreased tissue metabolism occurs in periulcerous areas (lower values of O_2 inversely related to CO_2 values) as compared to distal areas and this phenomenon is more evident in mixed ulcers than in venous ulcers

2) a higher LDF signal in the periulcerous area is probably a marker of desaturated blood stasis and a reduced LDF response to the thermal test can suggest a poor functionality of the newly formed vessels

3) The presence of a residual periulcerous oxygenation, the lack of acid catabolites and a good LDF thermic response seem to lead a better prognosis.

In conclusion, such tests seem to be very useful for in vivo assessment of periulcerous skin microcirculation.

REFERENCES

1) Mayrovitz HN, Larsen PB: Periwound skin microcirculation of venous leg ulcers. Microvasc. Res. 48(1): 114-23, 1994.

2) Cheatle TR, Stibe EC, Shahi SK, Scurr JH, Coledrige Smith PD: Vasodilatator capacity of the skin in venous disease and its relationship to transcutaneous oxygen tension. Br.J.Surg. 78 (5): 607-10, 1991.

3) Bongard O, Bounameaux H: Clinical investigation of skin microcirculation. Dermatology. 186 (1): 6-11, 1993.

4) Leu AJ, Franzeck UK, Bollinger A: Microangiopathies in Chronic Venous Insufficiency (CVI). Ther Umsch 48(10): 715-21, 1991.

Phlebology '95, D. Negus et al. (eds.). Phlebology (1995) Suppl. 1: 829-831

V/1.8

Varicectomy in Deep Vein Aplasia

I. Bihari, G. Tasnadi, L. Bohar, Z. Nagy, A. Szabo

Postgraduate Medical University, Budapest, Hungary

Introduction

In case of partial or total deep vein aplasia superficial veins play the role of the most important collateral pathways. Occasionally these veins dilate and become varicose, so that valves do not close and venous blood can flow not only in the direction of the heart but toward the ankle as well. In these cases, different complications of varicosity can develop. What is the solution in these cases ? Where will venous blood flow if varicose veins are ligated or removed ?

In our experience, varicectomy in postphlebitic chronic occlusion cases can be performed, if the third venous bed in the subfascial space, can drain sufficiently venous blood. These venous channels are sittuated in and between muscles (1,2). In the described case, presence of this subfascial collateral system could be proved with the help of a simple test, and ligation of varicose vein stems and limited varicectomy could be carried out with good results and without complications.

Case report

A 19 years old man was admitted to the Cardio-Vascular Surgical Clinic of the Postgraduate Medical University, Budapest with recurrent crural ulcer. Four years before he already had a crural ulcer, that responded to conservative therapy (compression bandage and local antiseptic treatment). In spite of continuous compression therapy, crural ulcer recurred two years later.

His complex vascular anomaly was recognised at his birth as a Klippel-Trenaunay syndrome. On his left lower limb wide-spread naevus vasculosus and varicosity could be observed. The varicosity was partly along the greater saphenous vein and partly along the persistent embrionic ischiadic vein. This later could be followed up to the left flank.

Arteriography was the first examination to reveal AV shunt, but it could not be detected.

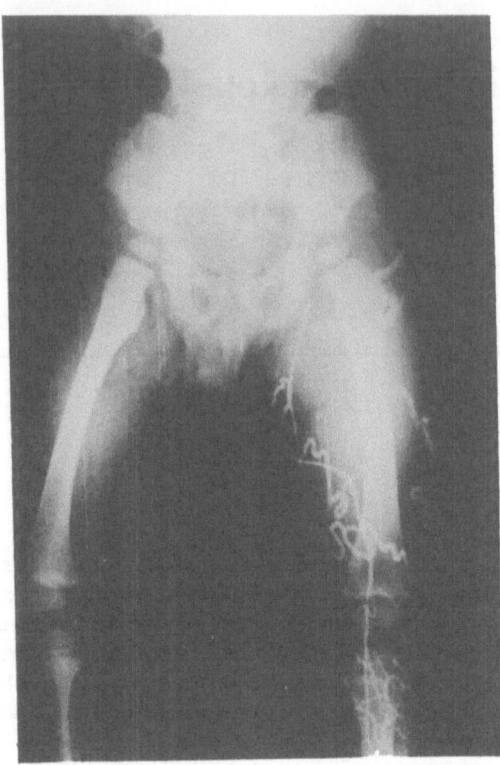

Fig. 1. Venography in his infancy - complete aplasia of deep veins including even the left iliac veins.

In his infancy venography was performed, and it was repeated now again - showed complete aplasia of deep veins including even the left iliac veins. The saphenous vein could be followed up to the groin and the recent venogram showed a spontaneous Palma arch joining to the opposite iliac vein. The ischiadic vein continues both to the flank and to the saphenous vein. A large bunch of varicose veins could be seen along the leg.

According to these findings it seemed, that the reflux in the varicose veins caused an increased peripheral venous blood pressure and this was the reason of crural ulcers. The task was to prove the existence and sufficient extent of subfascial venous drainage.

Duplex ultrasonography was performed but no anatomic or non anatomic venous channel could be detected.

Isotope venography delineated only the main venous pathway - that was the saphenous vein - spontaneous Palma arch - opposite iliac vein - route. It was the finding following bandaging of the limb as well.

The last and most important examination was a functional test - walking with an inflated tonometer cuff. It was placed below and later above the knee and inflated to 110 mmHg and the patient was asked to walk for 5 min. During this test the patient told us that his limb is lighter and no cyanosis could be detected. If the subfascial collaterals were

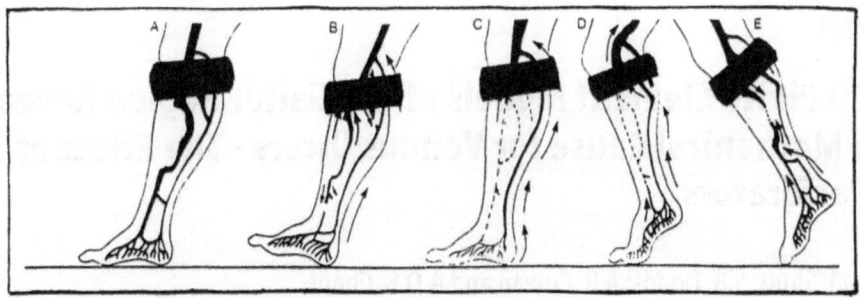

Fig. 2. A reliable method to examinethe subfascial venous collateral channels is the walking test with a tonometer cuff.

absent the patient would have reported complaints - heavy pain in the first minute and severe cyanosis could have been seen.

Following this examination an <u>operation was performed</u> (1993. nov.). The greater saphenous vein at the groin and the varicose, dilated lumbar veins were ligated and varices around the ulcer were removed. The later was performed using <u>a semiclosed method</u> with the use of a special knife called Smetana knife (3) which rolls up the veins beneath the skin in a 10 cm distance around from a 4 mm long stab wound, so the bleeding from AV microshunts could be controled without delay.

During the operation, lines were introduced into the central and peripheral veins of the limb to check the pressure changes following ligations. There were temporary high or increased pressures detected.

<u>After the operation the ulcer healed and there was no complication.</u> During the one year checkup the limb was in a farly good condition, without ulcer.

Conclusion

According to this case it seems that for the examination of subfascial collateral pathways the tonometer cuff test was the most reliable in a deep vein aplasia case. If it gives a negative result than varicose veins can be operated.

Literature

1. Bihari, I.: Un nouvelle et simple methode pur evaluer l`indication chirurgicale d`une varicose preocement apres une occlusion veinuse. In Davy A, Stricht J (eds): Phlebology`83, Vol.1. Bruxelles. Medical Media International. 1984. p.210.
2. Bihari I.: Can Varicectomy be performed if Deep Veins are Occluded ? J. Dermatol. Surg. Oncol.16:806-7. (1990)
3. Bihari I. et al.: Removal of varicose veins using Smetana`s saw kife. In Negus D, Jantet G (eds): Phlebology `85. London, John Libey Co. 1986. pp 182-4.

Phlebology '95, D. Negus et al. (eds.). Phlebology (1995) Suppl. 1: 832-834

P113

2D Finite Element Models of the Gaiter Region Reveal a Mechanical Cause for Venous Ulcers - The Effect of Perforators

A.M. Shutt, S.R. Dodds, A.R. Cowan and A.D.B. Chant

Department of Vascular Surgery, Royal South Hants Hospital, Southampton, UK

INTRODUCTION

Skin is a remarkable organ which performs many functions. It has a complex multicomponent microstructure comprising fibre networks of collagen and elastin, small blood vessels, lymphatics and nerve fibres [1]. In essence, skin is a viscoelastic, anisotropic, non linear inhomogenous time dependent material which demonstrates the properties of hysteresis, stress relaxation and creep [2]. Finite element analysis is a technique used to approximate solutions to complex mechanical problems [3]. There are limitations to this technique also, but it provides interesting insights into a possible mechanical cause for venous ulceration. Chant postulated a mechanical cause for ulceration based on elevated tissue pressure in a mechanically disadvantaged area of the lower limb, i.e. the gaiter region [4,5]. It is in an area close to venous perforators, which if incompetent, will lead to abnormally elevated hydrostatic and distending forces overlying it. In this paper, using empirically derived values for soft tissue cross sectional areas, we demonstrate one important factor, the effect of perforators on the stresses in the gaiter area.

METHOD

CT scans of lower limbs of subjects with proven deep venous insufficiency were examined to measure the various proportions of bone and soft tissue at 5 cm intervals above the medial malleolus to a level of 25cm. Scans were performed supine using a Somatom II scanner, (125kV, 4mm slices). A variety of measurements were taken from the scans, including bone and soft tissue areas. There was a total of 16 measurements for each level and 80 measurements in all for both limbs. Seven male subjects with six non affected and eight affected limbs were examined. Sixteen females with fourteen non affected and eighteen affected limbs were compared. The unpaired t-test was used to compare groups. Data from these scans were then used to construct a two dimensional finite element model of the medial gaiter region. This model was built using the Ansys® /ED Educational Finite Element Analysis package (Swanson Analysis Systems, Inc.) on a desktop PC. The modelling of the lower limb undertaken here assumes that within the limits set the viscoelastic substances behave in a linear fashion and are isotropic in nature. All stresses within the models are colour coded (Black and White for this paper) with identical scales for ease of comparison.

RESULTS

No significant differences could be found in the male group and are not considered further. Female non affected limbs differed from affected in total limb area and almost all levels of soft tissue area. (Table 1). The relative difference between affected and non affected limbs showed that the ratio between soft tissue area and bone area at 5cm above the malleolus in the female affected limb was 1.3 times larger.

Table 1. Comparison of Affected and Non Affected Limbs at Various Levels

LEVEL	FEMALE									
	5cm		10cm		15cm		20cm		25cm	
	Aff	Non	Aff	Non	Aff	Non	Aff	Non	Aff	Non
TBA	7.3	6.9	5.6	5.4	6.0	5.6	6.8	6.5	8.4	8.3
	(2.1)	(1.6)	(1.0)	(0.8)	(0.9)	(0.8)	(0.8)	(0.9)	(1.2)	(1.3)
TLA	48.2	37.1	58.1	46.9	77.8	63.0	99.4	84.6	109.3	91.1
	(15.8)	(7.6) **	(18.1)	(11.1) *	(21.0)	(13.9) **	(25.7)	(16.3) *	(24.5)	(16.1) **
STA	40.9	30.2	52.5	41.5	71.8	57.4	92.6	78.1	100.9	82.8
	(15.3)	(7.8) **	(17.7)	(11.2) *	(20.6)	(13.7) *	(25.4)	(16.0)	(24.1)	(15.3) **
SFT	1.0	0.8	1.5	1.1	1.6	1.1	1.4	0.9	1.6	1.2
	(1.0)	(0.5)	(1.0)	(0.5)	(0.9)	(0.5)	(0.7)	(0.3) **	(0.8)	(0.5) *

Aff = Venous Affected Limb, Non = Non Affected Limb, TBA = Total Bone Area, TLA = Total Limb Area, STA = Soft Tissue Area, SFT = Subcut. Fat Thickness. All areas in cm^2, thickness in cm. * $p < 0.05$, ** $p < 0.02$

Models

Five contrasting models have been produced. The first two consider the medial side of a normal leg with and without a perforator site. The third and fourth consider elevated pressures as seen in venous disease with and without a perforator site. The fifth model considers a stylised ulcer in the region of a perforator site. Within each model three different environments were compared. The first assumes standing with an unopposed pressure exerted along the fascial layer. The second considers a counterpressure applied on the skin surface, the order of magnitude comparable to a 30mmHg class II compression stocking. The third considers the limb to be supine, and for the purposes of the models presented here, effectively remove the fascial deforming pressure, whilst maintaining the counterpressure of the external stocking. The following diagrams illustrate some of the findings. Normal limb with perforator (a); venous limb with perforator (b); and without perforator (c). The differences to note are the forces appear greatest along the fascia, but also extend through the perforator defect.

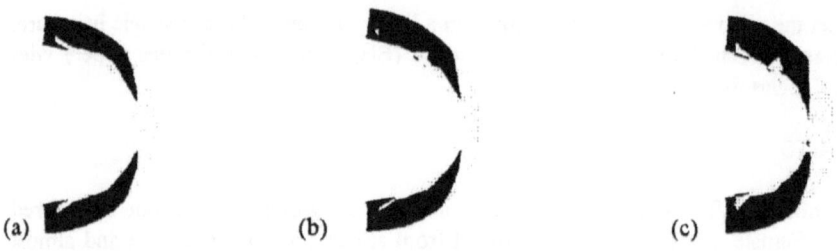

(a)   (b)   (c)

Lastly a stylised ulcer over the medial gaiter region can be shown. The effect of elevation and compression can be seen to reduce these forces.

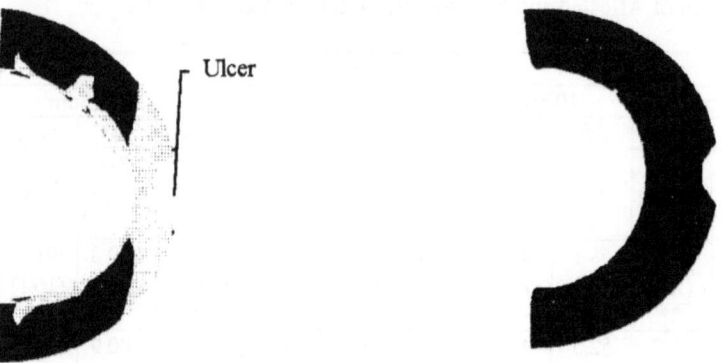

Ulcerated limb   Ulcerated limb with compression and elevation.

DISCUSSION
The CT cross sectional area study confirm significant differences between affected and non affected venous limbs within the female group with respect to total limb and soft tissue area. Using the values so obtained, possible scenarios have been modelled and the rationale of elevation and compression demonstrated. The simple 2D models presented here, support the idea that abnormal mechanical forces may be at work in the aetiology surrounding the formation of venous ulcers. The higher forces demonstrated in the ulcer base may also help to explain why ulcers persist. The beneficial effects of compressive forces are also demonstrated. Despite the reservations of the technique, they do reveal a fascinating aspect in the possible aetiology of venous ulcers.

REFERENCES

1.   Kenedi RM, Gibson T, Evans JH, Barbenel JC. Tissue mechanics. Phys Med Biol. 1975;20 (5):699-717.
2.   Tregear RT. Physical functions of skin. London: Academic Press, 1966:
3.   Zienkiewicz OC. The Finite Method in Engineering Science. New York: McGraw-Hill, 1977:
4.   Chant ADB. Tissue pressure, posture and venous ulceration. Lancet. 1990;336:1050-1.
5.   Chant ADB. Hypothesis: why venous oedema causes ulcers and lymphoedema does not. Eur J Vasc Surg. 1992;6:427-9.

Phlebology '95, D. Negus et al. (eds.). Phlebology (1995) Suppl. 1: 835-838

OP/6.2

Incompetent Calf Perforators in Venous Ulceration and Lipodermatosclerosis

M.R. Tyrrell, S. Arora and D. Negus

Department of Surgery, Lewisham Hospital, London, UK

INTRODUCTION

The ligation of incompetent calf perforating veins was popularised by Cockett's anatomical studies in the nineteen fifties[1] and encouraging results were reported in the sixties[2,3] and early seventies[4]. However, publications appearing in the seventies and early eighties not only shed doubt on the value of perforator vein ligation[5] but advised against all venous surgery in patients with deep venous incompetence[6]. Nevertheless combined saphenous and perforator surgery was still advocated by some[7].

Venous ulceration is probably a function of the relative contributions played by saphenous, perforator and deep venous incompetence. Calf perforator incompetence is not necessarily the sole or even dominant cause. A simple morphological classification of aetiology has been proposed by Darke[8]; I: isolated calf perforator incompetence; II: saphenous and calf perforator incompetence; III: primary deep venous incompetence (usually associated with saphenous and calf perforator incompetence); IV: post phlebitic damage. In this series, type II (in whom 90% were healed by saphenous surgery without perforator ligation) is the single most common morphological type associated with ulceration.

In order to re-examine Darke's hypothesis, we have conducted a retrospective review to determine the relative incidence of perforator incompetence, its haemodynamic significance and the effect of surgery.

PATIENTS AND METHODS

The records of 29 consecutive patients (33 legs) presenting to our vein clinic between March 1990 and September 1994 with ulceration and/or severe pre-ulcerative changes (but patent, competent deep veins) have been reviewed. We have noted the patient's age and sex, presenting complaint, Doppler or venographic assessment of perforator and deep venous competence. Where available, the haemodynamic significance of perforator incompetence was investigated by photoplethysmographic (PPG) measurement of venous refilling times with tourniquets placed above and below the perforator site, to produce a below perforator/below knee (BP/BK) ratio (a modification of Zukowski's method[9]). The same data points have been examined in the post operative follow-up period.

RESULTS

Seventeen men and 12 women, with a median age of 66 years (range 34-76) were investigated. Twenty-nine legs had demonstrable long saphenous incompetence (3 with co-existing short saphenous incompetence). Three legs had no identifiable saphenous reflux and none had isolated short saphenous disease. Thirty-one legs had calf perforator incompetence. In 3 legs this was the only identifiable venous abnormality. In 14 the haemodynamic significance of perforator incompetence was assessed (figure 1). The median BP/BK ratio was 1.1 (range 0.5-2.2). Seven legs demonstrated some degree of haemodynamic significance with a ratio greater than 1. In 5 this value was greater than 2 indicating that perforator incompetence contributed 50% or more of the reflux to that limb.

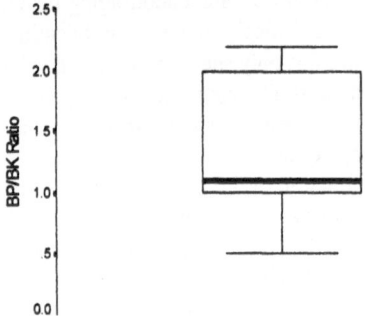

Figure 1. The relative venous refilling times (below perforator/below knee tourniquets). The median value (solid line), interquartile (box) and full range is shown.

Twenty-five legs have been operated on (22 by proximal ligation alone, 3 by combined proximal and calf perforator ligation) and follow-up data is available for 19.

Primary success (ulcer healing or improvement of lipodermatosclerosis) has been achieved in 18/19 at an average follow-up time of 10 weeks. Eleven had documented calf perforator incompetence post-operatively.

DISCUSSION

Venous hypertension has several possible aetiologies, including calf muscle pump failure, deep venous obstruction and deep and superficial reflux. Transmission of pressure to the corona phlebectatica (and thence ulceration) necessitates calf perforator incompetence (which transmits pressure via the posterior arch vein). This is usually associated with full length long saphenous reflux, deep venous incompetence or both.

Calf perforating vein incompetence is common (31 of 33 legs in the current series), but what is its clinical significance? A small perforator leak might have little influence on the overall functioning of the calf muscle pump. It might cause transient calf contraction-related superficial venous hypertension, but the overall calf venous pressure should fall with exercise providing the muscular and other venous components of the mechanism are intact. Conversely, a massive leak might reduce the efficiency of the pump by reducing effective calf ejection. This would cause both contraction-related hypertension and also reduce the pressure relieving effects of exercise, generating both exercise related and resting superficial venous hypertension. These very different physiological outcomes have at their core a single abnormality - calf perforator incompetence. Simple identification of the existence of perforator incompetence is therefore inadequate. This is borne out clinically by patients with isolated perforator incompetence complicated by ulceration (3 legs in the current series, 4% in Darke's series[8]) at one extreme and the common observation of uncomplicated perforator incompetence at the other.

We therefore suggest that Darke's type II patients comprise two distinct subgroups: saphenous reflux with (a). minor perforator incompetence (the majority) and; (b). major perforator incompetence. "Minor" and "major" are defined by the relative contribution to venous refilling time (BP/BK ratio) of the saphenous and perforator systems. In our series 3 patients had isolated calf perforator incompetence and a further five had a BP/BK ratio equal to or greater than 2. It is only by further detailed study of all patients with serious sequelae of peripheral venous hypertension that it will be possible to complete the categorisation of the wide spectrum of venous disease. This work is a vital first step towards the identification of appropriate patients for the various surgical strategies and also for meaningful comparative therapeutic trials.

REFERENCES

1. Cockett FB, Elgan Jones D. The ankle blow out syndrome; a new approach to the varicose ulcer problem. *Lancet* 1953;**1**:1-17.
2. Cranley JJ, Krause RS, Strasser ES. Chronic venous insufficiency of the lower extremity. *Surgery* 1961;**49**:48-58.
3. Arnoldi IC, Haeger K. Ulcus cruris venosum - crux medicorum? *Läkartidningen* 1967;**64**:2149-2157.
4. Field P, Van Boxall P. The role of the Linton flap procedure in the management of stasis dermatitis and ulceration in the lower limb. *Surgery* 1971;**70**:920-926.

5. Burnand KG, Lea Thomas M, O'Donnell E, et. al. Relation between post phlebitic changes in the deep veins and the results of surgical treatment of venous ulcers. *Lancet* 1976;**1**:936-938.

6. Browse NL, Burnand KG. The cause of venous ulceration. *Lancet* 1982;**2**:243-245.

7. Negus D, Friedgood A. The effective management of venous ulceration. *Br J Surg* 1983;**70**:623-627.

8. Darke SG, Penfold C. Venous ulceration and saphenous ligation. *Eur J Vasc Surg* 1992;**6**:44-49.

9. Zukowski AJ, Nicolaides AN, Szendro G, et. al. Haemodynamic significance of calf perforating veins. *Br J Surg* 1991;**78**:625-629.

Phlebology '95, D. Negus et al. (eds.). Phlebology (1995) Suppl. 1: 839-842

OP/19.1

Coagulation, Fibrinolysis and Kalikreinogenesis in Patients with Chronic Venous Insufficiency

Z. Rybak, P. Szyber and J. Garcarek

Department of Vascular Surgery and 2 Department of Radiology, Wroclaw Medical University, Wroclaw, Poland

INTRODUCTION:

Chronic venous insufficiency is the condition in which the entire venous return is impaired. This chronic state of congestion and of insufficiency of the deep vein system manifests itself in phlebectasias, inflammation, induration and ulcers (1). With destruction of valves in the deep venous system the pressure increases during calf muscle contraction is greater than that of the normal extremity or an extremity with superficial insufficiency alone. This pressure increase exceeds that of the saphenous vein by 30%. During rest however, the refilling time is more rapid due to reflux (2,3). Over a period of years the persistently raised venous pressure associated with this effect can lead to oedema, tissue damage and frequently, the formation of venous leg ulcers. On the other hand venous reflux produces stasis of blood, acidosis and multienzyme disorders. Recent studies have suggested that plasma kallikrein activated the extrinsic coagulation system. Activation of factor XII apparently initiates a series of events that lead to activation of several plasma protease systems including the coagulation, kinin, and plasmin systems. It also influences complement activation (4). It seems to be that the most significant factor in the development of chronic sequelae in the postphlebitic limb is the hydrostatic hypertension of venous incompetence. The aim of this study was to evaluate the role of venous hypertension on coagulation, fibrinolysis and kallikreinogenesis in normal and chronic venous insufficient patients.

PATIENTS:

57 patients and 28 controls were included in this study. Age of patients ranged from 25 to 68. Seventy five percent of the patients were between the 40 and 68 years and obesity was present in 55%. 28 patients had recently been treated for venous circulatory disorders by various procedures. In 15 patients both legs had been treated, in 8 only the right leg and in 5 only the left. 28 in-patients agreed to serve as controls. The patients were admitted to hospital for the following diseases: 12 with umbilical hernia, 16 with appendicitis. We distinguish three degrees of chronic venous insufficiency : Group I - 25 patients - corona phlebectatica. Group II 20 patients - hyperpigmentation or depigmentation with or without corona phlebectatica. Group III - 12 patients with florid or healed leg ulcer.

METHOD:

Pressure recordings were made with TESTAR 2000 which is microprocessor medical instrument designed for measuring venous pressure. The basis for diagnosis is observation and recording of vein pressure changes in a patient during a series of knee bends (muscle pump activation) and on standing still (5). Prekallikrein, kallikrein and antikallikrein was estimated according to Colman with TAMe substrate (6). Coagulation and fibrinolysis parameters were estimated routinely in the hospital laboratory (platelets, prothrombin, fibrinogen, plasminogen, fibrinolysis time, PTT, aPTT). For statistics Kolmogorow and correlation tests were used. Blood samples and pressure recordings were taken from the veins on the dorsum of the foot.

RESULTS:

Table 1 Mean values of post-exercise pressure and refilling time in group I,II,III patients and in controls.

Number of patient group	Pressure without cuff (mmHg)	Pressure with cuff (mmHg)	Refilling time without cuff (sek.)	RT with cuff (sek.)
Control n=28	9.2	6.5	27	35
Group I n=25	45.3	41.2	8.5	13.2
Group II n=20	59.3	44.1	6.8	11.5
Group III n=12	75.6	78.2	1	0

Table 2 Mean values of prekallikrein, kallikrein, antikallikrein, platelets, prothrombin, fibrinogen, plasminogen, fibrinolysis, PTT, aPTT.

Pts gr	PR	KL	AKL	Plat.	PT	Fibr.	Plas.	Lys-t	PTT	aPTT
Contr.	75.5	1.0	25.3	235	93	0.340	1.65	120.5	61	41.5
Gr-I	58.2	3.8	28.3	220	83	0.353	1.59	210	71	37
Gr-II	54.3	5.9	28.7	253	79	0.302	1.48	225	76	34.5
Gr-III	41.3	12.5	29.6	289	85	0.330	1.3	245	79	33

Platelets - y = n x 1000

There were marked differences between control and CVI groups of patients (p< 0.001). Post exercise venous pressure and kallikrein, fibrinolysis time, PTT and aPTT time correlations were significant.

Table 3 Correlation between venous pressure and kallikrein, fibrinolysis, PTT and aPTT.

	Kallikrein	Fibrinolysis	PTT	aPTT
Pressure	r=0.99148[*]	r=0.76983[*]	r=0.81466[*]	r=0.7814[*]

[*]p < 0.05

CONCLUSIONS:

High venous pressure in chronic venous insufficiency initiates coagulation, fibrinolysis and kallikreinogenesis.

REFERENCES:

1. Szydlowski Z., Szyber P., Dorobisz A., Zwierzchowska A., Rybak Z. Surgical treatment of the post-thrombotic syndrome. Pol. Tyg. Lek. 1992; 18-19:425-6.
2. Rybak Z. Phlebodynamometric evaluation of surgical treatment of varicose veins. Pol. Przegl. Chir. 1994; 66:699-704.
3. O'Donnell T.F., Shepard A.D. Chronic venous insufficiency, In: Jarrett F., editor. Vascular surgery of the lower extremity, St Louis: Mosby, 1985: 206-38.
4. Amundsen E. Role of the kallikrein-kinin system in shock, In:NIH Public. Chemistry and biology of the kallikrein-kinin system in health and disease. Bethesda, Maryland 1974;67:518-24.
5. Rybak Z. Dynamic measurement of venous pressure as alternative diagnostic method in limb veins diseases. Phlebol. Review, 1993; 1:19-30.
6. Colman R.W., Mason J.W., Sherry S. The kallikreinogen-kallikrein enzyme system of human plasma. Annals of int. Med. 1069;71:763-73.

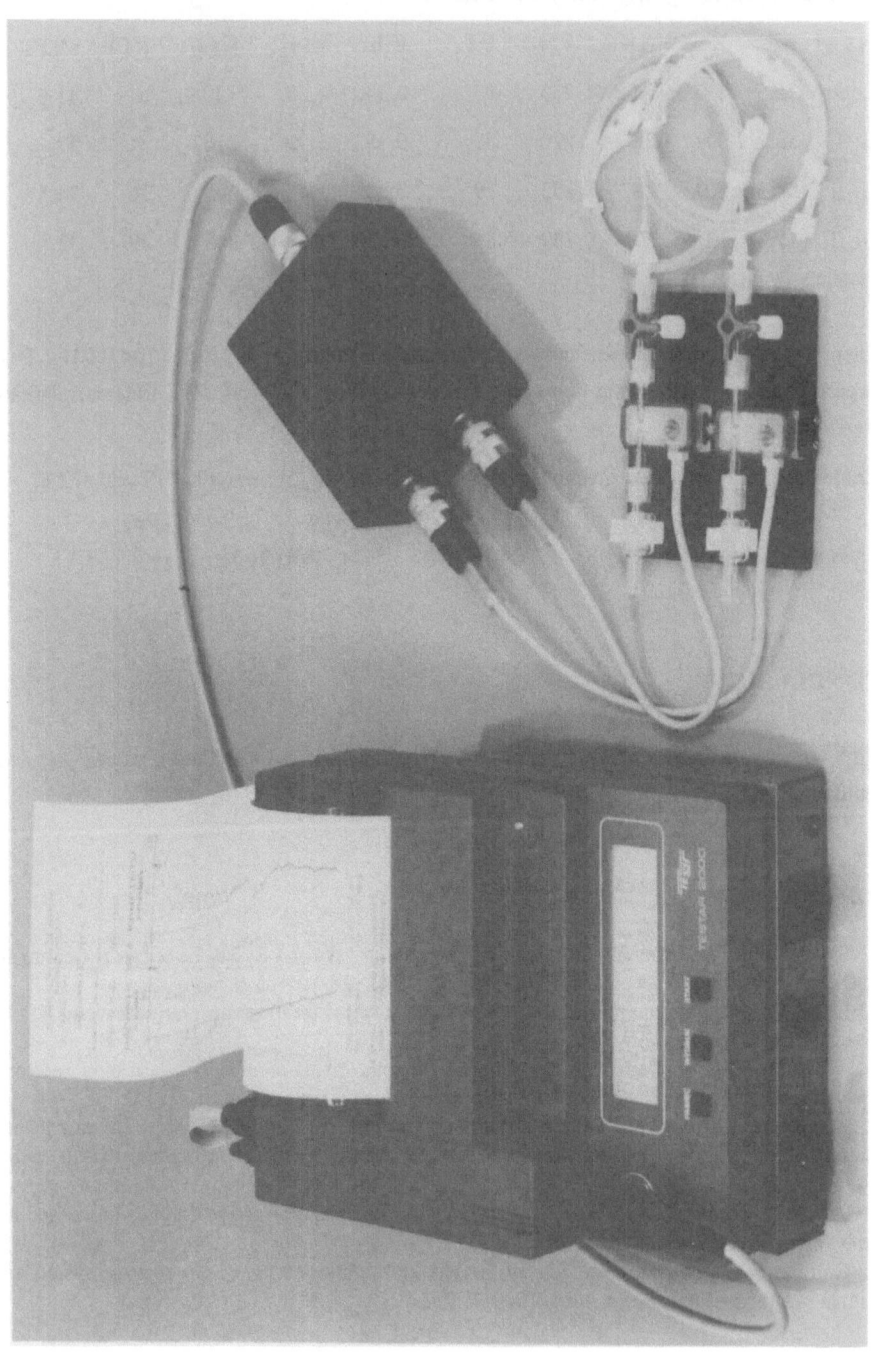

Phlebology '95, D. Negus et al. (eds.). Phlebology (1995) Suppl. 1: 843-845

OP/6.3

Correction of the Duplex and Physiological Abnormalities in Chronic Venous Insufficiency (CVI) Following Superficial Vein Surgery

C. Solomon, A.M. van Rij, R.A. Christie and G.B. Hill

Department of Surgery, University of Otago, Dunedin, New Zealand

INTRODUCTION

The association of venous reflux limited to the superficial veins and veinous ulcers has been established with the use of duplex ultrasound scanning and air plethysmography [1]. An implication of this is that superficial vein surgery assumes an important role in the management of venous ulcers. Such surgery, when used for dealing with simple varicose veins, has unfortunately been associated with significant failure rates [2]. Reasons for this have been attributed to diagnostic error, surgical error and true recurrence [3]. The impact and appropriatness of sugery can now be readily assessed non-invasively [4].

This study examines the effect of superficial vein surgery using duplex scanning and measurement of venous haemodynamics before and 2 weeks and 3 months after surgery.

METHODS

Patient selection and assessment

150 limbs of 106 consecutive patients undergoing superficial vein surgery for lower limb venous disease were included in the study. Preoperative venous assessment included: clinical examination and classification of limbs according to the SVS/ISCVS classes of chronic venous insufficiency (CVI); detailed duplex scanning (Acuson 128XP/5 scanner [Acuson, California]) and whole calf air plethysmography (APG) as routine clinical practice. Post operative assessments were similarly carried out at 2 weeks and 3 months. Subjective patient assessment of outcome and degree satisfaction were determined by self administered questionnaire at the 3 month assessment. Patients who could not be fully assessed due to mobility problems were excluded as were patients found to have significant arterial disease (ABI < 0.8).

Surgical procedures

Ligation of the saphenofemoral and saphenopopliteal junctions and incompetent perforators were performed as directed by the results of duplex scanning. Stripping of the long saphenous vein was attempted in all cases undergoing saphenofemoral ligation. Preoperative marking of visible varicose veins and avulsion of calf varices were performed routinely.

844

Analysis and statistical methods

Statistical analysis was performed using SPSS (Chicago, Illinois) on a Macintosh Power PC 7100. Chi- square tests were performed to test the significance of frequency differences. Continuous variables of venous function were compared by Student's paired t test or Mann-Whitney U test for normally and non-normally distributed data respectively. The level for declaring statistical significance was set at 0.05.

Mis-diagnosis was defined as the detection of reflux sites at the initial post operative assessment that were not previously noted. True surgical failure was defined as a persisting abnormality (reflux) at a site of surgical intervention which was present at the initial post-operative visit.

RESULTS

150 limbs [Class 1 (57) class 2 (37) and class 3 (56)] of 106 patients [M:F 1:1.65] were included. The age of class 1 patients [mean ± SD] (47 ± 16) was significantly less than class 2 (56±13) and class 3 (61±12) patients. The frequency of specific procedures performed to correct superficial vein reflux identified by duplex scanning was similar for all classes of CVI (p > 0.05). In addition, 13% and 19% of class 2 and 3 limbs respectively underwent subfascial ligation of incompetent calf perforators.

Duplex ultrasound assessments

Figure 1 shows the sites of reflux detected on duplex scanning before and after surgery.

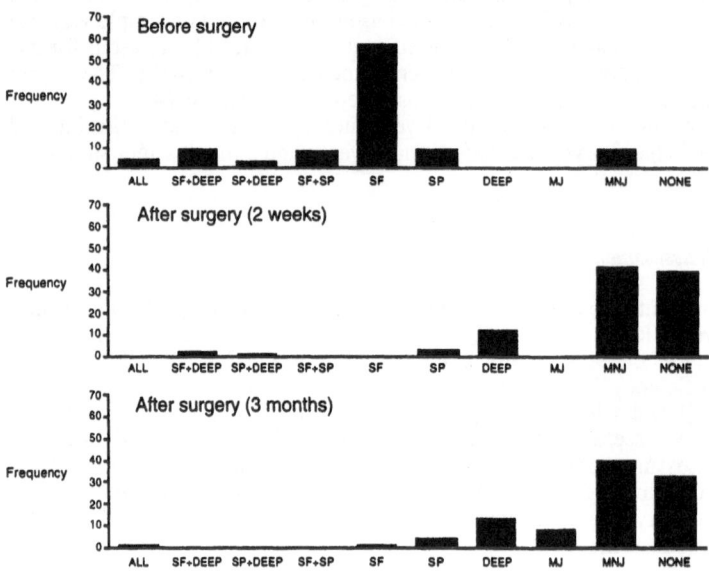

Fig 1: Histograms showing the frequency (%) of cases and sites of reflux before and after superficial vein surgery.
SF = reflux at the saphenofemoral junction
SP = reflux at the saphenopopliteal junction.
MJ = minor reflux at the SF or SP junctions
MNJ = minor non-junctional reflux.
All = reflux at the SF, SP junctions and deep system

Physiological effects of surgery

The haemodynamic measures of venous reflux and calf muscle pump function before and after surgery are shown in Table 1.

Table 1: The effects of superficial vein surgery on the physiological parameters measured by airplethysmography. († $p < 0.001$, * $p < 0.05$ from before surgery and 2 week values respectively)

	Before surgery	After surgery (2 weeks)	After surgery (3 months)
VFI(ml/s)	4.2 ± 2.7	1.9 ± 1.3†	2.0 ± 1.2*
VFT (s)	49.1 ± 33.3	90.3 ± 51.8†	81.3 ± 42.9*
VV (ml)	143 ± 53	126 ± 45†	124 ± 48
EV(ml)	66 ± 29	64 ± 26	63 ± 26
EF	0.47 ± 0.17	0.53 ± 0.17†	0.54 ± 0.19
RV(ml)	67 ± 35	45 ± 28†	42 ± 30
RF	0.46 ± 0.18	0.34 ± 0.17†	0.32 ± 0.17*
2 s outflow ratio	0.69 ± 0.13	0.65 ± 0.13†	0.64 ± 0.12
VFT/RF ratio	264 ± 1007	892 ± 2762†	885 ± 2580

While measures of venous reflux (VFI) and (VFT) and relative measures of calf muscle pump function (EF, RF) were significantly improved by surgery, calf vein volume was reduced but absolute calf muscle pump function given by the volume ejected during a single toe stand (EV) was not altered. At further follow up, a small but significant deterioration in filling indices (VFI, VFT) was noted.

Patient satisfaction

None of the patients in the study felt that surgery had worsened their condition but 10% felt little or only slightly improved overall effects. 90% felt that the surgical result was either 'excellent' or 'much improved'.

Venous haemodynamics (VFT, VFI, VFT/RF ratio) and patient satisfaction were significantly better in limbs without residual reflux (data not shown).

CONCLUSIONS AND DISCUSSION

Well directed superficial vein surgery has marked corrective effects on lower limb venous haemodynamics but does not alter absolute calf muscle pump function.

In this study, superficial vein surgery guided by duplex examination for all classes of CVI, was associated with low rates of both mis-diagnosis and immediate surgical failure. A large group of patients did, however, have minor residual reflux mainly in non-avulsed segments of vein remote from the saphenofemoral or saphenopopliteal junctions. While the significance of this finding is not clear, it was associated with slightly worse haemodynamic measures and lower patient satisfaction. Longer term follow up will be required to reveal if this abnormality is associated with the recurrence of varicose veins. It is possible that these might initially progress in a cephalad direction through branches of non-avulsed segments reopening larger connections with the deep system with ensuing reflux.

REFERENCES

1. van Rij AM, Solomon C,.Christie R. Anatomic and physiologic characteristics of venous ulceration. J Vasc Surg 1994; 20: 759-64.
2. Bradbury AW, Stonebridge PA, Callam MJ, Walker AJ, Allan PL, Beggs I, et al. Recurrent varicose veins: assessment of the saphenofemoral junction. BJS 1994; 81 373-5.
3. Royle JP. Recurrent varicose veins. World J. Surg 1986;10,944-53.
4. Christopoulos D, Nicolaides AN, Galloway JMD, Wilkinson A. Objective noninvasive evaluation of venous surgical results. J Vasc Surg 1988; 8: 683-7.

Phlebology '95, D. Negus et al. (eds.). Phlebology (1995) Suppl. 1: 846-848

PI/2.2

Pitfalls of Venous Ulcer Trials

H. Partsch

Dermatological Department, Wilhelminenhospital, A 1171 Vienna, Austria

INTRODUCTION

Randomized controlled trials entailing a parallel group design are necessary to provide scientific evidence of the effectiveness of a specific treatment modality. However, flaws in planning and evaluation of clinical studies may obscure the validity of trials. Table 1 contains the most important shortcomings of the methodology of ulcer-trials.

Table 1: Shortcomings of ulcer-trial methodology (1)
- Incomplete description of patient characteristics
- Randomization procedures
- Measurement of outcome
- Data-presentation

INCOMPLETE DESCRIPTION OF PATIENT CHARACTERISTICS

The underlying cause of the leg ulcer has to be specified as clearly as possible in every single case. If the study is restricted to venous ulceration, other possible causes have to be excluded (arterial, infectious, rheumatic etc). Especially arterial occlusive disease must be ruled out by non-invasive tests. Concomitant diseases should be mentioned (e.g. diabetes, haematological disorders etc) and the venous pathology has to be proven, such as refluxes, obstructions or both, and it is important also describe the localization and extent of the damage.

Major risk factors which affect the healing of a venous ulcer should be considered such as

previous deep vein thrombosis, trauma, treatment in the past, oedema and skin-changes.

Other contributory factors may be degenerative arthritis, ankylosis and related diseases, obesity, sitting or standing occuptions and inactive life-style, smoking habits, non-compliance and inability to participate actively in ulcer care program.

Daily activity and non-trial treatments such as dressings, bandages, and medication should be controlled and standardized.

In a prospective study we have compared patients whose ulcers were healed after 12 weeks of treatment with those which were not healed. We have worked out several clinical factors which obviously have a negative influence on ulcer-healing (2) (Table 2).

Table 2: Negative prognostic factors on ulcer healing.
- ulcers with long past history
- Long history of the present ulcer
- Large Patient's age
- Recurring ulcer area.

Additionally Skene and coworkers have also found deep vein insufficiency to also be a negative factor(3).

RANDOMIZATION PROCEDURES

Ideally all the factors affecting the trial should be equally distributed in the treatment groups before randomization.

Major variables should be controlled by stratification or by inclusion/exclusion criteria . A cross -over design is not appropriate, since the baseline for the second study-arm is not the same as for the first.

The study should be analyzed on an intention -to-treat basis, dropouts should be regarded as treatment failures.

MEASUREMENT OF OUTCOME

The primary end-point of ulcer trials is complete healing of all ulcers. An observation period of 6 months is usually adaequate.

Other parameters which can be considered are pain, frequency of dressing changes, and microcirculatory measurements.

Ulcers should be documented at each visit by tracing them on to a transparent sheet at short intervals. For the planimetric evaluation computer aid is helpful.

The time of healing and changing in ulcer size per week are not valid parameters as they depend on the primary size of the ulcer. Large ulcers take longer to heal than small ones.

The wound area reduction per day in mm or in percent changes during the course of the healing is higher in large ulcers and at the beginning of the treatment and much less in small ulcers and before healing. The calculation of a virtual radius and the report of daily radius reduction offers the possibility of comparing healing rates of large and small ulcers and of extrapolating the expected ulcer healing time by creating a linear function (4) (Fig. 1).

Prevention of ulcer recurrence by assessing cumulative re-ulceration using life-table analysis is an interesting approach to investigate therapeutic modalities (5).

DATA PRESENTATION

Reports of the results of ulcer healing trials should contain the absolute values of ulcer area and time of healing and not just percentage changes.
A second protocol analysis should be conducted , including data only on those patients who properly fulfilled the study protocol in order to confirm the validity of the intention-to-treat analysis (6).

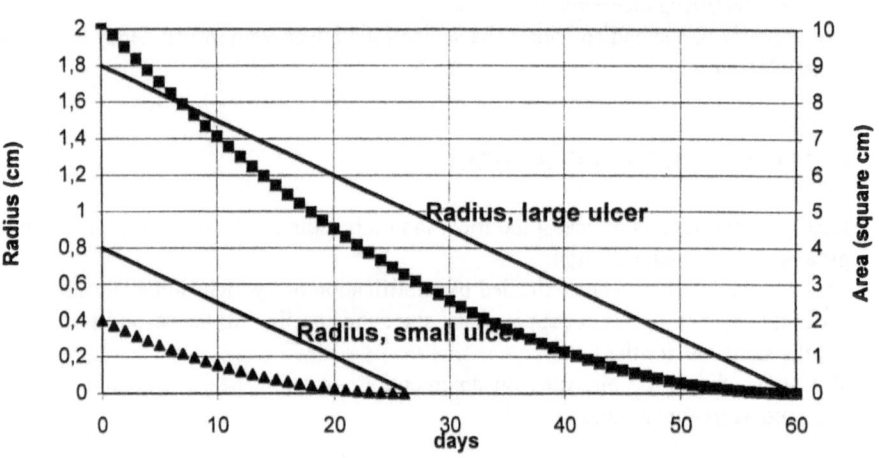

Decrease of area and radius of a large and a small ulcer
Equal healing rate, radius-reduction =0.03 cm / day

Fig. 1. Model of a large (upper curves) and of a small ulcer (lower curves) with equal healing rates. The straight lines represent virtual radius, the curved lines area. The larger ulcer takes longer to heal. Healing times may be extrapolated from the percentage change of the virtual radius but not from the area decrease.

REFERENCES

1. Van Everdingen J, Cullum NA. Compression bandaging as a therapy for venous ulcers-a systematic review of evidence. Oxford...
2. Mayer W, Jochmann W, Partsch H. Ulcus cruris: Abheilung unter konservativer Therapie. Eine prospektive Studie. Wien. med.Wochenschr.1994;144:250-2
3. Skene AJ, Smith JM, Dore CJ, Charlett A, Lewis JD. Venous leg ulcers: a prognostic index to predict time to healing. BMJ 1992;305:1119-21
4. Martin M. Dynamisches Wundheilungsprofil des venösen Ulcus cruris.VASA 1994;23:228-233
5. Wright DD, Franks PJ, Blair SD, Backhouse CM, Moffat C, McCollum CN. Oxerutins in the prevention of recurrence in chronic venous ulceration : randomized controlled trial. Br.J.Surg. 1991;78:1269-70
6. Breddin HK Browse NL, Coleridge Smith PD, Cornu Thenard A, Dormandy JA, Franzeck UK et al. Consensus paper on venous leg ulcers. Phlebology 1992;7:48-59

P004

DETECTION OF uPA, uPA RECEPTOR AND PAI-1 IN CHRONIC LEG ULCER BIOPSIES USING IN SITU HYBRIDIZATION

⁺Trengove N., *Stacey M.C. *Zheng M.,

✦ University Department of Surgery, Fremantle Hospital, W.A.
* University Department of Surgery QEII Medical Centre, W.A.

Objective: Plasminogen activators are thought to play a role in the underlying pathophysiology of venous ulceration. It was the purpose of this study to identify the cells producing urokinase plasminogen activator (uPA), uPA-receptor (uPA-R) and plasminogen activator inhibitor-1 (PAI-1) in non-healing and healing chronic leg ulcers.

Design: Comparative study of paired biopsy samples from patients with non-healing and healing chronic leg ulcers.

Patients: 1 patient (to date) admitted for skin graft of chronic leg ulcers.

Intervention: Tissue biopsy samples transecting the edge of the ulcer collected when patient first admitted to hospital (non-healing phase) and after 2 weeks bed rest in preparation for skin grafting (healing phase).

Measurements: Tissue biopsies (fresh frozen), were analysed for the expression of uPA, PAI-1 and uPA-R mRNA using *in situ* hybridization.

Results: The main location of cells expressing uPA and uPA-R were keratinocytes in the epidermis and generalised staining in the stroma. A similar staining pattern was observed for PAI-1 with additional localized staining immediately below the basement membrane zone. Obvious changes in expression were an increase in expression of uPA in the epidermis and stroma and a marked decrease in the expression of PAI-1 in the epidermis during the healing phase. The expression of uPA-R remained unchanged.

Conclusions:. The increase in uPA and corresponding decrease in PAI-1 during healing suggest that uPA may play a role in the adherence and migration of keratinocytes in the healing of chronic wounds.

P153

LIPOSCLEROSIS AND CUTANEOUS RETRACTIONS

Brizzio E O, Cumaldi A

Vascular Peripheral Laboratory -.965 San Martin St 1st floor, Capital Federal Buenos Aires Argentina
Argentine School of Phlebology of AMA.-1171 Santa Fe Av.Buenos Aires, Argentina

Introduction: Liposclerosis evolves from initial stages of lipoedema with initial lymphatic complications (lipolymphedemas) to an alteration reticular fibres around the adipose tissue and the capillaries. The alteration shows itself through an hyperplasia and an hypertrophy around the adiposite and pericapillaries fibres which generate micronodules and zones of tightness in the skin with the consequent cutaneous retractions.

Objective: To show the influence of fibrosis on cutaneous retractions, their way of action in dynamic of muscular contraction, the certain ecotopographic diagnosis and the minisurgical ecoguided strategy to be followed.

Number of Patients: 116 patients of feminine sex.

Design: 1) ectopographic diagnosis with lineal ecotomograph of 7 MHz. With dynamic comparative test of muscular relaxation against contraction. 2) Preoperative ecotomographic cartography. 3) Microsurgical operative technique consisting of a cut on retraction line.

Results: Diminution of skin tightness and pits

Conclusions: The right topographic diagnosis of the localisation retractions, their analysis under the dynamic muscular contraction, the preoperative cartography and the microsurgical cut of retraction improve the aesthetic result of treatments that may be applied to patients with liposclerosis.

OP15.7

THE USE OF HOME SEQUENTIAL GRADIENT PNEUMATIC COMPRESSION IN THE TREATMENT OF CHRONIC VENOUS INSUFFICIENCY

Arcelus JI, Caprini JC, Hoffman KN, Finke N, Pollard JC, Size G.
Department of Surgery, The Glenbrook Hospital, Glenview, IL and North western University Medical School, Chicago, IL, USA.

Objective: To evaluate the use of home sequential gradient pneumatic compression (SGPC) in the treatment of chronic venous insufficiency of the legs.

Design: Prospective study including a consecutive series of patients.

Patients: Twenty patients with symptomatic chronic venous insufficiency of the legs confirmed by duplex scanning and photoplethysmography (PPG).

Intervention: All patients were instructed to use SGPC at home for four hours a day, in addition to the use of elastic compression stockings, during six months.

Measurements: Clinical improvement was assessed by a scoring system completed by the patients before and after completion of the study. All patients underwent air plethysmography (APG) before compression and 1, 3 and months thereafter. The following APG indices were calculated: venous volume (VV), venous filling index (VFI), ejection fraction (EF) and residual volume fraction (RVF).

Results: The median total score was 20 (IQR 17, 2-20) before treatment and 13 (IQR 10-13) after SGPC treatment (Wilcoxon rank test, p<0.0001). The individual scores given by patients to symptoms such as swelling, pain, decreased physical activity and cosmetic problems were significantly reduced. Median APG indices VV, VFI and RVF did not change significantly. However, EF increased significantly after 3 and 6 months of compression (Wilcoxon rank test, p<0.05) compared to baseline.

Conclusion: The use of SGPC improved the ejection fraction, as measured by air plethysmography, in a group of patients with chronic venous insufficiency of the legs. This favorable hemodynamic response could explain the remarkable clinical response to this therapeutic modality.

OP/15.6

CLINICAL EVALUATION OF ELASTIC STOCKINGS

J C J M Veraart, G Pronk, H A M Neumann

Department of Dermatology, Academisch Ziekenhuis Maastricht, The Netherlands

Objective: Medical therapeutic elastic stockings are worldwide being used in the treatment of phlebological diseases, such as sclerotherapy and chronic venous insufficiency. They can be divided into four different classes I-IV according to their exerted pressure on a standard limb. A normal human limb does, however, resemble this standard limb. It was therefore our aim to investigate the pressure underneath stockings.

Design: Open clinical investigation.

Patients: 41 legs were evaluated. All patients were wearing elastic stockings for chronic venous insufficiency. All measurements were being performed within one month after wearing the stocking.

Measurements: Pressure recordings were being performed with an Oxford Pressure Monitor (OPM) (Talley, Oxford, Great Britain). Small cuffs are being inflated with air until counter pressure is given. 6 measurements were simultaneously being performed round the so called B-area (ankle).

Results: 40 measurements could be assessed. 48.5% (n=19) fell within its class and 52.5% (n=21) did not. All around measurements showed a big spreading; a maximum of 22.9% below (medial/lateral side) and 28.8% above (anterior/posterior side) the mean.

Conclusion: When prescribing elastic stockings they should be properly measured to the leg and one should realise the pressure difference markedly all around the leg according to Laplace's law. The results also advocate the use of pelottes.

OP/15.3

THE HAEMODYNAMIC EFFECTS OF GRADUATED COMPRESSION STOCKINGS.

Van Gerwen H.J.L, Braktce A.J.M., Kuiper J.P.

University Hospital Nijmegen, Dept. Dermatology
Postbox 9101, 6500 HB Nijmegen, the Netherlands

Objective: To study the haemodynamic effects of graduated medical compression stockings in patients with severe chronic venous insufficiency.
Design: The literature on the subject is reviewed. Venous pressure volume relations, calf muscle pumpfunction and venous reflux were measured both with and without stockings in patients with deep venous insufficiency.
Patients: 20 patients (30 legs), known to have deep venous insufficiency.
Measurements: Using the supine venous pump function test with strain gauge plethysmography, the venous pressure-volume relation, the expelled volume (Ve) and the ambulatory venous pressure fall (Pf) were determined. As a measure for venous reflux venous refilltime was measured by strain gauge plethysmography (SGP) and by digitalized photoplethysmography (dPPG). All measurements were made with and without class 3 made-to-measure stockings.
Results: In all 30 legs the pressure-volume relation measured with the stocking on was higher and steeper than measured without stocking. As a result of the compression the expelled volume Ve increased with 38 % from a mean of 0.94 to a mean of 1.31 % (p < 0.01, paired Student t-test). This resulted in an increase of Pf from a mean of 49 % to 55 % (in percentage 15 %; p < 0.01; normal values: > 70%). The refilltime increased from 11 to 13 seconds (SGP, p < 0.01) and from 9 to 11 seconds (dPPG, p < 0.01), as a result of the compression. The results correspond well with the results reported in the literature.
Conclusions: Elastic stockings reduce the venous volume, and increase the expelled volume. This however, leads to only a small increase of ambulatory venous pressure fall, which is the most important parameter to quantify the venous pump function. This apparent discrepancy can be understood as a consequence of the alinearity of the pressure-volume relation, which becomes steeper and higher as a result of the compression. The influence of compression on the venous reflux is also small and of only minor importance in the beneficial effect of elastic stockings in patients with venous insufficiency.

P042/P050

IN VIVO INVESTIGATIONS OF THE MICROCIRCULATION IN VENOUS ULCER IN VIEW OF THERAPEUTIC POSSIBILITIES

Steins A, Jünger M, Klyscz T, Hahn H, Galler S

University of Tübingen, Dep. of Dermatology, D-72076 Tübingen, FRG

How do capillary density, Laser-Doppler-Flux (LDF) and transcutaneous oxygen tension ($tcPO_2$) change in venous ulcer and adjacent areas during wound-healing? Is there an improvement of the known microangiopathy in these patients with severe chronic venous insufficiency (CVI)?
We examined 10 patients (4 women and 6 men; age $57,3\pm9,7$ (mean$\pm$SD) with CVI stage III according to Widmer, ulcer area $8,7\pm11,6$ cm^2) by means of capillaroscopy, transcutaneous oxygen partial pressure measurement and laser Doppler fluxmetry with local heating test. Measurements were taken at the beginning of the study and after complete wound-healing after $8,6\pm4,3$ weeks. The following results are given in medians. **Results:**

	before	after healing
-capillary density (ulcer) /mm²	5 (Q1=1;Q3=7,5)	21 (Q1=11;Q3=23)
-capillary density (adjacent area)	34 (Q1=20;Q3=36)	42 (Q1=29;Q3=55)
-tcPO₂ (adjacent area) mmHg	23 (Q1=7;Q3=30)	30 (Q1=20;Q3=47)
-tcPO₂ (prox. lower leg) mmHg	36 (Q1=31; Q3=45)	42 (Q1=35;Q3=50)

Capillary density and $tcPO_2$ increased during wound healing impressingly. Laser fluxmetry of the ulcer area showed an increase of vascular reserve to local heat after healing:

	before	after healing
-LDF (Heating, Ulcer) %	23.5(Q1=6.75;Q3=60.9)	35.5(Q1=13;Q3=48)

Conclusion: The healing of venous ulcer is associated with an improvement of skin microcirculation detected by these methods. We conclude that the value of therapeutic regimes in CVI can be assessed by investigations of the skin microcirculation during the healing process.

OP/10.1

SURGICAL FORMATION the DEEP (SUBFAS CIAL) LYMPHATICOVENOUS ANAS TOMOSIS IN POS TPHLEBITIC EDEMOTOSE SYNDROME

Zolotorevski V.

A.V.Vishnevski Institute, B.Serpukhovskaya 27, Moscow, Russia

Objective: To improve results of surgical treatment of the postphlebitic syndrome (PS) in patients with refractory leg edema.
Design: Information about new modification of the lynph draining operation.
Patients: Operated were 52 patients with leg edema due to incomplete recanalisation of iliac vein and disturbed permeability of inguinal and iliac lymphatic nodes proven by phlebography, ultrosound invastigation and rsdionuclide limphography.
Intervention: After conventional varicose vein techniques 1 or 2 limphaticovenous anastomoses were formed between the deep lymphatics and v.dorsalis pedis. Fenestration of fascia cruris (5x6 cm) was performed on medial surface in the muscle pump region.
Measurements: Clinical outcome, repeated circumferential of thigh, shin, foot were documented at 1, 6, 12 month after operation.
Results: In 4 petients were observed poor results. In 48 patients dimensions of operated extremity decreased by 50-80% in comperision with sound extremity. Cellulitis exacerbations ceased.
Conclusions: Technical problems for lymphodreining operations in surgical treatment the edemotose forms of PS needs further study. Special attention deserves edema of ancle segment.

PI/2.6

A RANDOMISED TRIAL OF SINGLE LAYER AND MULTI-LAYER BANDAGES IN THE TREATMENT OF CHRONIC VENOUS ULCERATION

Nelson EA, Harper DR, Ruckley CV, Prescott RJ, Gibson B, Dale JJ. Lothian and Forth Valley Leg Ulcer Study.
Royal Infirmary Edinburgh, Falkirk and District Royal Infirmary, University of Edinburgh

Objective
To determine whether a single layer system was as effective as a multi-layer elastic compression system.
Design
Randomised, parallel group, open clinical trial. Part of a multi-arm trial, other arms (dressing and oxpentifylline (Trental 400) vs placebo; double-blind) are reported in other communications.
Patients
Two hundred patients with pure venous chronic ulceration (range 2 - 240 months)
Intervention
Patients were randomised to a single layer regimen, i.e. Granuflex Adhesive Compression Bandage (Convatec, UK), or a multi-layer regime, i.e. Velband (Johnson and Johnson), Crepe (Smith and Nephew), Elset (Seton) and Coban (3M).
Measurements
The primary end-point was complete healing of all ulcers on the trial leg within 24 weeks. Sub-bandage pressures were also recorded.
Results
The multi-layer bandage healed 69 %, and the single layer bandage healed 49 % of ulcers in 24 weeks (Odds ratio 2.37; 95% CI = 1.3 - 4.2). Both regimes were capable of providing sustained compression.
Conclusion
The multi-layer regime tested healed significantly more ulcers than the single layer system.

P045

WHITE BLOOD CELLS TRAPPING IN THE MICROCIRCULATION: A POSSIBLE ROLE IN THE PATHOGENESIS OF VENOUS ULCERATION

Nikolovska S, Pavlova Lj, Dervendzi D, Starova A

Clinic of Dermatology, Medical Faculty, Skopje, Makedonija

Objective: To asses the role of white blood cells in the pathogenesis of chronic venous ulceration.

Design: Randomised parallel four groups open clinical trial.

Patients: Four groups of subjects were compared: normal controls, patients with uncomplicated primary varicose veins, patients with chronic venous insufficiency (CVI) with no active ulceration and patients with CVI and active ulcers.

Meassurements: Platlet counts, as well total and differential white cell counts were measured in the venous blood draining the foot of the patients in horizontal position and then during 60 minutes with the leg dependant.

Results: In patients with CVI we registrated a significant "loss" of white blood cells in the foot during dependency. This was 26% compared to 3% in the normal controls and patients with uncomplicated varicose veins (Paired Students t - test p < 0,01). There was a parallel loss of platelets which were not washed out after elevation of the foot.

Conclusions: Our results shows that patients with CVI have white blood cells "trapped" in the microcirculation of the dependant foot. This causes change in microcirculatory flow and the liberation of leukotrienes, proteolytic enzymes, oxygen - free radicals from the white cells and platelet aggregating factor from the platelets "trapped", leading to further nutrient capillary damage and tissue damage. This results suggest the benefit of hemorheological pharmacotherapy aimed to avoid this white blood cells and platelet "trapping".

OP/10.2

Influence of Venous Patency After Proximal Deep Venous Thrombosis on the Long Term Clinical Sequelae

Bauchart JJ, Thery CI, Asseman Ph, Loubeyre Ch.

Réanimation Cardiaque et Soins Intensifs
Hopital Cardiologique, Lille, France

In a prospective study, 98 patients, average age 44 (range 14 to 82) with a proximal deep venous thrombosis received Streptokinase intravenously (1000,000 U/hour) for an average of 2.8 days (0.7 to 7 days). All patients underwent a bilateral ascending phlebography before and after treatment.

In 70 patients, after a mean delay 34 months (range 25 to 45), the importance of clinical sequelae was determined according a severity score. We found that the patients discharged with complete lysis were more significantly free of sequelae than those with unsuccessful or partial lysis: 19/22 (86%) vs 16/48 (33%) p < 0,001).

854

OP/6.7

Phlebo - Oncology of the lower limbs

Rosli N., Lapid T., Sánchez V.

Centro de Flebologia Dr. Never Rosli, Córdoba, Argentina

OBJECTIVE: This work attempts to alert physicians who practise phlebology about the importance of the wide range of pre cancerous and cancerous lesions that, fixed on the lower limbs, may or may not be associated with some phlebopathy.

DESIGN: A retrospective study has been made of patients bearing ulcers in the lower limbs without determining their etiology.

PATIENTS: A total of 1.254 patients of whom 450 were men and 804 women.

MEASUREMENTS: This led us to normalize the study of the patients with

1. Thorough clinical checkup
2. Laboratory
3. Radiology
4. Ultrasound and TAC
5. Histopathology

Once malignity was confirmed, patients were immediately derived to an Oncological Centre This is why we have focused the study based on a wide classification that includes the most frequent processes within the diverse topographical possibilities of the lower members, adding to these a few cases which illustrate our experience.

RESULTS: The presence of malign lesions appeared in 7 cases out of the 1.254 patients, representing approximately 0.6%

CONCLUSIONS: We would like to emphasize these concepts on three fundamental points:

1. Keeping in mind in the practice of phlebology the possibility of coming across malign pathology.
2. The possibility of an ulcerous vein becoming malign is of 0.4%, according to TANOPYS and SILVERMAN
3. Faced with any suspicious ulcer and prior to the grafting of skin, it is imperative to perform a biopsy and histopathology.

P030

THE STATUS OF DEEP VEINS IN PRIMARY VARICOSIS

Zapalski S., Oszkinis G., Podstawski W., Pukacki F., Zielinski P., Krasinski Z.

Dept. of General and Vascular Surgery, Poznan, Poland.

Objective: The purpose of the study was to define the status of deep veins in patients with primary varicosis undergoing the stripping operation.

Design: Prospective investigation of a consecutive series.

Patients: 78 patients (127 limbs) with primary varicosis.

Measurements: All patients were investigated by venous photoplethysmography (without and with cuff) to assess venous refilling time (VRT). For 38 patinets (52 limbs) with an abnormal VRT with cuff (20 seconds), performed descending phlebography, for differentiation deep and / or perforator venous insufficiency.

Results: In the entire group of 52 limbs with deep and / or perforator venous insufficiency, valvular incompetence of deep veins was noted in 23 limbs (18.1%). The most commonly involved segment was the deep calf veins (15 of 23) followed by the popliteal vein - 6 limbs and superficial femoral vein - 2 limbs.

Conclusion: The results demonstrated the need for accuracy in examination of patients with primary varicosis. Some of them may be secondary, due to deep insufficiency. This suggests that a silent episode of thrombosis of deep veins may be present with minimal or no symptoms.

Deep Venous Reflux and Occlusion/Venous Ulcers

Treatment of Deep Venous Disorders and Venous Ulceration

Deep Venous Reflux and Occlusion/Venous Ulcers

Treatment of Deep Venous Disorders and Venous Ulceration
Conservative Treatment

Phlebology '95, D. Negus et al. (eds.). Phlebology (1995) Suppl. 1: 857-859

OP/7.1

Wound Care Knowledge in Community Nurses

L.A. Lambourne[1], A.C. Jones[1], P.J. Franks[2] and C.J. Moffatt[2]

[1] South Bedfordshire Community Health Care Trust, 1 Union Street, Luton LU1, Bedfordshire, UK
[2] Centre for Research & Implementation of Clinical Practice, London SW6 4UL, UK

INTRODUCTION

Community nurses spend between 10-60% of their time on the treatment of chronic wounds, most of which are chronic leg ulcers. In a study in South Bedfordshire 304/530 (57%) open wounds seen were chronic leg ulcers, giving a crude point prevalence of 1.1/1000 population [1]. These ulcers contributed 695 visits by community nursing staff to patients over a one week period, an average of 2.3 visits per patient per week, with average time spent treating them of 66 minutes. Over one week, 50 different wound care products were used on the patients with a cost of the products alone averaging out at £9.50 per patient per week. Despite the high use of resources in ulcer care, little is known of the appropriateness of these products in treatment of these patients and how this relates to community nursing staff training and knowledge of wound care products. With this in mind, a study was carried out to investigate the knowledge base of community nurses, the self assessed adequacy of training and the sources of reference for wound care products.

METHODS

All community nurses working within South Bedfordshire Community Health Care Trust were asked to complete a questionnaire on their wound care training. Questions were asked on the level of pre and post-registration training in wound care, and the nurses' satisfaction with their training in the assessment and treatment of wounds. In addition, questions were asked on the sources of information of wound care products and the nurses order of preference for each source of information.

RESULTS

Of the 84 responses to the questionnaire, 41 (49%) were district sisters with 28 (33%) enrolled nurses. The remaining 15 were either registered nurses (6) auxillaries (4) students (3) or others (2). Of the total, 39 (46%) stated that they had no formal post-registration training, whilst 29 (35%) estimated their training at less than one day in total. Only 4 (5%) had more than 10 days of training, these being nurses who attended a specific course in the assessment and treatment of leg ulceration [2]. Overall satisfaction with training in assessing and treating wounds was considered very good in only 9%, adequate in 40% and inadequate in 51%.

Table I. Sources of information for wound care products. Comparison of enrolled nurses and district nursing sisters.

	Total used	Enrolled	District sister	p
number	84	28	41	
1. Other Nurse	76 (90%)	25 (89%)	39 (95%)	0.656
2. Pharm. Rep.	54 (64%)	18 (64%)	31 (76%)	0.455
3. Nursing Journals	50 (60%)	12 (43%)	31 (76%)	0.012
4. Specialist Nurse	42 (50%)	14 (50%)	25 (61%)	0.512
5. Comm.Pharmacist	42 (50%)	10 (36%)	25 (61%)	0.069
6. British Formulary	30 (36%)	3 (11%)	23 (56%)	0.001
7. Gen. Practitioner	29 (35%)	7 (25%)	18 (43%)	0.177
8. Hosp. Pharmacist	13 (16%)	1 (4%)	11 (27%)	0.029

Table I illustrates the sources of information which the nurses used for their wound care knowledge. Clearly enrolled nurses and district nursing sisters had different sources of reference. Indeed, there were significant differences in the use of nursing journals, the British National Formulary and hospital pharmacists, with the use of community pharmacists approaching statistical significance. When recording the order of preference for the top three sources of information for all nursing staff, nursing colleagues were most frequently the first source of information, with pharmaceutical representatives and nursing journals used as subsidiary sources.

DISCUSSION

This study was initiated to determine the level of training in community nurses dealing with wounds on a daily basis. It has shown that there was a general dissatisfaction with training adequacy in the assessment and treatment of wounds. There was a high reliance on their nursing peers for their knowledge, together with pharmaceutical representatives. Enrolled nurses used fewer sources of reference, relying less on hospital pharmacists, the British Formulary and nursing journals.

At the time of this study the clinical nurse specialist was newly in post which may explain their relatively low use as a source of reference. It is expected that the specialist will become a key source of reference for all community nurses involved in the treatment of leg ulceration and other wounds. This study highlighted the dissatisfaction of community nursing staff with their post-registration training which has led to a wound care training programme in South Bedfordshire, led by the clinical nurse specialist to improve nurses awareness of assessment and treatment of wounds in the community. Through the process of re-audit it is hoped that the benefits of this training package can be realised in the improvement of patient care and professional satisfaction.

REFERENCES

1. Lambourne LA Moffatt CJ Jones AC Franks PJ:
Clinical community wound care audit: the south Bedfordshire experience.
Presented to the North Thames Clinical Audit Conference, London 1994

2. Moffatt CJ Karn EA: Answering the call for more education. Development of an ENB course in leg ulcer management. Professional Nurse 1994; 9: 708-12

Phlebology '95, D. Negus et al. (eds.). Phlebology (1995) Suppl. 1: 860-861

OP/1.4

Chronic Venous Insufficiency (CVI) and Occlusive Arterial Disease (OAD) in the Same Leg: Elastic Compression is Indicated?

A.I. Desogus, A. Rachele, M. Carta and M. Polo

Department of General and Emergency Surgery, "Marino" Hospital, Cagliari, Italy

INTRODUCTION:

Venous disease affects a large proportion of the population in Western society; appears more frequently with advancing age and is more common in women.
Arterial disease is more common in males with varicose veins and results from Framingham study suggest that both conditions have similar risk factors.
CVI produces a pathological condition of the skin and sub-cutaneous tissues, secondary to prolonged stasis of venous blood flow.
In the Basle study CVI was graded into three: grade I, dilated sub-cutaneous veins; grade II, hyper- or de-pigmented areas; grade III, open or healed leg's ulcer.

OBJECTIVE:

review our experience in the last 5 years to discuss clinical decision for prescription of elastic-compression (EC).

DESIGN:

two parallel groups of patients in open clinical trial.

PATIENTS:

90 patients (140 legs) whit association of CVI and OAD (35 male, 55 female - all over 65 years old - range 67,5). Diabetic pattern has been considered reason for exclusion; OAD are graded in I-II type of Fontaine scale. In 50% of these patients legs' venous ulcer were present. Patients were casually divided in two groups: 50 with EC, 40 without EC.

MEASUREMENT:

the inclusion and subsequent prescription (50 cases, 80 legs) of elastic socks (our preferred method) it was chosen the measurement of pressure index at tibial (posterior) artery level. Legs' venous ulcer were present in 25 patients (39 legs).

RESULTS:

Absence of flow (or continuous) at C.W. doppler examination in pedidia artery (65% of 50 cases) was not contraindication for EC. Clinical observation was prolonged over six months (2 controls/month) and included physical and doppler CW examination, dressing of ulcer, if present. Minimal or major peripheral vascular surgery was not performed during clinical trial. The two groups (50 with EC, 40 without EC) were homogeneous for sex, severity of venous disorders and general or local complications rates during the trial. Patients with EC reported significantly lower analgesic consumption, faster improvement in motor abilities, decrease of oedema and, in case of leg's venous ulcers, significantly faster recoveries (3 weeks with EC, 6 weeks in controls). In all patients we have used "low pressure" elastic socks during "work hours" (8.00 a.m. to 8.00 p.m.). We believe that 0.55 is the gold standard for the arterial pressure index (tibial post. artery) safety indicate EC in patients with contemporary CVI and OAD in same leg.

CONCLUSIONS:

clinical results appear encouraging in extensive treatment by EC with CVI and OAD, also in terms of control of venous insufficiency improvement of performance status and quality of life.

REFERENCES

1. Belcaro G., Laurara G., Cesarone M.R., Pomante P.: Elastic stockings in diabetic microangiopaty. VASA 21.193, 1992.
2. Bjordal R.I.: Studi emodinamici delle vene varicose e della sindrome post-trombotica. In J.T.Hobbs: Malattie delle vene-clinica e terapia; pag. 32; Ed. Il Pensiero Scientifico, Roma, 1981.
3. Bjordal R.I.: Flow and pressure studies in venous insufficiency. Acta Chir Scand Suppl
   544: 30, 1988.
4. Brand F.N., Dannenberg A.L., Abbott R.D., Kannel W.B.: The epidemiology of varicoses veins: The Framingham study. Am J Prev Med 1988, 4:96-101
5. Browse N.L., Burnand K.G., Lea Thomas M.: Diseases of the veins. Arnold Ed., London, 1988.
6. Camilli S., Guarnera G.: L'insufficienza venosa primaria; Ed. Piccin, Padova, 1993.
7. Gillot Cl.: La semelle de Lejars. Phlébologie 2:176, 1993.
8. Nicolaides A.N., Hussein M.K., Szendro G., Christopoulos D., Vasdekis S. and Clarke H.: The relation of venous ulceration with ambulatory venous pressure measurements. J Vasc Surg 2:414, 1993.
9. Raju S., Fredericks R., Lishman P., Neglén P., Morano J.: Observation on calf venous pump mechanism: determinants of post exercise pressure. J Vasc Surg 3:459, 1993.
10. Thulesius O.: Vein wall characteristics and valvular function in chronic venous insufficiency. Phlebology 3:94, 1993.
11. Van Cleef J.F., Ribreau C., Cloarec M.: Valvules parietals de la saphéne interne. Phlébologie 3:639, 1991.

Phlebology '95, D. Negus et al. (eds.). Phlebology (1995) Suppl. 1: 862-864

PI/2.5

The Effectiveness of Compression Stockings in Reducing Lipodermatosclerosis

Y.K. Vandongen, P. Rashid and M.C. Stacey

Department of Surgery, University of Western Australia, Fremantle Hospital, Fremantle, Western Australia

INTRODUCTION

Standard treatment for lipodermatosclerosis has been with elastic compression stockings. Fibrinolytic enhancing agents such as stanozolol[1,2] and defibrotide[3] together with compression stockings have also been evaluated as treatments for this condition. A significant reduction in area of lipodermatosclerosis using a combination of these agents was reported in these studies. However it remains uncertain what the precise role of elastic compression is in reducing lipodermatosclerosis. Liposlcerotic area was reduced in patients wearing stockings and receiving a placebo in these studies, however this reached significant levels in only one study[1]. No further analysis between these groups was reported and the effectiveness of stockings remains uncertain.

It was therefore the purpose of this study to assess the role of compression stockings alone in the treatment of lipodermatosclerosis.

METHODS

Patients in this study were participating in a larger study assessing the role of compression stockings in the prevention of ulcer recurrence. All patients had recently healed ulcers of venous aetiology and all remained in compression bandages until entering the study. Patients were randomized to receive either no stockings or were fitted with Venosan® 2003, below knee graduated elastic compression stockings (Venosan, Salzman AG, St Gallen, Switzerland). Patients were excluded if they were unable to manage the daily application of the stockings or had a history of non-compliance with compression therapy.

Measurement of Lipoderatosclerosis. The area of lipodermatosclerosis was determined both visually and by palpation. A line was drawn onto the skin along the border of the lipodermatosclerosis with a removable marker pen. This area was then traced onto a piece of polythene sheeting placed over the lipodermatosclerosis. The polythene sheeting was photocopied and the area measured using planimetry.

Lipodermatosclerosis was measured at the beginning of the study and repeated after six months and again at 12 months. The tracings were carried out by the same observer throughout the study.

Reliability of this method of measurement was assessed by repeating the tracings after two weeks. This was performed only in those patients remaining in compression.

Lipodermatosclerosis was not measured if reulceration occurred as these patients were then treated with standard compression bandaging for their ulcer.

Patients were withdrawn from the study if non-compliant with the treatment or for medical or personal reasons.

RESULTS

157 patients (169 limbs) were entered into the study. 72 patients were randomized to the stocking group (M=36, F=36) and 85 received no compression (M=40, F=45). Mean age in the two groups was 67 years and 66.8 years respectively.

Reproducibility   The mean change in 51 limbs remeasured at two weeks was 74.8cm^2 (range 0 - 684.9 cm^2).

In the initial six month period there was a reduction in mean area of lipodermatosclerosis in the group wearing stockings (69.1cm^2). Area of lipdermatosclerosis increased in the no stocking group over the same period of time (mean=32.7cm^2). In the patients in the stocking group who remained healed at 12 months the mean area of lipodermatosclerosis had reduced (98.2 cm^2) and had increased 29 cm^2 for the no stocking group.

These data were separately analysed for the two periods of time using a repeated measures ANOVA. A significant interaction between the two groups was found at six months (p=0.05) (Figure 1). Similarly there was a significant interaction between the groups when followed up 12 months after the commencement of the study (p=0.03) (Figure 2)

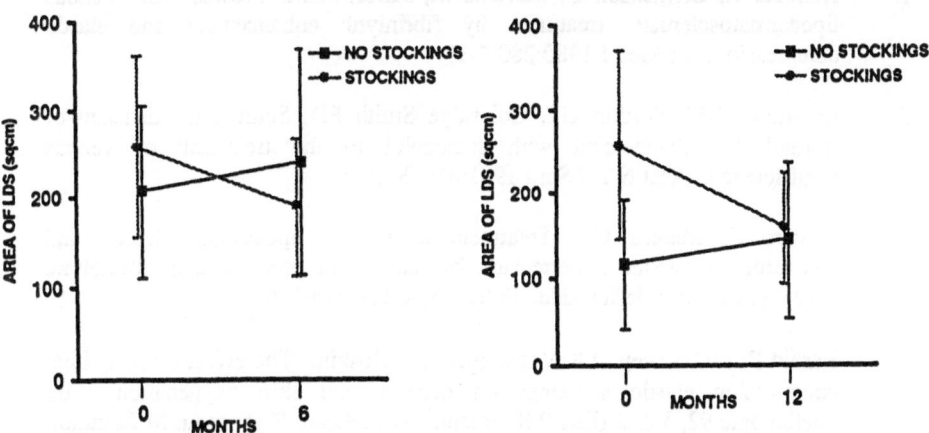

Fig 1. Area of lipodermatosclerosis after 6 months of treatment (means and confidence intervals).

Fig 2. Area of lipodermatosclerosis after 12 months of treatment (means and confidence intervals).

These data were further analysed to determine the nature of the changes within the individual groups. After six months of treatment the area of lipodermatosclerosis had reduced significantly in the stocking group (paired t-test, p=0.04). Area of lipodermatosclerosis in the stocking group patients followed up after 12 months was also significantly reduced (paired t-test, p=0.04). The changes in the no stocking group at each point in time were not significant.

DISCUSSION

This study has demonstrated that compression stockings alone are beneficial in the treatment of lipodermatosclerosis. The regular application of compression stockings significantly reduced the area of lipodermatosclerosis over a 12 month period and this was evident even after six months of treatment.

The no stocking group in this study also provided important information about the natural history of lipodermatosclerosis. This does not alter significantly in the 12 months period after healing of a chronic venous ulcer.

The measurement of lipodermatosclerosis is subjective and sometimes difficult. Data from only 10 patients have been available to suggest that this method is a reproducible procedure[1]. In this study repeated measures from 51 limbs produced a mean change of 74.8cm^2. The variablility in this data however indicates the need to examine a large number of patients to detect significant change.

This study has shown a clear benefit of wearing elastic compression stockings. Previously it has been shown that regular compression therapy does not increase tissue oxygenation[4] nor does it improve venous refilling time[5]. Reduction in liposclerotic area may therefore be one of the primary reasons, together with oedema control[4], why stockings help prevent ulcer recurrence.

REFERENCES

1.	Burnand K, Clemenson G, Morland M, Jarrett PEM, Browse NL. Venous lipodermatosclerosis: treatment by fibrinlytic enhancement and elastic compression. Br Med J 1980;280:7-11.

2.	McMullin GM, Watkin GT, Coleridge Smith PD, Scurr JH. Efficacy of fibrinolytic enhancement with stanozolol in the treatment of venous insufficiency. Aust N Z J Surg 1991;61:306-309.

3.	Belcaro G, Marelli C. Treatment of venous lipodermatosclerosis and ulceration in venous hypertension by elastic compression and fibrinolytic enhancement with defibrotide. Phlebologie 1989;4:91-106.

4.	Rashid P, MC Stacey, YK Vandongen, SE Hoskin. The effect of using high compression elastic stockings on oedema and skin oxygenation. In: Phlebologie 92, Vol 2 (Eds P Raymond-Martimbeau, R Prescott, M Zummo). John Libbey Eurotext: Paris, 1992:882-884.

5.	Vandongen YK, Rashid P, Stacey MC. The influence of graduated compression elastic stockings on venous refilling time. Primary Intention 1994;2:35-37.

Phlebology '95, D. Negus et al. (eds.). Phlebology (1995) Suppl. 1: 865-868

OP/1.5

Compression Treatment in Patients with Chronic Venous Insufficiency and Severe Ischemia

A. Faenza, S. Faenza, S. Selleri and A. Recordare

Department of Surgery Intensive Care and Transplantation, University of Bologna, Italy

INTRODUCTION

Conservative treatment of lower limb edema by Compression Bandaging (CP) is a well established form of therapy in patients with Chronic Venous Insufficiency (CVI) and Leg Ulcers but it is often considered hazardous if the patient has also an Arterial Insufficiency

We have already stated that CP is harmless and useful if ischemia is mild (I.W.>0,5) but it can be dangerous if it is critical [1] .
The aim of this paper is to present our further experience in cases with Leg Ulcers , CVI and severe ischemia (I.W.< 0,5).

MATERIAL AND METHOD

In a fifteen year period have we observed 15 patients with severe ischemia , various forms of CVI and different kinds of painful Leg Ulcers .
All had night pains and learned to sleep in the sitting position to improve the lower limb perfusion .All presented with severe edema .
A retrospective evaluation of the clinical history and of the morphology of the ulcer allows to distinguish three groups of patients :
A) Ischemic ulcers in patients with CVI
1 - *With acute onset* : 6 cases with a sudden appearance of a large area of ischemic necrosis , 5 in the anterior portion and one in the posterior portion of the lower limb .
CVI was for simple varicose veins twice and for a Post Phlebitic Syndrome (PTS) three times
2 - *With sub acute onset* : 3 patients with a round ulcer surrounded by normal skin beginning as small spot and progressively increasing in size .One was in the anterior portion of the lower limb and the two others were just above the external malleolus .
All the patients had simple varicose veins .

B) Venous Ulcers in patients with severe ischemia

6 patients with PTS had a typical venous ulcer in the middle of Pigmented Dermatosclerosis which had been complicated by the onset or worsening of the ischemia .

At first all the patients were given 5000 IU of subcutaneous heparin , put in bed with the affected leg 30 cm. above heart level and strictly monitored clinically and with a pocket Doppler .

RESULTS

The position was terribly painful in all the patients and in three of them (one in group A1 and two in group B) led , in less than 10 minutes to the disappareance of the Doppler sound and the loss of sensibility . They were directly assessed for surgical treatment . One was amputated and two had a femoropopliteal by pass with one success and one failure .

In the remaining 13 patients perfusion of the feet was satisfactory even in elevation and they were helped with medications to bear the position till the edema disappeared .

A Unna boot was then applied in all of them for the entire time of the treatment and changed once or twice a week .

No kind of harmful effect was ever noted with this type of compression .

The 5 remaining patients of group A1 had a remarkable improvement but some rest pains remained and they all had to be operated for the arterial disease . One patient, with a severe form of cardiac failure had an axillo bifemoral by pass : she died of her cardiac problems in the 20th post operative day when the ulcer was painless and half healed .Three had a femoropopliteal by pass with their dilated saphenous vein , with partial resection of its more diseased parts and sclerotherapy for the remaining varices. They all were finally cured .The last patient had a peripheral arterial disease not suitable for any direct surgery .He had first an unsuccesful Lumbar Sympathectomy then the application of a Spinal Cord Stimulator which finally cured him .

One of the3 patients in group A2 healed with only compression sclerotherapy and two , in whom the bandage had resolved the rest pains but not the ulcer , both had a stripping and an aortobifemoral by pass after which one was rapidly and the second very slowly cured (6 months) always by keeping the compression .

Of the last 4 patients in group B , 3 healed with compression sclerotherapy alone .The fourth was operated of aorto femoral by pass because healing was too slow with final success .

DISCUSSION

Tibbs states that in ischemic patients the elevation can be disastrous [2].

Mc Callum had 8 patients out of 600 with leg ulcers in whom the compression bandage was considered responsible of the worsening of limb perfusion and finally of the gangrene . The some author collected similar results from the Scottish experience[3,4] .

In our Departement , Phebology is performed in the middle of a large experience of Arterial Surgery which has allowed us to perform several observations :

1 - Severe acute ischemia can often be tollerated without irreversible changes for hours, often for days . Subcutaneous heparin is useful to avoid the progression of ischemia .

2 - If the perfusion of an ischemic limb worsens in elevation it happens at an early stage, within one hour , and if it surpasses this time limit it rarely occurs .
3 - Patients with critical ischemia often learn to rest with pendent limbs.
At the beginning this position is favourable because it allows a better perfusion but in a short time it is complicated by the onset of a severe edema which in itself is deleterious. As a matter of fact the experience has demonstrated that the resolution of this kind of edema can frequently be obtained with light analgesics and simple bed rest and in these cases it is followed by a drammatic improvement of the perfusion and of the pain .
The three previous points led us to think that a simple trial of putting in elevation patients with Leg Ulcers and critical ischemia could be performed without real danger if they were strictly monitored during the first hour of elevation .The position increases almost always the pain because both the infected ulcer and the ischemic lim react this way but a differential diagnosis betwen the two conditions is easy .
In fact three of them did not withstand the position for ischemia and this was obvious in a few minutes beacause of the paleness of the toes with disappearance of the Doppler pulse and decrease of sensibility : the trial was interrupted without permanent harm.
In none of the others we observed a late decrease of the perfusion under the bandage with Unna boot usually employed .
All our cases but one were treated as outpatients therefore often the initial period of elevation did not succeed in abolishing the edema. In those cases the bandage permitted always a further improvement with decrease of leg size. .
The old Unna Boot is still the best example of inelastic bandage which can be applied without tension and follows exacly the shape of the leg so that its does not produces any Resting Pressure and cannot worsen the resting perfusion .On the some time , as demonstrated by Partsh [5] and reported also by Stemmer [6] , the Ambulatory Pressure of any inelastic bandage theoretically improves arterial perfusion and as a matter of fact all our patients had some improvement of the ischemia with good symptomatic palliation of the pains in all .In several of them the improvement which followed this conservative treatment was not sufficient to heal the ulcer and an operation on the arteries was necessary and finally performed electively.
Conclusions : A severe edema in patients with advanced ischemia of the lower limbs worsens tissue perfusion and can sometimes be abolished with simple elevation and bandaging with clinical improvement and no danger because if the ischemia is so critical not to allow the trial this condition becomes evident within one hour .
To keep a swollen leg dry is favorable even in those patients and can be seen also as a good and harmless emergency treatment particulary useful if a contemporary CVI exists.
In some of our patients this treatment , and the abolition of the dilated superficial veins with Sclerotherapy , could cure the Leg Ulcers without the necessity of Arterial Surgery.
In those cases in whom arterial surgery was finally required it could be performed out of emergency .

REFERENCES

1.   Faenza M et al. Les ulceres de jambe d'etiologie mixte arterielle et veineuse : traitement du facteur arteriel.   Actes du 8eme Congres Mondial de l'Union Internationale de Phlebologie 1983, 382 .

2.   Tibbs D J Varicose Veins and Related Disorders   Oxford   Butterworth - Heinemann 1992 , 353 .

3. Callum M J Harper D R Dale J J Ruckley C V Arterial disease in chronic leg ulceration : un underestimated hazard Brit Med J 1987; 295,929 .

4. Callum M J Ruckley C V Dale J J Harper D R . Hazards of compression treatment of the legs from Scottish surgeons .Brit Med J 1987;295,1382 .

5. Partsh H Untersuchungen zur Wirsamkeit der Intermittirenden Kompression in: Die Intermittirende Kompression . Sanoz Schwartz . Manheim 1983 ,323 .

6. Stemmer R Bases theoriques et pratiques de la contention in : Phlebologie en Pratique Quotidienne Expansion Scientifique Francaise . Paris 1982 ; 294.

Phlebology '95, D. Negus et al. (eds.). Phlebology (1995) Suppl. 1: 869-871

OP/7.2

Wound Healing with a New Growth Factor Formula

A.H. Asselman MD[1], J.C.J.M. Veraart MD[1], H.A.M. Neumann PhD[1]
and E.H.B.M. Gronenschild PhD[2]

[1] Department of Dermatology and [2] Medical Statistics, Academisch Ziekenhuis Maastricht,
Postbus 5800, 6202 AZ MAASTRICHT, The Netherlands

Wound healing with a new growth factor formula

Venous leg ulcers still are a major socioeconomic burden. The prevalence has been estimated to be as high as 1% of the total population[1] . There is a marked increase in the prevalence of chronic leg ulceration with age. Beside high venous walking pressure, several theories about the final cause of the ulceration have been proposed, but still not yet elucidated the exact mechanism.

Uptil now there are no drugs available to treat venous leg ulcers, although many kinds of wound dressings, creams, ointments and foams are available to improve the wound-environment of the venous leg ulcers. They are applicated in addition to compression therapy of the lower leg and their aim is to accelarate woundhealing. Compression therapy is of great importance in the healing of venous leg ulcers, it gives an improvement of the microcirculation of the skin[2]. However, many of these wounds continue to be a burden for patient and doctor.

A new woundhealing gel has now been developed by Life Medical Sciences, Inc. This new treatment (Cariel ™ Dermal) is based on the hypothesis that woundcell proliferation depends upon the composition of the microenvironment. Also the vascularisation in the area below and around the wound is of great importance. Cariel ™ Dermal is a gel consisting of modified serum free cell culture medium, prepared in an alginale gel matrix, supplemented with growth hormone, Thyroxine, insulin and transferrin.

Previous research:
Toxicity studies were performed by CIT (Centre International de Toxicologie). No sings of toxicity were observed. Animal studies have shown an acceleration in woundhealing[3,4] and an uncontrolled human study has also been done[5] .
Based on the results of these studies, it seems to be justified doning a controlled study on humans.

Study objectives:
This a randomised, open label, active-controlled study designed to asses the clinical safety and effectiveness of Cariel ™ Dermal in the treatment of venous leg ulcers compared to a standard therapy, hydrocolloid dressing (Comfeel, Humlebaek, Denmark). We use hydrocolloids on the control group because today it is believed to be the best of all available wound dressings[6,7].

It is hypothesized that Cariel ™ Dermal will heal venous leg ulcers in more patients at the end of 12 weeks of treatment than standard treatment with a hydrocolloid Comfeel. ($p < 0.05$)

Additionally it is hypothesized that Cariel ™ Dermal will heal venous leg ulcers faster than Comfeel when used over a 6 month period and that it will provide better sustained wound closure of venous leg ulcers than with a standard hydrocolloid dressing.

Study design:

Study-population consists of a 120 patients between the age of 18 and 85 years with a venous leg ulcer that has a surface area of at least 1.5 cm^2 and not greater than 15 cm^2. Patients may not have diabetes or any other disease and may take no medication that may interfere with the ulcer healing process. Each ulcer is diagnosed as a venous leg ulcer by dopplersonography and light-plethysmography. In a wash-out period patients are treated during 1 week with a dry bandage only. Patients determined to be eligible are randomised into a Control group or a Study group. Both groups are treated at home every other day by a team of trained nurses. They receive the wound dressing and a non-elastic bandage for compression therapy of the leg. The Cariel ™ Dermal which fills up the wound, is covered by a polyurethaanfilm. Patients will be treated until complete wound closure occurs. After 12 weeks a blinded dermatologists will evaluate the wound.

The maximum study treatment period is 6 months for all patients. Every week patients are evaluated by a doctor (sub-investigator) and standerised slides are made. Quantitative planimetry measurements will be done with a specially designed Computerised Wound Image Analysis System.

Results:

An interim analysis of the study has been done in which 16 patients were treated with the new formula (Cariel ™ Dermal) and 14 with the hydrocolloid wound dressing (Comfeel).

After 4 and 8 weeks of treatment the study group showed a mean decrease in wound surface of 270.88 mm^2 and 577.97 mm^2. In the control group the figures were 158.66 mm^2 and 388.53 mm^2. Most patients treated with Cariel ™ Dermal showed an increase in granulation tissue in the woundbed already after a few treatments. At first some patients showed mild maceration around the ulcer. Later this problem was no longer present. No other side effects were seen, especially no systemic.

Conclusions:

The new growth factor gel Cariel ™ Dermal seems to be a new promising form of treatment in the healing of venous leg ulcers. The results show that it is at least as effective as the currently best available wound dressing.

References:

1. Callem M. Prevalence of Chronic Leg Ulceration and Severe Chronic Venous Disease in western countriesPhlebology Suppl. 1 (1992) 6-12

2. Tazelaar D.J., Neumann H.A.M., Veraart J.C.J.M., Korstanje M.J. Compressietherapie bij de behandeling van chronische veneuze insufficientie. NTvG 1994; 138: 1940-1944

3. Lindenbaum E.S. Personal communication.

4. E.S. Rosenbaum, M. Tendler, D. Beach. Serum-free cell culture medium induces acceleration of woundhealing in guinea-pigs. Burns 1995;21:110-5

5. Lindenbaum E.S., Ullman Y., Har Shay Y., Hirshowitz B., Tendler M., Beach D., (Sandiego 1993): Preliminary clinical application of cell culture medium in the treatment of wounds.

6. Moffart C.J. et al. A trial of a hydrocolloid dressing in the management of indolent ulceration. Journal of wound care september/october, vol 1. no 3, 1992

7. Gamborg Nielsen P., Munk Madsen S., Strömberg L.. Treatment of Chronic Leg Ulcers with a Hydrocolloid Dressing. Acta Derm Venerol. (Stockholm) supplementum 152

Phlebology '95, D. Negus et al. (eds.). Phlebology (1995) Suppl. 1: 872-873

OP/15.5

A Prospective Randomised Trial of Class 2 and Class 3 Elastic Compression in the Prevention of Venous Ulceration

D.R. Harper, E.A. Nelson, B. Gibson, R.J. Prescott and C.V. Ruckley

Lothian and Forth Valley Leg Ulcer Study. Falkirk & District Royal Infirmary, Royal Infirmary of Edinburgh, Edinburgh, Scotland

INTRODUCTION

Graduated compression is the mainstay of the treatment of venous ulcers [1,2]. This is supported by several physiological studies which have confirmed increased in femoral vein velocity [3,4], increased venous pressure [5], subcutaneous blood flow [3,6] and total blood flow [6,7]. Compression hosiery also is advised in patient management following leg ulcer healing but the optimum grade of compression required to prevent recurrence is not known.[6,8] In so far as grade 3 compression may be associated with poor compliance, particularly in the elderly, any advantage of high compression may be compromised by poor compliance. This trial was designed to investigate the recurrence rate and compliance associated with two strengths of compression hosiery.

METHODS

Three hundred patients with newly healed venous leg ulcers were recruited into this trial of class 2 and class 3 stockings. Upon entry into the trial, they were investigated using hand held Doppler to determine the nature and extent of venous disease present. They were measured and fitted for compression hosiery,and given verbal and written information on the care of their legs. Follow up appointments were arranged every 4 months for inspection of the leg,continued education on skin care,and re-measurement and supply of hosiery. The trial period was for 5 years. The patient continued to attend if a change in strength of stocking was required or after reulceration.

RESULTS

The results were analysed on an intention to treat basis. One hundred and fifty patients were randomised to each compression grade. Major recurrence within 36 - 60 months was found in 32% of the class 2 group and 21% of the class 3 group (p=0.034, Chi-square). Recurrence was significantly associated with non-compliance and class 2 stockings were tolerated by significantly more patients

DISCUSSION

Leg ulcers recurr after healing in the majority of cases [9,10]. Healing therefore represents an opportunity for secondary prevention either by conservative measures or venous surgery. It is logical to offer newly healed patients professionally fitted graduated compression.   The precise mechanism of action of compression therapy unknown.   Certainly swelling is inhibited and apporoximation of valve leaflets by the external compression has been suggested as a possible factor[11,12].   It is known to enhance venous function [3-8] but the significance of oedma in the aetiology of leg ulceration is not clear .

From this study of 300 patients, it would appear that the higher compression hosiery is more effective than the lower in preventing the recurrence of venous ulcers, but that patients find the higher compression difficult to tolerate.   Failure to comply predisposed to recurrence.   These results suggest that an effective strategy for secondary prevention is first to prescribe Class 2 stockings and encourage compliance, then on refitting offer the higher grade.   Any non compliers might then revert to Class 2 rather than abandon treatment altogether, while those that comply will enjoy enhanced protection.

REFERENCES

1 Blair SD, Wright DDI, Backhouse CM, Riddle E, McCollum CN. Sustained compression and healing of chronic venous ulcers. Br med J 1988;297:1159-1161.

2 Dale JJ, Gibson B. Compression bandaging for venous ulcers. Professional Nurse 1987;7:211-214.

3 Lawrence D, Kakkar VV. Graduated, static, external compression of the lower limb; a physiological assessment. Brit surg J 1980;67:119

4 Sigel B, Edelstein AL, Felix WR. Compression of the deep venous system of the lower leg dring inactive recumbency. Arch Surg 1973;106:38-43.

5 Somerville JJF, Brow GO, Byre PJ. The effects of elastic stockings on superficial venous pressures in patients with venous insufficiency. Br J Surg 1974;61:979-981.

6 Jones NAG, Webb PJ, Rees RI, Kakkar VV. A physiological study of elastic compression stockings in venous disorders of the legs. Brit surg J 1980;67:569-573.

7 Gjores JF, Thulesius O. Compression treatment in venous insufficiency evaluated with foot volumetry. Vasa 1977;6:364-368.

8 Dale JJ, Gibson B. Which compression stocking? Professional Nurse 1989;11:550-556.

9 Callam MJ, Ruckley CV, Harper DR, Dale JJ. Chronic ulceration of the leg: extent of the problem and provision of care. Br med J 1985;290:1855-1866.

10 Moffatt CJ, Dorman MC. Recurrence of leg ulcers within a community ulcer service. J wound care 1995;4:57-61.

11 Sarin S, Scurr JH, Coleridge Smith PD. Mechanism of action of external compression on venous function. Br J Surg 1992;79:499-502.

12 van Bemmelen PS, Beach K, Bedford G, Strandness DE, Jr. The mechanism of venous valve closure. Its relationship to the velocity of reverse flow. Archives of Surgery 1990;125:617-619.

Phlebology '95, D. Negus et al. (eds.). Phlebology (1995) Suppl. 1: 874-876

P156

Conservative Ambulatorial Treatment of Venous Ulcers: Analysis of Our Experience

M. Domanin, P. Bonadeo, R. Vitiello, M.R. Della Vedova and G.B. Agus

Institute of Vascular Surgery and Angiology, University of Milan, Italy

INTRODUCTION

Venous ulcers of the lower limbs are present in about 0.5-1% of the western adult population. About one third of the patients affected by chronic venous disease is exposed, within 10 years, to an ulcerative involvement which, in 60% of instances, is relapsing. Even if the medical literature does not give precise data on the actual rate of varicous or postphlebitic ulcers (VaU and PFU), these are valued from 40 to 60% of all the ulcerative lesions of the lower limbs.

The chronic venous hypertension is the primary etiopathogenetic moment to which venous ulcer is connected both for varicous and postphlebitic ulcers. This is essentially supported by three conditions of impaired venous functionality: 1) failure of the saphenous systems; 2) incontinence of the perforating veins; 3) valvular failure of the deep venous system.

The therapeutic strategy has to eliminate varicose veins (i.e. the reflux from the saphenous system) if present, to correct short reflux from the incompetence of the perforating veins (which is constant in the postphlebitic syndrome and frequent in the varicose syndrome) and to minimize the stasis oedema bound to the failure of the deep venous valvular system. In 90% of instances the treatment of venous ulcers is conservative i.e. ambulatorial, sometimes associated with sclerotherapy. In the remaining 10% of patients short hospitalization is needed for varicouse veins stripping and/or for subfascial ligature of perforating veins. The correct therapy does not consist only in healing of the ulcerative lesion but also in the prevention against possible and frequent recurrences.

MATERIALS AND METHODS

In the Ambulatorial Service of Institute of Vascular Surgery and Angiology of Milan University, 224 patients (240 legs) affected by venous ulcers were treated from October 1988 to November 1994; 16 patients had a bilateral lesion. The average age was 73 years (22-95) with a female prevalence (67,4%). The average time of lesion onset, at the first visit, was 3 months (1 month-2 years) with mean area of 3,5 cm2 (0.5-40 cm2); 89 patients (39,7%) reported previous recurrent ulcers. Each patient was submitted to an accurate anamnesis and a careful clinical evaluation in order to identify the etiopathogenesis of the lesion. In many instances the distinction between VaU and PPU is not so clear and for this reason we mainly carried out non-invasive diagnostic tests (U.S.Doppler and EchocolorDoppler) and, in a reduced number of patients, phlebography. We have submitted all the patients to a bacteriological examination in order to survey the presence of bacterial suprainfection and to begin selective antibiotic therapy; in presence of persistent ulcers exceeding one year from onset and characterized by hypertrophy with destroyed borderlines, we have performed biopsy on lesion margin.

On the ground of these data we have subdivided the lesions as follows: 144 (60,0%) PPU, 68 (28.8%) VaU, 28 (11,7%) other causes (3 hypertensive ulcers of Martorell, 14 post-traumatic ulcers, 7 venous ulcers with associated signs or symptoms of peripheric arteriopathy, 1 thalassemic ulcer, 2 neoplastic ulcer and 1 ulcer in course of rheumatoid arthritis).

In all the patients we have cleansed the lesion with hypoclorite solution or potassium permanganate 1:10000 or saline solution or fibrinolitic ointments or katadynic silver according to the local conditions and tolerance. Elasto-compression was always set up from the first moment through a mobile elastic bandage. When the cleansing is obtained we set up a fixed elastic adesive bandage under which we applied a zinc oxide bandage in order to improve the cutaneous trophism and avoid the appearence of allergic reactions; a Reston 3M sponge was moulded over the lesion to exert a greater compression and to absorb secretions: this bandage was renewed every 7-14 days. In case of overlying bacterial infection, dermatitis or when the daily cleansing of the lesion was necessary we continue to use a mobile elastic bandage with corticosteroids or fibrinolitic ointments. Sometimes we associate pentoxifylline to improve peripheral trophism and to quicken the healing of lesions. In other instance, expecially with pain, however, we used an occlusive hydrocolloid bandage which stimulates the recovery of the lesion and maintained a warm-moist microclimate.

On the basis of the data obtained from the non invasive tests we carried out a sclerotherapy of incompetent perforating veins and of the ectasic veins near the lesion in 34 (14,1%) patients. Twentyfive (10,4%) patients, with varices of the saphenous area, either primitive or secondary to deep venous thrombosis (DVT) with recanalization of the deep venous system or incompetent perforating veins were submitted to surgical interventions. When possible, we prefer to perform surgery after the recovery of ulceration, to prevent infection of the surgical wounds. In some instances the intervention was made with the lesion still open, limiting ourselves to a short stripping associated with post-operative sclerotherapy of the distal branches. After the healing we prescribed an elastic stocking; the patients were checked periodically (every 2 months) for an early individuation of eventual relapses.

RESULTS

During the treatment, 33 (14,7%) patients were lost and so them were cancelled from the study. On 191 patients we have obtained 164 healings (85,8%); of these 104 were PPU, 40 VaU, 14 post-traumatic ulcers, 4 mixed ulcers and 2 ulcers of other nature. The average recovery time was 91 days for PPU (7-330 days); 47 days

876

(10-120 days) for VaU and 79 (15-150 days) for the other ulcers. Nineteen patients are still under therapy, while 8 failed to heal for too much extensive area and will be submitted to plastic surgery. Forty (20,9%) had relapses (27 PPU, 5 VaU, 3 mixed ulcers, 4 post-traumatic and 1 thalassemic) at an average distance of 138 days from PPU recovery, of 195 days from VaU healing and of 60 days from the others. In 52.9% we obtained the secondary recovery. We noticed the presence of cutaneous neoplasia in 2 patients: the first was a basicellular epithelioma and the second a cutaneous localization of a lymphoma. Both were directed to an oncology center and excluded from surveillance.

CONCLUSIONS

Our experience leads us to assert that good results in the healing of venous ulcers can be obtained according to two fundamental moments: 1) Analysis of the conditions supporting venous hypertension; 2) Adoption of a personalized therapeutic strategy.
Ultrasonic methods, such as US Doppler and EchocolorDoppler, are necessary for an accurate study of the superficial and deep venous system in order to point out failure of the saphenous or of the deep venous system, the presence of a previous DVT and of the incompetent perforating veins. Therapy must corrects all the conditions of venous hypertension through the application, in all instances, of an elastocompression sometimes associated to sclerotherapy or surgery. On the other hand, the local topical therapy plays an important role to achieve good asepsis and cleasing of the lesion. Standardization of local therapy is difficult because the personal response and the frequent appearance of intolerance, often local but sometimes systemic, to the multiple pharmaceutical substances used. The maintenance of the results obtained is possible through the rigorous adoption of elastocompression with elastic stockings and the respect of hygienic-prophylactic rules such as a correct deambulation, a control of the overweight and an eventual passive mobilization. In conclusion we can assert that the correct application of these principles leads to satisfactory results on the grounds of costs, times of healing and prevention of recurrences. Hospitalization generally is almost never necessary in case of VU; so we think that ambulatorial treatment must be considered the treatment of choice.

REFERENCES

1) AGRIFOGLIO G., BONADEO P.: "Venous leg ulcers: conservative treatment". Proceedings of the Ist Mediterranean Congress of Angiology, 1988, May 29-June 3, Corfu' Minerva Medica Ed.
2) AGRIFOGLIO G., MONTORSI W., DONADI G.C.: "Flebologia". 1983 Masson Italia Editore, Milano.
3) CALLAM M.J., RUCKLEY C.V., HAPER D.R. et Al.: "Chronic ulceration of the leg, extent of this problem and provision of care. Br.Med.J. 1985;29:1855.
4) CIKRIT D.F., NICHOLS W.K., SILVER D.: "Surgical management of refractory venous stasis ulceration" J.Vasc.Surg. 1988;7: 473.
5) COLERIDGE SMITH P.D., THOMAS P., SCHRR J.H., DORMANDY J.A.: "Causes of venous ulceration; a new hypotesis". Br.Med.J. 1988;296: 1726.
6) CORNWALL J.V., DORIC C.J., LEWIS J.D.: "Leg ulcers" Br.J.Surg. 1986;73: 693.
7) NEGUS D.: "Leg ulcers. A practical approach to management" 1st Ed. Oxford: Butterworth-Heinemann : 1991.

Phlebology '95, D. Negus et al. (eds.). Phlebology (1995) Suppl. 1: 877-879

P157

Treatment of Leg Ulcers. The Effect of Dressing with a Hydrocellular Polyurethane

S. Massi, C. Ruggieri, A.M. Peccatori, G. Botta and S. Mancini

III Department of General Surgery and Pabisch Center of Phlebology, Faculty of Medicine and Surgery, University of Siena, Italy

INTRODUCTION

Many researchers have confirmed the beneficent effects of the occlusive treatments in the wounds healing both in the animal and in the man. In experimental wounds they seem to encourage the healing by different processes; an interesting hypothesis, recently expressed, based itself on the fact that in the wounds secretions many growth factor, able to modulate the tissue reparation, are present. The ulcers secretions, under occlusive treatment, create a microenviroment, favourable to the fibroblasts growth, as well as to the epidermic migration in vitro; this suggest that in a biologically occluded lesion a growth factors activation exist, whose accumulation may significantly cause the healing. Another important datum is that to get a ulcer epithelization is essential the preservation of a firm and gradual growth potential to start from margins, assuring a local blood flux.

The occlusive treatments, besides to improve the local blood sprinkling, work also on the derma level, causing the connective tissue regeneration. In the venous ulcers, in particular, these treatments, by the fibrinolysis stimulus and the angiogenesis stimulus, lead to a reduction of the perycapillary fibrin cuffes.

Clinical studies document a cleaning action, a stimulus to the granulation and to the re-epithelization from the occlusive treatment that therefore intervene positively in all phases of the cicatrization process of a ulcer.

Particular attention has to be put in the chronic ulcers treatment, inevitably colonized by the bacteria, in which the association between occlusion and infection complications takes place. In this case, in the occlusive treatment after a infection focuses drainage, uniting to the surgical cleaning a specific systemic antibiotictherapy cicle.

The traditional occlusive hidrocolloidal treatments are made by a internal absorbing stratum with hydrocolloi and by a polyurethane external stratum. Now to these a new occlusive hydrocellular treatment of polyurethane is added, particularly interesting, called Allevyn.

MATERIALS AND METHODS

For our research we have used the aforesaid occlusive hydrocellular treatment. Allevyn has a trilaminate frame of polyurethane, including a special tridimensional reticolum in the stratum in contact with the lesion, for his tridimensional particular frame results antisticking, the central hydrofilic stratum has an high absorption capacity and may absorb until ten times the same exudate weight; the extrernal stratum, then, being semipermeable, precedes the bacteria and fluids passage, however promoting the steam, oxigen and other gases passage to assure a good healing evolution.

We have used this product in the last 3 years on 80 patients suffering from lower limbs venous ulcers. 48 of these were females (60%) and 32 males (40%) with a middle age of 66 years (min.40-max.91). The venous ulcers diagnosis has been put on the ground of a precise clinical examination and of a strumental research with ultrasonography doppler c.w.

The ulcer valuation parameters have been the following: dimensions, deepth, seat, quantity and quality of the secretions, periulcerous tissue condition. Therefore morphometric remarks have been done on a millimeter transparent pellicle and also photographic remarks and secretions tampon for bacteriological examination.

After the lesion cleaning with physiological solution, we have applied Allevyn, making it be over one centimeter the ulcer border. The treatment has been fixed with a transparent pellicle of polyurethane (flexigrid), that, thanks to its peculiarities, protects the periulcerous tissue. The treatment may be ended with a rigid bandage application on the affected limb. The treatment has been renewed at the beginning every two days; then the time interval has been protracted until at most seven days with best remarks, because the lesion isn't subjected to continuous microtraumatism, due to its removal; the very secreting ulcer have requested homever a biweekly treatment renewal. During the removal the Allevyn seemed partly or totally imbued by the secretions, assuming in the external stratum a brownish colour, leaving in general the ulcer well clean, with a integral periulcerous tissue. In some patients we have been obliged to suspend the treatment for some weeks, because, probably owing to bacterial overinfections, an extreme exudate production happened with periulcerous tissue soaking and a regression of the same ulcers.

RESULTS

All the patients cured have refered a progressive reduction of the pain already from the first applications of the product. The healing has been got in 62 patients, in a middle time of 56 days (min.24-max.65). In 12 patients, in cure about 2 months, we have got a remarkable reduction of the ulcer dimentions, with a clear improvement of the local conditions. Four patients, suffering since 30 years from venous ulcers with big dimensions, have required the treatment suspension for some weeks.

We haven't allergies events to the product: the intollerance, evident in few cases, was not likely creditable to the product.

The results we have got, allow us the assertion that this new product is useful surely and therefore it may be included in the therapeutic luggafe of the lower limbs ulcer treatment, that represent the invalidating complication of a diffuse pathology as the chronical peripherical venous insufficiency.

SUMMARY

The lower limbs venous ulcers form an important reason of invalidating disease, with an high social cost, by the terms of lost working days.

In this work the Authors relete the preliminary results of the topical treatment of a group of patients suffering from lower limbs venous ulcers; it has been executed by a occlusive, absorbing, hydrocellular polyurethane dressing.

80 patients have been subjected to ambulatory treatments by by means of hydrocellular polyurethane plaques employment. It's a matter of 48 females (60%) and 32 males (40%), with a middle age of 66 yars (min.40-max.91).

The diagnosis of venous ulcer has been both clinical and instrumental, on the ground of the anamnesis, of the objective examination and of the ultrasonography Doppler c.w..

The morphometric remark of the ulcer have been executed before of the treatment and successively weekly, describing a lesion map on a millimeter transparent pellicle (flexigrid). Treatment application of polyurethane has been always preceded by a ulcer tampon for bacteriological examination and by the lesion cleaning by means of physiological solution. The treatment has been renewed, in the ground of ulcer quantity secretions, with variable intervals from 2 to 7 days. In all patients it has been associated a anelastic compressive bandage of the concerned limb.

About the 80 patients, 64 have reached the healing in a average time of 56 days (min.24-max:65. days), 12 are now cured and on the way of healing, while 4 have asked for the treatment temporary interruption.

The Allevyn has shown a good tolerance and it has not been found any allergy event.

REFERENCES

1   Eriksson G. Comparison of two occlusive bandages in the treatment of venous leg ulcers.Brit J Dermatol 1986; 114:227-30.
2.   Backhouse C.M., Blair S.D., Savage A.P., Walton J., McCollum C.N.:controlled trial of occlusive dressing in healing chronic venous ulcers. Br J Surg 1987;74:626-7.
3.   Williams D.L., Dykes P.J., Marks R. Effects of a new hydrocolloid dressing on healing of full thickness wounds in normal volunteers. An environment for healing; the role of occlusion. Ed T Ryan: Royal Society of Medicine. International Congress and Symposium Series No 88.

Phlebology '95, D. Negus et al. (eds.). Phlebology (1995) Suppl. 1: 880-882

OP/6.6

Treatment of Recalcitrant Venous Leg Ulcer with Retro-Grade Intravenous Infusion and PGE 1

N.G. Weindorf, T. Pfeil and A. Popp

Department of Dermatology, St. Elizabeth Hospital, Oberhausen, Germany

Introduction

In 1908 August Bier presented a new method to achieve local anesthesia in the extremities[1]. He used it for joint resection, necrectomy and amputation. In his publication we find remarkable descriptions which show that he foresaw future possibilities which go beyond simple regional anesthesia.

In the 1970's, Acevedo of Chile, revived Bier's method to treat patients with arterial occlusive disease[2]. With the aid of radioactive tracers, Partsch and his co-workers, demonstrated that retrograde intravenous pressure infusion in an arterial occluded segment of an extremity yielded a tissue concentration that is three times (3x) that using intraarterial injection and seven times (7x) that using standard i.v. infusion[3]. With urokinase as pharmacological agent, Partsch and Jochmann could obtain good therapeutic results in patients with chronic venous leg ulcers[4].
We decided to examine the efficacy of retrograde i.v. pressure infusion using prostaglandin E1 because of its known positive effects on nutritive blood flow, on function of platelets and leucocytes and on permeability of microcirculatory vessels. We were also impressed by the examinations of Pflug who had treated patients with different vascular diseases[5].

Patients and Methods

Six patients: three women and three men, 53-74 years of age, were treated. The duration of the ulcer was 1.5 to 3 years. Examination by Doppler ultrasound showed deep venous refluxes as a sign of intrafascial venous insufficiency in all cases. Digital photoplethysmography indicated muscle pump insufficiency that could not be improved by tourniquet test. The intravenous infusion was done into the dorsum of the foot of the arterial occluded extremity. 30 ml mepivacaine 1%, 20µg PgE1 (alprostadil) and 5.000 I.E.heparin were injected. The occlusion was maintained for 15 minutes. The treatment was for three times (3x) over five weeks. Transcutaneous pO_2 measurement was carried out before, during, and after the infusion. Measuring area was the inner aspect of the lower leg, electrode heating temperature was 44°C.

Results

The transcutaneous pO_2 values obtained at the end of the full treatment period revealed an increase compared with values measured at the start of therapy. The mean values were 38,2 +/- 9,8 mm Hg and 31,4 +/- 7,2 mm Hg respectively (see fig. 1). Four patients experienced healing of the ulcer.

Discussion

In our study which must be regarded as a pilot study, the retrograde intravenous pressure infusion showed positive clinical effects in two third of the patients. Thes increase of the transcutaneous oxygen pressure measurement after therapy probably indicates an improvement in the local microcirculation.

Using this method, there are some points which have to be taken into consideration:

- Local anesthetics with little systemic toxicity should be used . We do not use bupivacaine or etidocaine because of their long lasting activity and consequently higher systemic toxicity. In the United Kingdom, seven death have been recorded with bupivacaine using Bier's method.

- The occlusion time should not be below 15', otherwise there is a risk that higher amounts of the anesthesic will flood into the systemic circulation.

- The opening of the arterial occlusion should be done very slowly, i.e. over 3-5 minutes, for the above-mentioned reason.

- Following Bier's occlusion, patients should be carefully monitored via EKG, intermittent blood pressure controls performed and finally prophylactic application of oxygen.

- No absolute contraindication has been observed, however, the application of this method should be carried out with caution in patients with cardiac problems or convulsive disease.

Taken as a whole the retrograde intravenous pressure infusion with PgE 1 is a valuable additional method in conservative treatment. High tissue concentrations of the pharmacological agent may be obtained through this method, therefore making therapy more effective. Further studies including a control group will be necessary to confirm these previous data.

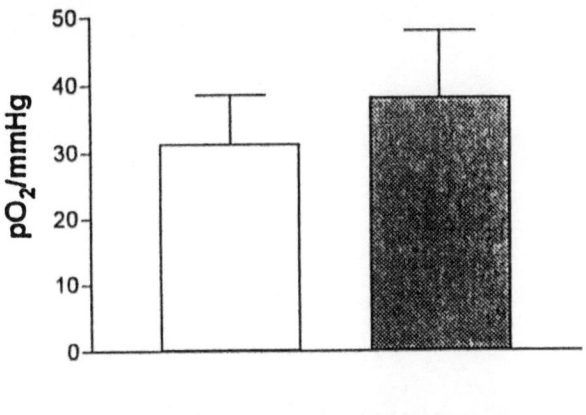

Fig. 1. Mean transcutaneous pO_2 values before starting the retrograde intravenous infusion therapy with PgE 1 and after five weeks of treatment.

882

References

1. Bier A, Über einen neuen Weg Localanästhesie an den Gliedmaßen zu erzeugen.Verh Dtsch Ges Chirurgie 1908;37:204-213.
2. Acevedo A, Schnell A, Persisting reactive hyperemia in the treatment of arterial insufficiency. J Cardiovasc Surg (Suppl): 433.
3. Partsch H, Jochmann W, Mostbeck A, Hirschl M, Nuklearmedizinische Untersuchungen zur Gewebekonzentration und hämodynamische Effekte von retrograden intravenösen Druckinfusionen. Wien Med WSchr 1993;143:172-176.
4. Partsch H, Jochmann W, Urokinase bei resistenten Unterschenkelgeschwüren: Therapie mit retrograder intravenöser Druckinfusion. Wien Med WSchr 1993;143:187-189.
5. Pflug J, Bier's intravenous method for Prostaglandin E treatment of critical ischemia of the leg. Vasa 1988;17:42-46.

Phlebology '95, D. Negus et al. (eds.). Phlebology (1995) Suppl. 1: 883-884

OP/15.8

A Study of Nurses' Bandaging Technique Using Elastic and Inelastic Bandages

E.A. Nelson[1,4,5], D.A. Brown[1], B. Gibson[2], J.J. Dale[1], J.C. Barbenel[4] and C.V. Ruckley[1]

[1] Lothian and Forth Valley Leg Ulcer Study, Royal Infirmary Edinburgh
[2] Falkirk and District Royal Infirmary
[3] University of Edinburgh
[4] University of Strathclyde
[5] University of Liverpool

Background

Nurses' bandaging techniques have been found to be poor, and to improve after training [1,2,3]. It was not known, however, if elastic bandages were easier to apply than inelastic, and if improvement in technique with training was different in the two types of bandage.

Objective

This study was designed to whether bandaging skill was influenced by the physical characteristics of the bandage.

Design

Comparative study of three bandages, one inelastic, the remaining two contain elastomeric fibres; Rosidal K (Lohmann), Setopress (Seton) and Tensopress (Smith and Nephew).

Subjects

48 trained community nurses attending leg ulcer study days.

Measurements

The nurses applied each of the bandages to one leg which had a pressure monitor attached. Sitting pressures were recorded and bandage placement noted. These were repeated after training in bandaging.

884

Results

The initial bandage pressure profiles were unsatisfactory, the most common reason was production of tourniquet at the calf .

Initial results

Bandage	mean calf / ankle pressure; (> 1 = tourniquet)
Rosidal K	1.343
Setopress	1.095
Tensopress	1.291

After training

After training the bandaging improved, the pressure gradient from the ankle to calf was improved in all bandages.

Bandage	mean calf / ankle pressure; (> 1 = tourniquet)
Rosidal K	1.17
Setopress	0.90
Tensopress	0.86

Conclusion

The most frequent problem in applying bandages was the production of a tourniquet at the calf. Bandaging technique with all bandages improved after training, however, the bandages without elastomeric fibres seemed to be more difficult to apply than those containing elastomers as a tourniquet effect was still a common fault.

References

1. Logan RA, Thomas S, Harding EF, Collyer G Bandage design and bandager experience: The effect on sub-bandage pressure. Phlebology, (1992): 7; 2, 89.

2. Millard LG, Blecher A, Fentem PH The pressure at which nursing staff apply compression bandages when treating patients with varicose ulcers. In Negus D, Jantet G. (Eds). Phlebology '85. John Libbey Co Ltd, 1986. p682-685.

3. Nelson EA, Ruckley CV, Barbenel JC. Improvements in bandaging technique following training. Journal of Wound Care1995: 4; 4: 181-184.

Phlebology '95, D. Negus et al. (eds.). Phlebology (1995) Suppl. 1: 885-887

P159

Hydrocolloid and Support Therapy in the Treatment of Venous Leg Ulcers

J. Gawrychowski, B. Lazar-Czyzewska and A. Romanski

Varicose Vein Clinic, 41-800 Zabrze ul. Gen. de Gaulle'a 60, Poland

INTRODUCTION

Chronic venous ulceration (C.V.U.) is a difficult problem for a therapeutist because of its chronic and recurrent characteristics. About 0.2 - 1.0% of the human population are affected with this disorder (6,7,11) but the percentage is higher (3.5 - 5.0%) in the group of elderly people, namely over 60 years of age (4,6,10, 20). Doppler's and venographic examinations showed that about 28 - 53% of the patients with C.V.U. had injuries to superficial venous system in extremities, about 32% had insufficiency both in superficial and deep veins and only about 15% had deep venous insufficiency. It seems that more than a half of them could benefit from surgical treatment (4,17,18).

The aim of our study was to review the results of management of patients with C.V.U. using hydrocolloid dressing and a compression by use of an elastic bandage.

MATERIAL AND METHODS

Out of 181 cases treated at the Outpatient Polyclinic of Zabrze between 15 June 1992 and September 1994, 156 patients were included in the study. The group consisted of 123 (78. 8%) women aged 36 - 88, mean 61 years, and 33 (21.2%) men aged 30 - 70, mean 57 years. 141 (90.7%) patients had been treated for a single or multiple inflammation of the veins, both superficial and deep, in the extremity affected. 118 (75.9%) cases were recurrences. Ulceration had lasted from 7 days to 22 years (mean 54 months) prior the first contact of these patients with our clinic. Nearly 85% of the ulcers were resistant to other kinds of ambulatory or hospital treatment (10%). Out of 156 patients, diabetes was diagnosed in 7 (4, 6%). Patients with atheromatous trophic changes were excluded. Intensity of C.V.U. was estimated by planimetric method. Ulcers were washed with isotonic salt solution and wrapped by turns with hydrocolloid dressing (Varihesive Hydroactive Dressing Squibb Corp.), extending 1 - 1.5 cm beyond their edges. The dressings were replaced every 6 - 7 days. Patients were instructed to stay in bed and wash the dressing surfaces with boiled water every day (1 - 2x) in order to remove any exudate that may have soaked through. Each time the dressing was replaced, "Codoban" elastic bandage of Trocomed, Łódź, was applied to the patient's leg.

Clinical evaluation of the treatment was performed in accordance with the following scale (1):

III	-	complete healing (100%)
II	-	significant improvement (60 - 99%)
I	-	improvement (30 - 59%)
0	-	no change (below 29%)
-I	-	deterioration.

RESULTS

In 112 out of 181 patients (61.9%), the above method resulted in the complete healing of the ulcerations (table 1.).

Tab. 1 - Results of treatment of 156 patients with 181 venous leg ulcers

Group % of healed extent	Nr of patients	Nr of ulcers	Ulceration extent from-to (mean) in cm^2	Duration of treatment (days) (mean)
III 100%	102	112	0.5 - 400 (34)	7 - 187 (68)
II 60-90%	12^x	15	5 - 324 (55)	91 - 183 (155)
I 30-59%	14^{xx}	18	12.5 - 600 (206)	78 - 426 (79)
0 (to 29%)	10^{xxx}	13	12 - 430 (84)	84 - 101 (88)
-I (deterioration)	4	5	8 - 620 (405)	1 x after 43 days
treatment discontinued	14	18	1 - 390 (16)	7 - 28 (14)

still under treatment
[x] - 9 patients
[xx] - 10 patients
[xxx] - 7 patients

The duration of the treatment was 7 - 187 days (mean 68 days) in this group. The mean extent of the ulcers healed was 336 cm^2 (0.5 - 400 cm^2). In 12 patients (7.7%) (15 lower extremities) with significant improvement, the ulceration extended from 5 to 324 cm^2 (mean 55 cm^2) where the treatment lasted 91 - 183 days (mean 155 days). In 14 patients (18 ulcers) classified in the 1st group, mean duration of the treatment was 79 days and the ulcers extended from 12.5 to 600 cm^2 (mean 206 cm^2). Only 10 patients [13 (7.2%) ulcers] had no improvement, whereas in 4 [5 (2.8%) ulcers], deterioration was observed (in 2 after 21, in 1 after 43 and in 1 after 51 days). In the latter group, the ulceration extent was 8 - 620 cm^2 (mean 405 cm^2). Fourteen patients discontinued the treatment (mean time - 14 days) in spite of the relatively small extent of the ulcers (mean 16 cm^2 - from 1 to 39 cm^2). 121 patients (78%) reported disappearance or significant reduction of pain soon after the ulceration had been covered with hydrocolloid dressing. 3 patients (1.9%) complained of pain intensification related to the application of the dressing. All of them discontinued the treatment. Complications included maceration of the skin around the ulcers (in 6.5% of patients) or flare and eczema (in 1.9% of patients).

REFERENCES:

1. Callam M.J., Eagistein W.H., Lynch D.J.: Meeting the challenge of leg ulcers. (S.L.Backhus ed.) Patient Care 1988, 22, 24-34
2. Clinical experience with DuoDerm in venous ulcers and clot resolution in experimental full-thickness wounds. Cherry G.W., Cherry C.A., Jones R.L., Ryan F., Ryan T.J., in: Cederholm - Williams S.A., Ryan T.J., Lydon M.J. eds. Fibrinolysis and angiogenesis in wound healing. Princeton, N.J.: Experta Medica 1988, 19-23
3. Cornwall J.V., Dove C.J., Lewis J.D.: Leg ulcers: epidemiology and aetiology. Br. J. Surg. 1986, 73, 693-6
4. Halbook T.: Leg ulcer epidemiology. Acta Chir. Scand. Suppl. 1988, 544, 17-20
5. Hansson C., Andersson E., Swanbeck G.: Leg ulcer epidemiology in Gothenburg. Acta Chir. Scand. Suppl. 1988, 544, 12-16
6. Sethia K.K., Darke S.G.: Long saphenous incompetence as a cause of venous ulceration. Br J. Surg. 1984, 71, 754-755
7. Shami S.K., Sarin S., Cheatle T.R., Scurr J.H., Smith P.D.C.: Venous ulcer and the superficial venous system. J. Vasc. Surg. 1993, 17, 487-490
8. Vollmer H.: Ulcus Cruris-ein Problem fur Patient und Arzt Z. Allg. Med. 1991, 67, 1791-1792

Phlebology '95, D. Negus et al. (eds.). Phlebology (1995) Suppl. 1: 888-891

OP/15.1

Reduction of Venous Reflux by Compression: A Comparison Between Short and Long Stretch Material

G. Menzinger, M. Horakova, W. Mayer and H. Partsch

Department of Dermatology, Wilhelminen-Hospital, Vienna, Austria

INTRODUCTION

Recent studies on the incidence of venous reflux after DVT showed that at the end of one year follow up nearly two thirds of the patients had developed valvular reflux. In more then 50% venous reflux was noted in the popliteal vein [1]. These refluxes cause ambulatory venous hypertension which may be followed by changes in the microcirculation leading to dermal damage and ulceration. Reduction or impedance of venous reflux are therefore important aims of therapy in patients with chronic venous insufficiency. In this study we examined the haemodynamic effects of long and short stretch compression in patients with popliteal reflux after DVT.

PATIENTS

A total of 46 patients with active or healed venous ulcers were investigated (median age 53, min 21 to max. 86 years). All patients had popliteal vein incompetence proved by Duplex (reflux time >0,5 sec).

METHODS

Duplex-scan (reflux-time in the popliteal vein with calf-decompression) and APG (venous filling index ,VFI) were used as quantitative parameters for the assessment of venous refluxes.

Two different kinds of experiments have been made:

A)   17 Patients which were treated by Sigvaris 503 compression-stockings and another 17 patients treated by short stretch-bandages were examined by APG with and without compression [2].

B)   In a group of 12 patients APG and Duplex examination was done without compression, with Sigvaris 503 below knee stockings (as a model for long stretch material) and with Rosidal   (short stretch bandages).

The sequence of examinations was as follows:

1.   Duplex scanning of popliteal veins and measurement of reflux time.

2.   Application of compression stockings class II (Sigvaris 503)

3.   Duplex-examination repeated

4.   Removal of stockings and application of short stretch bandages

5.   Duplex-examination

6.   APG (VFI)

7.   Removal of bandages and application of compression stockings

8.   APG (VFI)

9.   Removal of stockings

10.   APG (VFI)

The degree of compression exerted by the stockings and bandages was measured by a Talley-instrument and the pressure of the bandage was adjusted to the pressure of the stockings in every single case.

RESULTS

A)   VFI was reduced in average by 34% in the stocking- group and by 62% in the short stretch bandages group (both changes $p < 0,05$, Wilcoxon-test). Table 1 shows the results.

Table 1: VFI (ml/sec) before and after compression.

VFI without	Sigvaris	Diff %	without	Rosidal	Diff %
8,0+/-3,1	5,3+/-2,7	-34%	10,6+/-5,6	4,0+/-1,8	-62%

B)   Venous reflux time (Duplex) was increased by 52% (p<0,05)   after   Sigvaris and by 35%   with the non-elastic compression.   (Fig.2)

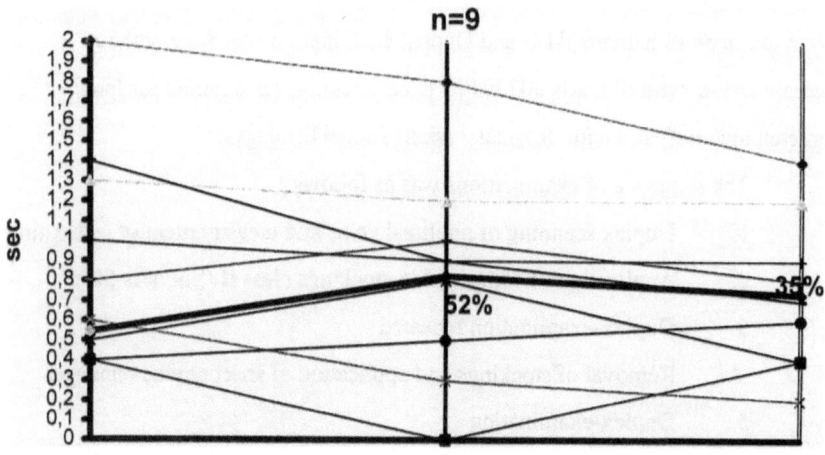

Fig. 2: Reflux time (Duplex), the bold bars represent mean-values (n=9)

Venous filling index (APG) diminished by 32% with the elastic compression stockings and by 55% by the short stretch bandage   (p<0,05)   (Fig.3).

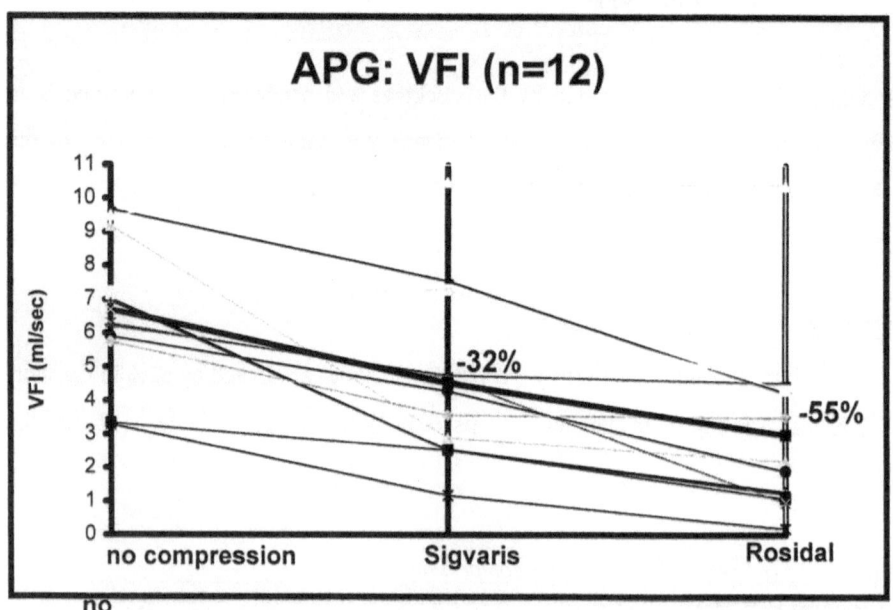

Fig. 3: Venous filling index without compression, with long stretch (Sigvaris) and short stretch (Rosidal) compression.

DISCUSSION

Reflux time in the popliteal vein measured by Duplex indicates valvular incompetence in this segment.

Compression revealed variable changes of this parameter which are difficult to explain and which also might be influenced by several technical difficulties.

On the other hand APG showed a diminution of VFI in every single case. This parameter which reflects global refluxes in the superficial and deep veins is affected more by inelastic than by elastic compression material.

CONCLUSION

It may be concluded that with equal compression-pressures short stretch bandages which do not give way to swelling during standing exert a more pronounced effect concerning the impedance of venous refluxes than elastic material.

REFERENCES

1.   Markel A., Manzo RA, Bergelin RO, Strandness DE. Venous reflux after DVT. Incidence and time occurence. J Vasc Surg 1992; 15:377

2.   Partsch H., Horakova M. Compression stockings for the   treatment of venous leg ulcers. Wien.med.Wochenschr. 1994; 144: 242-7.

Phlebology '95, D. Negus et al. (eds.). Phlebology (1995) Suppl. 1: 892-894

P163

Defibrotide Treatment of Venous Ulcers of the Leg

M. Cospite and G. Milio

Department of Angiology, University of Palermo, Italy

INTRODUCTION

Venous ulcers of the leg are a common cause of illness in the community; the condition has a prevalence of 1% and it recurs chronically (1). Failure to heal a leg ulcer is usually the result of inappropriate care of the wound.

Ulcers of the leg are expensive to treat. The cost of illness include evaluation, diagnosis, treatment regular dressing, time off work and disability. Improvement in healing time could achieve substantial savings.

In the hospital's point of view relevant costs are those incurred during the hospital stay. For instance, the hospital welcomes drug therapy that can reduce the lenght of stay and/or other services (2).

Venous hypertension is the final common pathway leading to venous ulceration in most cases. It arises as a result of incompetence of the valves and associated phenomenon of venous reflux or retrograde flow. Raised venous pressure produces disorganization of microcirculation that, in turn, causes venous ulceration (3). A number of hypotheses have been advanced in attempts to link these observed facts to the ethiology of leg ulcers. They include pericapillary fibrin deposition, localized microvascular ischemia, white cell adherence, white cell activation and the activity of inflammatory mediators such as oxygen free radicals, cytokines, and proteases (4-7).

Defibrotide (Prociclide ®, Crinos) has been found to have fibrinolytic effects, antithrombotic and anti-ischaemic actions due to its ability to selectively increase prostaglandins I_2 levels, to increase tissue plasminogen activator and decrease plasminogen activator inhibitor function (8). Defibrotide also influences the behaviour of white cells, reducing the production of superoxide anions induced by stimulatory agents in neutrophils and monocytes (9-10). In a previous study defibrotide showed some effects on the healing of venous ulcers (11).

It therefore seemed reasonable to verify the time to heal of venous ulceration of the leg in patients treated with defibrotide in addition to a standardized method of bandaging in comparison with bandage alone.

METHODS

The trial design was a prospective, randomized, open, parallel group of 40 consecutive patients with clinical evidence of uncomplicated venous ulceration of the leg.

Inclusion criteria were venous ulceration, ratio of ankle to brachial systolic pressure above 0,9, no contraindication to the prescription of defibrotide. Echo-color-Doppler was used to characterize the venous cause of the ulcer.

Exclusion criteria were insulin dependent diabete mellitus, anticoagulants, antiplatelet agents and non-steroidal anti-inflammatory drugs, poor patients' compliance due to concomitant disability.

Consecutive eligible patients were randomized to receive either defibrotide (600 mg i.v. infusion twice a day for 30 days followed by 800 mg by mouth twice a day for two months or until the ulcer healed if this occured sooner) in addition to a standardized method of bandaging or the same method of bandaging alone. At the initial visit the largest ulcers were selected to be monitored as the reference ulcer for the duration of the study. Patients were evaluated after 20, 40, 60 and 90 days of treatment.

The statistical methods included the χ^2 test and the long rank test, which were used to compare the two treatment groups for overall healing of ulcers.

RESULTS

40 patients (27 females and 13 males range of age 41-78 years) were randomized to the two treatments. There were no differences in the characteristics of the patients between treatment groups. 20 patients suffered from varicose veins and 20 patients had history of post-thrombotic syndrome. All patients had one or more chronic venous ulcers.

By the end of the study all the reference ulcers had healed. Complete healing of the reference ulcer occured sooner in the patients randomized to receive defibrotide.

After 20 days 45% (9 patients) of reference ulcers had healed in patients treated with defibrotide compared with 10% (2 patients) in those treated with bandage alone.

Within 60 days all the ulcers had completely healed in the defibrotide group compared with 60% (12 of 20) in those treated with compression bandage alone (Table 1). This result was significant. (Log Rank Test: $\chi^2 = 3,398$, p<0.01).

Days	20	40	60	90
Defibrotide	9 (45%)	15 (75%)	20 (100%)	20 (100%)
Control	2 (10%)	7 (35%)	12 (60%)	20 (100%)

Table 1: Patients with ulcers healed at each visit. In brackets the percentage of patients with reference ulcers healed

The results shown in Figure 1 give the percentage of ulcers healed at each visit.

No side effects were observed attributable to defibrotide and the tolerability was excellent.

Treatment with defibrotide was able to induce a more rapid and valid healing of chronic ulcers.

These data confirm that drug treatment in addition to compression bandage improves healing time and plays a role in the management of ulcer disease.

894

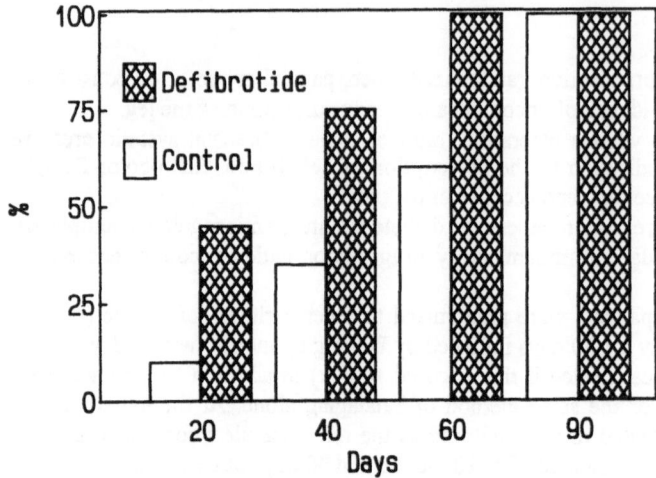

Fig. 1. Percentage of patients with healed ulcers at each visit

REFERENCES

1. Callam MJ, Ruckley CV, Harper DR, Dale JJ. Chronic ulceration of the leg: extent of the problem and provision of care. Br Med J 1985; 290: 1855-6
2. Larson LN. Cost determination and analysis. In: Bootman JL, Townsend RJ, Mc Ghan WF, eds. Principles of Pharmacoeconomics, Cincinnati, Harvey Whitney Books Company 1991, 35-49
3. The Alexander House Group. Consensus Paper on Venous Leg Ulcer. J Dermatol Surg Oncol 1992; 18: 592-602
4. Browse NL. Venous ulceration. Br Med J 1983; 286: 1920-2
5. Browse NL, Burnand KG. The cause of venous ulceration. Lancet 1982; ii 243-5
6. Thomas PRS, Nash GB, Dormandy JA. White cell accumulation in dependent legs of patients with venous hypertension: a possible mechanism for trophic changes in the skin. Br Med J 1988; 296: 1693-5
7. Coleridge Smith PD, Thomas P, Scurr JH, Dormandy JA. Causes of venous ulceration: a new hypothesis. Br Med J 1988; 296: 1726-8
8. Palmer KJ, Goa KL. Defibrotide: A Review of its Pharmacodynamic and Pharmacokinetic Properties and Therapeutic Use in Vascular Disorders. Drugs 1993; 45 (2): 259-294
9. Cirillo F, Margaglione M, Vecchione G, Ames PRJ, Coppola A et al. In vitro inhibition by defibrotide of monocyte superoxide anion generation. A possible mechanism for the antithrombotic effects of a polydeoxyribonucleotide - derived drug. Haemostasis 1991; 21: 98-105
10. Di Perri T, Laghi Pasini F. Ceccatelli L, Pasqui AL. Defibrotide inhibits Ca^{2+} dependent neutrophil activation: implications for its pharmacological activity in vascular disorders. Angiology - The Journal of Vascular Diseases 1991; 971-976
11. Belcaro G, Marelli C. Treatment of venous lipodermatosclerosis and ulceration in venous hypertension by elastic compression and fibrinolytic enhancement with defibrotide. Phlebology 1989; 4: 91-106

Phlebology '95, D. Negus et al. (eds.). Phlebology (1995) Suppl. 1: 895-896

P165

The Influence of Low Molecular Weight Heparin to the Healing of Chronic Foot Ulcers

M. Kucharzewski, R. Macyszyn, A. Niemiec and M. Paliga

II Department of General Surgery, Silesian Medical Academy, Bytom, Poland

INTRODUCTION

Leg ulcers are a common problem, the point prevalence of open ulcers known to healthcare profesionals is in the range 0,11- 0,30 per cent (2,7).Most patients suffer from their ulcers several months or even year (1,2).The treatment of chronic foot ulcers is most difficult, especially if the arterial circulation of the region is impaired (4).The factors like hypercoagulation and fibrynolysis might contribute to the impaired healing process (6).Heparin, which increase the fibrynolitic activity and has antithrombotic effect (3) might therefore be of value in the treatment of the ulcers.

METHODS

Twenty men with chronic ulcer of one foot since a mean time of 10 months (range 6-15 months) were investigated.Mean age was 52,8 years (range 47-76 years).All patients had clinical signs of peripheral arterial occlusive disease, and 11 men suffered from intermittent claudication, and seven had rest pain.Ankle blood pressure measurements showed peripheral acclusive disease in all patients (ankle/arm pressure ratio≤ 0,6).The nutritional skin microcirculation of the toes and around the foot ulcers was evaluated by vital capillaroscopy.The structural apperance and blood filling of the capillaries were classified according to a three graded scale (5).The ulcers area was estimated according planimetry.All men had previously conventional treatment during 10-16 weeks (6), without any noticeable improvement on ulcer healing.After conventional treatment, all men were given 7500 U. AXa IC low molecular weight heparin (Fraxiparine® ,Sanofi Wintrop, France) subcutaneously one a day for five weeks.

RESULTS

The ulcers area decrease significantly in 17 patients of which twelve healed the ulcers completely, whereas five men showed a decreases of the ulcers area.The ulcers area was unchanged in three patients after treatment.No significant changes were seen in ankle/arm pressure ratio during the investigation period.The macrocirculation were unchanged in all patients, whereas the nutrional capillary circulation improced in 17 men.

Table 1.
Classification of the structure and blood filling of the nutritional skin capillaries.

	Capillary stage	Before treatment	After treatment
Normal	Small dot or comma shaped Slightly dilated	4	12
No or minor risk necrosis	Widely dilated Indistinct capillaries	11	5
High risk of skin necrosis	Capillary hemorrhages	5	3

CONCLUSIONS

We suggest that Fraxiparine® postitively influences on healing process of chronic foot ulcers.

REFERENCES

1. Ahroni JH, Boyko EJ, Pecoraro RE.Diabetic foot ulcer healing: Extrinsic vs. intrinsic factors.Wounds 1993; 5: 245-5.
2. Baker SR, Stacey MC, Sing HG, Hoskin SE, Thompson PJ.Aetiology of chronic leg ulcers.Eur J Vasc Surg 1992;6: 245-51.
3. Berqvist D.Review of clinical trials of low molecular weight heparin.Clinical review.Eur J Surg 1992; 158: 67-8.
4. Callam MJ, Ruckley CV, Harper DR, Dale JJ.Chronic ulceration of the leg, extent of the problem and provision of care.Br Med J 1985; 290: 1855-6.
5. Fagrell B, Lundberg G. A simplified evaluation of vital cappilary microscopy for predicting skin viability in patients with severe arterial insufficiency.Clin Physiol 1984;4: 403-6
6. Hansson C. Optimal treatment of venous (stasis) ulcers in elderly patients.Drugs Aging 1994;5: 323-334
7. Nelzen O, Berqvist D, Linghagen A. Venous and non-venous leg ulcers: clinical history and apperance in population study.Br J Surg 1994;81: 182-7.

Phlebology '95, D. Negus et al. (eds.). Phlebology (1995) Suppl. 1: 897-899

P167

Myths and Truths in the Treatment of Venous Ulcers

C.F. Sánchez[1,2], E. Altmann-Canestri[1,2], U.P. Tropper[1,2], F.F. Pace[2,3], L. Báez[1] and A. Torassa[1]

[1] *Phlebological Clinic,* [2] *John F. Kennedy University,* [3] *Medical Center*

INTRODUCTION

When patients with leg ulcers come to us, we tend to indicate cleansing and disinfection as a first measure. These terms are not synonymous and, though generally associated, they must be considered as two separate procedures. Ulcers must be cleansed first, and then disinfected only when considered necessary.

By definition, every wound, including ulcers, is an injury to body integrity, and any additional trauma will delay the repairing process. These traumas may be classified as: mechanical (brushing) and chemical (physiologically incompatible substances).

CLEANSING OF WOUNDS

The products used for cleansing wounds may be separated in two: the active principle and the excipient. In general, the excipient or "carrier" is supposed to be inactive. This is a great mistake because most "carriers" commercially used are extremely toxic by themselves.

Regarding the active principles of the cleansers, inasmuch as a cleansing must be achieved, the limit between the tissue and the bacteria and particles of dirt must be broken by reducing the superficial tension in order to extract those particles from the wounds. Tensioactive substances which have that property, are classified according to their charge into cationic (when the charge is positive: benzalkonium chloride, Gillot solution, DG6 quaternary ammonium compound); anionic (when it is negative: detergents and regular soaps) and amphoteric (when they have both charges, positive and negative, in their molecules: TEGO 103).

Research carried out has shown that substances with chemical charge are toxic for tissues. These charged materials interact with the cellular membrane, disturbing it. The membrane loses permeability, which produces its death. Therefore, all these agents are toxic for the tissue defenses and they inhibit the healing of wounds.

DISINFECTION OF WOUNDS

Many doctors are paranoid where bacteria are concerned. They believe they must do even what is impossible in order to eliminate all bacteria from wounds. To do this they resort to antiseptic agents, not considering that all these substances, besides killing microorganisms, are lethal to the cells in the wound and should not be used.

Iodine is the disinfectant most indiscriminately used, as well as peroxides, permanganates, acetic acid, Datkin solution, etc., which were proved to have the same noxious effect.

Our team carried out this simple experience: some bacteria are added to a tube of saline solution; they will be seen to float freely, exposed and vulnerable. If we add some drops of povidone-iodine, the bacteria will die immediately. But this is not the real situation happening in wounds. When we add pus, protein, serum, blood and devitalized tissues to the same tube to make the content more similar to a wound, then the povidone-iodine will not kill any of those bacteria. Litter describes povidone-iodine as an effective disinfectant for the surgical field but not indicated in the cleansing of wounds because it turns inactive in contact with organic matter.

Although the effect is void, what we deal with in this study is the fact that povidone-iodine, as well as the other disinfectants, are not only ineffective but harmful. To prove this we propose this simple test, easily reproducible, which anybody may carry out. Just take an empty tube, put a blood sample in it and add povidone-iodine 1 to 1, or any other of the many disinfectants. Take it to the hematologist for a cell count. If you use an isotonic saline solution for control, you will obtain a normal count of red and white cells and no hemoglobin suspended in the solution, while in the tube with disinfectant, all the red and white cells will be instantly lysed and traces of hemoglobin will remain in the solution. Therefore, these agents not only produce no benefit, but they are toxic.

Another interesting experience may be made with an infected wound model. This model is very simple and requires two incisions made on either side of the back of a Guinea pig. In this way, the same animal acts as its own control. Both wounds are contaminated with a previously known number of bacteria, one of the wounds being treated with saline solution and the other with any disinfectant. Both wounds are covered and then the defensive action of the tissues against the bacterial attack is observed. The results obtained in the control wound support much of the basic knowledge we have regarding natural defense of tissues. This proves that wounds have an exquisite ability to protect themselves against the attack of bacteria when their natural defenses are not inhibited.

"In vitro" studies show the harmful effect of antiseptics on fibroblasts, whose presence and integrity are fundamental for the healing process, as well as on granulocytes and monocytes which clean wounds and eliminate bacteria and foreign bodies. The response is similar for all of them: a very important dilution of the antiseptic is needed to eliminate the toxicity of these defensive cells [1, 2].

Our team described, a few years ago, the method we used as a routine for cleansing ulcers by brushing and with powder antiseptic [3, 4]. Presently, we only use it exceptionally and in very contaminated ulcers, but instead of antiseptics we use physiological solution with the only purpose of sweeping away necrotic tissues. Then we use, according to the type of ulcer, heterografts (membranes with different characteristics commercially available), autografts, Unna bandages, etc., always with the principle of moving bandages very little to avoid damaging the delicate growing tissues.

In order to evaluate the importance of preserving the physiological microenvironment as a stimulus for angiogenesis and regeneration of granulation tissue in ulcerous lesions, our team carried comparative studies during one year on two series of 80 patients each, subject to a two-month treatment.

METHOD

The study group was subjected to cleansing with physiological solution for the first 7 days and then occlusive techniques to preserve the microenvironment of the lessions (Group A).
The control group received daily brushing and antiseptic washing (Group B).

CONCLUSIONS

We believe the rapid healing of ulcers consecutive to preservation of the microclimate in 30 days (84% of the ulcers) in relation to the control group (34%) is a consequence of preserving the growth factors and the aerobic flora which induces granulation and epithelization.

Number of patients	Age	Sex	Number of ulcers	Complete healing in 30 days	in 60 days	50% healing in 60 days
6	<40	F	8	7	1	
5	<40	M	7	6	1	
23	40-60	F	32	29	2	1
18	40-60	M	25	22	3	
17	>60	F	27	21	5	1
11	>60	M	19	14	3	2
80			118	99	15	4

Group A

Number of patients	Age	Sex	Number of ulcers	Complete healing in 30 days	in 60 days	50% healing in 60 days
7	<40	F	10	3	4	3
5	<40	M	7	2	3	2
25	40-60	F	34	15	11	8
19	40-60	M	28	9	12	7
14	>60	F	26	7	11	8
10	>60	M	19	6	7	6
80			124	42	48	34

Group B

REFERENCES

1.   Connoly J C and Gilmore O J A. A study of the effect of povidone-iodine on polymorphonuclear leukocyte chemotaxis. Brit J. Exp. Path. 1979; 60: 662-666.
2.   Lineweaver W, Howard R, Soucy D, Mc Morris S, Freeman J, Crain C et al. Topical antimicrobial toxicity. Arch Surg. 1985; 120: 267-279.
3.   Sánchez C, Altmann-Canestri E, Tropper U P. Preparación del lecho ulceroso. Injerto de piel ambulatorio. Manual de Escleroterapia y Flebectomía Ambulatoria. Buenos Aires: Editorial Celcius, 1992: 335-337.
4.   Sánchez C F. Preparación del lecho ulceroso. Úlcera. In: Altmann-Canestri E, Sánchez C F, Tropper U et al. Tratado de Flebología y Linfología. Buenos Aires: Fundación Flebológica Argentina, 1995: 244.

Phlebology '95, D. Negus et al. (eds.). Phlebology (1995) Suppl. 1: 900-903

P168

Clinical Improvement in Patients with Chronic Venous Incompetence (CVI) With an Intensified 6-Week-Long Physical Training Programme

T. Klyscz[1], M. Nicolaus[2], C. Mohr[2], T. Horstmann[3], A. Steins[1], M. Hahn[1] and M. Jünger[1]

[1] Department of Dermatology, [2] Department of sports Medicine and [3] Department of Orthopaedics University of Tübingen, D-72076 Tübingen, Germany

INTRODUCTION

Primary varicosis and postthrombotic syndrome are often accompanied by macrocirculatory and microcirculatory disturbances and trophic changes of the skin, especially in the inner ankle region, mainly as a result of disturbed haemodynamics. Venous congestion is thought to be the pathogenic mechanism for both the trophic skin changes and the damage of further anatomical structures, especially of the upper and the lower ankle joint. Schmeller (5) has shown that in elderly people mobility of the upper ankle joint is always reduced, even more so in patients with chronic venous insufficiency (CVI).

Sufficient dorsalextension in the upper ankle joint, however, is one of the most important mechanisms for the venous drainage of the legs, since it is closely linked to the activity of the calf muscle pump. Although patients with CVI often claim adequate physical exercise from daily walking they always have a severely deficient physiological walking pattern. Put simply, their unnaturally cautious gait is haemodynamically insufficient.

METHODS

The therapeutic aim, therefore, must be a reduction of the increased ambulatory venous pressure by improving calf muscle ankle joint mobility and strengthening the calf muscle pump. A special, intensified 6-week-long exercise training programme was developed for patients with CVI in order to improve the function of the calf muscle pump, strengthen the calf muscles and improve upper ankle joint mobility with physical exercises and the use of a newly developed exercise machine (4) (Pat. pending). Training intensity for the training group was 1 hour 2 times a week for 6 weeks. The exercise programme was supervised by experienced trainers and physicians in a gymnasium at the University Hospital of Tübingen.

The 1-hour lesson was divided into 4 parts each devoted to a different therapeutic aspect. Training started with a 15-minute warming-up period, followed by walking exercises and pedal ergometry training using our own specially developed multi-purpose pedal ergometer (4). Each patient's individual exercise load was chosen to correspond to 80% of his or her maximum tolerance. The training programme was designed to increase strength; in other words, fewer repetitions and greater exertion.

The final quarter hour was spent on games and relaxation exercises. After the exhausting parts of the lesson the patients had to elevate their legs to facilitate venous drainage.

PATIENTS

16 patients suffering from CVI stages I-III according to Widmer were included. There were 10 patients in the training group (TG): 5 women and 5 men with a mean age of 54,8 years. Six patients were examined in the control group (CG): 2 men and 4 women with a mean age of 51,3 years with no additional exercise programme. To exclude severe coronary heart disease an exercise electrocardiogram was required before participation in the patients' training group. All patients had to wear compression bandages or stockings during training lessons.

MEASUREMENTS

Measurements were performed before (examination 1) and after the 6-week training period (examination 2). Calf muscle pump function and venous drainage were measured by phlebodynamometry and DPPG, skin microcirculation by transcutaneous oxygen tension (tcpo$_2$, 37°C), and upper ankle joint mobility by dorsal extension and plantar flexion (in °) and isokinetic forces (LIDO-System, Loredan Biomechanical Inc., Davis, USA).

RESULTS

		Examination 1	Examination 2	Difference	Signif.
Dorsalextension	VG	7,7 ± 6,6	11,5 ± 5,5	+3,8 (49,4%)	*
Dorsalextension	KG	23,0 ± 3,7	21,5 ± 3,0	-1,5 (-6,5%)	n.s.
Plantarflexion	VG	26,7 ± 6,2	29,0 ± 5,5	+2,3 (8,6%)	n.s.
Plantarflexion	KG	31,8 ± 3,4	29,8 ± 3,6	-2,0 (-6,3%)	n.s.

Table 1: Upper ankle joint mobility (in °)

		Examination 1	Examination 2	Difference	Signif.
TcPO, at rest	VG	28,1 ± 15,1	38,5 ± 13,6	+10,4 (37%)	*
TcPO, at rest	KG	36,0 ± 7,2	32,7 ± 7,3	-3,3 (-9,2%)	n.s.

Table 2: TcPO,-values at rest at the distal limb in supine position (37°C)

		Examination 1	Examination 2	Difference	Signif.
Isometric forces	VG	54,2 ± 31,9	71,0 ± 35,9	+16,8 (30,9%)	*
Isometric forces	KG	58,1 ± 18,7	56,5 ± 18,7	-1,7 (-2,7%)	n.s.

Table 3: Isometric forces (Nm) during plantarflexion

		Examination 1	Examination 2	Difference	Signif.
Isometric forces	VG	28,7 ± 11,0	36,6 ± 14,1	+7,9 (27,5%)	*
Isometric forces	KG	25,7 ± 13,8	28,7 ± 10,7	+3,0 (11,6%)	n.s.

Table 4: Isometric forces (Nm) during dorsalextension

In the TG there was an improvement in subjective complaints (oedema and pain), a significant improvement in dorsal extension, a significant improvement in tcpo$_2$ values measured at the distal part of the limbs in the supine position and increased isokinetic forces during dorsal extension and plantar flexion, in contrast to the non-significant changes in the control group (CG). Phlebodynamometry and DPPG values increased in the training group, although they did not appear to be significant by the end of the six-week training period. Thus both macro- and microhaemodynamics were improved at the end of the training period.

CONCLUSION

There is a close correlation between improvement in subjective complaints and venous haemodynamics and skin microcirculation in patients with CVI in a physical exercise programme. Improvements in plantar flexion, dorsal extension and transcutaneous oxygen tension in the skin could already be documented after a 6-week-long intensified training programme, whereas there was no improvement in the control group. Isokinetic forces increased significantly during the training period, which mirrors the improvement in calf muscle activity and its strengthening during the exercise training programme. There was a therapeutic benefit in all the patients included in the training programme.

Our experience with this therapeutic concept is very promising. We had no complications at all and no worsening of clinical symptoms or subjective complaints. Costs for the training participants are still covered by the patients' health insurance companies under the German „Behindertensportabkommen" which was last revised in 1993.

Physical exercise training should become an integral part of therapy for chronic venous incompetence. The formation of out-patient training groups should be supported by phlebologists.

1. Gaylarge PM, Dodd HJ, Sarkany I. Venous leg ulcers and arthropathy. Br J Rheumatol 1990;29 (2):142-144.
2. Jamieson WG. State of the art of venous investigation and treatment. Can J Surg 1993;36 (2):119-28.

3. Jünger M, Jünger I, Klyscz T, Geiger H, Hahn M, May B, Schiek B. Improvement of clinical symptoms and hemodynamics by physical training in patients with chronic venous incompetence (CVI). Int J Microcirc Clin Experimental 1993;12(2): 215.
4. Klyscz Th, Jünger I, Jung M, Mohr C, Hahn M, Jünger M. Clinical improvement in patients with chronic venous incompetence (CVI) by physical exercise training using a new developed exercising machine. European Journal of Applied Physiology and Occupational Physiology. Suppl. 1994;69(3):40.
5. Schmeller W. The significance of ankle joint movement in lower leg venous function. In: Orfanos CE, Stadler R, Gollnick H (eds) Dermatology in Five Continents. Proceedings of the XVII. World Congress of Dermatology, Berlin, May 24-29, 1987. Springer, Berlin.1988.
6. Welkie JF, Comerota AJ, Kerr RP, Katz ML, Jayheimer EC, Brigham RA. The hemodynamics of venous ulceration. Ann Vasc Surg 1992;6 (1): 1-4.

Phlebology '95, D. Negus et al. (eds.). Phlebology (1995) Suppl. 1: 904-906

P169

Therapy of Non-Healing Venous Stasis Ulcers with Autologous Growth Factors

S. Bort, H. Reutter, M. Hahn, T. Klyscz, A. Steins, W. Schippert and M. Jünger

Department of Dermatology, University of Tübingen, Liebermeisterstr.25, D-72076 Tübingen, Germany

INTRODUCTION

The rationale behind treating venous ulcers with platelet-derived wound healing factors (PDWHF, Procuren[R]) is the severe cutaneous microangiopathy which characterizes severe chronic venous insufficiency (CVI). The superficial capillaries responsible for skin nutrition are dilated, arcuate, branched, and glomerulate, producing functional shunts for nutritients. Above all, these nutritive capillaries are **rarefied** in severe CVI.

PDWHF act by directing fibroblast proliferation and migration, collagen synthesis and **endothelial cell migration and mitosis to produce capillaries**. In the initial phase of the healing process macrophages and platelets have been demonstrated to be the primary regulatory cells. Platelets release locally acting growth factors, and similar factors are produced later by the macrophages.

Platelets are easily obtained from blood, in contrast to macrophages, which are difficult to procure. Although it has not been demonstrated that the growth factors from platelets are identical to those obtained from macrophages, their biological activity is exactly the same. Platelet-derived wound healing factors are released when platelets are exposed to thrombin. There are several growth factors released from platelets, including platelet-derived growth factor (PDGF), platelet factor-4 (PF-4), transforming growth factor-beta (TGF-beta) and beta-thromboglobulin (beta-TG)-related peptides. PDGF acts on fibroblasts, smooth muscle cells and glial cells. PF-4 is a chemoattractant for neutrophils and monocytes. It also interacts with the blood-clotting cascade. TGF-beta influences the synthesis of fibrin-collagen and stimulates a local increase in macrophages. Beta-thromboglobulin is chemotactic for fibroblasts, which are involved in the formation of granulation tissue.

Here patients suffering from persistent venous ulcers were treated with PDWHF (Procuren[R]). We were primarily interested in the efficacy and safety of PDWHF. In addition, we examined skin microcirculation during the treatment period.

METHODS

Patients

So far 4 patients (3 f, 1 m; age: 70.5 years) have been treated with Procuren and an additional 10 patients (8 f, 2 m; age: 68.5 years) have given their consent to participation in a multicenter placebo-controlled double-blind study. In the „Procuren" group, ulcer duration was 27 months, as opposed to 37 months in the placebo-controlled study group. At the beginning the ulcers were 41.8 cm^2 large in the Procuren group and 93 cm^2 in the placebo-controlled study group. All figures given here are medians.

Patients with peripheral arterial occlusive disease, diabetes mellitus, malignant ulcers and osteomyelitis were excluded from the study.

Treatment

At the first clinic visit the wounds were thoroughly debrided of all soft necrotic tissue. At each subsequent clinic visit, all wounds were inspected and debrided of any necrotic material or fibrin which had developed in the meantime. The wounds were treated with PDWHF after all superficial purulence and necrotic tissue had been eliminated. Patients were generally treated on an outpatient basis. They were examined and treated in the clinic every other week.

Preparation of PDWHF

Platelets used to prepare PDWHF were obtained from approximately 200 ml of whole blood drawn from the patient at the time of screening. If necessary, additional blood was drawn after about 8 weeks of participation. The blood was immediately put on ice for transport from the clinic to the laboratory (Curative Technologies GmbH, Zum Schurmannsgraben 12, 47441 Moers, Germany). PDWHF was prepared in HEPES platelet buffer solution after thrombin release of the platelet alpha-granules under aseptic conditions. Each 10 ml dose of PDWHF contained a 1:100 dilution of the concentrate. The placebo consisted of sterile HEPES platelet buffer solution. The placebo and PDWHF solutions and their containers were identical in appearance.

As standard care in CVI every patient wore compression bandages on the lower leg.

PDWHF application

The patients were instructed to apply a thin layer of the PDWHF salve (usually 1 container per day) to the entire surface of the wound. This was covered with petroleum-impregnated gauze and a sterile gauze dressing. The PDWHF was left on for 24 hours, after which it was removed.

Laboratory

Intravital capillaroscopy

By means of intravital microscopy with epiillumination the cutaneous nutritive capillaries were examined in vivo at a magnification of 80 x (Leitz „Bollinger" microsope). Each dermal papilla usually contains 1 to 3 of these superficial capillaries, which are responsible for skin nutrition. Reliable information about nutritional cutaneous blood flow can only be achieved by capillaroscopic methods

The microscope is fixed to a heavy support in order to avoid vibration-related artefacts, but it can be moved along 3 axes to reach any desired skin area. The capillaroscopic examination is documented on video tape. Capillaries are counted (normal: > 40 cap./mm^2) and morphometry is performed by computer-aided analysis of the video sequences

Transcutaneous oxygen partial pressure (tcPO$_2$)

tcPO$_2$ was measured in the ulcer border area (normal: > 40 mmHg; Radiometer, Copenhagen). The electrode core temperature was 43°C.

Laser Doppler flux (LDF)

Measurement of LDF was made by a laser with a 632.8 nm spectrum (Periflux PF2, Fa. Perimed, Stockholm). The technique itself has been evaluated by Nielsson and Tenland, who gave a detailed description.

The skin surface is illuminated by a low power laser beam, which is reflected by moving blood cells. The back-scattered light, detected by an optical system, is Doppler-shifted in proportion to the velocity of the blood cells.The Doppler shift, interpreted as flux, is the product of the number and mean velocity of the moving blood cells.

The LDF can be used as a measure of the overall blood flow of the examined site. Although the LDF is a measure of the overall blood flow in the examined site, it mainly reflects blood flow in the deeper subpapillary plexus and not in the nutritive compartment of the skin.

Course of examination

Patients were examined in a supine position.

A transparent film was put over the ulcer and the border of the ulcer was marked on the film. Later the size of the ulcer was determined by means of planimetry.

A drop of oil rendered the skin area of interest more transparent.

The border of the ulcer and the ulcer itself were examined by means of intravital capillaroscopy in order to describe morphological characteristics and to determine capillary density.

Simultaneously measurements of $tcPO_2$ and of LDF were performed close to the ulcer in the border area. The LDF was also determined in the center of the ulcer.

Statistics: All data are given as median values.

RESULTS

Since the double-blind study has not yet been finished, the results presented here apply only to the 4 patients who were treated with PDWHF.

Patients were treated for 17 weeks (median).

Ulcer size:

In 1 of the 4 patients the ulcer healed and was completely covered with new epithelium.

If we look at the group of patients as a whole, the ulcer became smaller by 9%.

Skin microcirculation:

The number of capillaries increased at the border of the ulcer from 10.6 to 19.9 cap./mm^2.

At the end of the treatment period a $tcPO_2$ of 23 mmHg was measured, compared to the initial value of 16 mmHg.

The LDF decreased from 72 to 66 AU at the border of the ulcer and in the ulcer from 595 to 517 AU.

DISCUSSION

If we bear in mind the extreme persistence of the ulcers before treatment with PDWHF was started, the healing achieved here in 1 patient can be termed a clinical success. At the same time the ulcers healed and improved, the number of nutritive capillaries and the transcutaneous partial pressure increased. This finding confirms the close relationship between skin perfusion and healing processes. The desired healing can probably only be initiated if capillaries grow into the wound. It is, however, not an increase of the overall blood flow in the skin, but an improvement in the perfusion in the nutritive compartment, in the nutritive capillaries, because the LDF, a measure of the total blood flow in the skin, actually decreased during the healing process. The latter finding means that luxus hyperperfusion and the maldistribution of blood flow disappeared to a certain extent.

To assess the clinical value of PDWHF for the treatment of chronic venous stasis ulcers further data have to be gathered and analyzed. Hopefully the placebo-controlled double-blind study presented here will help determine the clinical benefit which can be achieved by PDWHF in CVI.

REFERENCES

1. Knighton DR, Fiegel VD, Austin LL, Ciresi KF, Butler EL: Classification and treatment of chronic nonhealing wounds. Annals of Surgery 1986; 204: 322-330.
2. Haselbach P, Vollenweider U, Moneta G, Bollinger A: Microangiopathy in severe chronic venous insufficiency evaluated by fluorescence video-microscopy. Phlebology 1986; 1: 159-169.
3. Jünger M, Hahn U, Bort S, Klyscz T, Hahn M, Rassner G: Bedeutung der kutanen Mikroangiopathie für die Entstehung von Stauungsdermatosen bei chronischer Veneninsuffizienz (CVI). Wien. med. Wochenschr. 1994; 144: 206-210.
4. Nilsson GE, Tenland T, Öberg PA: Evaluation of a Laser Doppler Flowmeter for Measurement of Tissue Blood Flow. IEEE Trans Biomed Eng 1980; 27: 597-604.

Phlebology '95, D. Negus et al. (eds.). Phlebology (1995) Suppl. 1: 907-909

OP/18.3

Clinical Efficacy of Compression Therapy and its Influence on Cutaneous Microcirculation

S. Galler, T. Klyscz, M.F. Jung, A. Steins, S. Bort, M. Hahn and M. Jünger

*Department of Dermatology, University of Tübingen, Liebermeisterstr.25,
D-72076 Tübingen, Germany*

INTRODUCTION

Chronic venous insufficiency (CVI) results from disturbances in venous macro- and microhemodynamics. Primary varicose veins or a history of deep venous thrombosis are the most common clinical entities provoking either venous hypervolemia in the leg or an increased resistance to the backflow of blood towards the heart. Compression therapy is considered to be the standard treatment for these common diseases. Elastic bandages and stockings support the venous flow in the lower extremities by compressing the superficial vein lumen and supporting valvular function and the muscle pump. It is also effective in reducing and preventing edema.

In recent years attention has been turned to the microcirculatory aspects of CVI (2). Microangiopathy has been examined by intravital capillaroscopy (2,3), which revealed changes in the superficial capillaries responsible for skin nutrition. They are dilated, arcuate, branched, and glomerulate, producing functional shunts for nutritients. These nutritive capillaries are rarefied in severe CVI. Nevertheless a luxus hyperperfusion affecting the subpapillary plexus characterizes the chronically congested skin e.g. in the inner ankle area. Thus a maldistribution of the cutaneous blood flow between the subpapillary plexus and the nutritive compartment of the skin is an important part of the pathophysiology in CVI. Laser Doppler flux is correlated with blood flow to the skin (4), but mainly reflects the perfusion of the subpapillary plexus.

The aim of the present study was to determine how a four-week-long compression treatment affects skin microcirculation.

METHODS

Patients

Included in the study were 20 patients with CVI, 10 men and 10 women, with a mean age of 54.9±9.5 years. According to Widmer, 7 patients belonged to stage I and 13 to stage II. 3 patients had had a deep venous thrombosis in the past. All patients had palpable pedal pulses with an ankle/brachial index of > 1.0. The average venous refill time measured by LRR was 20±12 sec. Examination by Doppler ultrasound showed an insufficiency of the deep veins in 7 patients. 12 patients had insufficient superficial veins, 6 incompetent perforating veins.

Compression treatment and examinations

Compression therapy consisted of two parts: after compressive bandaging of the lower leg for two weeks with elastic bandages ("Comprilan"), the patients were treated for another two weeks with made-to-measure class 2 compression stockings, or class 3 for patients with PTS.

Examinations were done before therapy (E1), after treatment with bandages (E2), and finally after wearing stockings for an additional two weeks (E3).

At the beginning of every examination the patients were asked to rate their subjective symptoms with regard to pain, tautness, swelling, itching, and feelings of coldness, heat or restriction, on a scale of 0 (no complaints) to 3 (maximal complaints).

The LDF probe was placed at two skin sites: on the forefoot and above the medial ankle region. At every visit the same sites were chosen for laser Doppler fluxmetry.

Measurements were taken with the patients in a supine position after they had rested for at least 20 min.

Laboratory

Calf volume
A special paper tape measuring system (Fa.Jobst) was used to register shank circumferences at 11 distinctive sites 1.5 inches apart. Calf volume was determined using the formula for calculating frustums.

Laser Doppler flux
Measurement of LDF was made by a laser with a 632.8 nm spectrum (Periflux PF2, Fa. Perimed, Stockholm). The technique itself has been evaluated by Nielsson and Tenland, who gave a detailed description (4).

The skin surface is illuminated by a low power laser beam, which is reflected by moving blood cells. The back-scattered light, detected by an optical system, is Doppler-shifted in proportion to the velocity of the blood cells. The Doppler shift, interpreted as flux, is the product of the number and mean velocity of the moving blood cells.

LDF was taken at rest and after arterial occlusion for three minutes. The relative LDF-increase after arterial occlusion is a measure of cutaneous vascular reserve. „Biological zero" (1) means the minimum LDF during arterial occlusion. Here, data are presented both as measured and after correction by the „biological zero".

Statistics
Statistical analysis including Student's t-test was performed by SAS (statistic analysis system). All data are given as median values with 25% (Q1) and 75% quartiles (Q3).

RESULTS

Clinical symptoms:
In the course of therapy subjective complaints in all the patients decreased, except for the feeling of coldness, which increased when stockings were worn. None of the patients complained about a feeling of restriction after the second part of therapy.

Calf volume:
After wearing compression bandages for two weeks the patients' calf volumes had been reduced significantly (p<0.0001) from 3004.5 (2719.4/3249.9) ml to 2850.8 (2574.4/3127.8) ml. During therapy with stockings calf volume increased slightly, but still ended up lower than the starting level.

LDF values:
In the inner ankle area the luxus hyperperfusion receded: before therapy 29 AU (Q1 19 AU, Q3 50 AU) were measured. After 2 weeks of compression bandages LDF had dropped to 22.5 AU (Q1 12.5 AU; Q3 35.5 AU). After another 2 weeks of wearing compression stockings LDF was 20 AU (Q1 18 AU; Q3 38 AU).

After correction for the so-called biological zero the resulting LDF values were: at E1 20 AU (Q1 15 AU; Q3 42 AU), at E2 14 AU (Q1 9 AU; Q3 24 AU) and at E3 15.5 AU (Q1 10 AU;Q3 30 AU).

DISCUSSION

Clinical improvement was caused by a significant reduction in calf volume, which means that hypervolemia and edema had been successfully treated by the compression therapy chosen here. Both the bandages and the stockings were suitable for achieving the clinical goal.

Our interest was focussed on skin microcirculation. In the inner ankle area, in which venous congestion usually plays a major role, luxus hyperperfusion was reduced, as indicated here by laser Doppler flux. Malperfusion may also have been influenced in a positive manner: compression bandages and stockings reduce hyperperfusion in the subpapillary plexus, and the nutritive blood flow of the superficial capillaries is probably improved at the same time. The latter has to be examined by intravital capillaroscopy (3).

REFERENCES

1. Caspary L, Creutzig A, Alexander K: Biological zero in laser Doppler fluxmetry. Int J Microcirc Clin Exp 1988; 7: 367-371.
2. Haselbach P, Vollenweider U, Moneta G, Bollinger A: Microangiopathy in severe chronic venous insufficiency evaluated by fluorescence video-microscopy. Phlebology 1986; 1: 159-169.
3. Jünger, M., Hahn, U., Bort, S., Klyscz, T., Hahn, M., Rassner, G. Bedeutung der kutanen Mikroangiopathie für die Entstehung von Stauungsdermatosen bei chronischer Veneninsuffizienz (CVI). Wien. med. Wochenschr. 1994; 144: 206-210.
4. Nilsson GE, Tenland T, Öberg PA: Evaluation of a Laser Doppler Flowmeter for Measurement of Tissue Blood Flow. IEEE Trans Biomed Eng 1980; 27: 597-604.

Phlebology '95, D. Negus et al. (eds.). Phlebology (1995) Suppl. 1: 910-912

P170

Hyperbaric Oxygen Therapy of Varicose Ulcers

O. Andoniades[1], R. Mirabella[1], M. Conzi[1], J. Liendo[1], N. Subbotina[2], C. Gulo[2] and J. Pisarello[2]

1 Department of Surgery, Section of Phlebology and Lymphology, Hospital B. Rivadavia, University of Buenos Aires Medical School, Buenos Aires, Argentina
2 Hyperbaric Center, Sanatorio Modelo Quilmes, Quilmes, Pcia. de Buenos Aires, Argentina

INTRODUCTION

Varicose ulcers represent 70% of all vascular ulcers, are potentially incapacitating, and frequently constitute a difficult medical problem and a therapeutic challenge

Hyperbaric oxygen therapy (HBOT) is a relatively new therapeutic modality that has been utilized in the treatment of wounds resistant to therapy. These include diabetic foot lesions, radionecrotic ulcers, vasculitic ulcers, etc. Oxygen breathing at pressure produces a variable increase in the mean oxygen partial pressure of all tissues. Tissue hyperoxia is a potent physiologic event resulting in various biochemical and physiologic phenomena, some of which result in a therapeutic effect [1]. Results of the use of HBO in specific groups of refractory wounds are encouraging [2]

In this paper we report our experience in the treatment of 46 cases of varicose ulcers which failed to heal after at least two months of conventional therapy. HBOT was then added to the treatment regime .

After 30 HBOT sessions, 91% of the patients demonstrated objective improvement. In 39%, this improvement was prominent, with more than 50% reduction of the size of the ulcer; 28% of all patients healed completely.

METHODS

Patients. Patients had been treated by a phlebologist for a minimum of 2 months with surgical debridement, local cleansing solutions, compression dressing, creams, and ankle joint physical therapy. HBOT was added to the treatment when there was no evidence of granulation tissue or decrease in the size of the lesion. Table 1 describes characteristics of the group.

HBOT. The hyperbaric treatment consisted in breathing oxygen continuously at 1.7-1.9 ATA for 60-75 minutes daily . Initially, 20 treatments were given daily on weekdays. Additional 10 treatments were given after a period of 3-4 weeks, during which periodic evaluation continued as described below

Evaluation. Ulcer size was conventionally assessed measuring the two major diameters with a caliper, regardless of the location of the diameters previously measured. Data is reported as the average of the percentages in variation of the major diameters from the initial to the final measurement. Measurement of the lesions and photographic documentation was obtained weekly.

RESULTS

After 30 HBOT, patients were divided in two groups according to clinical outcome: Group A) (42 patients: 91%) the general appearance of the lesion improved, with reduction of edema and diminution of pain, as well as a measurable reduction in the surface of the wound. In group B) (4 patients: 9%) there was no improvement or reduction in the surface of the ulcer. Group A) was divided in two subgroups: A1) reduction of ulcer >50% (18 patients: 39%) and A2) reduction of ulcer <50% (24 patients: 52%) (table 1)

CONCLUSIONS.

Our results show that the addition of HBOT improves the clinical outcome of venous stasis ulcers treated conventionally as described. These results are somewhat unexpected, considering that HBOT is in general thought to produce modest improvement of varicose ulcers. HBOT has been formally recommended only for selected cases of varicose ulcers [3].

The majority of patients in our series showed improvement of the lesions, and 13 (28%) healed completely. Even the 24 patients who experienced less improvement (group A2) showed different degrees of development of granulation tissue to the extent of making possible the consideration of skin grafting and potential complete resolution.

Analysis of our data suggests that addition of HBOT can improve the clinical outcome in the majority of cases of conventionally treated refractory varicose ulcers . Patients younger than 60 y.o. with a recent ulcer and less signs of chronic venous insufficiency have a better chance of healing as a result of HBOT. It is interesting to observe that duration of chronic venous insufficiency was similar in the three groups. HBOT should constitute a therapeutic consideration for refractory varicose ulcers.

Table 1. Characteristic of the groups defined by clinical outcome

Parameter	A1	A2	B	total
number	18	24	4	46
male:female	7:11	7:17	1:3	15:31
age (years)	63.7	70	67.5	67.4
age>60 y.o.	13 (63.3%)	22 (91.6%)	4 (100%)	39 (84.8%)
years of CVI@	19.75(n=8)	25.67(n=15)	26.75(n=4)	24.08 (n=27)
signs of CVI$	14%	36%	75%	30.8%
years of VU&	5.02 (n=10)	7.3 (n=14)	17(n=4)	7.85 (n=28)
observation period (months)	4.8	3	4.6	3.8
initial ulcer size				
d*1xd*2 (mm)	47x31	70x42 +5 gigantic	38x27 +1 gigantic	
reduction in ulcer size	81% (51-100)	10.2% (0-50)	-14% (-33-0)	

@ Chronic venous insufficiency
$ Pigmentation, edema and induration
& Varicose Ulcers
* Diameter

REFERENCES

[1] Strauss MB, Hargens AR, Gershuni DH, Greenberg DA, Crenshaw AG, Hart GB, Akeson WH: Reduction of skeletal muscle necrosis using intermittent hyperbaric oxygen in model compartment syndrome. J. Bone Jt Surg 65 - A.656-662,1983.

[2] Bass, BH The treatment of varicose leg ulcers by hyperbaric oxygen. Postgrad Med J 46:407, 1970

[3] Hyperbaric Oxygen Therapy : A Committee Report: Undersea and Hyperbaric Medical Society. Bethesda. 1992.

Phlebology '95, D. Negus et al. (eds.). Phlebology (1995) Suppl. 1: 913-914

OP/7.3

A Randomised Trial of a Knitted Viscose Dressing and a Hydrocolloid Dressing in the Treatment of Chronic Venous Ulceration

E.A. Nelson[1,4], C.V. Ruckley[1], D.R. Harper[2], B. Gibson[2], J.J. Dale[1] and R.J. Prescott[3]

[1] Lothian and Forth Valley Leg Ulcer Study, Royal Infirmary Edinburgh, [2] Falkirk and District Royal Infirmary, [3] University of Edinburgh, [5] University of Liverpool

Background

It is recognised that compression bandaging is the single most important element in the treatment of venous leg uceration, however, it has not been established definitively that choice of dressing can improve healing trates, although two recent studies seem to indicate that there may be some benefit in choosing occlusive dressings over non-occlusive ones [1,2].

Objective

To compare the healing rates using a knitted viscose dressing, NA (Johnson and Johnson) and a hydrocolloid, Improved Formulation Granuflex, (IFG) (Convatec) in the treatment of chronic venous leg ulcers.

Design

Two hundred patients with chronic venous leg ulceration (duration range 2 - 240 months) were recruited to this randomised, parallel group, open clinical trial.

Inclusion criteria were; age > 18, informed written consent, signs of venous disease. Exclusion criteria included; severe concurrent concurrent disease, ABPI < 0.8, diabetes, serological positive rheumatoid arthritis, participation in a concurrent clinical trial, taking vaso-active drugs, warfarin or steroids.

The bandage study was part of a multi-arm trial, other arms (bandage and oxpentifylline (Trental 400) vs. placebo) are reported in other communications.

Intervention

Patients were randomised to either an NA dressing or Improved Formulation Granuflex. Dressings were changes weekly, or more frequently due to exufdate leakage. Compression was provided by either single-layer or multi-layer bandages as dictated by the randomisrtion in the other arm of the trial. Additionally, patients received either Trental (3*400mg daily) or placebo.

914

Measurements

Monthly tracing of all ulcers on the trial leg until complete healing of ulcers or trial complete at 24 weeks.

Results

Healing rate was 59.8 % in 24 weeks with the IFG dressing and 57.1% with the NA dressing . The difference in healing rates was not significant (Odds ratio 1.12; 95% CI=0.64 - 1.96).

Conclusion

The two dressings healed similar proportions of leg ulcers when used in combination with high compression bandaging.

References

1. Callam MJ, Harper DR, Dale JJ, Brown D, Gibson B, Prescott RJ,Ruckley CV Lothian and Forth Valley Leg Ulcer Healing Trial, Part 2: Knitted viscose dressing versus a hydrocellular dressing in the treatment of chronic leg ulceration. Phlebology 1992: 7; 4 142-45.

2. Moffatt CJ, A trial of a hydrocolloid dressing in the management of indolent ulceration. J Wound Care, 1992: 1; 3; 20-22.

Phlebology '95, D. Negus et al. (eds.). Phlebology (1995) Suppl. 1: 915-916

PI/2.6

A Randomised Trial of Single Layer and Multi-Layer Bandages in the Treatment of Chronic Venous Ulceration

E.A. Nelson[1,4], D.R. Harper[2], C.V. Ruckley[1], R.J. Prescott[3], B. Gibson[2] and J.J. Dale[1]

[1] Lothian and Forth Valley Leg Ulcer Study, Royal Infirmary Edinburgh, [2] Falkirk and District Royal Infirmary, [3] University of Edinburgh, [5] University of Liverpool

Background

Previous work has demonstrated the efficacy of multi-layer, elastic, high compression regimen in the treatment of chronic venous leg ulcers (1). This study was designed to determine whether a single layer elastic system was as effective as a multi-layer elastic compression system.

Design

Two hundred patients with chronic venous leg ulceration (duration range 2 - 240 months) were recruited to this randomised, parallel group, open clinical trial.

Inclusion criteria were; age > 18, informed written consent, signs of venous disease. Exclusion criteria included; severe concurrent concurrent disease, ABPI < 0.8, diabetes, serological positive rheumatoid arthritis, participation in a concurrent clinical trial, taking vaso-active drugs, warfarin or steroids.

The bandage study was part of a multi-arm trial, other arms (dressing and oxpentifylline (Trental 400) vs. placebo) are reported in other communications.

Intervention

Patients were randomised to a single layer regime, i.e. Granuflex Adhesive Compression Bandage (Convatec, UK), or a multi-layer regime, i.e. Velband (Johnson and Johnson), Crepe (Smith and Nephew), Elset (Seton) and Coban (3M). The Elset and Granuflex bandages were applied in a figure of eight manner, all other bandages were applied using a simple spiral technique. Bandages were renewed weekly, or more frequently if necessary due to exudate leakage.

The primary dressing was either a knitted viscose dressing, or a hydrocolloid dressing, as determined by randomisation in the other arm of the trial. Patients were also randomised to either Trental (400mg three times daily) or placebo. For the purposes of analysis the three trials are considered separately.

916

Measurements

Ulcer tracings were taken every 4 weeks until all ulcers on the trial leg were healed or until the end of the trial at 24 weeks. The primary end-point was complete healing of all ulcers on the trial leg.

Results

The multi-layer bandage healed 69 % of reference ulcers, and the single layer bandage healed 49 % of reference ulcers in 24 weeks (Odds ratio 2.37; 95% CI = 1.3 - 4.2).

Conclusion

The multi-layer regime tested healed significantly more ulcers than the single layer system.

Reference

1. Callam MJ, Harper DR, Brown D, Gibson B, Prescott RJ, Ruckley CV. Lothian and Forth Valley Leg Ulcer Healing Trial. Part 1: Elastic versus non-elastic bandaging in the treatment of chronic leg ulceration. Phlebology 1992; 7: 136-141.

Phlebology '95, D. Negus et al. (eds.). Phlebology (1995) Suppl. 1: 917-918

OP/6.5

A Randomised, Double-Blind Placebo Controlled Trial of Oxpentifylline in the Treatment of Venous Leg Ulcers

J.J. Dale, C.V. Ruckley, D.R. Harper, B. Gibson, E.A. Nelson and R.J. Prescott

Lothian and Forth Valley Leg Ulcer Study, Vascular Studies Unit, Royal Infirmary of Edinburgh, UK

INTRODUCTION

Leg ulcers have an estimated prevalence of about 1% in Great Britain. Younger people as well as the elderly are affected and ulcers may remain unhealed for months or even years. Most ulcers will heal with adequate compression bandaging and suitable dressings but there are few drugs which have been shown to enhance conservative treatment. Oxpentifylline is a vaso-active drug which reduces leucocyte adhesion and has mild fibrinolytic effects. It has been suggested that treatment with oxpentifylline might reverse some of the effects observed in the occurrence of venous ulcers, namely the formation of pericapillary fibrin cuffs and white cell trapping.

This trial, which is part of a multi-arm study of compression bandaging, dressings and pharmacological treatment for leg ulcers, examines the effects of oxpentifylline on pure venous ulcers.

PATIENTS AND METHODS

Two hundred patients were entered into the pure venous arm of the trial. Inclusion criteria were; **age:** over 18 years, **ulcer duration:** at least two months, **size:** at least one centimetre in diameter, **aetiology:** purely venous. Exclusion criteria included: patients with diabetes, rheumatoid arthritis, an ankle/brachial arterial pressure index of <0.8, a history of recent cardiac, liver, renal or malignant disease, immobility, recent treatment with anticoagulants, systemic cortico-steroids, cytotoxic and other drugs which might affect healing. Sloughy ulcers and local infections were treated before randomisation.

Patients meeting the criteria were randomised sequentially to receive either slow-release oxpentifylline 400mg three times daily or an outwardly identical placebo, in combination with a standardised dressing (knitted viscose or hydrocolloid) and compression treatment (elastic single layer or multilayer bandages). One leg only for each patient was designated as the trial leg. Dressings were renewed weekly. Ulcers were traced and compliance checks were made at four-weekly intervals for 24 and weeks or until all ulcers on the trial leg were healed (i.e. fully epithelialised).

RESULTS

One hundred and one patients were treated with oxpentifylline and 99 with the placebo. The groups were well matched for age, sex, initial ulcer size and duration and other aetiological factors. Analysis on intention to treat showed that 65(64%) of those given oxpentifylline and 52(52%) of those given the placebo had completely healed ulcers within 24 weeks. [Odds ratio (95% CI)=1.67(0.94-2.99), p = 0.08].

Table 1 shows the patients who completed the trial according to the protocol.

TABLE I:
COMPLETE HEALING IN THE PURE VENOUS ULCER GROUP.

	Oxpentifylline	Placebo
Healed	61 (66%)	49 (53%)
Not healed	31 (34%)	44 (47%)
Total	92	93

[Odds ratio (95% CI) = 1.77 (0.98-3.20), p = 0.059].

After logistic regression analysis to compensate for the influence of bandage and dressing the results become statistically significant in favour of oxpentifylline.
[Odds ratio (95% CI) = 1.86 (1.01-3.42), p = 0.046].

CONCLUSIONS

The benefits of treating venous ulcers with oral oxpentifylline, although small, are useful in dealing with an intractible problem.

Phlebology '95, D. Negus et al. (eds.). Phlebology (1995) Suppl. 1: 919-921

V/3.8

Unna's Rigid Bandages as a Useful Method of Ambulatory Treatment of Vast Varicose Leg Ulcers

K. Twardowska-Saucha, Z. Fiutek, D. Czaczka and W. Saucha

Varicose Vein Clinic "Medservice", Zabrze, Poland

INTRODUCTION

The most frequently used type of wound dressings in the case of varicose ulcers of lower extremities are hydrocolloids dressings [1]. They are the method of choice in the treatment of small and medium ulcers in outpatient procedure, because they are easy to apply by the doctor as well as by the patient at home. They reduce pain quickly and may be left on for several days.

The treatment of big ulcers with accompanying inflammation, oedema, great ooze meets many inconveniences in outpatient procedure. In these ulcers the dressings should be changed frequently, sometimes every day. Another basic condition of successful treatment of leg ulcers is the use of proper compression [2].This is difficult especially in the patients unable to visit ambulatory very often and a lot of them are unable to change the dressing properly by themselves either.That's why these patients are treated predominantly in hospital.

The economical aspect of the matter is important too, since hydrocolloid dressings are expensive and the cost of treatment often exceeds the financial possibilities of the patient.

We were looking for the optimal method of treating this type of ulcers in outpatient procedure. So, an attempt was made to investigate the efficacy the forgotten method of treatment by Unna's rigid paste bandages (URPB). URPB was described for the first time in 1854 [3]. Since there are some inconveniences for medical staff when putting it on, it is hardly used. Both the components of the paste, the possibility of keeping it longer (7-10 days) and above all the possibility of applying constant compression, as well as much lower cost of treatment spoke for the use of URPB in this type of ulcers..

MATERIAL AND METHODS

URPB was used in 45 patients, i.e. 9 men, age $\bar{x}=61.6 \pm 8.24$ and 36 women, age $\bar{x}=60.2 \pm 9.8$ with vast, oozing ulcers, with accompanying inflammation and oedema, lasting from 1-25 years; one case 42 years. The size of the ulcers was estimated according to 4 grade score: I° - microulcers to $4cm^2$, II°- below $16cm^2$, III°- 16–$64cm^2$, IV°- above $64cm^2$. According to this score, there were: 3 patients with the II°, 24 ones with III°, 16 ones with IV° including 2 patients with the ulcers above $200cm^2$. In 42 patients we found varicose ulcers, in 3 patients mixed ulcers. Out of the last three, two patients were diabetic. URPB was used in the case of side effects or no reaction to the treatment used before. URPB was changed mostly every 7-10 days.

URPB composition: Zinci oxidati 60.0, Glycerini 100.0, Gelatini 60.0, Aquae destilatae 200.0 M.f. collodium.

Since URPB is of solid consistency, it was warmed up in a water bath until it achieved liquid consistency. Two or three cotton bandages were soaked with URPB and the leg was wound up from the foot to the knee. The ulcer was carefully cleaned with H_2O_2 before. Before the dressing was applied the patient kept his leg raised above the heart level for 1-$1^1/_2$ h. Oral antibiotics were applied in the cases of intensive inflammation. After 7-10 days the progress of the treatment was checked.

After the treatment with URPB was over, i.e. when there was no oedema, inflammation, oozing, when the surface of the ulcer was decreased, we used another method of treatment (absorbent or occlusive dressings or surgical treatment).

RESULTS

In 48.8% of patients URPB was used 3 or 4 times. In 17.7% of patients, it was sufficient to apply URPB only twice. 28.8% of patients required changing of URPB 5 or 6 times. In two patients (4.4%) in whom the surface of the ulcer exceeded $200cm^2$ URPB was changed 15 times.

In 40 patients, our treatment caused the complete healing of ulcers. It must be stressed that in 11 patients out of 45, URPB was used already during the 1st visit, because of marked inflammation and oozing. In 34 patients, URPB was applied because other treatment was ineffective.

In one patient with circular ulcer, above $64cm^2$ with circulatory insufficiency, and in 2 patients with ulcers above $200cm^2$, significant decrease of ulcer surface was achieved, however, no complete healing followed so far. One patient died before the end of the treatment for other reasons. In patient, with the ulcer of 35 cm^2 no complete healing was achieved because of his lack of co-operation with medical staff. In 7 patients surgical treatment was performed. Three of them underwent surgery before total healing of ulcer (quick healing of the ulcer followed).

DISCUSSION

URPB dressings appeared to be very effective form of treatment of vast varicose leg ulcers in the system of outpatient procedure. The efficacy of this treatment results from the several facts.

URPB dressings fulfil the basic condition of the proper ulcer treatment, i.e., constant compression. It works because it is set into a semi-hard cast which acts as a very effective form of external compression. The paste simply allows the bandage to mould to the shape of the limb. This is difficult in the case of hydrocolloid dressings.

URPB dressings absorbs the exudate, excess of which may easily pass through the dressing. This facilitates the quick ulcer cleaning. Hydrocolloid dressings do not give us this possibility in the cases of vast, oozing ulcers. The excess of the exudate seeps beside the dressing. This involves the necessity of frequent, even daily, change of the dressing at home by the patient, who is unable to do it properly.

URPB dressings do not limit the normal activity of the patient although he is forced to frequent keeping the leg in the horizontal position.

Between 1991-1994 Varicose Vein Clinic „Medservice" in Zabrze treated 312 patients with varicose vein ulcers. Out of them 45 (14.4%) required URPB use. In all those patients suffering from vast ulcers with inflammation, oozing and oedema URPB gave very good therapeutic effect.

CONCLUSIONS

URPB dressing is not very popular in Poland because of many technical inconveniences for medical staff. However, the application of this method in the case of vast ulcers allows much quicker healing process. Its combination with other methods of treatment creates the possibility of outpatient procedure. It is a very convenient method of treatment for disabled and/or elderly patients, living alone or in the patients who for many reasons are unable to visit a phlebologist frequently.

From our point of view the outpatient procedure makes it possible to achieve good results in leg ulcer treatment and a lot of patients consider this kind of therapy more comfortable then hospitalization.

REFERENCES

1. Browse NL, Burnard KG, Lea Thomas M. Diseases of the veins. London: Edward Arnold, 1988, 411-422.
2. Partsch H. Recommendation for compression therapy. Phlebologia Houston 91;302-325. PRM Editions, Dallas, Texas, USA.
3. Unna PG. Veber Paraplaste eine neue form medikaneutoser Pflaster.1854 Wien Med Wochenschr 1896; 46:1854-6.

Phlebology '95, D. Negus et al. (eds.). Phlebology (1995) Suppl. 1: 922-924

P175

The Treatment of the Extensive Venous Ulcers

G.R. Askerhanov, G.N. Emirov, G.M. Makhatilov and Z.G. Luguev

Surgical Clinic Dagestan Medical Institute, Makhachkala, Russia

INTRODUCTION

Extensive venous ulceration of the leg is one of the most serious complications of postphlebitic disease [1,2]. It depends on incompetence of the deep vein valves and pathological blood circulation in the perforating veins [3]. The traditional application of the proteoclastic enzymes, antiseptics, ointment bandage with the purpose of preparing the ulcer surface for autodermoplasty doesn't satisfy surgeons because of its duration and lack of efficacy [4]. Serious infective complications may follow surgery at an unprepared site.

The purpose of this investigation is the study of the efficacy of a new method of biological stimulation of the regenerative processes (MBSRP) and less traumatic surgical operations in patients with chronic venous insufficiency, complicated by the extensive ulceration.

METHODS

90 patients with extensive venous ulcers were examined. Dynamic plethysmography, Doppler ultrasound, phlebography , phlebomanometry, microbiological, histopathology, pH-meter testing of wound secretion were included in the investigation.

The patients were divided into two groups:

1. For the first group (55 patients) the proteoclastic enzymes, antiseptics and ointment bandages were applied.

2. MBSRP was used on 35 patients.

The MBSRP is based on the application of a combination of drugs in following concentrations: pepsinum - 2 parts, betaini chlorhydrate - 2 parts, methyluracilum - 1 part, dissolved in 5 parts of physiological solution. Gauze tampons were soaked and put on the wound twice a day. The suggested combination was used in exudative ulcers and in the early granulation phase of the ulceration process.

RESULTS

While using MBSRP positive changes in the ulcer process was observed from the first day of treatment. After 3-5 days ulcers were cleaned from a purulent appearance to active granulation and the epithelium appeared at the wound edges.

Microbiological investigation and histopathology of the contiguous tissue the ulcer became sterile after 5 days treatment. By this time a rapid change from a necrotic process to regeneration was marked. A considerable increase of the macrophages in the phase of active phagocytosis as well as the rapid growth of granulation tissue (profibroblast and fibroblast) were also noticed.

Autodermoplasty in combination with reconstructive surgery of the veins was performed after 15.7±4.3 days for second group of patients. Complete skin cover was obtained with 31 patients and partial cover in 4. (Table 1)

Table 1. The comparative indices of autodermoplasty results.

The timing and results of autodermoplasty	First group of 55 patients	Second group of 35 patients
Timing of autodermoplasty	24.3 ± 5.1 days	15.7 ± 4.3 days
Ulcer healing		
- complete	44 (80%)	31 (88.6%)
- partial	11 (20%)	4 (11.4%)

924

Autodermoplasty in 83 patients was combined with reconstructive venous surgery. Subfascial clipping of incompetent perforating veins by Linton's and Cockett's methods was performed in 61 patients. Suppuration of wounds in the postoperative period was noted in 6 (9.8%) of patients, necrosis of the wound edge in 9 (14.8%), lymphoedema in 3 (4.9%). Late ulcer recurrence was found in 5 (8.2%) patients.

Subfascial electrocoagulation or clipping of perforating veins through small incisions was employed in 22 patients with perforator incompetence. This method of subfascial disconnection through small incisions is considerably less radical than the Cockett and Linton's procedure. Efficacy of this operation was confirmed by quantitative assessment of the venous system using Doppler ultrasound and dynamic plethysmography in the immediate post operative period and during later follow up.

Decrease of the speed of reverse blood flow in the deep and perforating veins was marked after Cockett operation only in 38.5%, after Linton operation in 85.7% and in subfascial disconnection of perforating veins through small incisions in 72.9%. The total reverse blood flow was reduced to 76.4%, 9.2% and 88.5% of the pre-operative measurements. Using this method of operation on perforating veins greater improvement of the muscular-venous pump was observed. Post operative complications in this group comprised 4.5% of patients. Long term healing was obtained in 90.9% of patients.

CONCLUSION

The application of MBSRP combined with subfascial disconnection of perforating veins reduces the period of treatment required in patients with extensive venous ulcers.

REFERENCES

1. Browse N L, Burnand K G, Lea Thomas M. Diseases of the veins. Pathology, diagnosis and treatment. London: Edward Arnold, 1988.
2. Negus D. Leg Ulcers: A Practical Approach to Management. Oxford: Butterworth/Heinemann, 1991.
3. Hansson C. Studies on Leg and Foot Ulcers. Acta Derm Vener 1988; Suppl. 136: 1-45.
4. Blair S D, Wright D D I, Backhouse C M, Riddle E, McCollum C N. Sustained compression and healing of chronic venous ulcers. Br.Med.J. 1988;297;1159-61.

Phlebology '95, D. Negus et al. (eds.). Phlebology (1995) Suppl. 1: 925-928

P181

Comparative Study of Venous Leg Ulcer Treatment by a Local Use of Hypolipemics, Esters of Aryloxycarbonic Acid (Clofibrate, Fenofibrate and Bezafibrate)

M. Gligora

Private practice, Dermatovenerologist, Croatian Phlebological Society, A. Kovacica 22, 51000 Rijeka, Croatia

INTRODUCTION

In medical practice hypolipemics, esters of aryloxycarbonic acid (AOCA) derivatives have been solely used in the treatment of hyperlipidaemia peroraly: Clofibrate, Fenofibrate, Bezafibrate etc. [1,2]. We patented the use of these derivatives locally in the treatment of dermatological diseases [3,4]. Our ten years of local use of hypolipemics in patients with venous leg ulcer gave us possibility to compare results of double blind trials with 2% ointment Clofibrate, Fenofibrate and Bezafibrate. Further analysis showed that these substances stimulated various cells of mesodermal origin including lymphocytes, the principal cells of the immune system [5].

METHODS

There have been treated 40 patients in each group with 2% ointment Clofibrate, Fenofibrate (Procetofen) and Bezafibrate, along with the same number in the control groups with placebo. In the first two groups the placebo was white vaseline, while in the group with 2% Bezafibrate the placebo was certain epithelization ointment. Ointment was applied in thick layer on the venous leg ulcer twice a day. Treatment lasted from four weeks up to six months.

Laboratory findings

All subjects underwent the standard haematological and biochemical blood investigations prior to, during and after the therapy, as well as urine examinations. The AOCA (clofibric acid) in the serum was also examined in three patients before, during and after the therapy using spectrophotometry. Biopsy was carried out in 10 venous leg ulcer patients prior to and after the epithelization. All 10 subject underwent histopathologic research and ultramicroscopic examination.

RESULTS

Healing or reduction of venous leg ulcer was determined in 62% of patients treated with the 2% ointment Clofibrate, in 58% treated with Fenofibrate, and 56% in the group of patients treated with 2% ointment Bezafibrate. Side effects or allergic manifestations in not even one patient were determined during the whole treatment if ointments were applied in mentioned concentrations. The first sign of the treatment's positive results is disappearance of the pain after 3 or 4 days, and the first signs of epithelization are noticed during the second week of the treatment. The two types of epithelization, the centripetal and the insular, were very seldom seen simultaneously. Laboratory studies of standard haematological and biochemical examinations, as well as the urine tests have not shown alterations of normal values [3].

Clofibric acid was absent in the serum in the patient with venous leg ulcer before the therapy, but it increased from 0.3-0.71 µg/ml between third and eight day of local application of the drug, and never exceeded 1.60 µg/ml, even in patient with the largest leg ulcer after six months therapy (Table). This is only one third of the 4-5 µg/ml which results from moderate oral dosage [3].

T a b l e

No.	Patient	Sex	Age	Time of treatment	Serum concentration of clofibric acid in µg/ml
1.	V. R.	f.	31	3 days	0.30
2.	M. T.	f.	66	2 months	1.48
3.	J. P.	f.	65	6 months	1.60

Histopathological preparations of biopsy material, taken before the therapy and stained with haematoxylin-eosin lack fibrin show residual necrotic cells and cell nuclei. After epithelization the hyperplastic epidermis with hyperchromic nuclei and parakeratosis were found. Numerous newly formed blood capillaries in the corium, extending like a finger towards the epidermis, are observed after Mallory's staining [3].

In the ultramicroscopic examinations, the picture of the collagen fibers before the therapy is hazy, unclear and only their contour is seen (Figure 1.), After the therapy we could see fibroblasts rich with organellae and newly created collagen fibers and bundles together with numerous mast-cells (Figure 2.).

Depending on the concentration some derivatives of AOCA stimulate or suppress the proliferative response of lymphocytes, pointing to the possible use of these drugs as immunomodulators in clinical practice as well. We succeeded in demonstrating the proliferative response of peripheral blood lymphocytes to Bezafibrate, measured through the incorporation of [^{3}H]thymidine. In concentrations between $2x10^{-6}$ mg/ml and $2x10^{-3}$ mg/ml, Bezafibrate increase the proliferation of these principal cells of the immune system [5].

On the basis of the clinical experience, histopathologic, ultramicroscopic and immunological findings, and on the basis of pathogenetic notion about forming of venous leg ulcer, we think as older authors did, that the primary damage in venous leg ulcer is one that originates in mesenchyma, that is in blood vessels and collagen fibers of the dermis, caused by defect of microcirculation.

927

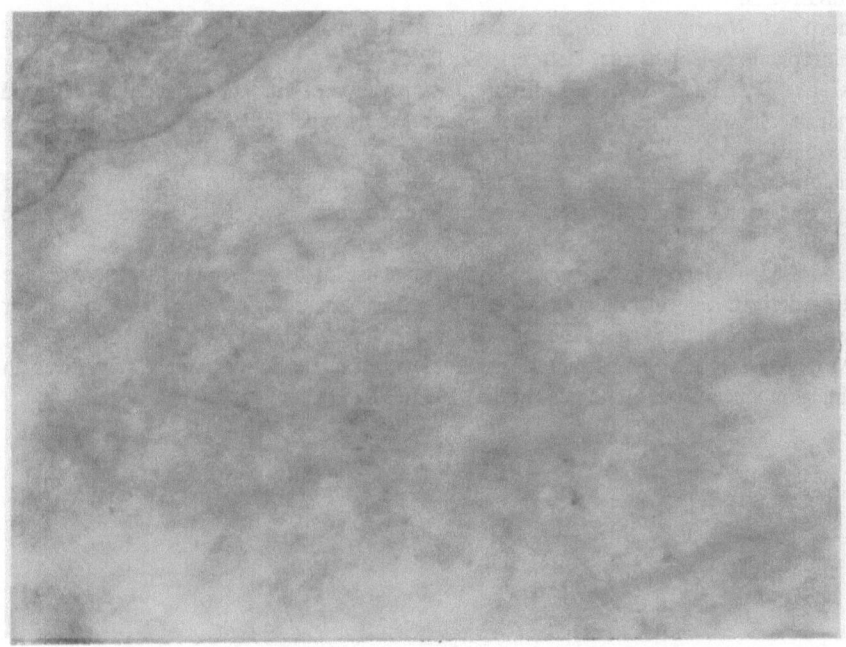

Figure 1.

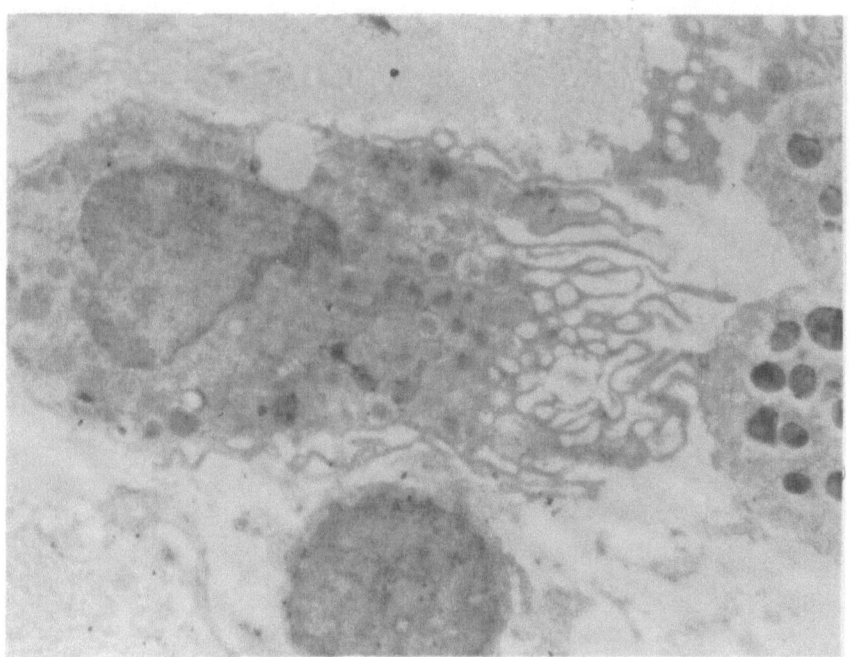

Figure 2.

REFERENCES

1. Thorp JM, Waring WS. Modification of metabolism and distribution of lipids by ethyl chlorophenoxy-isobutyrate. Nature 1962; 194:948-9.
2. Monk JP, Todd PA. Bezafibrate; A review of its pharmacodynamic and pharmacokinetic properties, and therapeutic use in hyperlipidaemia. Drugs 1987; 33: 539-576.
3. Gligora M. Regeneration of mesenchyma by a local use of hypolipemics, esters of aryloxycarbonic acid derivatives, in various dermatoses. J. Appl. Cosmetol. 1989; 7: 49-60.
4. Gligora M. Regeneration of mesenchyma by a use of hypolipemics, aryloxycarbonic acid derivatives, in mucocutaneous diseases, neurologic diseases, locomotor disturbances and diseases of the eye. Croatian patent 1993. No P 931105 A.
5. Dorić M, Gligora M. Further possibilities of using aryloxycarbonic derivatives in clinical practice. Folia Biologica (Praha) 1991; 37:131-3.

Phlebology '95, D. Negus et al. (eds.). Phlebology (1995) Suppl. 1: 929-931

OP/7.4

The Effectiveness of Compression in Healing Chronic Venous Ulcers

M.C. Stacey, Y. Vandongen, N. Trengove, S. Hoskin, P. Thompson and C. Pearce

University Department of Surgery, Fremantle Hospital, Fremantle, Western Australia

INTRODUCTION

The methods used to treat venous ulcers have not advanced dramatically for several centuries, apart from having available a large number of dressings to place on the ulcers. There has been no conclusive evidence that any particular agent, be it a dressing, a systemic drug or a topical agent, can speed up the healing of chronic venous ulcers.

The mainstay of treatment of venous ulcers is the provision of compression bandages to the leg[1]. These are thought to improve the venous return of the leg and as a consequence to improve the healing process[2]. Descriptions of compression methods have existed for several centuries[3]. In spite of this there is no clear evidence available to indicate whether compression does in fact improve the healing of chronic venous ulcers, and if so to what extent. Venous ulcers do at times heal without the use of compression bandages, and many patients find the bandages to be cumbersome and very limiting to their normal activities[4].

The aim of this study was to assess the influence of compression bandaging on the healing of chronic venous ulcers.

METHODS

This study was designed as a randomised controlled trial of compression bandaging compared to a local bandage only in the healing of chronic venous ulcers. Patients entered into this study had presented to the leg ulcer clinic at Fremantle Hospital. Only patients with proven venous ulceration and no other contributing cause for the ulceration were entered into this study. Investigations performed to assess ulcer aetiology were - arterial Doppler pressures, photoplethysmography, haemoglobin, urea and electrolytes, blood glucose, rheumatoid serology, and autoantibody screen.

After consenting to enter the study, patients were randomised to one of two groups. The dressing used in each group was identical - a hydrocolloid dressing (Duoderm, Convatec). If the skin surrounding the ulcer became macerated the dressing was changed to Allevyn (Smith and Nephew). Patients in the compression group had two short stretch bandages (Comprilan, Beiersdorf) applied to the leg from the base of the toes to just below the knee, and a stockingette placed over this to keep the bandages in place (Tubigrip, Seton). The no compression group had only a piece of stockingette placed over the region of the dressing in order to prevent it from lifting or moving. Patients attended the leg ulcer clinic weekly for dressing changes and review. If the ulcer was producing a lot of exudate which required more frequent dressing and bandage/stockingette changes, the dressings were performed two or three times per week as necessary.

Patients were continued in the trial until the ulcerated leg had healed or for a maximum of three months. Patients who had a rapid increase in ulcer size, or whose ulcer doubled in size during the course of the trial were regarded as having failed the trial and alternative therapy was instituted.

RESULTS

Eighty three patients have been randomised to this study. There were 40 females and 43 males, and the median age was 71 years.

Table 1 outlines the numbers of patients in each treatment group. Twenty two percent of patients withdrew from the no compression group compared to 9% from the compression group. The reasons for withdrawal were unrelated to ulcer healing - admission to hospital for another illness, noncompliance with the treatment method and personal reasons. In the compression group 28 patients (67%) had healed their ulcers by three months, compared to 9 patients (26%) in the no compression group.

No. of limbs	Compression	No compression
Randomised	46 (41 patients)	45 (42 patients)
Withdrawn	4	10
Healed	28	9
Failed to heal	14	26

Table 1. Outcome for ulcerated limbs in each treatment group.

The times taken to total healing of the limbs were evaluated by Cox Regression analysis, taking into account other variables such as ulcer size, patient age, duration of ulcer history and duration of the current ulcer. Compression therapy had a highly significant influence on the time to total healing of the ulcerated limbs. The β coefficient, Wald statistic and levels of significance of these different variables are shown in table 2 .

	Regression coefficient(β)	Wald statistic	p-value
Compression	0.597	9.092	0.003
Ulcer size	-0.038	1.734	0.188
Age	0.015	1.103	0.294
Ulcer duration	0.001	0.198	0.657
Ulcer history	-0.022	2.143	0.143

Table 2. Results of Cox regression analysis taking into account different variables.

The difference in healing times between the two groups is demonstrated graphically in Figure 1 which represents Kaplan-Meier survival curves for the two groups.

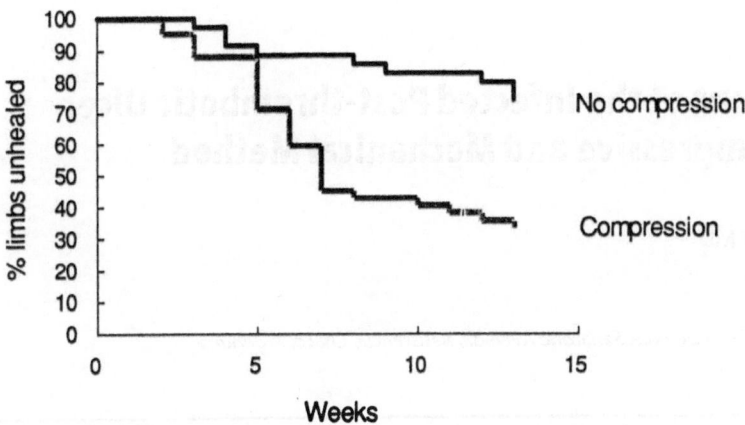

Figure 1. Kaplan-Meier survival curves for patients treated with and without compression therapy.

DISCUSSION

This study has demonstrated that effective compression therapy with short stretch bandages does significantly improve the rate of healing of chronic venous ulcers. This provides objective evidence for what to date has been only a generally held impression.

In addition this study has demonstrated that some patients are able to heal their venous ulcers in a relatively short time without requiring compression therapy. This implies that there may be a possibility of selecting those patients who will and those who will not require compression therapy. This would be of considerable practical advantage since patients are markedly limited in their activities by wearing compression bandages.

Other specific variables such as ulcer size, the age of the patient and the duration of the ulcer have not been found to significantly affect the time to ulcer healing in this study.

Clearly any potential advantages of modern dressings will not be maximised in patients with venous ulcers unless adequate compression therapy is instituted.

REFERENCES

1. Alexander House Group. Consensus paper on venous leg ulcers. Phlebology 1992; 7: 48-58.
2. Van der Molen HR, Toth LM, Collard JJ, Balmus KJ. Hemodynamic effects of elastic and non-elastic compression. Lymphokinetics1979; 33: 99.
3. Wiseman R. Severall Chirurgical Treatises. London, Royston & Took, 1676.
4. Baker SR, Stacey MC, Jopp-McKay AG, Hoskin SE, Thompson PJ. Epidemiology of chronic venous ulcers. Br J Surg 1991; 78: 864-7.

Phlebology '95, D. Negus et al. (eds.). Phlebology (1995) Suppl. 1: 932-934

OP/7.5

Treatment of the Infected Post-thrombotic Ulcer with Compressive and Mechanical Method

E.O. Beskow MD

Department of Phlebologie, Sanatorio Avenida, Resistencia, Chaco, Argentina

Living and working in the hot part of a country where the average monthly salary is around $ 150 dollars, and where a basic ten day antibiotic treatment cost arround $ 100 ,it is very difficult to perform an ideal medical practice. In addition the health insure pays $ 5.50 Dollars no more than two times monthly.

In these conditions we must seek simple, practical and affordable methods to treat the average patient, as it is explained in the following paragraphs.

REQUIRED MATERIALS:
- -REGULAR GARDEN TYPE WATER HOSE
- -THREE 20 CENTIMITERS WIDE, PLAIN GAUZE BANDAGES, 3 METERS LONG.
- -WALL PAPER COVERING, VINILIC TYPE GLUE
- -TUBULAR COTTON STOCKING .50 CENTIMITERS
- -TUBULAR ELASTIC COTTON STOCKINS , 50 CENTIMITERS
- -ANGLED SISSORS.
- -CONTAINER FOR THE VINILIC ADHESIVE GLUE
- -POLYURETANE FOAM (the bath type)

COST:

The gauze must be a linneal one and the nine meters cost $ 2.50
The wall paper covering vinilic glue comes from 1 kilogram, 10 and 20 kilos bucket. The cost of each is $ 0.30 the cost of 50 centimiters is. $ 0,60 and the elastic tubular $ 1.50. The polyuretane foam $ 0.10

The cost of the first bandage is around $ 5.10
The next bandage cost around $ 3.50

The social security pays $ 9.00 dollars each boot and most of them, are changed weekly. very few every 5 days. In especial circumnstances.

METHOD

In order to treat the local infections the patient must apply a high pressure jet and hitting on the ulcer surface during half an hour 3-4 times a day. favorable results are seen 5 to 30 days depending on the severity of the infection. The high pressure imparts a double effect:

a) mechanical cleaning of the infecting organisms and debris.

b) local stimulation of blood and lymph circulation.

In the case when Pseudomonae species are the etiologic agents a characteristic secretion is detected as bluegreen color and we apply cooking vinegar wich contains acetic acid. The latter causes a low ph in the area wherein the specific organisms can not survive.

Once the infection is overcame then is ready for the compressive treatment wich is recognized as highly efficient.

Our modification of the compressive treatment consists in the material utilized.

The ulcer is first covered with a gauze. Over the gauze we apply the poliuretane foam (we employ the type one used for upholstery) shaped a little larger than the ulcer surface.

In the next step the leg is wrapped around with a cotton bandage or cotton stocking up to the knee.

Finally the leg is wrapped around from distal to proximal up to the knee with three layers of overlapping gauze bandages.

The latter are previously immersed in the vinilic glue (liquid or Paste depending on the country). Blow-dryer can be use in cold places to accelerate the drying process.

After this put on the elastic cotton stockings or the elastic bandage.

The result is a semirigid bandage resembling a cast but relatively flexible in order to allow normal walking.

The bandage boot is removed between 5 to 7 days depending on the amount of secretion produced by the ulcer bed. The removal is done with am angled pair of scissors. When it is posible catch the free and unwrap it out.

The patient is encouraged to walk as much as possible during the treatment since the mechanism of action of this method is based on the effect of the muscle-pump and the venous return off the leg.

Most of the patients had been laying in bed for weeks or months under different treatments and therefore the possibilty of walking is greatly appreciatd by them.

The healing process of the ulcer advances at a rate of approximately 1 to 2 mm per week in a concentric manner.

We found that with the application of the compressive method and in the absence of infecction. any posthrombotic ulcer can be healed with perseverance.

If during the comppresive treatment infeccion recurs, discontinue the bandage and repeat the water impact treatment.

In patients when the surgical treatment with auto grafts failures we use sintetic grafts (PROTEITA)

934

Other uses may be given to this type of bandage such as
inmobilization in orthopedic injuries for instance, wrist
or ankle enthorsis and inmobilization of different types of
wounds, skin grafts , etc.etc.

ERWIN OMAR BESKOW   M.D.
SANATORIO AVENIDA
AV. SARMIENTO 391
3500 RESISTENCIA
CHACO -ARGENTINA

P150

THE ROLE OF PROTEIN-FREE CALVES' BLOOD EXTRACT IN THE MANAGEMENT OF CHRONIC VENOUS CRURAL ULCERS.

FAROUK A. MOLOKHIA (MD,FACS)

Dept. of Surgery, Faculty of Medicine, Alexandria University - EGYPT.

Objective   : To evaluate the role of protein-free extract of calve's blood in healing of chronic venous leg ulcers.

Design   : Clinical trial.

Patients   : 20 legs with clincally chronic post-phlebitic ulcer.

Intervention: Drug given intramuscular and topically applied with leg elevation and elastic compression.

Measurements: Regular observations for signs of healing.

Conclusions : All ulcers healed within an average of 42 days. No side effects were noted.

P036

EARLY TREATMENT OF THE LOWER LIMBS OEDEMA FOLLOWING INGUINO-ILIAC NODAL DISSECTION FOR METASTASES OF MELANOMA

Zanolla R, Balzarini A, Pirovano C, Martino G.

Physical Therapy and Rehabilitation Department, National Cancer Institute, Milan, Italy

Objective: To evaluate the efficacy of early rehabilitative treatments of the oedema of the lower limbs following inguino-iliac nodal dissection for metastases of melanoma.

Design: Prospective study of a consecutive series.

Patients: 60 patients with nodal metastases of melanoma.

Intervention: Starting from the first day after surgery, elastic compressive bandage. Heparinic treatment (Calciparine 0.2 ml t.i.d.) in cases with deep venous thrombosis (DVT). In the other patients, from the fifth day, passive and active mobilization and assisted walk. At the discharge from hospital, in cases with medium or severe diffuse oedema, hypoproteic and hypolipidic diet, 3 courses of manual or ultrasonic lymphatic drainage or mechanical pressure therapies every four months and made to measure elastic sleeve. In cases with slight and/or localized oedema only diet therapy and elastic sleeve.

Measurements: In all cases articular and muscular examination, centimetric measurements of both limbs, repeated every four months for a year. In cases with clinical signs of DVT Echocolordoppler (ECD), repeated after pharmacological treatment.

Results: Immediately after surgery there was, in all the patients, the appearance of oedema, localized or diffuse and ranging from slight to medium/severe, associated with algic functional limitations. In 6 cases there was DVT, confirmed by ECD. The pharmacological treatment allowed, in all of them, the whole recovery of venous flow but not the disappearance of the oedema. In the 27 patients with slight or localized oedema the diet therapy and the regular use of elastic sleeve led to disappearance or sharp reduction of lymphostasis. In the 33 cases with medium or severe oedema, including those caused by vascular damage, early draining therapies enabled us to stabilize or to reduce of about 30% the oedema size. In no cases there were functional or algic sequelae.

Conclusions: Early rehabilitative treatments have proved to be efficacious in reducing the oedema size and in preventing its impairment.

P154

DIFFERENCE IN WOUND HEALING BETWEEN CONVENTIONAL TREATMENT AND NEW GROWTH FACTOR FORMULA

Maessen-Visch MB, Asselman AH, Veraart JCJM, Neumann HAM

Department of Dermatology, Academisch Ziekenhuis Maastricht, The Netherlands

Objective: Many different types of wound dressings are available to stimulate healing of different types of wounds. To improve wound healing we developed a wound gel, containing amino-acids, vitamins, sugars, inorganic salt, trace elements, growth hormone, insulin, triiodothyronine and transferrin called Cariel. The gel is normally used for culturing keratinocytes.
Design: Pilot study
Patient: 19 donorsites from punchgraft biopsies taken from one patient on the upper leg were treated with conventional therapy (unitule) and 19 donorsites from punchgraft biopsies were treated with the new wound formula. Surroundings of the wound were protected with zinkzalf. Dressing changing took place every day.
Measurements: Evaluations were made the third, sixth and ninth day. Standard slides of the wounds were made. Different stages of wound healing were compared.
Results: There was a remarkable difference between the donorsites treated with the new wound formula and the control group. Donorsites treated with the new formula healed much faster than with conventional therapy.
Conclusions: The new growth factor gel Cariel Dermal seems to be an effective form of stimulating wound healing.

V/3.6

CAUSATIVE THERAPY OF LEG ULCERS

Dr Marte-Rotter, Elizabeth

Institut für hypostat. Beinleiden, A-5020 Salzburg, AUSTRIA

The concept, method and results of a causative therapy of leg ulcers as it was developed and practised by Dr Hans Rotter are summarised in a video. The principle of this therapy makes use of accelerating the blood flow in the legs by compression bandages as introduced by H Fischer. The refined original Rotter-method employing individually modelled bandages is demonstrated; examples of cases with hypostatic diseases (acute and chronic) are being presented and their clinical outcome is visualised. The results in 1408 fully treated chronic cases indicate cure without recurrence in 1294 patients (92%), cure with recurrence in 98 (7%) and improvement, but no cure in 16 patients (1%). The ratio of patients who discontinued the treatment prematurely was 192 of 1600 (12%).

P158

THE RESISTENT ULCUS CRURIS IN THE AMBULATORY CARE

Stahel H.-U.

Stadelhoferstr. 8, CH-8001 Zürich,
Switzerland

The resistent ulcus cruris is often representing a therapeutical problem because of its multiple sources. A good clarification is the basis for the therapeutical concept.
The therapy is conformed to the aetiological factors and to the local treatment, at which the treatment of the ulcus, inclusively manual lymphdrainage, is taking up a key-position.

P161

IN WHICH PATIENTS COMPRESSION STOCKINGS MAY CURE VENOUS ULCERATION?

Horakova M., Mayer W., Partsch H.

Dept of Dermatology, Wilhelminen Hospital,
A-1171 Vienna, AUSTRIA.

Objective: To compare the treatment of venous ulcers by elastic stockings with short stretch bandages and to evaluate causes for non-healing. **Design:** In a prospective trial 25 patients were treated by Sigvaris stockings and 25 by Rosidal-bandages. **Results:** After 3 months 21 (84%) ulcers were healed in the Sigvaris-group and 13 (52%) in the Rosidal-group. The reason for the better results with Sigvaris was mainly the fact that in the Rosidal-group more severe and resistant cases had been included. Negative predictive factors for non-healing of ulcers were: higher age, longer duration and larger size of venous ulceration and a positive Stemmer's sign on the foot. **Conclusion:** Patients who do not present with these conditions are potential candidates for therapy with compression stockings.

P171

RESULTS OF A RANDOMISED, DOUBLE-BLIND, PLACEBO CONTROLLED TRIAL OF OXPENTIFYLLINE IN THE TREATMENT OF ARTERIAL LEG ULCERS.

Prescott RJ, Ruckley CV, Harper DR, Gibson B, Nelson EA, Dale JJ, Lothian and Forth Valley Leg Ulcer Study: Falkirk and District Royal Infirmary, Royal Infirmary Edinburgh, University of Edinburgh. Scotland.

Objective

To compare oxpentifylline (Trental 400 mg, three times daily) with placebo, in the healing of arterial leg ulcers.

Design

Randomised, parallel group, two-centre, open clinical trial. Part of a multi-arm trial, other arms (compression bandages for venous ulcers and dressing) are reported in other communications.

Patients

Forty one patients with arterial impairment and arterial leg ulceration were randomised to receive either oxpentifylline (Trental 400 mg slow release tablets three times daily) or placebo, in the arterial limb of a larger study of 286 ulcer patients, with additional randomisation for type of dressing.

Measurements

The primary end-point was complete ulcer healing within the treatment period of 24 weeks.

Results

Seven of 22 (32%) patients in the Trental arm healed their ulcers compared to one of 19 (5%) patients on placebo (Odds ratio 8.4; 95% CI = 0.87 - 399; p = 0.07). There were similar numbers of adverse events in the two groups.

Conclusion

Treatment with oral oxpentifylline (400 mg three times daily) was well tolerated and gave encouraging results with regard to complete ulcer healing, though just failing short of achieving statistical significance at the conventional 5% level.

P191

SURGICAL TREATMENT OF VARICOSE LEG ULCERATION IN DAY SURGERY.

Piutek Z., Twardowska-Saucha K., Czaczka D., Wygoda Z.

Varicose Vein Clinic "Medservice", Zabrze, Poland.

Objective: The efficacy of surgical varicose ulceration treatment.

Design: Retrospective evaluation of treatment results.

Patients: 48 patients with leg ulcer with patent but not always sufficient deep system and long saphenous vein and/or short saphenous vein insufficiency and/or incompetent perforating veins.

Intervention: Conservative leg ulcer treatment preceded surgery. In 50% patients surgery preceded final ulcer healing. Methods: limited stripping, phlebectomy, ligation of insufficient perforators.

Measurements: Evaluation of healing time, trophic changes, edema and pain disappearance, remission frequency (after 6 months).

Results: Group operated before final - ulcer healing: complete healing after 2 weeks. No complications or remissions were observed in both groups.

Conclusions: Surgery accelerated healing process, caused the disappearance of oedemas and pain and the decrease of trophic changes.

P086

MERCURY PRESSOTHERAPY IN THE TREATMENT OF LIPODERMATOSCLEROSIS

Louis Grondin, Ron Young, Lilly Wouters
The Grondin Medical Center, Calgary, Canada

The importance of compression as the silent healer of veno-lymphatic disorders is presently well accepted (1). At present the international effort of standardisation (2) of support garments offers to both the therapist and the researcher unsurpassed tolls in broadening the field of application of compressive therapy. Mercury pressotherapy as a new therapeutic modality (3) has offered further assistance in the management of chronic edema and lymphoedema (4).

Lipodermatosclerosis (5) has been described as an intermediate state of chronic venous insufficiency leading to further complications such as bouts of acute hypodermatitis and recurrent stasis ulcerations. Its treatment besides the daily use of compression garments has included various agents such as pentoxiphillin (6) and dapsone (7). Pentoxiphillin has the disadvantage of requiring several weeks before improvement may be observed (6), and dapsone has definite toxic side effects which limits its use and indications (7). Finally fibrinolytic agents such as stanozol (8) and other products (9) have been found effective in reversing chronic lipodermatosclerosis and its complications.

In our experience mercury pressotherapy has demonstrated to be an excellent therapy for lipodermatosclerosis in not only reversing the underlying condition without chemotherapy, but also in preventing and reversing its complications namely, acute dermatitis and stasis ulcerations.

References: (1) Bassi, Stemmer (1983): Traitement Mecaniques Fonctionnels En Phlebologie Editions Piccin; (2) Gummistrumpfe, EV, Schattauer. (1989). The Medical Compression Stocking. Gutezeichengemeinschaft Medizinischer; (3) Cartier, CJ (1983): Traitment Des Oedemes Vasculaires Des Membres Par Bain De Mercure. Hour. Des Mal. Basc, 1983 P. 297-300; (4) Schadech M (1991) Mercury Bath Pressotherapy on Lympho-venous Disorders. Proceedings of the Canadian Sceeity of Phlebology, Whistler 1991; (5) Caille. (1985): Phlebologie en Pratique Quotidienne. Expansion Scientifique Francaise; (6) (1988): Haemorheologie Et Agregation Erythrocytaire. Deuxieme Symposium International, Paris; (7) Lack, Edward (1989): The Use Of Dapsone In The Treatment of Lipodermatosclerosis. Proceedings of the Phlebology Society of America. (8) Layer, TT et al (1986): Stanozol And The Treatment Of Venous Ulceration. Phlebology, December 1986; (9) Belcaro, G, Marelli C (1989): Defibritide, Elastic Compression and Lipodermatosclerosis. Phlebology, June 1989.

P172

TOPICAL APLICATION OF PGE2 IN TREATMENT OF VENOUS ULCERS

Pavlova Li, Nikolovska S, Dervendzi D, Starova A, Grivceva-Panovska V
Clinic of Dermatology, Medical Faculty, Skopje, Makedonija

Objective: To evaluate the benefit of topical applicated PGE_2 in the treatment of venous ulcers.

Design: Randomised open clinical trial.

Patients: 50 outpatients with venous ulcers; 32 with ulcus cruris hypostasicum and 18 with ulcus cruris postphlebiticum.

Intervention: After prior complex investigative procedures (photoplethysmography refilling tests, doppler ultrasound examination and bacteriological indentification) PGE_2 on gel - foam carrier was topically applied. This therapeutical scheme was continuously repeated every 3 - 4 days.

Measurements: The assesment was clinically done by a skilled dermatologist. The following criteria were taken into consideration: clinical withrowal of inflamation, clinical time between the first signes of granulomatous tissue up to epithelisation and tolerability of the treatment.

Results: Complete epithelisation was documented in 29 vs 32 patients with hypostasic venous ulcers in a period ranged from 14 up to 40 days in dependency with the ulcer extension. In the group of 18 patients with venous postphlebitic ulcers, complete epithelisation was diagnosed in 9, while 6 had significant granulations and 3 were non - responsive in 40 days follow - up. In 6 months follow - up period we did not find recidiving ulcers.

Conclusions: The presented data strongly suggests that this therapeutical approach shortens the duration of treatment, attain a stable and lasting closure of the wound completly respecting the comfort of the patient.

P173

LOW FREQUENCY ULTRASOUND OF CHRONIC VENOUS LEG ULCERS IN AN OUTPATIENT THERAPY

Peschen M, Vanscheidt W

Department of Dermatology, University of Freiburg, Germany

Objective: To review the preliminary clinical experience of a new method in local treatment of chronic venous leg ulcers when given in addition to conventional therapy.
Design: Randomised parallel group open clinical controlled study.
Patients: Twelve patients with chronic ulcerations of the leg due to chronic venous insufficiency.
Intervention: Patients were randomised to conventional therapy with topical application of fibrinolytic agents and compression therapy or conventional therapy with additional ultrasound treatment for 12 weeks. The ultrasound treatment consisted of 10 minutes of foot bathing with application of 30 kHz ultrasound 100 mW/cm^2 three times a week.
Measurements: The ulcer area was measured by planimetry before treatment and after treatment and after 2, 4, 6, 8, 10 and 12 weeks therapy. Colour photographs of the ulcers were taken under standard conditions at the same time. After each treatment local findings and side effects were recorded.
Results: After 12 weeks treatment the ultrasound group (6 patients) showed a significant better response to therapy than the control group. While the control group showed a mean decrease of 9% in the ulcerated area, in the ultrasound group the mean ulcerated area decreased by 65% ($p < 0.05$). There were only minor side effects of mild erythema and occasionally small pinhead sized bleedings.
Conclusions: The application of low frequency ultrasound seems to be a helpful treatment option in chronic venous leg ulcers, especially if they are not responding to conventional ulcer treatment.

OP/22.5

EMBOLISATION OF INSUFFICIENT PERFORATORS IN PATIENTS WITH VARICOSE ULCERATION

Garcarek J, Rybak Z, Szyber P

Department of Vascular Surgery and Radiology.
Wroclaw Medical University, Wroclaw, Poland

Objective: To review the preliminary clinical experience of a new method of treatment incompetent perforators with an embolisation.
Design: Review of patients underwent embolisation of insufficient perforators with Gianturco-Wallace and Amplatz coils.
Patients: Seven (11 legs with open ulceration) were undergoing this study. Diagnosis was stated by phlebology, venous pressure recordings and doppler examination.
Intervention: After localisation of insufficient perforators and elimination of deep vein thrombosis with a puncture of the superficial vein of the leg Gianturco-Wallace coil was inserted to the place of insufficient perforator. At the same time Amplatz coil was placed just below sapheno-femoral junction to prevent extension of thrombus to the deep system or pulmonary embolism.
Measurements: 7 to 8 phlebograms in two projections were performed before and following procedure which was fluoroscopic controlled. Using the same needle venous pressure recordings were performed with TESTAR 2000 as well as doppler examination.
Results: Early results are promising. Ulcerations were healed within 4 weeks. Any complications were observed. Venous pressure decreased about 15 mm Hg following procedure.
Conclusion: This procedure is an alternative for Linton operation in high risk patients.

OP/1.6
LOHMANN'S THREE PHASE WOUND MANAGEMENT SYSTEM FOR LEG ULCERS

Horakova A M

Mosnova 25, 15000 Praha, Czech Republic

Objective: The study will demonstrate that the treatment of leg ulcers according to Lohmann's three phase wound management heals faster and in a more economical manner in comparison with the conventional treatment with traditional wound pads. In the exudative phase the Lohmann's three phase wound management uses an absorbent wound pad (Oprasorb), in the granulation phase a Hydrogel (Opragel) according to the principle of the moist wound treatment and in the final epithelisation phase a polyurethane film (Opraflex) which further contains the moisture in the wound environment.

Design: Randomised study with a test and control group.

Patient: 15 test groups with leg ulcers. 15 control groups with leg ulcers.

Intervention: Just patients with leg ulcers. Leg ulcers must be in the exudation phase, max. size 9 x 9 cm. Basis therapy with compression bandages. No use of additional medication during the treatment.

Measurements: Measuring of the size of the wound and photo documentation every week.

Results: The study will be finalised in February 1995. It reveals that the wound treated according to the Lohmann's three phases wound management really heal faster in comparison with the use of traditional compression bandages.

Conclusion: The result is that this treatment of leg ulcers according to the three phases saves costs expensive wound dressings are used.

P179
Antibiotic Policy in Leg Ulcer Management

Mr. I. G. Schraibman

Department of Surgery
Birch Hill Hospital
Rochdale.

Objective - To determine the need for antibiotic therapy in leg ulcers in relation to the type of organism present.

Setting - Dedicated Leg Ulcer Clinic

Subjects - 508 patients seen over 10 years (1983-93)

Design - retrospective analysis of bacteriological swabs identifying four grops of organisms - Staphylococcus aureus, enterobacteria, anaerobes and Beta haemolytic streptococcus (BHS)

Main outcome measure - proportion healed related to the presence of bacterial groups.

Statistics - life table analysis

Result - there was significant decrease in proportion of ulcers healed associated with the presence of BHS but not with any other bacteria.

Conclusion - there is an indication to treat BHS if present in leg ulcers but this does not apply to staph aureus, enterobacteria or anaerobes.

P180

Ten year personal experience of a Leg Ulcer Clinic (L.U.C.)

Mr. I. G. Schraibman

Department of Surgery
Birch Hill Hospital
Rochdale.

552 new patients were seen in the Rochdale LUC 1983-93. The records of 508 were examined. 21% were referrals from outside Rochdale; the incidence p.a. was 0.018%. The largest diagnostic group were venous ulcers (51%). Overall healing rate was 60% (upto 80% in some categories) with a low recurrence rate of 12%. A group of Non-V, Non-A ulcers seen distinct. Foot pulses impalpable in 46% of the whole group but in only 13% was arterial disease confirmed by A/A ratio. As previously reported, Beta haemolytic streptococcus was present in 19.3% of swabs and was associated with a significantly delayed healing time. The LUC was cost-effective with a saving of £28,000 in the first year, rising to £50,000 over 5 years.

P087

TREATMENT OF VENOUS ULCERS AND VENOUS INSUFFICIENCY WITH NON-ELASTIC SUPPORT. (CIRCAID LEGGING)

Gonzalez C.A.

2834 N. Milwaukee, Chicago, IL 60618.

Objectives: Evaluate role of non-elastic support as a means of healing venous ulcers and improvement of venous insufficiency.

Design: Patients using conventional therapy with elastic supports and patients with non-elastic supports. Measure compliance and comfort associated with healing of the ulcer and improvement of the quality of life.

Patients: 8 on elastic supports, 11 on non-elastic supports.

Results: Healing rates with elastic supports were lower and compliance very poor due to difficult and painful application of the stockings.
After healing of the ulcer, compliance with elastic stockings improved due to greater cosmetic acceptability.

Use of non-elastic supports resulted in good compliance due to the easy and comfortable application to the ulcerated leg, and no need for special application devices. Results are optimal and superior in every aspect regarding elastic supports.
After healing compliance decreased due to cosmetic reasons. Consequently we advise to switch to elastic supports at this stage.

Conclusion about non-elastic supports:
Superior performance.
Better compliance.
Low rate of recurrence.
Easy application.
No need for special application devices.
Excellent durability.

OP/6.4
30-kHz ultrasound treatment of chronic leg ulcers

M.Weichenthal, P.Mohr and E.W.Breitbart

Dermatologisches Zentrum

Am Krankenhaus 1, D-21614 Buxtehude, Germany

Objective: To evaluate the effect of ultrasound treatment in chronic leg ulcers of either veneous or of arterial or diabetic etiology.

Design: Comparison of two controlled studies.

Treatment: Patients receiving a standard conventional ulcer therapy were randomly assigned to receive additional ultrasound treatment receiving approx. 100mW/cm^2 for 15 minutes 3 times weekly.

Measurements: The ulcers surface was calculated by planimetry once weekly, and healing was compared between both treatment groups. Additionally, perfusion was monitored by Laser Doppler blood flow measurements after ultrasound exposure.

Results: In comparison to controls, additional 30 kHz ultrasound treatment 3 times weekly significantly improved wound healing. This effect was more pronounced in outpatient treatment as compared to a hospital based study. While the latter study was only performed on veneous ulcers, new data show that arterial or diabetic ulcers may also have benefit from ultrasound treatment. Thus, the mechanisms of ultrasound treatment seem not to be related to venous hypertension alone. Improvement of perfusion could be shown by Laser Doppler blood flow measurements after ultrasound exposure which may account for the effects of treatment .

P185
TOPICAL APPLICATION OF GROWTH FACTORS: A NEW THERAPY IN CHRONIC VENOUS DISEASE

F Schellhammer, G Raderschadt, A Gaitsch

II Dep of Surgery, University Cologne (Dir. H Troidl, PhD)

Purpose: Approximately 1 percent of the whole population is suffering from chronic venous crural ulcers. Prolonged ulceration not only causes an individual psychological burden, but also significant socio-economic expense, our purpose was to observe the use of topical application of growth factors in order to accelerate wound healing.
Method and Materials: Patients with chronic crural ulceration were treated with growth factors (PDGF, PF-4, PDAF, TGAF-B, PDEGF) prepared from homologous platelets. Each treatment was initiated by surgical debridement and compression bandage therapy. Inclusion criteria were chronic venous crural ulcers of more than 8 weeks, or presentation for amputation. Pregnant patients were excluded and also patients suffering from any kind of carcinoma or infectious disease.
Results: 9 patients with 13 ulcers, grade 2 to 5, were treated. 4 patients suffered from a postphlebitic limb, 5 had gravitational ulcers. Ulcer histories averaged 13 months with a range of 3 to 36 months. We achieved epithelialisation in 11 cases with a mean 7 weeks of therapy (range: 3 to 12 weeks), without operative treatment. However, in two cases, treated for 26 weeks, no wound-healing was achieved since the wound floor consisted entirely of hypertrophied fascia. Cockett's procedure lead to improvement in one non-responding case.
Conclusion: Topical application of growth factors has been reported to be useful in the treatment of chronic diabetic wounds. Wound healing was shown to be accelerated, resulting in a more stable scar. In addition, a therapy using growth factors seems to be reasonable. We believe growth factors to be a new powerful tool in the therapy of chronic venous ulcers. However, we understand, that our preliminary data does not represent a proper clinical study, which has yet to be done.

Deep Venous Reflux and Occlusion/Venous Ulcers

Treatment of Deep Venous Disorders and Venous Ulceration
The Surgical Treatment of Deep Venous Disorders and Leg Ulcers

Phlebology '95, D. Negus et al. (eds.). Phlebology (1995) Suppl. 1: 945-948

OP/6.9

"Shave-Therapy" of Lipodermatosclerosis: A New Treatment for Chronic Venous Ulcers

W. Schmeller and S. Roszinski

Department of Dermatology and Venereology, Medical University of Lübeck, Germany

INTRODUCTION

Lipodermatosclerosis (LDS) means induration of dermis and subcutis in the legs of patients with chronic venous insufficiency (CVI) (1). Computed tomographic scanning, magnetic resonance imaging (4) and 20 MHz-ultrasound (7) showed, that it is a consistent feature of the tissue around and under venous ulcers; it is characterized by typical morphological (6) and functional (3, 5) changes. Because the removal of circumscribed areas of LDS had proved to be beneficial in the treatment of venous ucers (2), we used a special surgical procedure in patients with ulcers resistant to therapy and extensive forms of LDS, that covered vast areas of the lower leg.

PATIENTS

In the last 18 months in the Department of Dermatology in Lübeck 3 men and 5 women (average age 68,8 years) were treated with a new therapeutic procedure. In these 8 patients 10 legs showed chronic and recurrent venous ulcers, that were treated without success for long periods, some for more than 20 years. 5 patients had a history of deep vein thrombosis. In all of them a deep venous insufficiency was revealed by Doppler ultrasound.

METHOD

In spinal anesthesia the ulcers together with all surrounding sklerotic areas in the lower legs were removed in layers with the

Schinkel humby knife. Often these areas covered the whole circumference of the lower leg. According to the amount of lipodermatosclerosis the "shaving"-depth reached the superficial or deep layers of the fibrotic subcutis. Grafting with meshed split skin from the thigh was done immediately afterwards.

RESULTS
More than 90 percent of each graft was taken. Clinical examination after 3 and 6 months showed very good results (Fig. 1a and 1b).

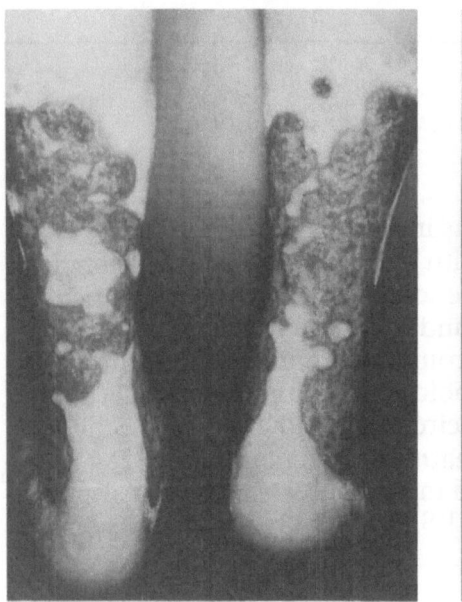 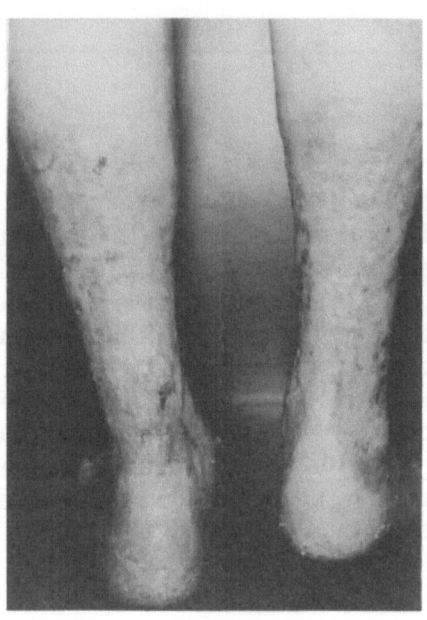

1 a   1 b

Fig. 1 79 year old patient with deep venous insufficiency in postthrombotic syndrome a) before and b) 3 months after "shave"-therapy

Measurements of different parameters of microcirculation were performed in healthy appearing skin in the proximal third of the lower leg and at the ulcer border before and 3 months after surgery. In addition to established methods of microcirculation the intracutaneous oxygen pressure (icpO2) was examined with steel shafted needle probes as described earlier by our group (3). The results are shown in table 1. Significant differences were found post-operatively in the grafted areas in the parameters transcutaneous (44°C) and intracutaneous oxygen pressure and Laser Doppler flow (p<0,05, Wilcoxon Matched-Pairs Signed-Ranks Test).

Table 1

	healthy skin before operation	healthy skin after operation
tcpO$_2$ 37°C	12 +/- 4	9 +/- 5
tcpO$_2$ 44°C	66 +/- 8	65 +/- 16
icpO$_2$	47 +/- 8	44 +/- 6
LDF	13 +/- 6	16 +/- 10
a (colorimetry)	4,7 +/- 1,4	4,9 +/- 1,8
temp	31,1 +/- 1	31,7 +/- 1

	ulcer border before operation	grafted ulcer after operation
tcpO$_2$ 37°C	0,5 +/- 1	1,0 +/- 1,5
tcpO$_2$ 44°C	3,0 +/- 3,5	19 +/- 15
icpO$_2$	15 +/- 8	23 +/- 6
LDF	172 +/- 92	99 +/- 91
a (colorimetry)	13,6 +/- 4,4	12,3 +/- 2,5
temp	32,3 +/- 1	33 +/- 1

CONCLUSION

"Shaving" of lipodermatosclerosis is a simple and quick surgical procedure and seems to be very effective in the treatment of venous ulcers, that are resistant to other therapeutic modalities. Long time follow up studies and experiences with large numbers of patients are still missing.

948

REFERENCES

1. Kirsner RS, Pardes JB, Eaglstein WH, Falanga V. The clinical spectrum of lipodermatosclerosis. J Am Acad Dermatol 1993; 28:623-627

2. Lehnert W, Winter H, Bellmann KP. Radikale Ulkus-Narben-Faszienexzision bei schweren und schwersten Formen der chronischen Bein-Beckenveneninsuffizienz. Tagungsbericht der Deutschen Dermatologischen Gesellschaft. Zbl Haut Geschl Kr 1993; 62 (Suppl):204

3. Roszinski S, Köser T, Wilhelm KP, Schmeller W. Untersuchungen der Oxygenierung von Dermis und Subkutis bei Dermatolipo-sklerose. Vasa 1993; 22 (4):297-305

4. Schmeller W, Gmelin E, Rosenthal N. Veränderungen des Retromalleolarraums bei chronisch venösem und arthrogenem Stauungssyndrom. Phlebol Proktol 1989; 18:175-181

5. Schmeller W, Maack A. Multilokuläre Sauerstoffpartialdruck-messung ("oxygen mapping") an der unteren Extremität Venengesunder und Venenkranker. Akt Dermatol 1990; 6:181-186

6. Tronnier M, Schmeller W, Wolff HH. Morphological changes in lipodermatosclerosis and venous ulcers: light microscopy, immunohistochemistry and electron microscopy. Phlebology 1994; 9:48-54

7. Welzel J, Schmeller W, Plettenberg A. Dermatoliposklerose in der 20 MHz-Sonographie. Hautarzt 1994; 45:630-634

Phlebology '95, D. Negus et al. (eds.). Phlebology (1995) Suppl. 1: 949-951

PI/10.3

Venous Valvuloplasty with Angioscopy

S. Hoshino, A. Tsuda, H. Satokawa, H. Midorikawa, S. Takase, T. Ogawa and T. Igari

Department of Cardiovascular Surgery, Fukushima Medical College, Fukushima, Japan

INTRODUCTION

Over the past two decades, many surgical procedures have been done for chronic venous incompetence in the lower extremities. Valvuloplasty techniques are especially applicable in patients with primary deep vein incompetence. However ,an incision in the vein wall is necessary for the internal technique of valvuloplasty. In the external techniques, the degree of plication tightness is decided according to surgeon's feeling and experience. With this in mind, we recently employed a new technique using angioscopy to precisely evaluate incompetent venous valves and further performed valvuloplasty under direct observation during surgery.

METERIAL AND METHOD

Subjects : 23 superficial femoral veins (SFV) and 51 long saphenous veins (LSV) with chronic venous incompetence detected by duplex scanning and descending phlebography.

Angioscopy : An angioscopic system, OLYMPUS OES angioscope,AF type 28C, was used and the angioscopic images were recorded with a VTR system. The angioscope was inserted through a branch of the long saphenous vein and venous valves were observed in retrograde by flushing of heparin added saline solution from the angioscope flush lumen.

Morphology : Morphology of the incompetent valves was classified into 3 types I , II , III as follows (Fig. 1); valves with elongated and atrophic cusps-type I , valves with expanded and depressed comissures with cusp changes-type II , and valves which had cusps with other deformities-type III [1,2] .

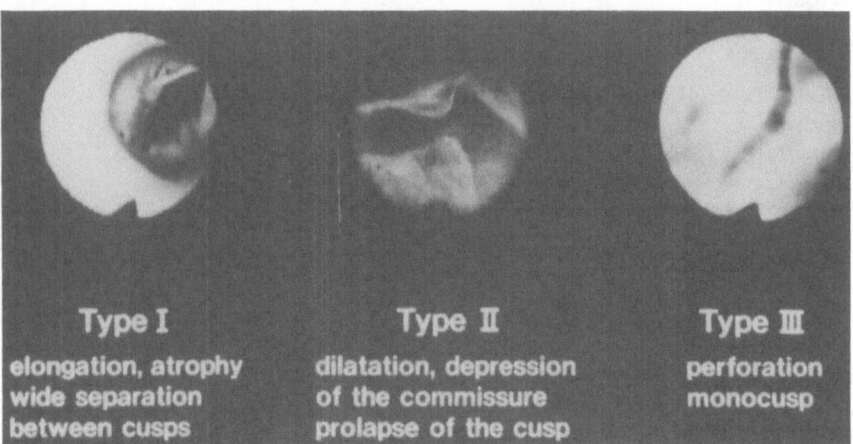

Fig.1 Classification of the Venous Valve by Angioscopy

Technique : The techniques of valvulopasty are shown in fig.2. Incompetent valves were observed and repaired using the angioscope through a branch of the LSV. Our surgical techniques consisted of total plication by running sutures (I), banding using autogenous femoral fascia or silastic cuff (II) and plication of commissures including cusp edges using horizontal mattress suture (III) [3~7]

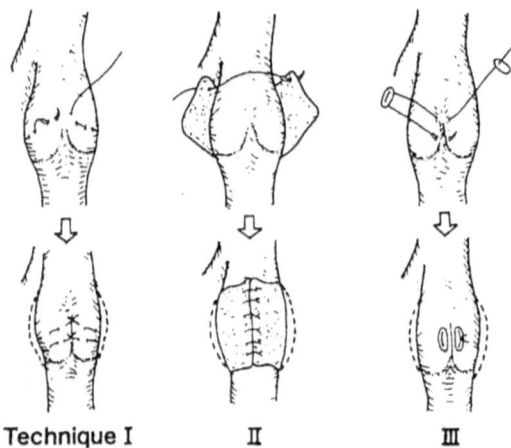

Fig.2 The techniques of Valvuloplasty

Results : Angioscopic valvuloplasty was performed in 23 SFV and the reflux disappeared in 21 SFV (91%) at 2-35 month (mean 22) follow-up. Reflux was recognized in 2 SFV (9%), but there was no tendency of increased regurgitation at 1.5 and 2 year follow-ups respectively. Reflux dissappeared in 47 out of 51 LSV (92%). At 1-49 months (mean 31), there were 2 LSV with occlusion (4%) and 2 LSV which required sclerotherapy due to recurrence of varicose veins (4%).

Conclusions : The application of intraoperative angioscopy is useful in diagnosing incompetent valves and in performing angioscopic valvuloplasty, which may lead to improved surgical results.

REFERENCES

1. Satokawa H, Iwaya F, Igari T, Abe T, Hagiwara K, Tanji M, et al, Morphological studies of the venous valves by angioscopy. J Jap Coll Angiol. 1992: 395-401.

2. Hoshino S, Satokawa H, Iwaya F, Igari T, Hagiwara K, Tanji M, et al, Diagnosis and surgery of venous insufficiency : valvuloplasty using intraoperative angioscopy. Jpn J Phlebol 1993;4 : 1-8.

3. Hoshino S, Satokawa H, Ono T, et al, Surgical treatment for primary varicose veins of the legs using intraoperative angioscopy. In : Phlebologie 92. Paris : John Libbey Eurotext, 1992 : 1083-1085.

4. Satokawa H, Iwaya F, Igari T, Tanji M, Wtanabe M, Midorikawa H, et al, Endoscopic venous surgery. Jpn J Vasc Surg 1994;3 : 613-618.

5. Satokawa H, Iwaya F, Igari T, Hagiwara K, Tanji M, Watanabe M,et al, Endoscopic surgery for venous disorders. Jpn J Vasc Surg 1994;3 : 411-416.

6. Satokawa H, Iwaya F, Igari T, Hagiwara K, Tanji M, Watanabe M, et al, Surgical treatment for the patients with varicose veins of the lower extremities using intraoperative angioscopy.Jpn J Phlebol 1992;3 : 75-81.

7. Hoshino S, Satokawa H, Iwaya F, et al, Valvuloplastie externe sous controle angioscopique pre-operatoire. Phlebologie, 1993;46 : 521-530.

Phlebology '95, D. Negus et al. (eds.). Phlebology (1995) Suppl. 1: 952-955

P162

Aspect Echo-Doppler des Récidives Variqueuses Après Traitement Chirurgical de la Saphène Interne

F. Vin and F. Chleir

Départment de Phlébologie, Hopital Notre Dame de Bon Secours, 75014 Paris, France

Echo-Doppler Findings of Varicose Recurrences after Surgery of the Long Saphenous Vein

SUMMARY

The authors study by duplex scanning the cause of postoperative recurrences of varicose veins in 82 patients treated surgically.

ASPECT ECHO-DOPPLER DES RECIDIVES VARIQUEUSES APRES TRAITEMENT CHIRURGICAL DE LA SAPHENE INTERNE

F.VIN, F.CHLEIR
Département de Phlébologie Hopital Notre Dame de Bon Secours 75014 PARIS FRANCE

INTRODUCTION

Le traitement chirurgical des varices des membres inférieurs avec crossectomie et stripping a longtemps été considéré comme radical.Les échecs et récidives rencontrés, étaient souvent mises à tort sur le compte d'une erreur de technique opératoire ou d'un traitement incomplet(1).

De nombreuses études récentes ont montré que la fréquence des récidives post-chirurgicales était de 15 à 40% à 5 ans (2) (3) (4) . Notre étude porte sur 82 patients opérés par des chirurgiens vasculaires et controlés par écho-doppler afin de mettre en évidence l'aspect morphologique des récidives variqueuses.

MATERIEL ET METHODE

82 patients présentant pour une récidive variqueuse post-opératoire ont été examinés.La majorité d'entre eux n'avait pas eu de suivi phlébologique systématique.

Un examen clinique a été réalisé avec la recherche d'un reflux veineux superficiel au doppler de poche au niveau du 1/3 supérieur de la cuisse. Il a toujours été précédé d'un interrogatoire qui a cherché à mettre en évidence la présence d'une symptomatologie fonctionnelle, des antécédents familiaux de varices, ou l'existence de facteurs de risque ayant pu être à l'origine de la récidive (station professionnelle debout, grossesse, traitement hormonal).

Un écho-doppler pulsé a été réalisé à titre systématique avec un appareil de type ESAOTE AU 530 avec une sonde de 10 Mhz. Il avait comme objectif de confirmer le reflux et d'en localiser la source. Les troncs veineux profonds ont également été étudiés à titre systématique à la recherche d'une séquelle de thrombose.

RESULTATS

Parmi les 82 patients étudiés, il y avait une majorité de sexe féminin (70 femmes, 12 hommes). Ils étaient agés de 23 à 85 ans pour une moyenne de 70 ans.133 membres présentaient une récidive variqueuse entre 1 et 37 ans après crossectomie et stripping saphène SI. La récidive était dans 51,8 % des cas à gauche et dans 48,2 % à droite.

31 patients (37,8 %) avaient une récidive unilatérale sur un stripping unilatéral, 51 patients (62,2%) avaient une récidive bilatérale sur un stripping bilatéral .20 membres sur 133 (15%) avaient eu deux cures chirurgicales du territoire saphène interne du même membre.

L'intervalle moyen en la première et la deuxième intervention était de 11 ans.

L'intervalle entre la deuxième intervention et la consultation était également de 11 ans.

Lorqu'il y avait eu une seule intervention l'intervalle moyen entre la cure chirurgicale et la consultation était de 15,33 ans (minimum 1 an- maximum 37 ans). 2 patients sur 82 avaient des séquelles de thrombose veineuse.

ORIGINE DES RECIDIVES

Plusieurs types échographiques de récidive avec la présence d'une varice et d'un reflux ont été retrouvés au niveau de la région inguinale. Dans certains cas, il s'agissait d'un moignon de crossectomie avec abouchement d'une ou plusieurs petites collatérales responsables de la récidive. Dans d'autres cas, il a été retrouvé une saphène interne en position anatomique avec un reflux sans que l'on puisse déterminer son étiologie. L'existence d'une perforante avec une communication avec la veine fémorale superficielle au 1/3 moyen, au 1/3 supérieur de cuisse est une autre source de récidive. Dans certains cas, une ou plusieurs collatérales incontinentes peuvent s'aboucher directement dans la veine fémorale commune et responsables d'une saphène antérieure ou d'une saphène postérieure de cuisse. Les carvernomes ou lacis veineux indéfinisables sont caractérisés par la présence d'un réseau veineux anarchique siègeant au niveau de la zone de crossectomie ou autour de la fémorale commune. Enfin dans certains cas , des collatérales incontinentes n'avaient aucune connexion avec la veine fémorale commune ou la veine fémorale superficielle et provenaient d'un réseau veineux superficiel par une veine sous-cutanée abdominale, circonflexe iliaque superficielle, ou par des varices vulvo-périnéales.Sur 133 malades étudiés, il a été retrouvé 151 origines différentes décrites dans le tableau I.

Tableau I

Type I	Récidive sur moignon	32 cas	21%
Type II	Saphène en place	26 cas	17,2%5
Type III	Perforantes communicant avec la veine fémorale superficielle au 1/3 moyen ou au 1/3 supérieur de cuisse	18 cas	12%
Type IV	Collatérales s'abouchant dans la fémorale commune avec saphène antérieure ou saphène postérieure	37 cas	24,5%
Type V	Cavernomes ou lacis indéfinisables	7 cas	4,6%
Type VI	Collatérales ne s'abouchant pas dans la fémorale commune	31 cas	20,5%

De nombreuses études ont déja mises en évidence les récidives variqueuses post-opératoires (5) (6). Il est toujours difficile à postériori de savoir s'il s'agit d'un traitement incorrect et incomplet ou d'une évolution de la maladie.
Certains auteurs comme G. FRANCO classent les reflux selon l'importance de leur taille : les reflux majeurs ou la taille de la fuite est égale à une crosse saphènienne, les reflux modérés où la taille de la fuite est habituellement inférieure à celle de la crosse saphènienne et les reflux mineurs essentiellement dus au micro-cavernomes ou néogénèse constitués de fins chevelus de veinules immatures criblant la lame lympho-ganglionnaire. Pour M. PERRIN, les reflux majeurs seraient secondaires à une crosse restante par crossectomie incomplète.Les reflux modérés dont la taille est inférieure à celle d'une saphène seraient en rapport avec une néo-crosse par néo-jonction saphèno-fémorale macroscopique.Les reflux mineurs seraient en rapport avec une microgénèse par néo-jonction saphèno-fémorale de type microscopique.
D'autres comme D.CRETON définissent les récidives également en fonction de l'importance du reflux. Des récidives de type hémodynamique, sont souvent issues de fautes chirurgicales avec une pression de reflux inguinal residuelle importante.
Des récidives de type angiogénèse associées à un reflux mineur inguinal et des varices diffuses.

L'écho-doppler pulsé avec codage couleur est certainement le meilleur examen qui permet d'apprécier l'origine, la morphologie de la récidive et l'importance du reflux.
Il existe incontestablement des erreurs de techniques chirurgicales ou la saphène interne reste en situation anatomique avec dans d'autres cas la persistance d'un moignon dans le lequel s'abouche une veine collatérale.Parfois, il s'agit de branches saphèniennes antérieures ou postérieures qui s'abouchent directement dans la veine fémorale commune et qui auront été négligées. Afin l'existence de petites veines collatérales présentant un reflux et s'abouchant dans une fémorale commune ou la présence d'un lacis veineux tourtueux de type carvernome témoigne d'une évolution de la maladie et la présence d'une angiogénèse.

Reste le problème des perforantes situées au 1/3 supérieur ou au 1/3 moyen de la cuisse alimentant un réseau variqueux des sources de récidive.Il est dans ce cas difficile de savoir s'il s'agit d'un traitement incomplet ou d'une évolution de la maladie.En effet lors du stripping,certaines perforantes ont pu être arrachées, se sont thrombosées et reperméabilisées réalimentant un réseau variqueux secondaire.Dans d'autres cas l'évolution de la maladie est telle que le développement d'une collatérale qui était inexistante lors de l'intervention a pu développer le réseau variqueux récidivé pathologique.
La maladie variqueuse est une maladie chronique et évolutive.Un bilan écho-doppler systématique est indispensable avant toute cure chirurgicale afin de localiser les autres sources de reflux possible que celles provenant de la jonction saphéno-fémorale ou de ses collatérales. Le traitement chirurgical ne peut être considéré comme un traitement définitif, même s'il est réalisé par un chirurgien vasculaire exclusif. L'étude présentée sur 82 patients et 133 membres opérés contrôlés par écho-doppler met en évidence les différents types de récidive variqueuse possible. En fonction de l'aspect morphologique, hémodynamique et échographique, il est possible de distinguer des crosses restantes avec crossectomie incomplète en rapport avec un erreur de technique chirurgicale, les néo-crosses par néo-jontion saphèno-fémorale macroscopique et les micronéogénèsses par néo-jonction saphèno-fémorale microscopique.
Cette étude est une analyse qualitative de la récidive variqueuse et non pas quantitative.

REFERENCES

1- NEGUS .D Recurrent varicose veins : a national problem
Br J SURG 1993 Jul 80(7) 823-824

2 -CAMPBELL W.A Sapheno-femoral reconnection in recurrent varicose veins advances in medical and surgical treatement of venous disorders
7th annual meeting of the North American Society of Phebology MAUI 1994

3 - JUHAN.C, HAUPERT.S, MITGEN G et al Recurrent varicose veins
Phlebology 1990,5 : 201-11

4 - SARIN.S, SCURR J.M, COLERIDGE SMITH PD. Assessment of stipping the long saphenous vein in the treatment of primary varicose veins Br J Surg 1992 Sep 79(9) 889-93

5 - GLASS J.M Pré-jonction of recurrent sapheno-femorale incompetence after surgery of varicose veins. Br .J.SURG 1989 76 : 1210

6 - THIBAULT.PK, LEWIS WA. Recurrent varicose veins.Evaluation utilizing duplex venous imaging J Dermatol Surg on-col 1992, Jul 18(7) 618-24

Phlebology '95, D. Negus et al. (eds.). Phlebology (1995) Suppl. 1: 956-958

P191

Surgical Treatment of Varicose Leg Ulceration in Day Surgery

Z. Fiutek, K. Twardowska-Saucha, D. Czaczka Z. Wygoda and M. Filipowski

Varicose Vein Clinic "Medservice", Zabrze, Poland

INTRODUCTION

Venous ulceration is a troublesome and disability causing complication, which remains one of the most difficult problems to treat. The principal physiological abnormalities besides the ulceration are: increased venous pressure in the lower limb caused by varicose veins, deep vein reflux produced by deep vein thrombosis, primary valve failure or isolated incompetence of perforating veins [1].

The fundamental approach in leg ulcers associated with chronic venous insufficiency treatment is the permanent control of pathological pressure, which is primarily achieved by means of phlebosurgery, sclerotherapy and/or conservative compression therapy. Scott found that about two-thirds of patients presenting the symptoms of chronic venous insufficiency had only superficial venous disease [2].

Neither is the single type of venous operation applicable to all cases of venous leg ulceration, nor should the surgery be regarded as an alternative stand-alone therapy.

It must be integrated into a comprehensive plan of management that includes compression therapy, which should be confirmed post operatively.

Simple procedures should be done before more complicated operations are attempted.

Full correction of insufficiency of superficial veins and/or perforating veins should always be carried out prior to considering surgery for deep venous insufficiency.

MATERIAL AND METHODS

Between October 1993 and December 1994 48 patients (41 female and 7 male) underwent surgical treatment in Varicose Vein Clinic "Medservice". Their age ranged from 28 to 61 years (mean 45). Before admission to the Clinic all the patients had active leg ulcers from 3 months until 9 years (mean 21 months).

Ulcer area was determined by multiplying the maximum horizontal and vertical diameters. When patients had more than one ulcer the ulcer sizes were added to each other, to reflect the total area of ulceration.

All the patients were instructed to rest and sleep with legs raised about 10-15 centimetres above heart level. Duo-Derm and compression dressing and/or Unna's boot were applied before surgery. In our clinic patients were treated in this way from 2 weeks until 3 months. Operations were carried out in 14 cases before complete healing of leg ulcer.

Limited stripping of long saphenous vein (LSV) and stripping of short saphenous vein SSV and local phlebectomy were performed in 10 patients. 34 patients underwent limited stripping LSV and local phlebectomy. Full stripping LSV and local phlebectomy were carried out in 3 cases. 1 patient was treated by SSV ligation and phlebectomy.

At the day of planned surgery the ulcer is usually covered with the new Duo-Derm dressing. All varicose veins are precisely marked with indelible dye.

Patients were premedicated with 5 - 10 mg of intravenous Diazepam and then they were placed in Trendelenburg position and the operation area was prepared. This was followed by the femoral nerve block applied by means of 0,5% Xylocain. Sometimes intravenous Pentazocine from 15 to 30 mg was administered. Long saphenous vein and /or short saphenous vein were removed with the invagination technique (Van der Stricht). All the marked varices were then removed by means of special hooks set which operated through the very small incisions.

Compression dressings were applied from the base of the toes to a thigh for 2-6 days, then replaced by graduated compression elastic stockings.

RESULTS

In the group with active leg ulcer complete healing was achieved in two - three weeks time after surgery. There were no serious infectious complications. There were no recurrent ulcers during 6-months follow-up. Postoperative pain was not very serious, only in 6 cases patients required oral analgesics administration from 2 to 6 days after intervention.

Labropoulus [3] estimated frequency of reflux presence among patients with veins thrombosis in the past. They found that skin changes and leg ulceration are mainly connected with reflux in superficial veins. Retrograde blood flow in deep veins has no influence on the development of such changes.

The important aspect of stab avulsion technique is, that by removing the varicose tributaries any distal incompetent perforators must be disconnected from the superficial veins and therefore there is no need to locate them.

Avulsion of varices, which almost always involve tributaries of the main trunk of the long or short saphenous veins, stops all leakage from distal perforating veins, but does not prevent leakage through incompetent sapheno-femoral or sapheno-popliteal valves. The stab avulsion technique is therefore only the part of the successful treatment of the majority of varicose veins and leg ulcers. It must be combined with flush proximal ligation of the major valves if ultrasound examination demonstrates their incompetence [4].

The method of leg ulceration treatment accompanied by LSV or/and SSV insufficiency that we have presented is very well tolerated by patients, safe and giving a chance of permanent remission, but prophylaxis in the form of compression stockings should follow the active surgical treatment anyway.

REFERENCES

1. Corwall J.V. Leg ulcers; epidemiology, aetiology. Br J Surg 1986;73: 693.
2. Scott H.J. Venous disease: investigation and treatment fact or fiction?
   A.R. Coll Surg Engl 1990;72:189-92.
3. Labropoulus S. Venous reflux in patients with previous deep venous thrombosis;
   correlation with ulceration and other symptoms. J Vasc Surg 1994;20:385.
4. Large J. The treatment of varicose veins: a personal review. Phlebology 1990;5:
   141-146.

Phlebology '95, D. Negus et al. (eds.). Phlebology (1995) Suppl. 1: 959-961

OP/17.6

Perforating Veins Insufficiency: Long Term Results in 4494 Cases with Different Surgical Techniques

R.A. Lacour, J.R. Cigorraga, M. Sala Haedo and J.A. Cigorraga

Department of Phlebology, Hospital de Clinicas, University of Buenos Aires and Department of Vascular Surgery, Haedo Surgical Institute, Buenos Aires, Argentina

INTRODUCTION

Perforating veins insufficiency of the lower limbs generally causes different trophic troubles in lower third of the affected legs. To interrupt the reflux through these veins we have been used different surgical therapies from 1956 up to now. This one is a summary of our general and specific results with each type of technic.

METHODS

From 1-3-56 up to 1-3-94 we have performed 4494 operations in 4371 patients with peerforating veins insufficiency. Those operations were carried out by two different teams using standardised surgical techniques.

In 1562 cases (34,8%) there was primary or posthrombotic deep venous incompetence (DVI); in 2932 cases (65,2%) the diagnosis was primary varicose veins with normal deep venous system (PVV).

To obtain the correct diagnosis we used clinical examinations, phlebography, bidirectional Doppler ultrasound, photopletysmography or Dupplex Scanning.

In 3250 limbs the "valve technique" was performed. This technic was published by Cigorraga J.R. et all (1) in 1958 and their results were shown in the 17th World Congress of The International Union of Angiology in April 1995 (2).

In 1206 cases the perforating veins insufficiency was solved by subfascial operations that using long vertical incisions. Linton's technic (3) was used in 591 limbs, Felder's modification (4) in 103 limbs and Cockett's technic (5) in 512 limbs. In the 38 remaining cases extrafascial techniques were performed.

INDICATIONS

In general, we avoid the incisions that involve trophic troubles areas; for this reason we prefer the "valve technic". This operation destroys the perforating veins from an incision done in the upper third of the medial aspect of the leg, by the subfascial passage of a metallic valve. We usually reserve this operation for patients with trophic troubles and/or ulcers that do not exceed half of the leg circumference.

We have chosen Cockett's or Linton's operations only in a limited amount of cases because they frequently cause healing troubles and necrosis of the wound edges. Now we only use Cockett's operation in patients with small lesions when we can perform the incision on suitable tissues.

Linton's technic has been utilized in cases of perforating veins insufficiency in the lateral aspect of the leg, where the intermuscular fascias avoid the use of the "valve technic". We have also performed it when associating ulcer extirpation with consecutive plastic repairing was necessary.

Felder's operation has been exclusively used when the perforating veins insufficiency involved both surfaces of the leg.

To end with, we have used extrafascial techniques in cases of perforating veins insufficiency with no trophic troubles.

RESULTS

Results have been evaluated by clinical methods; lately non invasive resources have been associated with equal purpose.

Evaluation included 3718 cases (82,7%). Deep venous incompetence (DVI) was present in the 91,7% and primary varicose veins (PVV) was present in the 77,4%. The follow up time varyed from 1 to 38 years. There was no mortality due to the operations.

Immediate results were good in the 89,2 % of the cases treated with "valve technic" (DVI= 83%; PVV= 94%). On the oposite, the number of good results was minor in patients with low vertical incisions (Linton= 52,6%; Felder= 53,4%;

CHART 1

TECHNIC	OPERATIONS			IMMEDIATE GOOD RESULTS		
	No.	DVI	PVV	No.	DVI	PVV
VALVE	3250	1235 38%	2015 62%	2919 89,2%	1025 83%	1894 94%
LINTON	591	231 39,1%	360 60,9%	311 52,6%	128 55,4%	183 50,8%
FELDER	103	46 44,7%	57 55,3%	55 53,4%	22 47,8%	33 57,9%
COCKETT	512	154 30,1%	358 69,9%	306 59,7%	79 51,3%	227 63,4%
EXTRA FASCIAL	38	---	38 100%	36 94,7%	---	36 94,7%
TOTAL	4494	1666 37%	2828 63%	3627 82,8%	1254 75,2%	2373 83,9%

CHART 2

	FOLLOW UP			LONG TERM GOOD RESULTS		
	No.	DVI	PVV	No.	DVI	PVV
VALVE	2665 82%	1146 92,8%	1519 75,3%	2161 81,1%	779 68%	1382 91%
LINTON	501 84,7%	210 90,9%	291 80,8%	385 76,8%	143 68,1%	242 83,1%
FELDER	91 88,3%	39 84,7%	52 91,2%%	66 72,5%	24 61,5%	42 80,7%
COCKETT	435 84,9%	134 87%	301 84%	343 78,8%	94 70,1%	249 82,7%
EXTRA FASCIAL	26 68,4%	---	26 68,4%	24 92,3%	---	24 92,3%
TOTAL	3718 82,7%	1529 91,7%	2189 77,4%	2979 80,1%	1040 68%	1939 88,5%

Cockett= 59,7%) (Chart 1). Bad immediate results were
generally related to postoperative complications of the
wound (skin and subcutaneous necrosis, infections,
hoematomas).

Long term results (Chart 2) were good in the 81,1% of the
cases of "valve technic" (DVI= 68%; PVV= 91%). Patients
with low vertical incisions have had less positive results
but the difference was not significant (Linton= 76,8%;
Felder= 72,5%; Cockett= 78,8%). Bad long term results were
related to reappearance of ulcerous pathology.

Such immediate and late results suggest that both groups
of operations are equal for removing perforating veins.
Therefore, both have similar long term effectiveness. On
the other hand, short term effectiveness is greater with
the "valve technic" because with this one complications
related to wound location are not frequent.

REFERENCES

1. Cigorraga JR et all.. El tratamiento quirurgico de la
   insuficiencia de venas comunicantes. Tecnica de la sec-
   cion subaponeurotica de comunicantes. Bol. y Trab. de
   la Soc. Arg. de Cirujanos, 1958;19:281.
2. Cigorraga JR, Lacour RA, Saliva J, Cigorraga JA.
   Original technic for the section of the perforating
   veins. Results in 3250 operations. 17th World Congress
   of The International Union of Angiology. London, 1995.
3. Linton R.. The communicating veins of the lower
   legs and the operative technic for their ligation. Ann.
   Surg., 1938;107:582.
4. Felder D, Murphy T., Ring D. A posterior subfascial
   ap-proach to the communicating veins of the leg. Surg
   Gyn
   and Obs, 1955;100:730.
5. Cockett F. The pathology and treatment of venous ulcers
   of the leg. Br J Surg 1955;43:260.

Phlebology '95, D. Negus et al. (eds.). Phlebology (1995) Suppl. 1: 962-964

P224

Embolisation of Insufficient Perforators in Patients with Varicose Ulceration

J. Garcarek[1], Z. Rybak and P. Szyber

[1] Department of Vascular Surgery and Radiology, Wroclaw Medical University, Wroclaw, Poland

INTRODUCTION

Pollack and Wood (1949) established for the first time that an abnormal superficial venous hypertension was the basic physiological fault in varicose veins and venous ulcers. The anatomy of the Hunters canal perforating vein was described by Boyd and Dodd and the group of ankle perforating veins were investigated by Linton and Cockett. It was shown that this veins were the main venous drainage pathway of the ulcer bearing area of the ankle. The importance of the valve in these small perforators, which prevented the considerable venous hypertension in the deep veins from reaching the delicate venules of the ankle skin was appreciated, and it was shown how breakdown of this valve established a hypertensive leak straight into the ankle capillaries - leading to ulceration [1].Leg ulcer is a common problem in old people. Most patients suffer from their ulcers for years. They were treated often unsucessfuly for months by different specialists and sometimes they do not belive to achieve healing [2,3].

METHODS

Seven patients (11 legs with ulceration) were undergoing this study. Inclusion criteria were venous ulceration of more than 6 months duration, age above 45 years, ulcer area above 1.0X2 normal foot pulse, ankle/arm pressure index above 1.0, and disability to surgery. Exclusion criteria were history of evidence of peripheral arterial disease, age below 45, history of surgical treatment in the past. Diagnosis was stated by phlebography, venous pressure recordings and Doppler examination.

Intervention

After localisation of insufficient perforators and elimination of deep vein thrombosis with a puncture of the superfitial vein of the leg Gianturco-Wallace coil was inserted to the place of insufficient perforator. At the same time Amplatz coil was placed just below sapheno-femoral junction to prevent either extension of thrombus to the deep system or pulmonary embolism.

Measurements

7 to 8 phlebograms in two projections were performed before and following procedure which was fluoroscopic controlled. Venous pressure recordings with TESTAR 2000 as well as Doppler examination were made before, and 30 days following embolization [4].

RESULTS

Early results are promising. Ulcerations were healed within 4 weeks. Any complications were observed. Venous pressure decreased about 15 mm of mercury - fig. 1. Effect of embolization is shown in fot.1 and 2.

Fig. 1. The mean venous pressure before and after embolisation of insufficient perforators

Number of legs	Mean pressure before embolisation	Mean pressure after embolisation mm Hg
11	64 +/- 6	49 +/- 5
With cuff	59 +/- 4	51 +/- 2

CONCLUSION

This procedure is an alternative for Linton operation in high risk patients.

1. Cockett F.B., A historical outline of varicose vein surgery up to the present day. Flebolinfologia 1990; 1:3-5.
2. Baker SR, Stacey MC, Jopp-McKay AG, Hoskins SE, Thompson PJ, Epidemiology of chronic venous ulcers. Br J Surg 1991; 78:864-7.
3. Callam MJ, Harper DR, Dale JJ, Ruckley CV, Chronic ulceration of the leg: clinical
   history. Br Med J 1987;294:1389-91.
4. Rybak Z, Dynamic measurement of venous pressure as an alternative method in limb vein diseases. Phlebol Reviev 1993;1:19-30.

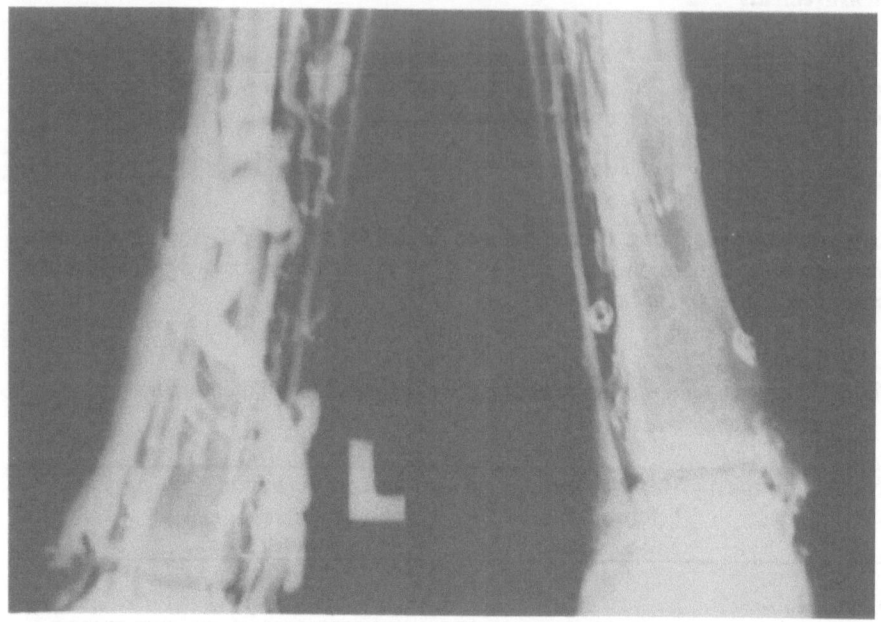

1. Antero-posterior view of the leg before and after embolisation.

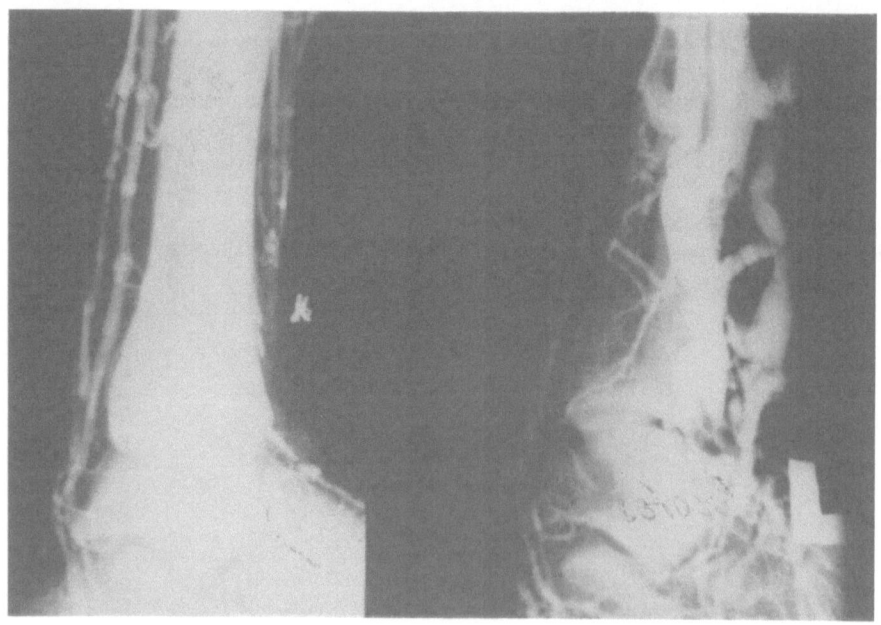

2. Side view of the leg before and after embolization of perforators.

Phlebology '95, D. Negus et al. (eds.). Phlebology (1995) Suppl. 1: 965-967

V/1.11

New Methods of Correction Circulation Disorders in Limb and Pelvic Veins in Patients with Post-Thrombophlebitic Disease

A.N. Vedensky[1,2,3], Y.M. Stoiko and V.V. Sabelnikov

Postgraduate Education Academy, St.Petersburg, Russia

INTRODUCTION

Postthrombotic change of pelvic and lower limb veins are usually accompanied by severe disturbances of blood outflow. The results of treatment of 989 patients with such disturbances are analyzed. In 326 cases with unilateral iliac vein occlusions cross autovenous shunting was performed. On 721 patients with trophic changes in the soft tissues of the distal 1/3 of their lower legs the occlusion of the posterior tibial veins (according to Vedensky) was done. Both operations were performed in a new way consecutively in 58 cases. The favourable outcome was achieved in 94% of patients. The length of the follow-up was from 8 to 24 years.

METHODS

Our rather lengthy (from 1962 till 1984), and cross shunting not consistently successful experience of 160 operations revealed the main factors, determining the preservation of good shunt functioning. Indications for this operation were specified, as well as good, satisfactory and bad conditions for its performance.

During the last 10 years 100 operations were done under good conditions, and 66 under satisfactory ones. In 89 cases it was decided to with hold from the operation due to bad conditions for it.

The principal factor, creating good conditions for the operation, is the availability of a suitable autograft. Usually it is a uniformly distended v. saphena magna, 8-10 mm in diameter, which to a considerable degree lost its ability to contract due to phlebosclerosis. To prevent further shunt ectasia, it is placed into a lavsan spiral (according to Vedensky).

The conditions are considered satisfactory when the autograft is narrow (5-6 mm), or has not lost its ability to undergo a spasm. This group also includes cases in which the shunt is formed out of two saphena magna veins longitudinally sewn together. Here the risk of the shunt obstruction with a thromb amounts to 30%, and it is discussed with the patient before the operation. The unfavourable outcome of surgery is not connected with a remarkable deterioration of the disease manifestations.

Bad conditions for surgery may be the reason for withholding from it. Usually they implicate a small diameter of the supposed autograft (4-5 mm), the dispersed type of v. saphena magna structure, and their completely preserved ability to undergo spasms. In some cases these veins were removed earlier.

On 58 patients their surgery was performed in two stages, cross shunting being the first one. It decreased the length, the extent and the severity of the operation and promoted patients' earlier mobilization. All this lessened the probability of thromb formation within the shunt. The second stage – posterior tibial vein occlusion in the distal 1/3 of the lower leg – may be performed on various terms after the first operation (from 3-6 up to 27 months).

The posterior tibial vein occlusion was performed on 721 patients with trophic changes of lower leg soft tissues. This surgical intervention consists in revealing the vessel plexus behind the medial malleolus, ligating both posterior tibial veins, their transacting, and introducing obturating material into the lumen. For the purpose we usually use strips of the tissue 2-3 mm in width cut out of the wall of v. saphena magna. They are introduced into the lumen of both veins for 12-17 cm in the region of soft tissue trophic changes. After that both veins are ligated, fixing at the same time the tissue introduced into them. The wound is closed with two sutures. This operation eliminates the pathological blood flow through the supramolleolar perforating veins and the blood reflux into the deep veins of the foot. There is no need in having surgical cuts within the regions of the trophically changed tissues. Other inconsistent perforating veins are ligated over the fascia through small surgical wounds. Some patients are in need of the perforating vein ligation on the border of the lower leg middle and distal thirds. This vein is connected with gastrocnemius muscle venous sinuses, and is not excluded out of the circulation after the obturation of the tibial veins.

DIAGNOSIS

Roentgen-contrast phlebography was performed before the operation and on various terms after it through a percutaneous punction of the femoral or the popliteal vein. At the same time dopplerography, and occlusion pletysmography were done.

RESULTS

Among 160 previously operated patients 70-50% had episodes of shunt thromboses in different years with a tendency to the improvement of the results. Out of 100 patients on whom the operation of cross shunting was performed under good conditions excellent results were achieved in 94%, and out of 66 patients with satisfactory conditions – in 70% of cases. In 75-78% of patients the obturation of the posterior tibial veins provided in 2-8 years a considerable decrease of skin hyperpigmentation with the restitution of its normal coloring in 7% of cases.

CONCLUSION

Besides a good autograft necessary for faultless shunt functioning, the pressure gradient is created due to the ligation of collateral. The arteriovenous fistulae formation is not necessary. The refusal from subfascial approaches increased the esthetic effect of surgery, the threat of marginal tissue necroses disappeared. The obturation of the posterior tibial veins substantially improves the function of the lower leg muscle – venous pump.

REFERENCES

1. Vedensky A.N. Plastic and reconstructive surgery on magistral veins. Leningrad, "Medicina", 1979, 224p.
2. Vedensky A.N. Varicose disease. Leningrad, "Medicina",1983, 238p.
3. Vedensky A.N. Postthrombotic disease. Leningrad, "Medicina", 1986, 242p.

Phlebology '95, D. Negus et al. (eds.). Phlebology (1995) Suppl. 1: 968-970

OP/17.1

Surgical Results on Recurrent Leg Ulcers in Primary Deep Vein Insufficiency Treated by Valve Repair

M. Perrin[1], J.L. Calvignac[1], B. Hiltbrand[2] and J.M. Bayon[2]

[1] Chirurgie Vasculaire, Lyon, France
[2] Angiologie, Clinique du Grand Large, Decines Charpieu, France

MATERIAL AND METHODS

From 1988 to 1992, twenty nine out of sixty extremities (46 patients) were operated for recurrent leg ulcers by valvuloplasty of the femoral vein.

All had a failure of conservative treatment and 18 have had previous surgical procedures (18 strippings and 2 perforator ligations). Preop investigations were ascending and descending phlebographies, AVP and (or) PPG, Duplex Scanning. Reflux was assessed by measurement of VRI.

When considering etiology, 18 extremities were classified isolated Primary Deep Vein Incompetency (PDVI) and 11 extremities combination of proximal PDVI and distal Post-Thrombotic Syndrome (PTS).

Preop hemodynamics were as follow :
. Reflux (Descending Phlebogram) :
    Grade 4 all except two grade 3.
. Refilling Time (AVP and/or PPG) :
    Average 9 sec (-9, + 6).
. Pressure Drop Measurement :
    All less than 38 %.
. VRI : Average 1.1 (0.8 to 3).

SURGICAL PROCEDURES

29 valve repairs were performed in the proximal part of the superficial femoral vein (Internal valvuloplasty as described by SOTTIURAI).

Additional procedures on the deep veins were associated in 3 cases (external valve repair) at the popliteal level and on the superficial or perforatoring veins (14 strippings - 16 ligations of perforators - 3 ligations of gastrocnemius veins).

Four instances of post operative thrombosis (4/29 = 13.8 %) were identified by ascending venography performed in the first 36 post operative hours. All had a combination of PDVI and PTS.

Post op monitoring consisted in clinical and hemodynamical exam (PPG, Descending Phlebography and/or Duplex Scan) each year. The average follow-up of the group was 43 months (24 - 74 M). 27 ulcers healed and only three recurred (figure 1 and 2).

In the PDVI (18 extremities) we found only one transient recurrence. In the PDVI + PTS (11 extremities) we found 2 non healing ulcers and 2 recurrences (p > 0.01).

NO ULCER RECURRENCE

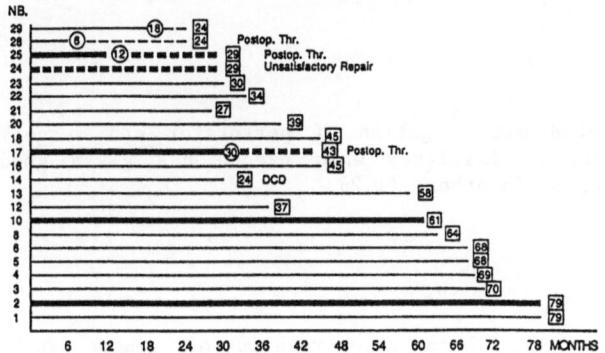

Figure 1

ULCER RECURRENCE

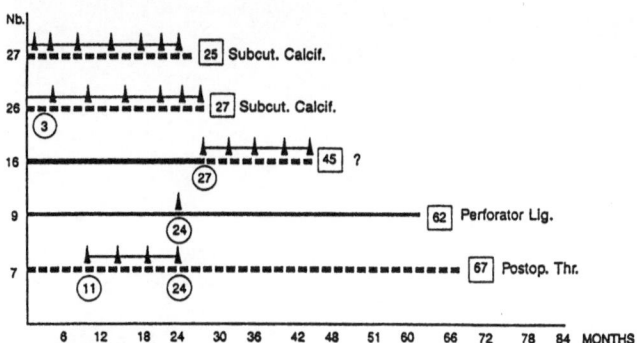

Figure 2

LEGENDS

——— PDVI Competent Valve Repair
▬▬▬ PDVI + PTS Competent Valve Repair
- - - - PDVI Incompetent Valve Repair
▪▪▪▪ PDVI + PTS Incompetent Valve Repair

45 Duration of follow-up
(24) Time of Ulcer recurrence
↑ Ulcer recurrence
↑——↑ Duration of Ulcer Recurrence

Correlation between ulcer persistence or recurrence and competency of valve repair was checked and found.
24 extremities without ulcer : Twenty competent valve repair.
5 extremities with persistent or recurrent ulcer : Four incompetent valve repair.
Clinical outcome was strongly correlated with patency of valve repair (p > 0.01).

DISCUSSION

These results are similar to Kistner's series (1) which has a longer follow-up (four to twenty-one year) on two points :
. Results are better in isolated PDVI compared to PDVI + PTS.
. There is a strong correlation between efficiency of valve repair and non recurrence of ulcer.

CONCLUSION

Valve repair associated with ligation of perforator and surgery of superficial venous insufficiency when needed has given good results in this series as in others (1,2).

REFERENCES

1 Masuda EM, Kistner RL. Long term results of venous valve reconstruction : A four to twenty-one year follow-up. J Vasc Surg 1994 ; 19 : 391-403.
2 Sottiurai VS. Surgical correction of recurrent venous ulcer. J Cardiovasc Surg 1991 ; 1 : 104-109.

Phlebology '95, D. Negus et al. (eds.). Phlebology (1995) Suppl. 1: 971

V/2.9

Surgical Technique of Valvuloplasty in the Deep Vein

M. Perrin

Chirurgie Vasculaire, 9 Cours Général Giraud, Lyon 69001, France

Three techniques have been described for Internal Valve Repair (KISTNER, RAJU, SOTTIURAI).

The technique depicted in this video is basically the procedure described by SOTTIURAI with minor modifications.

The femoral veins (Common, Superficial, Deep) are exposed through a longitudinal incision. The sapheno femoral junction is ligated when incompetent.

The vein adventitia is infiltrated with a papaverine solution to avoid spasm.

The proximal valve of the superficial femoral vein is identified and its incompetence checked by Milking Test and Valsalva maneuver. After systemic heparinization (Heparin 50.000 UI) silastic loops are placed on the common, superficial and profunda veins proximal and distal to the valve. All their tributaries must be controlled. A transverse phlebotomy is made on the superficial femoral vein, one cm superior to the commissures of the valve cusps after identification.

A vertical venotomy starting from the middle of the transverse phlebotomy is made downwards using right angle POTT's scissors. The valve cusps are carefully examined and their redundance objected by injection of heparinized solution. The flaps of the phlebotomy are retracted by 6-0 polypropylène.

Repair of the first commissure is undertaken. The needle of a double ended suture 7-0 polypropylene is inserted from superior to inferior to transfix both cusps at the commissure before exiting the vein wall. A similar stich is made in the opposite direction using the needle from the opposite end of the suture. Ties are placed on the external wall of the vein.

Two to four tackings are needed to stretch the free borders of the valve. The same procedure is done on the opposite commissure.

The valve cusp opposition is checked. Sometimes one extra suture can be necessary on one or both commissures.

The phlebotomy (vertical and transversal) is closed by running sutures.

The efficacy of the valve repair is checked by Milking Test after release of vascular loops.

The same procedure can be done on the profunda femoral vein or the popliteal veins.

Phlebology '95, D. Negus et al. (eds.). Phlebology (1995) Suppl. 1: 972-974

P267

Surgical Treatment for Lower Limb Chronic Venous Thrombosis

A. Diaz[1] and K. Diaz[2]

*[1] Instituto de Angiologia, Chirugía Vasculare e Impotencia Sexual
Av de la República 770 y Eloy Alfaro, Quito, Ecuador*

INTRODUCTION

In phlebological practice,accidentaly is frequent to discover,some compensated or not compensated venous damages. Just after to complete clinical study,including Doppler, echography,gammagraphy and plebography procedures,we are able to determine the appearance of venous post-thrombotic pathology,compensated or not. Observing those natural venous reconstruction changes,we accept to perform,with certain success,venous and veno venous grafts and by-pass.
We began fourteen years ago, to do these procedures. Well understood that in past decades reconstructive and functional vein surgery,has been exceptional procedure,and it was limited for it´s great number of failures;but durig the last years,this kind of procedures arises due: 1.Adequate sellection of the type of venous pathology upon which we can work with good possibilities of success: thrombosis and extraluminal compression. 2. Good knowledgement of appropiate material to use in this kind of procedure.3. A great advance in management and knowledgement of coagulation,anticoagulation,plate aggregation and reological circulatory features.
4.Improvement in surgical technique in different areas of human body,where pathological frequence is greater;and, 5. knowledgement of the different kind of procedures to be used as:anatomical and extra-anatomical by-passes and transpositions.

DIAGNOSIS AND DIVISIONS:

Diagnosis is difficult,clinical anamnesis and physical examination give us about 70% . There are multiple auxiliary procedures to improve diagnosis and those are divided into: routine and special tests,which give us the last 30% diagnosis,those are:doppler,echography gammagraphy and specially phlebography,which permits us,in a best way,to have conviction of a clear and precise diagnosis,and also it help us as a comparative basis for an adequate treatment and definitive prediction.

According anathomical topography location,we divide deep venous thrombosis of lower limb into: foot,leg,thigh and ilio-cava areas,and in conformity,with this,we execute our treatment as follows: a) On foot area,we only perform clinical treatment and we divide it in two parts:basic and anticoagulant. Basic means: elastic contention,physiotherapy, anti-static position plus medication:as anti-inflamatory and anti-aggregating drugs. For anticoagulant treatment we use Heparine and Natrium Warfarine. b) On leg venous thrombosis we just recommend the same clinical treatment. c) At thigh level and due to the shortness of the deep venous network system,we believe at the importance of compensation and dis compensation, "our own concept".

The compensation state may be both: radiological or physiological. The radiological and physiological compensation states may co-exist together;but,in some cases, radiological compensation state may co-exist with physiological discompensation state.

There is a physiological compensation state,when venous insufficiency symtomatology is not present and when distal venous pressure is within normal limits. Discompensation state will be,the one,in which appear a venous insuffici - ency symtomatology,as edema,cianosis,venous turgescence, pain,venous dilatation and distal venous hipertension.

Those concepts are very important for the treatment of ilio-femoral or femoro-popliteal venous thrombosis by grafts or by by-pass or venous transposition. Physiological compensated state do not need any kind of surgical treatment. d) Ilio-cava venous thrombosis have been divided in four groups: 1. Iliac bilateral venous thrombosis,in which we advise to perform a surgical treatment with one or bilateral axilo-femoral grafts (we have not any case performed). 2. Iliac one side venous thrombosis,in which we perform femoro femoral or sapheno-femoral derivations, according palma´s technique,plus our modifications. 3. One side ilio-femoral thrombosis in which we execute sapheno-femoral, contra-lateral derivations associated with sapheno-poplitea venous by pass and sometimes varicotomies and ligatures. 4. One or bilateral iliac-venous thrombosis plus spontaneous discompensated recanalization in which the elective treatment is valvular transplantation. (we did not have any case). Now,I must tell you that: " we call disconnecting surgery to all procedures of disconnection of superficial axis from deep axis,such as: partial ligatures,scaled ligatures perforating ligatures and vein-extraction. On the other hand,we call con- necting surgery to all procedures for re-establish venous circulation such as: by-passes,and transpositions".

SURGICAL TECHNIQUE

In one side lateral iliac or ilio-femoral thrombosis we perform sapheno femoral or sapheno-sapheno-venous by-pass with Palma´s technique,modified in some way by us.

In femoro-popliteal obliterations,we perform venous transposition technique,which means to cross saphenous vein behind sartorious muscle.

In femoral or femoro-popliteal thrombosis,we had performed 7 sapheno femoral derivations by transposition of saphenous vein to the popliteal or femoral vein,and only 3 cases of femoro-femoral free grafts.

In one lateral iliac or ilio-femoral thrombosis we have performed 33 connecting operations,20 of them,were sapheno-femoral and 13 were sapheno-saphenous by-pass.

27 procedures were made in males and 6,in females. We have 15 singles connecting operations,12 singles connecting ope - rations plus dis-connecting,and 6 connecting operations plus elastic contention.

We have had 24 iliac venous thrombosis and 9 ilio-femoral venous thrombosis.

Phlebolography control showed us,at the post-operatory phase:27 permeable cases,4 obliterated cases and 2 without control.

After 24 months,20 were permeable,4 obliterated and 9 wi-thout control.

CONCLUTIONS

1. Anatomical ethiological classification is necessary
&&2. Phlebographic tests are extremely important.
3. Knowledge of surgical technique is recommeded.
4. Expecience in handling anti-coagulation,anti-aggregation and reological features is required.
5. Arterio-venous fistulae is not indispensable

Phlebology '95, D. Negus et al. (eds.). Phlebology (1995) Suppl. 1: 975-977

OP/17.3

Linton Approach and Vein Reconstruction Procedures for Chronic Vein Insufficiency - Analysis of Own Material

S. Otto, A. Szubert, P. Wozniak and J.A. Polanski

3rd Department of Surgery, 2nd Faculty of Medicine, Warsaw Medical School, Warsaw Poland

Chronic vein insufficiency (CVI) of the lower extremity is a common clinical problem. Approximately 1% of the European population is affected by venous leg ulceration [1]. High ambulatory pressures transmitted from deep venous system via incompetent perforating veins to superficial veins play a major role in the pathogenesis of the disease [2,3,4]. Subfascial ligation of perforating veins since its introduction by Linton in 1938 has become a generally accepted and widespread way of treatment for venous stasis ulcers [3,4,5]. Over the last decade more interest has been focused on deep vein incompetence. Surgical reconstructive procedures directly addressing the existing pathology within deep veins have been evolved and constitute nowadays the approved way of surgical treatment for CVI [3,6,7,8,9].

The objective of this study is to evaluate early and late postoperative results after surgical procedures performed by us for CVI.

MATERIAL AND METHODS

From 1980 to 1994 77 patients were subjected to surgery for CVI due to post-thrombotic syndrome. They were 41 women and 36 men, of median age 56 years. If present all leg ulcerations were mandatory healed before admission. 57 patients (74%) had a history of deep vein thrombosis.

Up to 1988 all patients were studied mainly on the basis of clinical examination (tourniquet-tests). Since 1989 when we started routine phlebographic examinations, ascending and descending phlebography, vein pressures measurements and Doppler ultrasound have been carried out.

67 patients were subjected to subfascial ligation of incompetent perforating veins using the Linton approach combined with stripping of the long and short saphenous veins.

Since 1989 10 patients underwent vein reconstruction procedures. They were qualified to reconstructive surgery on the basis of the following criteria: patent deep veins, ambulatory vein pressure more than 60 mmHg, refilling time less than 15s, deep vein incompetence- 2-4 grade of Kistner classification.In 7 patients valvuloplasty of the highest superficial femoral vein valve was performed (in 6 cases according to Kistner and Raju technique and in 1 case a new valve was created with autogenous vein and fascia tissue),2 patients had a vein valve transplant and 1 patient underwent superficial femoral vein transfer operation. In 7 cases subfascial ligation of perforating veins was additionally carried out as well. All patients after surgery were applied with compressive stockings.

RESULTS

LINTON APPROACH PROCEDURES.

Early postoperative results in all cases were satisfactory.However wound infection and marginal skin necrosis occurred in 15% of cases.

Late postoperative results were evaluated in 47 cases. The follow-up ranged from 6 to 60 months.Recurrent ulcers developed in 10 cases (21%),mainly due to deep vein thrombosis and incompetence of perforating veins.

VEIN RECONSTRUCTION PROCEDURES.

During the follow-up period ranging from 6 to 36 months satisfactory results with haemodynamical improvement were achieved in 9 patients. In 1 case vein valve transplant occluded due to thrombosis. The diagnosis was confirmed by radionuclide phlebography. This patient is under our control and presents with no recurrent ulceration.

DISCUSSION

Results after subfascial ligation of incompetent perforating veins using the Linton approach are quite controversial. Wound complication rate of up to 58% and ulcer recurrence rate of 40% have been reported [3,4,5]. However, many authors described good and excellent long term results with recurrence rate of 10%-15% and wound healing complications not exceeding 17% [3,10,11]. 21% of ulcer recurrence in our material is in our opinion a satisfactory result. Recent development of percutaneous, endoscopic technique of subfascial perforator veins ligation seems to bring a new attractive surgical approach. The results of this minimally invasive surgery are very promising as the reported complication rate of 7.5% and recurrence rate of 2.5% are relatively low [3,4].

Should deep vein insufficiency with valve incompetence and vein reflux occur valve reconstructive surgery is indicated [6,7,8,9]. These recently evolved methods consisting on valvuloplasties, vein valve transplantations and venous transposition operations aim to correct the venous reflux and restore normal activity of calf pump function [3,6,7,8]. The results are very encouraging and 69-90% of clinical success is reported [6,7]. Valvuloplasties are mainly performed in primary deep vein insufficiency. Most of our patients were operated on for CVI due to post-thrombotic syndrome, however we found valve repair possible. Usually, in such cases vein valve transplantations appeared to be more suitable.

Our experience in vein reconstructive surgery is initial. However, on the basis of our early postoperative results we consider this type of surgery justified. In selected cases reconstructive surgical procedures on deep veins could be safely performed together with superficial vein surgery with satisfactory postoperative results.

REFERENCES

1 Baker SR, Stacey MC, Jopp-McKay AG, Hoskins SE, Thompson P.J. Epidemiology of chronic venous ulcers. BR J Surg 1991; 78: 864-7.
2 Negus D, Friedgood A. The effective management of venous ulceration. Br J Surg 1983; 70: 623-627.
3 Wittens CHA, Pierik RGJM, van Urk H. The surgical treatment for incompetent perforating veins. Eur J Vasc Endovasc Surg 1995; 9: 19-23.
4 Pierik EGJM, Wittens CHA, van Urk H. Subfascial endoscopic ligation in the treatment of incompetent perforating veins. Eur J Vasc Endovasc Surg 1995; 9: 38-41.
5 Szostek M, Skorski M, Zajac S, Kowicki A, Zlotorowicz W, Fraczak M. Recurrences after surgical treatment of patients with postthrombotic syndrome of the lower extremities. Eur Vasc Surg 1988; 8: 191-197.
6 Taheri SA, Cullen J, Wormer T. Venous reconstruction in chronic venous insufficiency. Vasc Surg 1989; 6: 470-477.
7 Perrin M, Bayon JM, Castells-Ferrer P, Hiltbrand B. Resultats de la chirurgie restauratrice dans le reflux veineux profonds a l'etage sous-inguinal (A propos de 93 interventions). Phlebologie 1995; 45: 315-330.
8 Wilson NM, Rutt DL, Browse NL. Repair and replacement of deep vein valves in the teatment of venous insufficiency. Br J Surg 1991; 78: 388-394.
9 Psathakis DN, Psathakis ND. How to select and operate on patients with deep venous insufficiency of the lower limb. Vasc Surg 1989; 2: 102- 114.
10 Negus D. Prevention and treatment of venous ulceration. Ann R Coll Surg Engl 1985; 67: 144-148.
11 Cikrit DF, Nichols K, Silver D. Surgical management of refractory venous stasis ulceration. J Vasc Surg 1988; 7: 473-478.

Phlebology '95, D. Negus et al. (eds.). Phlebology (1995) Suppl. 1: 978-979

OP/20.3

Microsurgical Modified Technique for Correction of Incompetent Venous Valves

V. Krylov, E. Shifrin and B. Morag

Department of Vascular Surgery, Sourasky Medical Centre, Tel-Aviv University, Tel-Aviv, Israel

In patients with primary valvular insufficiency of the lower extremities (without previous history of thrombophlebitis) incompetent venous valves can be repaired using a microsurgical technique. The complete diagnosis can be made by modern duplex technique, which allows visualisation of the leaflets of the valves in the common (superficial) femoral and in the popliteal veins. In some, but not all cases, retrograde phlebography is necessary to confirm the diagnosis. A comparison carried out in 35 cases, confirmed the accuracy of the duplex technique for the diagnosis of valvular insufficiency and provided the information for strict indications for reconstructive microsurgical intervention.

MATERIAL

Forty patients with primary valvular insufficiency of the lower extremities were operated on. The group was selected using the following criteria:
1. Clear demonstration of the insufficient valves in the common, superficial or popliteal vein by colour duplex scanning.
2. No previous history of deep thrombophlebitis.

METHODS

Our technique of microsurgical correction of the valvular insufficiency has two steps:

Step 1:   If there was insufficiency of the superficial venous system and especially of the sapheno-femoral junction (confirmed by duplex and Doppler studies), this was eliminated by ligation and stripping of the great saphenous vein and dividing its branches.

Step 2:   Was a direct approach to the valves in the common/superficial femoral vein. After exposure of the segment of the femoral vein with incompetent valve, the circumference of the vein was measured and the diameter calculated, and correspondingly, the necessary length of valve leaflet. A longitudinal venotomy was made under the microscope in the sinus of the valve in order not to damage the leaflets. The length of the venotomy was 10-12 mm. In some cases stay-stitches were applied and both leaflets became open to inspection and measurement. After measurement, the leaflets were shortened to the desired length with two stitches with 8/0 Prolene under x 12 magnification of the operating microscope (Carl Zeiss). The venotomy was closed with a continuous suture using 8/0 Prolene.

After completion of this stage, two circular purse-string sutures were applied through the adventitia above and below the valve to prevent widening of the valve ring. For evaluation of the reconstruction result the 'milking test' was performed after restoration of flow to confirm the adequate function of the reconstructed valve. The patient was allowed to walk the second postoperative day. After operation all patients underwent duplex confirmation of the competency of the reconstructed valves.

RESULTS

In 33 out of 40 cases the repaired valves in common/superficial femoral vein remained competent (Group 1).
In 4 cases there was a partial failure with short duration (2-3 seconds) regurgitation during Valsalva manoeuvre (Group 2).
In 3 cases the insufficiency remained unchanged (Group 3).

There was no surgical morbidity in this series.

CONCLUSION

This modified microsurgical technique to repair the insufficiency of the valves in the femoral veins with direct microsurgical reconstruction of the leaflets is a promising method in terms of the better control of valve insufficiency in the lower extremities.

Phlebology '95, D. Negus et al. (eds.). Phlebology (1995) Suppl. 1: 980-982

OP/17.2

Evolving Surgical Approaches for Venous Ulceration

Ralph G. DePalma, MD, FACS

Department of Surgery, University of Nevada School of Medicine

INTRODUCTION

Venous hypertension causes dermatitis, liposclerosis and ultimately lower leg ulceration. Conventional approaches described by Linton [1] and by Dodd and Cockett [2] noted that perforating vein and saphenous interruption offered the potential for mitigating these effects. Recently the role of the foot perforators and distal saphenous vein has been underscored by Negus.[3] Ultimately, if transmission of venous hypertension to the skin and subcutaneous tissue is reduced ulcer healing can occur.

METHODS

The author has modified surgical treatment for venous ulceration. Modifications include "safe" skin line incisions, excision and grafting of ulcers with correction of axial saphenous incompetence at one operation.[4,5] The availability of Doppler, Duplex scanning, and refined techniques of venography improved the precision of varying elements of these procedures. Ultimately, extrafascial shearing via a skin line incision over the posterior arcade origin with ligation of Boyd's perforator [6] perforator shearing in the axis of the posterior arcade, subfascial ulcer excision with local perforator ligation and skin grafting, and saphenectomy with submalleolar vein interruption characterized a complete procedure for reflux. (Figure 1)

When needed, patients were admitted for intensive treatment of infected ulcerations for 2-3 days. As previously described [4] strict bed rest and elevation were enforced with the leg elevated prior to surgery; ulcers were treated with wet to dry dressings and systemic antibiotics. This made possible a comprehensive operation done in one stage. Whenever possible outpatient treatment was used to control ulcer infection and the majority of patients are now admitted on the same day as the planned surgery.

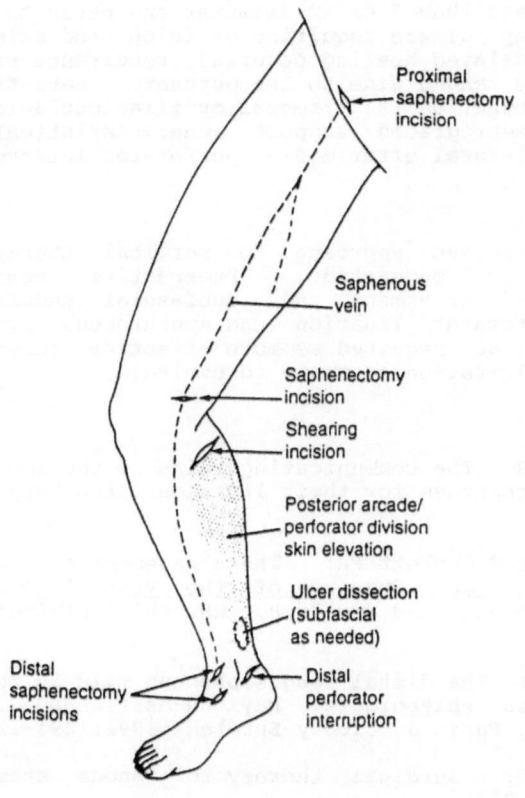

Proximal
saphenectomy
incision

Saphenous
vein

Saphenectomy
incision

Shearing
incision

Posterior arcade/
perforator division
skin elevation

Ulcer dissection
(subfascial
as needed)

Distal
saphenectomy
incisions

Distal
perforator
interruption

Legend Procedure used for saphenous incompetence, perforator interruption with dissection and grafting of ulcer. Note interruption of distal saphenous and submalleolar foot perforators. [3]

RESULTS

Since 1980, 75 extremities in 63 patients with refractory venous ulceration were treated. Two staged Palma procedures for iliac vein occlusion (3%) and three synchronous valveplasties (4%) for severe deep reflux were also done. Thirty five long and four short saphenous veins were excised. With the extrafascial shearing procedure, hospital stays averaged three to four days for ulcers less than 3 cm in diameter and seven to eight days for larger or deep ulcers requiring excision and skin grafts. One instance of delayed healing occurred; recurrence rates up to two to five years ranged nine to ten percent. Late failures related to caval obstruction (3) femoral or iliac occlusion (3), and/or failure to wear graded support. Characteristically recurrence tends to be lateral after medial perforator interruption.

ASSESSMENT

A more aggressive approach to surgical therapy for venous ulceration is suggested. Prospective comparisons with "conservative" treatment and subfascial endolaparoscopically assisted perforator ligation and synchronous bypass or valve plasties will be required as more effective surgical procedures for venous ulceration continue to evolve.

REFERENCES

1. Linton RR: The communicating veins of the lower leg and the operative techniques for their ligation. Ann Surg 1938; 107:582-593.

2. Dodd H and Cockett FR: The management of venous ulcers in The Pathology and Surgery of the Vein of the Lower Limbs Edinburgh, London and New York, Churchill-Livingstone 1976:269-296.

3. Negus D: The distal long saphenous vein in recurrent venous ulceration In Phlebologie, Raymond-Martinbeau P, Prescott R. Zummom (Eds), Paris J. Libbey-Eurotext 1992:1291-1293

4. DePalma RG: Surgical therapy for venous stasis. Surgery: 1974; 76:910-917.

5. DePalma RG: Surgical Therapy for venous stasis: results of a modified Linton operation Ann J Surg 1979; 137:810-813.

6. DePalma RG: Surgical treatment of chronic venous ulceration In: Venous Disorders. Bergan JJ and Yao (Eds) Philadelphia, W.B. Saunders Co, 1990;396-406.

Phlebology '95, D. Negus et al. (eds.). Phlebology (1995) Suppl. 1: 983-985

PI/10.2

Valve Repair in Deep Veins of the Lower Limb. Techniques, Indications and Results

M. Perrin[1], B. Hiltbrand[2], J.M. Bayon[2] and J.L. Calvignac[1]

[1] *Chirurgie Vasculaire, Lyon, France*
[2] *Angiologie, Clinique du Grand Large, Decines Charpieu, France*

INTRODUCTION

In severe Chronic Venous Insufficiency (CVI), deep vein reflux is involved in 22 to 77 % of limbs (1). The most frequent types are Post Thrombotic Syndrome (PTS) and Primary Valve Incompetence (PVI). But in some patients the disease pattern can be identified as a combination of PVI in the proximal part of the limb and PTS in the distal part (2). The purpose of this article is to :
. Review the different techniques of valve repair.
. Report the long term clinical, hemodynamic results of valve repair in 60 limbs operated on from 1988 to 1992.

TECHNIQUES

INTERNAL VALVE REPAIR

The first deep vein valve repair was performed by KISTNER in 1968. Through a longitudinal phlebotomy, he repaired each valve by interrupting a series of sutures placed at each commissure. In 1993, RAJU proposed a supravalvular incision and a continuous suture to shorten the valve leaflets in a curtain-like fashion. In 1988, SOTTIURAI using a supravalvular T-shaped phlebotomy tacked the valve cusp to the vein wall with double-ended sutures at each commissure.

EXTERNAL VALVE REPAIR

In 1990, KISTNER again proposed to restore valve competence without phlebotomy by placing an external row of sutures along the diverging margins of the valve cusp insertion.
In 1991, GLOVICZKI added the use of angioscopy to improve the accuracy of external valve repair.

MATERIAL AND METHODS

From January 1988 to December 1992, we treated 60 limbs (48 patients) by valvuloplasty of the deep veins.
The sex ratio was (M : 22 - F : 26) and mean age fifty (27-77). Clinical severity was graded class 3 in 54 limbs, class 2 in 6 limbs. Twenty nine patients (48.3 %) had previous or active ulcer, 54 lipodermatosclerosis, six isolated edema. All had failure of conservative treatment.
The disease patterns identified by phlebography were :
PVI : 44 - Combination of PVI (proximal) and PTS (distal) : 15 - Klippel-Trenaunay : 1.
Pre-op hemodynamics were as follow :
Reflux : Descending phlebogram grade 4 : All (except three grade 3).
Refilling Time : AVP or (and) PPG : 9 sec (-9, +11).
Drop Pressure Measurement : APG : Less than 40 %.
Venous Reflux Index : Duplex-Scan : 1.1 (Average).

SURGICAL PROCEDURES

34 limbs out of 60 had had previous surgery of the superficial system (34 strippings + 1 perf ligation). Valvuloplasty was performed on the femoral veins (57 internal - 2 internal + external - 1 external). Concomittant surgery of the superficial system (23), ligation of perforators (21) was undertaken few days before when needed.

RESULTS

In the immediate post operative period, thrombosis was checked by ascending phlebogram (1st p.op day) and Duplex-Scan (before discharge). We registered 6 immediate p.op thrombosis (10 %) : 2/44 in PVI group (5 %) and 4/15 in PVI + PTS group (27 %).
The average follow-up of the group is 43 months (24-74 M).
Clinical results are always difficult to assess except when patient have had an ulcer.
- 29 patients had a previous ulcer before valvuloplasty : 26 healed and only two recurred.
- In the PVI group (18 extremities) we found only one recurrence.
- In the PVI + PTS (11 extremities) we observed four non healing ulcers or recurrences (p > 0.01).
- Correlation between ulcer persistence or recurrence and competency of valve repair was checked and found.
24 extremities without ulcer : Twenty competent valve repairs.
5 extremities with persistent or recurrent ulcer : Four incompetent valve repairs.
Clinical outcome was strongly correlated with patency of valve repair (p > 0.01).

Hemodynamic results of the entire group were assessed by :
Duplex-Scan :
- Reflux (55 patients checked) :
Patent no reflux : 40 (72 %) - Patent mild reflux : 5 - Patent major reflux : 4 - P.op thrombosis : 6.
- VRI (47 patients checked) : Normal : 36 (77 %).
PPG :
- Refilling Time (51 patients checked) :
Normalised : 32 (62 %) - Improved : 16 - Worse or unchanged : 3.

CONCLUSION

These results are matching with other previous studies published (KISTNER (2), ERIKSSON (3), RAJU (4,5), SOTTIURAI (6)). Valve repair is an efficient procedure in selected cases particularly in PVI after failure of conservative treatment.

REFERENCES

1 O'Donnel TF. Popliteal vein valve transplantation for deep venous valvular reflux : Rationale method and long term
   clinical, hemodynamic and anatomic results. In Bergan JJ and Yao JST editors. Venous disorders. Philadelphia. WB SAUNDERS. 1991 : 273-295.
2 Masuda EM, Kistner RL. Long term results of venous valve reconstruction : A four-to twenty-one year follow-up. J Vasc Surg 1994 ; 19 : 391-403.
3 Eriksson I, Almgren B. Influence of the profunda femoris vein on venous hemodynamics of the limb. Experience from 31 deep vein recontructions. J Vasc Surg 1986 ; 4 : 390-395.
4 Raju S, Fredericks R. Valve reconstruction procedures for non obstructive venous insufficiency. Rationale, techniques and results in 107 procedures with 2 to 8 years follow-up. J Vasc Surg 1988; 7 : 301-310.
5 Raju S. Multiple valve reconstruction for venous insufficiency: Indications, optimal technique and results. In Veith FJ ed. Current critical problems in vascular surgery. Quality Medical Publishing. ST LOUIS. 1992 ; 4 : 122-125.
6 Sottiurai VS. Surgical correction of recurrent venous ulcer. J Cardiovasc Surg 1991 ; 1 : 104-109.

P270

LATE RESULTS IN PTS DEEP VENOUS SURGERY

Dall'Aglio,O;Canestri,E;Lapertosa,E.

Calle 11n°1018-La Plata,Bs.As.(1900)
República Argentina

Objectives:To present aur late result deep venous
surgery and to show the fallacy between global -
vs/discriminative results
Patients:Fron 1970 we perform 151 procedures.60
in Persistent occlution of the deep venous sys-
tem(PODVS)and 91 in Avalvulation(AV)
Interventions:In PODVS we use Derivative by pass
and we categorized 4 groups according to the pathology and surgical possibilities.
    In AV we use Contensive methods;V●
nous Transposition;V.Transplant;V.Valvuloplasty;
Combinated Procedures and Other.Iven into each -
group we use different tecniques accordin to the
findings and tactical possibilities.
Results;Also in PODVS and in AV,global methods
show 50% results comparing 100%success and 100%
unfortunate events.Discriminative ones show that
iven into a same item,results could be different
according to a lot of factors we will going to -
discuss
Conclutions;Global and ᴰiscriminative results -
must to be presented together in order to be con
gruent with any surgical possibilities.

P271

AUTOGENOUS VEIN VALVE TRANSPLANT USING TWO
SEGMENTS OF SAPHENOUS VEINS WITH COMMON OSTIUM

Molokhia F

Dept of Surgery, Faculty of Medicine, Alexandria University, Egypt

Calibre mismatch is a major problem in venous reconstruction. The concept of using two venous segments of the greater saphenous vein tailored to have one common wide ostium at both ends is introduced, with creation of a temporary AVF using the prolene loop procedure. The technique can correct obstructive and regurgitative veins conditions. It can solve the problem of calibre mismatch since the width of the ostium can be adjusted to the needed diameter. Furthermore, the load of the venous drainage of the lower extremity is divided on more than one valve and thus prevent latter fatigue and function deterioration and obviate the need for external support of the transplanted vein, allowing the normal physiological factors.

V/3.9

THE CORRECTION OF DEEP VENOUS REFLUX WITH VENOCUFF

Botta G, Lorenzi M, Intermite R, Mancini St, Mancini S
III Department of General Surgery and Pabisch Centre of Phlebology-
Director Prof. Sergio Mancini
Faculty of Medicine and Surgery, University of Siena, Italy

Objective: To correct the deep venous reflux surgically.

Design: Discussion of a clinical case of deep venous reflux, corrected with the technique of external valvuloplasty of the common femoral vein with VenoCuff.

Patients: N.E., of 33 years, came to us for varices of the left lower limb. She was operated in March 1991 for external preterminal valvuloplasty of the greater saphena with Mancini's technique. After 3 years of follow-up the patient presented with recurrent varices. The descending phlebography revealed a venous reflux, of both superficial and deep femoral veins.

Intervention: In March 1994 the patient was operated again for external valvuloplasty of the common femoral vein, with the use of the VenoCuff, associated with stripping of the greater saphena and exeresis of the insufficient medial collateral veins of the thigh.

Results: The clinical, instrumental and phlebographic controls one year after the operation show a good result, with the absence of clinical disturbances initially presented by the patient.

Conclusions: The technique of external banding with VenoCuff of the common femoral vein at the level of the insufficient valve has proved to be effective in the revival of the valvular continence and therefore in the abolition of deep venous reflux.

P160

SURGICAL TREATMENT OF VENOUS LEG ULCERS

Rück F., Agostini M., Giansiracusa G.

Surgical Department, General Hospital, Lovere, Italy

Objective: To evaluate the results of the surgical treatment of venous leg ulcers.

Design: Retrospective review of a consecutive series.

Patients: Seventy patients with leg ulcers underwent the surgical treatment after phlebography.

Intervention: The treatment consisted in the removal of the ulcer with the surrounding scar-tissue; the ligation of insufficient venae perforantes; the covering of the defect by free skin-graft; the compression therapy with elastic bandage.

Measurements: The swellings healed in a range of time varying from three weeks up to six months.

Results: Results were positive in 90% of cases and the ulcers disappeared.

Conclusions: The high percentage of positive results confirmed that this method was really efficacious for the treatment of leg ulcers.

P166
LINTON OPERATION IN THE END OF THE TWENTIETH CENTURY - ANALYSIS OF 30 CONSECUTIVE CASES

Pereira A, Castro J M, Duarte J N, Carvalho S, Farrajota A

Vascular Surgery Unit - H St Marta Lisboa Portugal

Objective: There are great discussions about the validity of the Linton operation and about its indication. The authors review their clinical experience in a series of consecutive cases.
Design: Retrospective review of a consecutive series.
Patients: 28 consecutive patients (30 legs) with venous stasis syndrome were studied (between 6/1990 and 6/1991), with Duplex scan and in case of doubts with venography (ascendant and descendent). 13% have active ulcers and have superficial venous insufficiency with or without involvement of the profound venous system.
Intervention: Only 3% of the cases were operated with classic Linton Technique. Most of them were operated with one of the variants of this operations that was our preferential option, and all were combined with superficial venous surgery. The patients in post operative were observed every 3 months and all were submitted to sclerotherapy of residual varicose veins.
Results: In 1/1995 all patients were submitted to a Duplex scan to analyse their venous state. 86% have good results, no recidence of ulcers and no important recurrence of varicose veins. 2% have important profound venous insufficiency or recanalization and have recidence of varicose veins but no apparition of their stasis syndrome because they were controlled with sclerotherapy.
Conclusion: The authors concluded that the Linton Operation and its variations associated to post operative sclerotherapy are a technical and beneficial option to treat patients with venous stasis syndrome.

PI/10.4
DEEP VEIN VALVE REPAIR; A NEW TECHNIQUE AND EARLY RESULTS.

Akemoto K, and Ueyama T,

Department of Cardiovascular Surgery, National Hospital of Kanazawa, KANAZAWA, Japan.

Objective: A review of clinical experience of our new method. It is an external sinus plication that is not necessary of venotomy and anti-coagulation.
Design: Retrospective review of a consecutive series.
Patients: 28 patients who have severe reflux from common femoral vein(CFV) towards ankle region detested by descending phlebography at semi-up light position. They complained severe skin change as, pigmentation 12, ulceration 8, and reccurent varicose veins 10 cases.
Investigations: The valves which were detected by preoperative descending phlebography were exposes under epidural anesthesia. The valves are thinned and expanded at the site of incompetent points. The competence of the valve is checked by milking test. The wall is then plicated with 5-7 interrupted sutures (7-0 polypropylene) from the outside of the vein without venotomy.
Results: The valve competence recovers completely. This situation is investigated by intraoperative angioscope and postoperative phlebography. All deep venous reflux had disappeared completely.
Conclusions: Technical procedure and early results of our new method are presented and no recurrence is observed.

OP/22.5

Embolisation of insufficient perforators in patients with varicose ulceration

Garcarek J., Rybak Z , Szyber P

Department of Vascular Surgery and Radiology, Wrocław
Medical University, Wrocław, Poland

Objective: To review the preliminary clinical experience of a new method of treatment incompetent perforators with an embolisation.

Design: Review of patients underwent embolisation of insufficient perforators with Gianturco-Wallace and Amplatz coils.

Patients: Seven patients (11 legs with open ulceration) were undergoing this study. Diagnosis was stated by phlebography, venous pressure recordings and doppler examination.

Intervention: After localisation of insufficient perforators and elimination of deep vein thrombosis with a puncture of the superficial vein of the leg Gianturco-Wallace coil was inserted to the place of insufficient perforator. At the same time Amplatz coil was placed just below sapheno-phemoral junction to prevent extension of thrombus to the deep system or pulmonary embolism.

Measurements: 7 to 8 phlebograms in two projections were performed before and following procedure which was fluoroscopic controlled. Using the same needle venous pressure recordings were performed with TESTAR 2000 as well as doppler examination.

Results: Early results are promising. Ulcerations were healed within 4 weeks. Any complications were observed. Venous pressure decreased about 15 mm Hg following procedure.
Conclusion: This procedure is an alternative for Linton operation in high risk patients.

OP/22.6

DEEP VEIN RECONSTRUCTIVE SURGERY

Prof. Roberto Simkin, Ruben Bulloj MD. A Fuentes MD

Malabia 3166 (1425) Buenos Aires, Argentina
Buenos Aires University

In this work we are presenting the surgical experience in the Deep Vein pathology.
We are making a difference between the primary valve insufficiency and the secondary valve insufficiency.
We are also making a description in detail of the different techniques used to this day by the different authors and the results obtained with these techniques.
The surgical treatment of the primary valve insufficiency was carried out with the technique proposed by Kistner in 3 cases; and with a technique called Intraluminal Valvuloplasty created by the author (Simkin) in 4 cases. In the secondary valve insufficiency the following techniques were used: Venous transposition in 15 cases; interposition (Tahery) 6 cases; Axillary interposition: 3 cases femoro-femoral by pass: 19 cases, plus a.v.f 7 cases; Palma Operation: 19 cases, plus avf (arterio-venous fistulae) 8 cases. The results of these surgeries were: femoro-femoral bypass: 5 occluded, femoro-femoral plus avf: 3 occluded, femoro-femoral 14 permeable.
The failures in this kind of surgery were due to a bad surgical indication; recurrent reflux; residual or remnant drifts; lack of treatment of the internal saphenous vein; lack of treatment of collaterals of incompetent or defective accessory.

P183

LINTON'S OPERATION IN THE SURGICAL TREATMENT OF POSTPHLEBITIC SYNDROME

Lorenc Z, Oczkowicz G, Malczyk M, Kusmierski S

I Department of Surgery Silesian Medical Academy - Katowice, Szpital Górniczy, 41-200 Sosnowiec, Poland

From 1986 till 1992, 266 patients ill of post phlebitic syndrome received ambulant treatment, among which 170 wre diagnosed, during the course of treatment, to have had venous ulceration and in 104 cases it was found out that the ulceration was of a recurrent character. In the diagnosis of the post phlebitic syndrome, except close clinical examination, the Doppler's and phlebographic examinations wee carried out. Using both examinations it was discovered that the reason for the ulceration of 121 patients were insufficient vessels intersecting under thigh. 68 patients of this group were operated and the rest 53 ones were treated pharmacologically. The goal of this paper is the evaluation of the results in the treatment of patients with type I of the post phlebitic syndrome. Considering the degree of the advance of the morbid process, patients were allotted to one of two groups (I-62, II-59 patients). The period of observation figured at least two years. The total healing of ulceration and the lack of return in the period of next 18 months were considered, by the authors, to be a good effect of the treatment. Apart from the Linton's operation, less complete operations, e.g. 'limited' saphenectomy with suprafascial ligation of the perforating veins or 'lifting' of ulceration by Madden-Kimm's method were performed among a chosen group of patients. In the group of 53 patients treated pharmacologically, only in 12 cases the return of disease during the period of observation was not ascertained. In the group of operated patients the best results were recorded in the first group of advancing (two returns). 'Limited' saphenectomy with suprafascial ligation of the perforating veins in this group of patients, including 5 patients after the Linton's operation. **Conclusion:** The Linton's operation among patients with type I of postphlebitic syndrome is the best conduct. Early evaluation as fit for operation gives bigger possibility of permanent cure.

P273

VALVE REPAIR. RESULTS IN 68 PROCEDURES.

PERRIN M., CALVIGNAC JL.

Clinique du Grand Large - LYON - FRANCE.

From 1988 to 1993, sixty eight extremities with deep vein reflux were treated by valve repair. Clinical severity was graded class 3 in sixty four extremities including thirty two recurrent ulcers (47 %). Preoperative and postoperative evaluation consisted in physical examination, ascending, descending phlebography or Duplex-Scanning, ambulatory venous pressure or photoplethysmography.
Patterns of etiology were classified in 2 groups : Primary Deep Vein Incompetency (PDVI) or combination of Post-Thrombotic Syndrome (distal) and PDVI (proximal). Associated procedures (previous or concomittant) were performed in association with internal valve repair: Stripping and ligation of perforators.
The mean duration follow-up was forty-two months (12 months to 74 months). Clinical outcome was correlated with competence of valve repair. 82,5 % of ulcers remained healed.

Hemodynamic results were as follows :
. Refilling time was normalised in 62 % (PPG).
. Reflux was abolished in 72 % (Duplex-Scanning).
These results are in accordance with previous others studies (KISTNER, SOTTIURAI, RAJU, ERIKSSON).

V/2.10

VIDEO-ENDOSCOPIC SURGICAL TREATMENT OF PERFORATING VEINS.

Gasbarro V.M.D., Pozza E.M.D., Viaggi R.M.D., Vettorello G.F.M.D., Pollinzi V.M.D., De Anna D.M.D.*. Derwish A.M.D., Donini I.M.D.
Institute of Clinical Surgery-Ferrara-Italy.
* Institute of Surgical Pathology-Sassari-Italy.

The AA describe their experience related to the videoendoscopic legature of incompetent perforating veins of the legs according to G.HAUER Technique; it consists in isolation and resection of all incompetent perforating veins of the legs, using an operative optic introduced under the muscle fascia through a cold light tube. This surgical procedure has the same indications as the traditional surgical treatment: 1) Recurrent or primary varicose veins due to incompetent perforating veins with major trophic lesions 2) Venous ulcers not-cured by medical therapy or compressive bandages. The only contraindications is DVT. Advantages are the mini-incisions distant to the ulcerative or dermatologic lesions, the short operating time and precocious deambulation of the patient. Since January 1994 in our institute 14 patients have undergone legature of incompetent perforating veins by video-endoscopic approach. Investigated preoperatively by echo-doppler and ascending phlebography. All had grave dermal affections of low extremeties with incompetent perforating veins of legs. 3 patients with clinical post-phlebitic syndrome. In 10 cases was associated a short stripping of the long saphenous vein, in only one case a revision of the sapheno-femoral junction was done. In all the patients we have got the absence of the symptomatology by venous stasis, without any immediate post-operative complication. Follow-up was made for one year by echo-doppler every 3 months.

Venous Dysplasis

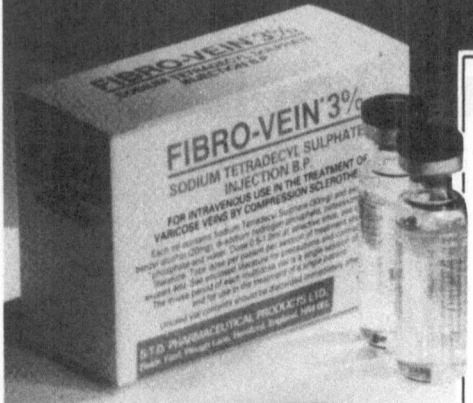
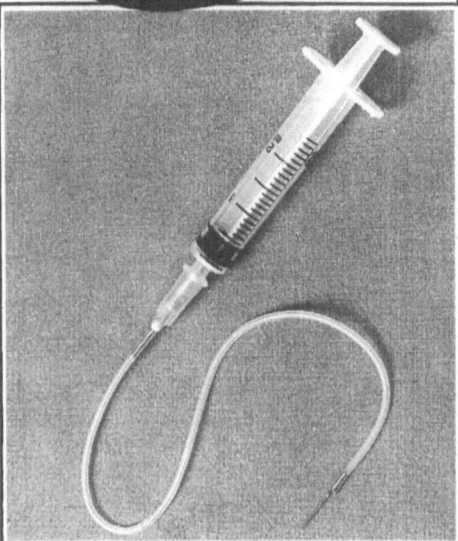
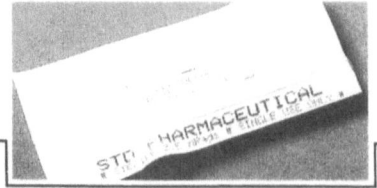
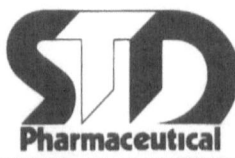

Phlebology '95, D. Negus et al. (eds.). Phlebology (1995) Suppl. 1: 995-997

V/3.1

A Case of Klippel-Trenaunay Syndrome Associated with Cerebellar Dysfunction

N. Uchida[1], M. Sakuma[1], T. Furuuchi[1], H. Satoh[1], K. Furukawa[1], N. Suzuki[2] and T. Yamawaki[2]

[1] Department of Surgery and [2] Department of Neurology, Mito Red Cross Hospital, Mito, Japan

INTRODUCTION

The three clinical findings of a cutaneous nevus, varicose veins and hypertrophy of bone and soft tissue affecting one or more limbs was first described as a single disease entity by Klippel and Trenaunay in 1900 [1] . Afterwards there are some case reports of Klippel-Trenaunay syndrome (KTS) associated with neurological disorders such as mental retardation or myelopathy. However, this is the first case report (to our knowledge) linking this diagnosis with cerebellar dysfunction.

CASE REPORT

Patient 52-year-old Japanese male

Presentation

This patient consulted our hospital because of jerky and poorly controled movements which have been present since adolescence and have worsened with age. Extensive varicose veins and hypertrophy of the left lower extremity have been present since birth. As shown in Fig.1 the affected left leg is 3cm longer than the right;the thigh and calf circumferences are 5 and 8 cm larger, respectively. No port-wine nevus is apparent.

Neurological Findings

Ataxia of gait, nystagmus, dysarthric speech and urinary incontinence are noticeable. Choreiform movement is present on the whole body. There are no cranial nerve palsies. Deep tendon reflexes are normal. Babinski's and Chaddock's signs are positive on the left leg. Dysdiadochokinesis is noticed bilateraly. Romberg's and Barre's signs are negative. There is no other abnormality such as paralysis, seizures or visual distubances. Patient is of normal intelligence.

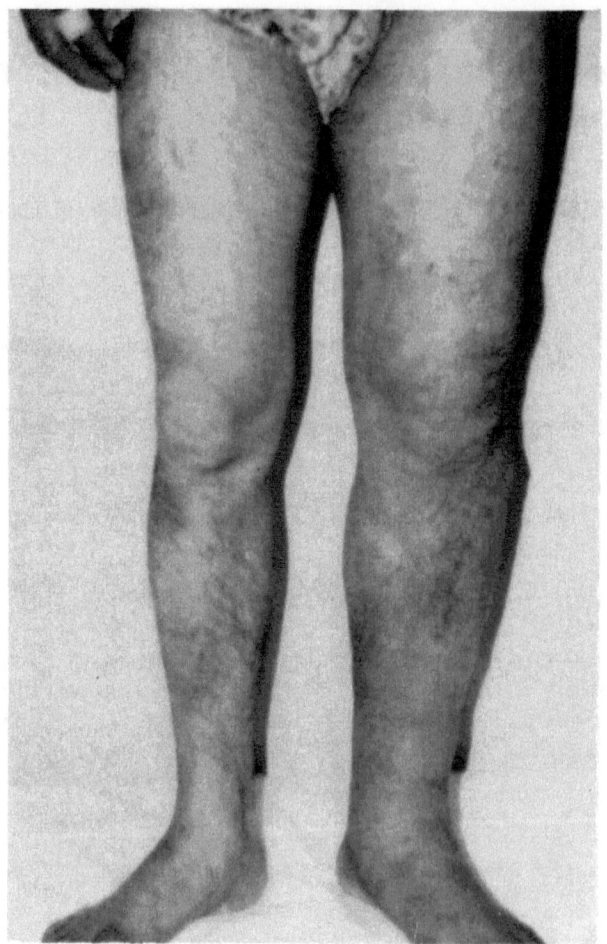

Fig. 1

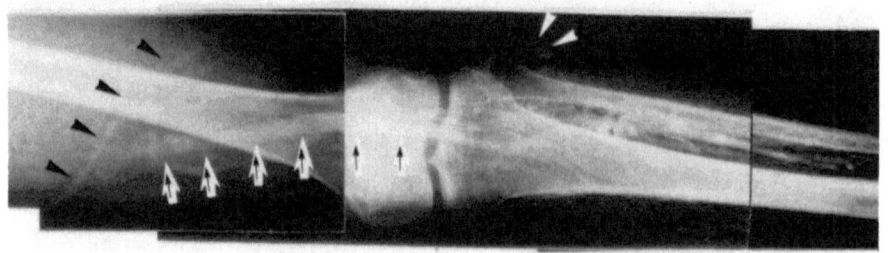

Fig. 2

Diagnostic Studies

No biochemical abnormality has been defined. Phlebography revealed lateral marginal vein (Fig.2 arrow heads) and varicose veins particularly pronounced in the calf. Deep veins (Fig.2 arrows) were patent. Digital subtraction angiography visualized incompetent type persistent sciatic artery. There was no apparent arterio-venous fistula. No significant findings were detected by cranial CT and MRI except mild atropy of the cortex. Electroencephalogram at rest showed fast wave and no α wave. Reaction to the eyes-opening-closing test and hyperventilation was not clear.

DISCUSSION

The above findings suggest a diagnosis of KTS associated with cerebellar dysfunction. Klippel and Trenaunay classified another group of patients who had only two of the three classic characteristics as *forme fruste*. Our case belongs to this category because it lacks port-wine nevus. Altough there are some case reports of KTS associated with anomalies of fingers and toes such as syndactyly or polydactyly [2] , our case has no other anomalies. A few cases of familial KTS have been described [3] , however no family members of our case had limb hypertrophy or port-wine nevus and varices. This patient's father also had involuntary movement,but detailed information is not available. Our case is strongly suspected of hereditary cerebellar ataxia, and further examinations including chromosomal study are recommended.

On the one hand there are some case reports of hereditary cerebellar ataxia combined with malformation [4] , and on the other hand there are some case reports of KTS associated with nerological disorders such as microcephaly, cerebral and spinal arterio-venous fistulas, brain stem angiomas and ischemic infarcts [5,6] . However, this is the first case report (to our knowledge) linking KTS with cerebellar dysfunction. Although there are some case reports of KTS which are treated surgically, we think that a careful explanation, psychological support and good elastic stockings are the most effective approaches in the management of this patient.

REFERENCES

1. Klippel M, Trenaunay P. Du naevus variquex osteo-hypertrophique. Archives Generale de Medicine (Paris)1900;3:641-72.
2. McGrory BJ, Amadio PC, Dobyns JH, Stickler GB, Unni KK.Anomalies of the fingers and toes associated with Klippel-Trenaunay syndrome. The Journal of Bone and Joint Surgery 1991;73:1537-46.
3. Aelvoet GE, Jorens PG, Roelen LM. Genetic aspects of the Klippel-Trenaunay syndrome. British Journal of Dermatology 1992;126:603-7.
4. Katzman R. Degenarative and heredodegenerative diseases. In: Merritt HH,editor. A textbook of neurology. London:Lea and Febiger,1979:535-49.
5. Goldstein SJ, Lee C, Young AB, Guidry GJ. Aplasia of the cervical internal carotid artery and malformation of the circle of Willis associated with Klippel Trenaunay syndrome:case reprt. J Neurosurg 1984;61:786-9.
6. Jaksch H, Bewermeyer H, Dreesbach HA, Heiss WD. Cerebral hemorrhage in arterio-venous malformation associated with Klippel-Trenaunay syndrome. J Neurol 1986; 233:48-50.

Phlebology '95, D. Negus et al. (eds.). Phlebology (1995) Suppl. 1: 998-1000

P094

Venous Aneurysms of the Greater and of the Lesser Saphenous Veins: The Color-Doppler Point of View

A. Pieri, A. Vannuzzi, S. Michelagnoli, F. Marcelli and G. De Saint Pierre

III Cardiology Unit-Diagnostic Angiology Module ((Dir. Prof. G. De Saint Pierre), Azienda Ospedaliera Careggi - Firenze, Italy

Venous aneurysms of the greater (GSV) and of the lesser (LSV) saphenous veins have been considered since nowadays as the expression of angiodysplasias (1) or of a perforator vein's reflux directed towards the venous wall. Venous dilatation would have been secondary to refluxes' direction against venous walls and the perforator vein would have been located in the center of the aneurysm in the deep face of the vessel. C.W. doppler findings of an high velocity pattern strongly supported this interpretation.

Color-Doppler (CD) allows to denie such point of view in most cases showing that facts are quite different (2,3).

Venous aneurysms of the saphenous veins are frequent in varicose disease of the lower limbs and occur mostly at thigh level. They are preferentially located at the upper and lower third of the thigh (mostly below ostial, pre-ostial and middle saphenous valves of the GSV) and at the upper third of the leg just below sapheno-popliteal junction of the LSV (fig. 1).

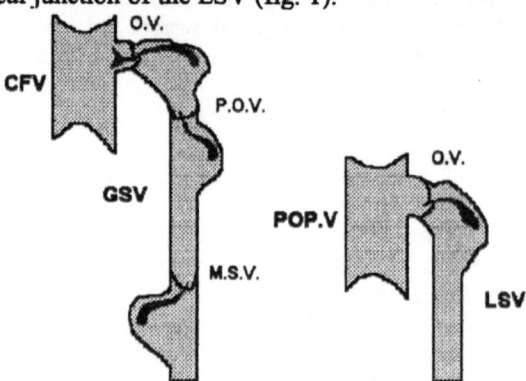

Fig. 1 - Favourite sites of venous aneurysms: transvalvular jets' directions determine venous wall bending. (CFV=common femoral vein, O.V.=ostial valve of sapheno-femoral and of sapheno-popliteal junctions, P.O.V.=pre-ostial valve, GSV=greater saphenous vein, POP.V=popliteal vein, M.S.V.=middle saphenous valve, LSV=lesser saphenous vein).

Generally their shape is of a saccular aneurysm. By ultrasounds investigation we can observe that at their proximal end there is a venous valve that shows a mild incontinence owing to valvular edges' defect or dilatation.

CD shows the presence of a narrow shaped, fast reflux through valvular edges directed towards the saccular enlargement of the wall. (fig. 2)

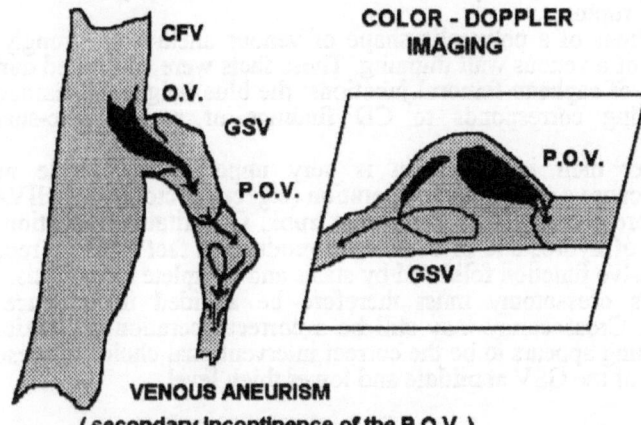

VENOUS ANEURISM
(secondary incontinence of the P.O.V.)

Fig.2 - Proximal venous aneurysm of the greater saphenous vein (GSV), located just below the pre-ostial valve (P.O.V.).(CFV=common femoral vein, O.V.=ostial valve of sapheno-femoral juncion)

Visual impression is that the wall bends itself to receive the reflux, in order to smooth off its violence. Inside the saccular dilatation of the vein wall we can see fast turbulences directed forward and reverse, following aneurysm's shape, before flowing into the distal varice.

Venous aneurysms are so to be considered as true post-stenotic aneurysms (in the sense of venous flow direction), similar to arterial ones. They are expression of the strong resistence that saphenous valves oppose to the progression of the varicose disease and are secondary to proximal saphenous vein's incontinence. Sometimes a mild defect of valvular limbs' insertion may be in cause.

Quite different patterns are showed by the venous aneurysms originating by perforator veins' refluxes: they are spindle-shaped and they are located just above a venous valve or in a non valvulated tract of GSV.

All of them however must not be confused with normal venous ectasias surrounding normal venous valves (fig. 3).

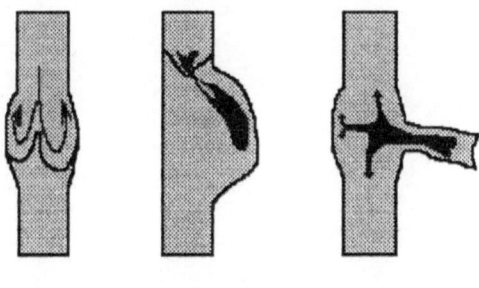

a   b   c

Fig. 3 - Different shapes of superficial venous ectasias: a) normal venous valve; b) saccular aneurysm located just below a slightly incompetent valve; c) spindle-shaped aneurysm, secondary to a perforator vein's reflux. Their shapes appear to correspond to the different ways of genesis.

A complete pre-operatory CD study of the whole GSV and LSV must always be performed because the detection of venous aneurysms is foundamental owing to vein's walls thinning: an accurate dissection may avoid intraoperatory aneurysms' ruptures.

CD findings of a polyciclic shape of venous aneurysms strongly suggest the possibility of a venous wall thinning. These facts were confirmed during accurate dissections of sapheno-femoral junctions: the blue bulging appearance of venous wall thinning corresponds to CD findings of a polyciclic-shaped venous aneurysm.

Moreover their identification is very important to decide interventional strategy because a conservative operation (e.g. crossectomy or CHIVA) can result in a full thrombosis of the saphenous trunk. Quantitative reduction both of the reflux and of hydrostatic pressure may produce in fact a partial recovery of the proximal valve function followed by stasis and complete thrombosis.

CHIVA's crossotomy must therefore be avoided in presence of venous aneurysms. Crossectomy may still be a correct operation in proximal ones but short stripping appears to be the correct interventional choice in presence of such aneurysms of the GSV at middle and lower thigh level.

REFERENCES

1 - Pearce W.H., Yao J.S.T., Baxter B.T., McCarthy W.J.: Venous angiodysplasia and venous malformations. In Bergan J.J., Yao J.S.T.: Venous Disorders - Philadelphia, W.B.Saunders Company, 1991: (Chapt.25), 360-371.

2 - Pieri A., Vannuzzi A., Duranti A., Vin F., Benelli L., Michelagnoli S., Caillard Ph., De Saint Pierre G.: Rôle central de la valvule pré-ostiale de la veine saphène interne dans la gènese des varices tronculaires des membres inférieurs. Démonstration diagnostique par echo-doppler couleur. Phlébologie 1995: (47), 2 in press.

3 - Pieri A., Vannuzzi A., Duranti A.: L' incontinence primitive de la valvule pré-ostiale dans la gènese des varices: demonstration par doppler couleur. J Mal Vasc 1994: 19, (suppl. B), 246

Phlebology '95, D. Negus et al. (eds.). Phlebology (1995) Suppl. 1: 1001-1002

P238

Medical and Surgical Treatment of a Stasis Ulcer in Kippel Trenaunay Syndrome (KTS)

S.J. Simonian

Department of Surgery, Georgetown University Medical Center, Washington, DC, USA

INTRODUCTION

The purpose of this study was to determine for a venous stasis ulcer the interdependent roles of medical and surgical treatments in a patient with KTS [1-5].

METHODS

DP is a 58 year old male, PhD, physicist, who was first seen on July 29, 1993 with a non-healing venous stasis ulcer on the medial ankle for 1 1/2 years on his left KTS leg, despite wearing 30-40 mm Hg graduated compression stockings (GCS). The patient had stopped playing tennis.

In 1965, Servelle et al explored and wrote him up as the first case of KTS with agenesis of the left external iliac vein [6].

Clinical examination showed KTS in the left lower extremity with hypertrophy, prominent bulging veins, angiomata, pigmentation, lipodermatosclerosis and ulceration, 80 mm x 10 mm in the left medial ankle.

Phlebography revealed absent deep veins: popliteal, superficial femoral, common femoral and external iliac. Venous drainage from the popliteal vein was through a competent superficial large (50 mm diameter) protruding vein from the distal anterior thigh to the left groin, then going across the pubis to the other (right) side common femoral vein. Color duplex confirmed the above, plus showed incompetent deep anterior and posterior tibial veins. Air plethysmography showed a venous filling index of 7.3 ml/sec, high (normal below 2.0 ml/sec), ejection fraction of 25%, low (normal over 60%) and ambulatory venous pressure of 61 mm Hg, high (normal below 35 mm Hg). Continuous wave Doppler confirmed incompetent tributaries of the long saphenous and perforator veins below the knee.

Diagnosis was KTS with non-healing ulcer secondary to deep, superficial and perforator vein incompetence despite wearing GCS.

INTERVENTIONS

Two 30-40 mm Hg GCS, one on top of the other, were worn for 6 weeks. Followed by ambulatory phlebectomy of incompetent superficial varicose and perforator veins on October 28, 1993.

RESULTS

The ulcer healed after six weeks of wearing double GCSs. Following the phlebectomy, only one GCS has been worn. The patient resumed tennis and the ulcer has remained healed during a period of 1 1/2 years follow up.

DISCUSSION

Ten per cent of patients with KTS develop venous stasis ulcers from incompetence of deep or superficial and/or perforator veins as they age [1-6]. Besides GCS, surgical excision of superficial and perforator incompetent veins is the treatment of choice to heal the ulcers.

CONCLUSION

A 58 year old male patient with KTS, had deep, superficial and perforator vein incompetence and non-healing venous ulcer, despite wearing GCS. Double GCSs healed the ulcer in six weeks and surgical excision of the superficial incompetent saphenous and perforator varicosities maintained the healing of the ulcer during the 1 1/2 years follow up period.

REFERENCES

1. Klippel M, Trenauny P. Du noevus variquex et osteo-hypertrophique. Arch Gen Med (Paris) 1900;185:641-72.

2. Servelle M. Klippel-Trenaunay's syndrome. Ann Surg 1985;197:365-73.

3. Lindenhauer SM. The Klippel-Trenaunay syndrome. Ann Surg 1965;162:303-14.

4. Baskerville PA, Ackroyd JS, Lea Thomas M, Browse NL. The Klippel-Trenaunay syndrome: Clinical radiological and hemodynamic features and management. Br J Surg 1985;72:232-36.

5. Villavicencio JL. Treatment of varicose veins associated with congenital vascular malformations. In: Bergan JJ, Goldman MP, editors. Varicose veins and telangiectasias. Diagnosis and treatment. St Louis, Quality Medical Publishing, Inc., 1993:329-42.

6. Servelle M, Zolotes E, Soulie J, Andrieux J, Cornu C. Syndrome de Klippel et Trenaunay malformations des veines iliaques, femorale et poplitee. Arch des Mal de Coeur 1965;8:1187-97.

Phlebology '95, D. Negus et al. (eds.). Phlebology (1995) Suppl. 1: 1003-1005

OP/18.5

Therapeutic Management and Results of Congenital Angiodysplasias

P.B. Dimakakos[1], K. Katsenis[1], B. Arapglou[1], M. Papasava[1] and A. Antoniou[2]

[1] Vascular Surgical Department of the 2nd Surgical Clinic and [2] X-Ray Department
University of Athens, Athens, Greece

INTRODUCTION

Congenital vascular malformations (CVMs) are rare lesions of uncertain etiology with structural disorders of the vascular system, nondegenerative and noninflammatory in origin, which occur during embryologic development. They constitute a heterogeneous group of diseases which are also often accompanied by other congenital syndromes.

In co-existing arteriovascular communications the "combined" therapy of surgical and non-surgical methods, is considered as the treatment of choice [1]. Early ligation of the feeding arteries restricts embolization which often requires more therapeutic sessions.

Prior to commencement of treatment the therapeutic plan must be laid out for every case by an experienced team which mainly decides whether treatment will be embolization, surgical or conservative (symptomatic) [1].

MATERIAL AND METHODS

Sixty patients with CVMs were seen during the period of 1980-1994. Of these 17 were arteriovenous fistulas (AVF), 14 had the Klippel Trenaunay syndrome, 1 had Kasabach Merritt and 28 had venous hemangiomas.

a. AVF constitute a "surgical" angiodysplasia due to local and general complications. Our material comprised 11 males and 6 females, aged 20 months to 59 years, who were studied angiographically by coloured Doppler, peripheral plethysmography and peripheral pressure indices.

Tables 1 and 2 show the localization and our surgical tactics.

Follow-up for 8.5 years (min. 1 yr - max. 14 yrs) showed a clinically and angiographically relapse in 35% of the patients (6/17), all were type II according to Vollmar [2] (3 embolizations and ligation and 3 with ligation and excision) extending to the muscles and bones.

Table 1. Localization of 17 AV fistulas

Localization	No of cases
Upper extremities	7
Lower extremities	6
Neck/face	2
Intraperitoneal cavity	1

Table 2. Surgical treatment of 17 AV fistulas

Surgical treatment	No of cases
Ligation + Excision	8
Skeletonization	4
Embolization + Ligation	4
No treatment	1

b. Klippel Trenaunay syndrome. This constitutes a venous but not a surgical angiodysplasia. Fourteen cases studied by intraarterial and radioisotopic arteriography and phlebography. Hypertrophy in 43.2% (6/14), acromegaly in 21.6% (3/14), 3 with agenesia of the deep venous system. Six with excision of varicose veins and 3 with sclerotherapy, relapsed. The treatment of choice was symptomatic therapy which had a good evolution in all the patients.

c. Venous angiomata. The study of 28 cases was carried out by means of phlebography, measurement of O_2 saturation, arteriography, ankle-brachial pressure indices and plethysmography. Nine patients were managed therapeutically for cosmetic reasons with Laser, 4 with sclerotherapy and compression and 2 with excision.

CONCLUSIONS

Treatment of congenital angiodysplasias still remains a problem. Due to the multiformity of this disease entity, individual evaluation is required which predisposes experience, morphologic and hemodynamic analysis as well as highly specialized surgical ability.

REFERENCES

1. Loose D. Combined treatment of congenital vascular defects seminal. In: Vascular Surgery. E.B.Saunders, 1993:4:260-5.

2.   Vollmar JF, Nobble FR. Arteriovenoese fisteln und dilatierende Arteriopathien. Stuttgart: Thieme Verlag, 1976:66-76.
3.   Loose DA, Belov S. Chirurgische therapiemoeglichkeiten bei angeborene peripheren gefass-dysplasien. In: Loose DA, editor. Periodica Angiologica No 11. Hamburg: Einhorn Presse, 1985:55-84.

OP/22.1

AN EXPERIMENTAL STUDY OF PREPARING AND GRAFTING OF THE HUMAN UMBILICAL VEIN

Chen Weipei, Guo Guangjin, Yao Changle.

Department of Applied Anatomy and Operative Surgery, Third Military Medical College, Chongqing, China.

Objective: To evaluate the effect of grafting the human umbilical vein(HUV).

Design: Study on the preparing and grafting of the HUV. 12 dogs in this experiment.

Measurements: The histologic, biochemical, physical and antigenic properties of HUV treated with different agents and their usage in the grafting to aortae.

Results:The histologic change in 10% formalin-treated umbilical vein is smaller than in the glutaraldehyde-treated specimens.The protein content(Kjeldahl's method)in 10% formalin treated specimen was the lowest in all groups(P< 0.01). Next was the 0.5% glutaraldehyde-treated groups (p< 0.05) . Both the fresh umbilicus and treated HUV with formalin or glutaraldehyde have identical elasticity coefficients and breaking strengths measured by the pulling force device. The double agar diffusion showed a positive reaction from fresh HVU, but not at the treated groups. All the grafts treated with 10% formalin and 0.5% glutaraldehyde had good patency rate (91%)in 1-24 months.The neoendothelium grew into the umbilical vein and substituted really the fibrinous membranes after 60-120 days after transplantation.

Conclusion:The umbilical vein have several merits for middle and large arterial grafts. such as:mild reactivity, good patency rate, and greater flexibility.

P237

ANGIODYSPLASIAS AND CONGENITAL ARTERO-VENOUS FISTULAS: OUR CLINICAL EXPERIENCE.

Fregonese V,Gonano N,Santarelli R,Biasi G,Andolfato G,Pfeiffer P,Mozzon L.

Vascular Surgery Unit, Udine Regional Hospital, 33100 UDINE (ITALY)

OBJECTIVE: To review the clinical experience of a recently constituted Vascular Surgery Unit.To report a case of A-V fistula successfully treated by surgery.

DESIGN: Retrospective review (January 1992-December 1994).

PATIENTS:16 patients affected with congenital angiodysplasias:2 Klippel-Trenaunay Syndrome,3 Phleboangiomatosis of limbs,6 A-V Fistulas(1 associated to left Inferior Vena Cava),1 Venous aneurysm,3 dysplastic arterial aneurysms,1 Marfan Syndrome with multiple venous and arterial aneurysms.

TREATMENT:Appropriate surgical or endovascular therapy in according to clinical features was performed.

CASE REPORT (poster presentation):A male child,preterm born at 31st pregnancy week (birthweight 1,540g-APGAR index 3-6) clinically examined after 5,7,12,22 months because of a pulsatile mass of the right elbow.EchoDoppler and angiographic evidence of a single direct fistula connecting brachial artery (much enlarged) and cephalic vein,with high flow pattern.No peripheric steal or venous stasis.No cardiac decompensation.Percutaneous endoluminal embolization wasn't applied for the large (1.5 cm)diameter of fistula. Anomalous duct was excised after a double ligation,on May 1994. At present,the patient is in perfect health:no residual circulatory or hemodynamic defect has been noted.

CONCLUSIONS:For selected cases of angiodysplasia,surgical treatment can play a conclusive role,before a severe worsening of local or systemic circulatory status could develop.

P272

KLIPPEL TRENAUNAY SYNDROME ANGIODYSPLASIA

Simkin R, Bulloj R, Fuentes A

Malabia 3166 (1425) Buenos Aires, Argentina

The authors present their experience in the treatment of Klippel Trenaunay Syndrome from 1970 to date.
There is a bibliographical review on the topic and a consecutive series of the works published by the authors. (Simkin)
316 Klippel Treanaunay Syndrome cases were studied from 1970 to 1994, finding the following pathologies: varicose veins in 316 cases; chronic venous insufficiency 32 cases; differences in the size of the bones: 312 cases: arteriovenous fistulae: 313 cases; pigmentary nevus in 194 cases; polydactylia: 16 cases; macrodactylia: 12 cases; diffuse angioma: 14 cases; and neurological anomalies in 6 cases. The treatment used on these patients was: epiphisiodesis in 17 cases; venous resection only in 29 cases; venous resection plus espiphisiodesis in 17 cases; venous resection only in 29 cases; venous resection plus espiphisiodesis 25 cases; regional segmentary.
Skeletization plus venous resection 142 cases; foot angioma 6 cases and dorsal angioma 6 cases; these last ones, relate to another surgery.
The results were good in 70%; fairly good in 22% and bad in 8%.
As a conclusion we consider the treatment of Klippel T. syndrome with this technique to be of great help for these children to reduce considerably the elongation of a limb respect to the other.

P243

A NEW TREATMENT OF VENOUS ANGIOMATOSES

Coget J M, Breviere J P, Beregi J P

61 Rue de Turenne 59000 Lille, France

The treatment of venous angiome is often difficult, because they are spread out. The sclerosis gives bad results, because, it includes many inflammation and always a repermeation. The surgery is also difficult because the wall of the vena is delicate. The cryo-surgery of the venous network is a good technique and present the destruction of the subcutaneous venous network with two cuts of the skin. We introduce a case with a good result proved clinically and with RMN.

P244

POSTNATAL DEVELOPMENT OF THE LOWER EXTREMITIES
IN SOME FORMS OF VENOUS MALFORMATIONS
Tasnádi G., Acsády Gy.

Heim Pál Hospital for Children and
Univ.Clinic Cardiovasc.Surgery, Budapest

One of the most important factors of development, growth of the extremities is the systemic circulation. On the basis of our researches, and literary data we found out, that the circulation of the extremity changes with age.

The physiologic, biochemical and pathologic features after standing up, during walking are approaching to those measured in adulthood.

The change of the characteristics are influences by the vascular malformations of the extremities.

On the basis of our observations in the cases of predominant venous truncular malformations, the total and nutritive blood flow is decreasing, the oxygen consumption is on the increase, the activity of the LDH is decreasing, the venous pressure is increasing, minimal hypertrophy - or porther hypertrophy the extremity develop.

In the cases of diffuse phlebectasia, phlebangiomatosis, the venous pressure is decreasing /!/ beside similar physiologic, biochemical data, a shortening, deformity of the bones, so called pseudohypertrophy comes into being.

By, in adequate are performed corrective operations - resulting mostly the equalization of the venous pressure - the decompensation of the circulation of the extremity, the progression of its consequences are avoidable. /Case reports/

According to our experiences the data of the surgical treatment plays a very important role in its success. In the venous malformations of the extremities it is suitable to operate during the period of compensation or subcompensation, that is at the age of 3 to 7 years.

Axillary, Subclavian and Arm Venous Disorders

There is an attractive alternative for your patients

- Clinically proven graduated compression
- Wide range of fabrics and styles
- Standard sizes and made to measure

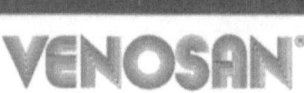

Phlebology '95, D. Negus et al. (eds.). Phlebology (1995) Suppl. 1: 1011-1014

OP/5.8

Venous Problems in Thoracic Outlet Syndrome

J.D. Gruss

Department for Vascular Surgery, Kurhessisches Diakonissenhaus, Kassel, Germany

INTRODUCTION

The Thoracic Outlet Syndrome comprises all compression syndromes of the venous, arterial and nerval structures at the thoracic outlet. Usually neurological, arterial, and venous symptoms overlap so that diagnosis is often made pretty late or when complications arise. However, there are cases where the neurological, the arterial or the venous signs are predominant. Venous symptoms can arise from chronic venous compression, from acute subclavian vein thrombosis, in the most severe cases presented as phlegmasia cerulea dolens, and disabling postthrombotic syndrome. It seems important to remind that 1 - 2 % of lethal pulmonary embolisms origin from subclavian vein thromboses and that about 10 % of previous subclavian vein thromboses result in an insurance relevant upper extremity postthrombotic syndrome.

PATIENTS AND METHODS

This report is based on the evaluation and treatment of 1,545 patients presenting with upper extremity symptoms or vascular complications of thoracic outlet syndrome from 1976 to 1994. During this period of time 594 operations to decompress the neurovascular bundle at the thoracic outlet were performed. More than 20 % of these interventions were necessary on behalf of acute arterial or venous complications, with a ratio of 3 - 1 in favour of the venous complications. 177 operations were done because of a mainly venous indication. In this group 40 suffered from chronic venous compression, 93 patients had acute subclavian vein thromboses and 44 presented with a severe postthrombotic syndrome.

DIAGNOSIS AND TREATMENT

Diagnostic evaluation includes a thorough history, examination and assessment of occupational and recreational activities. In addition to palpation of pulses and auscultation for bruits at neutral, adduction and abduction-external rotation all patients were evaluated with the abduction elevation stress test (AEST). This test is not done if an acute subclavian vein thrombosis is supposed. In these cases we only perform an ascending phlebography of the diseased arm for documentation of the thrombosis. The first aim of treatment is the restauration of the venous flow. This can be accomplished by venous thrombectomy or by fibrinolysis. It is of utmost importance to repeat the phlebography after the successful reopening of the subclavian vein by either method and to visualize the subclavian vein in normal as well as in abduction and elevated position either to confirm or to exclude the compression at the thoracic outlet. This additional phlebography is performed immediately after thrombectomy usually at the day of operation or in case of fibrinolytic therapy 4 days after the starting of this treatment. When we are able to document and underlying causal venous compression at the thoracic outlet we perform the transaxillary exarticulation of the 1st rib within 24 hours. This operation includes also the resection of a cervical rib or the removal of any fibromuscular bands. All patients are maintained under anticoagulation and are supported with a class 3 compressive arm stocking for 6 months postoperatively.

In patients with chronic venous compression presenting with a bluish discoloration of their arms in the morning, increasing pain and heaviness during the day and venous congestion during over-head working as well as patients with postthrombotic syndrome showing a swollen arm with dark pigmentation and secondary varicose veins at the arms, the shoulder, the chest-wall undergo a complete workup like patients with a mainly arterial or neurological TOS. This includes the visualization of the subclavian artery and vein in normal and elevation-abduction position, and a neurological evaluation with electromyographical measurement of the proximal ulnar and median nerve conduction times. It includes also x-rays of the cervical spine in 4 dimensions as well as a special x-ray of the upper thoracic outlet. In cases showing ischemic symptoms a complete visulatization of the arteries of the upper extremity including the digital arteries is mandatory.

We think in patients with a postthrombotic syndrome phlebography should show under abduction and elevation of the arm not only the compression of the recanalized subclavian vein but also a more or less complete compression of the collaterals.

RESULTS

The best results were achieved in the group with chronic venous compression. 39 out of 40 patients are completely symptom-free. 1 patient suffered from wound infection and later from scar problems.

In the group of 93 patients with an acute subclavian vein thrombosis 83 showed phlebogaphically long-term permeability but 89 were symptom-free. Only 3 patients suffered from severe postthrombotic syndrome. 1 patient with a phlegmasia cerulea dolens died from pulmonary embolism. There was no difference between patients treated primarily with thrombectomy and patients treated primarily with fibrinolysis.

The interpretation of the results in the last group - 44 patients with postthrombotic syndrome - is difficult because there is no. complete restitution possible. However, 14 patients became completely symptom-free, 26 showed a significant reduction of pain, swelling and heaviness and only 4 remained unchanged.

During the same period of time there was a small group of 34 patients treated with thrombectomy or fibrinolysis alone, because we could not document a venous compression by the second phlebography. In this group only 15 patients showed a patent subclavian vein at the follow-up examination 19 veins were reoccluded. We must conclude that at least in part of cases the causal compression due to unsatisfactory diagnostic techiques was not detected.

REFERENCES

1.   Bergan JJ, McCarthy WJ, Vogelzang R, Peck JJ. Thromboses veineuses axillo-sous-clavières. In: Kieffer, E. (ed): Les Syndromes de la Traversée Thoraco-Brachiale. AERCV, Paris 1989; 199.
2.   Dunant JH. Trauma als ätiologischer Faktor beim Schultergürtelsyndrom. Vasa 9, 74, 1980.
3.   Dunant JH. Thoracic outlet Syndrome: Treatment of vascular complications. Vasa 14 (1), 51, 1985.
4.   Eklof B. Thromboses veineuses axillo-sous-clavières. In: Kieffer, E. (ed): Les Syndromes de la Traversée Thoraco-Brachiale. AERCV, Paris 1989;189.
5.   Gruss JD, Bartels D, Kawai S, Karadedos C, Tsafandakis E, Straubel H, Ohta T. Das Thoracic outlet Syndrom. Angio 2, 77, 1980.
6.   Gruss JD, Bartels D, Karadedos C, Tsafandakis E, Straubel H, Ohta T. Unser Behandlungskonzept beim akuten Verschluß der Vena subclavia. Phlebol. u. Protokol 10, 25, 1981.
7.   Gruss JD, Vargas-Montano H, Bartels D, Simmenroth H, Haidar A. Results achieved in the surgical treatment of the thoracic outlet syndrome. Intern.Angiology 2, 179, 1984.
8.   Gruss JD, Kozuschek W. Der Schulterschmerz als Leitsymptom angiologischer Erkrankungen. In: Breitenfelder J und Yücel M (eds): Der Schulterschmerz. Georg Thieme Verlag, Stuttgart, New York, 1986; 63-68.
9.   Gruss JD, Hiemer W, Bartels D. Klinik, Diagnostik und Therapie des Thoracic outlet Syndroms. VASA 16, 337, 1987.
10.   Gruss JD. Thrombectomie veineuse axillo-sous-clavière. In: Kieffer E (ed): Les Syndromes de la Traversée Thoraco-Brachiale. AERCV, Paris 1989; 195.
11.   Gruss JD, Geissler C, Hiemer W. Zweiteingriffe bei Thoracic outlet Syndrom. Vortrag: International Vascular, Workshop XI 24.-31.3.1990, Obergurgl.
12.   Gruss JD, Geissler C. Aktueller Stand von Klinik, Diagnostik und Therapie der Kompressionssyndrome an der oberen Thoraxapertur (TOS). Vortrag 25. Jahrestagung der Österreichischen Gesellschaft für Gefäßchirurgie, 16.-18.9.1993, Wien.
13.   Gruss JD. Die chirurgische Behandllung des Thoracic outlet Syndroms. Vortrag 10. Jahrestagung der Deutschen Gesellschaft für Gefäßchirurgie, 11.-14.5.1994, Düsseldorf.
14.   Gruss JD, Geissler C. Venöse Komplikationen bei Kompressionssyndromen an der oberen Thoraxapertur. Vortrag 23. Jahrestagung der Deutschen Gesellschaft für Angiologie, 7.-9.9.1994, Dresden.
15.   Gruss JD. Zweiteingriffe bei Kompressionssyndromen an der oberen Thoraxapertur. In: Hepp W (ed): Neurovasculäre Kompressionsyndrome. Blackwell Wissenschaftsverlag Berlin (im Druck)
16.   Kieffer E. Les syndromes de la traversée thoraco-brachiale. Editions AERCV, 1989.
17.   Lindgren SHS, Ribbe EB, Norgren LEH. Two years following of patients operated on for Thoracic outlet Syndrome. Effect on sick-leave incidence. Eur. J. Vasc. Surg. 3; 411-413, 1989.
18.   Machleder HJ. Complications and Recurrences;. 205. In: Machleder HJ (ed): vascular disorders of the upper extremity. Futura Publishing Company Inc., New York, 1989.
19.   Mercier, C, Huguet JF, Piquet P. Syndrome de compression intermittente de la veine sous-clavière. In: Kieffer E (ed): Les Syndromes de la Traversée Thoraco-Brachiale. AERCV, Paris 1989; 183.

20.   Roos DB. Thoracic outlet syndrome;. 367. In: Najarian JS, Delany JD (eds): Vascular Surgery. Thieme, Stuttgart, 1978.

21.   Roos DB. Thoracic outlet syndromes; 91. In: Machleder HJ (ed). Vascular Disorders of the upper extremity. Futura Publishing Company Inc. New York, 1983.

22.   Roos DB. Recurrent thoracic outlet syndrome after first rib resection. Acta Chir. Belg. 79, 363, 1980.

23.   Roos DB. Thoracic outlet syndromes: Update 1987. Am. J. Surg. 154,568, 1987.

24.   Roos DB. Récidives postopératoires des syndromes de la traversée thoraco-brachiale; 317. In: Kieffer E (ed): Les syndromes de la travesée thoraco-brachiale. AERCV, Paris, 1989.

25.   Roos DB. Overview of Thoracic outlet syndromes. In: Machleder H (ed): Vascular Disorders of the upper extremity, Second Revised Edition, Futura Publishing Company Inc. Mount Kisco, NY, 1989; 155.

26.   Sanders RJ, Haug CE, and Pearce WH:. Recurrent thoracic outlet syndromes. J.Vasc.Surg. 4; 390-400, 1990.

27.   Schulze-Bergmann G. Das Paget-von Schrötter-Syndrom, Med. Welt 43: 1952-1956, 1975.

28.   Urschel HC, Razzuk MA, Albers JE. Reoperation for recurrent thoracic outlet syndrome. Ann.Thorac.Surg. 21.19.1976

Phlebology '95, D. Negus et al. (eds.). Phlebology (1995) Suppl. 1: 1015-1018

V/3.2

Phlébectomie Esthétique des Veines des Mains

J.M. Trauchessec[1] and R. Vergereau[2]

1 Dermatologiste à Paris, France
1 Angéiologue à Chamalieres-Royat, France

Cosmetic Phlebectomy of the Veins of the Hand

SUMMARY

The authors describe the technique of microphlebectomy applied to the veins of the dorsum of the hand.

PHLÉBECTOMIE ESTHÉTIQUE DES VEINES DES MAINS

J.M. TRAUCHESSEC[1], R. VERGEREAU[2]

[1] Dermatologiste à PARIS FRANCE
[2] Angéiologue à CHAMALIERES-ROYAT FRANCE

INTRODUCTION

Nos patientes nous demandent parfois une solution efficace et esthétique pour se débarasser définitivement des veines dilatées, disgracieuses qui apparaissent sur le dos des mains.

Cet outrage des ans n'avait trouvé jusqu'à présent aucune solution thérapeutique simple, reproductible.

Nous avons eu l'idée d'adapter la technique de l'exo-éveinage esthétique aux veines du dos des mains et nous apportons notre expérience qui nous semble être la solution de référence actuelle dans ce domaine.

ANATOMIE DES VEINES DU DOS DE LA MAIN

Le sang veineux des doigts est drainé par les veines digitales collatérales. Ces dernières apparaissent à la base de la première phalange se réunissant parfois sur le versant digital de l'articulation métacarpophalangienne en une arcade digitale (1).

La collatérale interne du cinquième doigt prend le nom de veine salvatelle :
elle circule le long de la face postérieure du muscle abducteur du petit doigt. La veine salvatelle se draine dans la veine cubitale superficielle au poignet. Elle reçoit fréquemment une veine perforante entre l'extrémité inférieure du cubitus et l'os pisiforme.

Les veines de drainage du pouce se collectent dans la veine céphalique du pouce, qui circule le long de l'axe du premier métacarpien en regard des tendons du long extenseur et du court extenseur du pouce. La veine céphalique du pouce se jette dans la veine radiale superficielle.

Les veines digitales, de manière directe ou par l'intermédiaire d'une arcade, se poursuivent en veines métacarpiennes.

Les veines métacarpiennes par des variétés courtes ou longues se jettent dans une arcade dorsale à l'extrémité inférieure, et à terminaison supérieure en dedans la veine cubitale superficielle, en dehors dans la veine radiale superficielle.

Il existe parfois des anastomoses diagonales entre veines radiales et veines cubitales.

Les veines perforantes reliant le système superficiel au système profond sont nombreuses, volontiers sur l'ensemble de la périphérie du dos de la main.

LA TECHNIQUE DE PHLÉBECTOMIE ESTHÉTIQUE

L'orifice cutané se réalise par perforation à l'aiguille, telle qu'elle a été décrite pour la première fois par R. Vergereau pour éviter l'incision. L'autre main du chirurgien pince et soulève la peau entre le pouce et l'index pour parer à une lésion des gaines du tendon extenseur sous-jacent. Un crochet affûté, introduit à travers l'orifice cutané, aggripe la veine souvent associée à des tissus fibreux, parfois sous croisée par des filets nerveux.

La connaissance précise de l'anatomie et l'expérience de l'esthétique dans la phlébecto-mie, permettent de maîtriser les difficultés liées à la topographie.

Les trousseaux collagènes inextensibles, mats, gris-marron, sont disséqués de l'adven-tice avec une pince fine, puis sectionnés.

Parfois, ils sont séparés et sectionnés simultanément par la lame du bistouri en cas d'individualisation à la simple traction.

Les filets nerveux sensitifs, fins, discrètement tractables, de teinte proche de l'ivoire, sont délicatement séparés dans l'adventice sans traumatisme.

L'exo-éveinage se poursuit sur le trajet veineux au moyen d'orifices cutanés partiqués à la demande en fonction de la laxité, de l'élasticité des tissus et des branches de bifurca-tion veineuse.

Les perforantes directes seront interrompues au ras des veines profondes, par torsion axiale sans nécessité de ligature ou par ligature-section.

DISCUSSION

1) L'exo-phlébectomie des veines du dos des mains était déjà mentionnée dans notre ouvrage de 1989 (2).

Les patientes que nous avons opérées nous ont gratifié d'un indice de satisfaction élevé, en rapport avec la forte motivation esthétique.

Les remarques les plus surprenantes tiennent au fait que les patientes pensaient ce geste techniquement impossible, le corps médical leur ayant jusqu'alors opposé de mul-tiples refus.

Les travaux d'un dermatologue et d'un angéiologue démontrent qu'actuellement l'exo-phlébectomie des veines du dos des mains a droit de cité dans le cadre de notre pratique de la chirurgie veineuse esthétique, en toute sécurité et innocuité (3).

2) Les autres traitementes sont grevés d'insuffisance ou de dangers

a) L'endo-phlébectomie des veines du dos des mains

Décrite par Fournier en 1987 (4), la méthode nécessite des instruments allongés supplé-mentaires introduits dans la lumière des veines. Ils augmentent le temps opératoire, ne peuvent pas suivre les bifurcations, et ignorent les perforantes.

b) La sclérose

Le liquide sclérosant fuit par les veines perforantes dans les veines profondes du dos de la main avec le danger de phlébite profonde du membre supérieur.

CONCLUSION

L'exo-éveinage esthétique est un procédé de choix dans l'ablation des veines du dos de la main sous couvert d'une connaissance précise de l'anatomie dermatologique et d'une dextérité confirmée dans la gestion de l'exo-phlébectomie.

BIBLIOGRAPHIE

1. Bouchet A., Cuilleret J. -"Anatomie" Tome 3. Editions Simep-Villeurbanne, 1985.
2. Trauchessec J.M. - In : "Dès Belles Jambes pour la Vie". Editions Encre - Paris, 1989.
3. Trauchessec J.M., Vergereau R. - Exo-éveinage esthétique des veines du dos de la main. Communication à la 9° Réunion de la Société Européenne de Phlébectomie, 1993, 38 à 54.
4. Fournier P.F. - "Historiques et techniques de rajeunissement ou d'embellissement des mains : Le Filling des mains". La revue de chirurgie esthétique de langue française, N° 47, Tome 12, 1987, 59-65.

Phlebology '95, D. Negus et al. (eds.). Phlebology (1995) Suppl. 1: 1019-1021

P277

Transaxillary First Rib Resection in Subclavian Vein Effort Thrombosis

M. Dlugaj, K. Ziaja, M. Blaszczynski, T. Drazkiewicz and M. Tochowicz

Department of General and Vascular Surgery, Silesian School of Medicine, Katowice, Poland

The pathogenesis of subclavian vein thrombosis (Paget-Schroetter syndrome) is unclear. It is suggested that thrombosis is caused by some sort of mechanical trauma, in spite of the absence of obvidious injury [2, 3, 4, 5].

The uncertainty of pathogenesis of this syndrome has produced various terms such as: primary, idiopathic, traumatic vein obstruction, or effort thrombosis [1, 8]. In these patients phlebography and Doppler sonography are diagnostic procedures of choice.

When there is venous occlusion, phlebograms should be obtained on both sides [6].

Some authors also argue that acute venous thrombosis should also be treated by early operation with management of the underlying anatomical abnormality and with thrombectomy [7].

This requires early diagnosis of the venous thrombosis and a high level of surgical skill and experience.

This series presents the operative results in 18 patients with subclavian effort vein thrombosis.

Patients and methods:

18 patients (12 males, 6 females) with subclavian vein effort thrombosis were treated operatively in our Clinic in years 1980-1993. There were clinical symptoms of thrombosis of subclavian vein and signs of thoracic outlet syndrome (signs of ischaemia, positive neurovascular tests, positive Doppler sonography examinations) in all patients. In all patients phlebography confirmed the presence of compression of the vein. At admission all patients suffered from pain, oedema, cyanosis, and dilated superficial veins of the extremity. There were also dilated veins in anterior surface of the chest.

5 patients were given streptokinase intravenously (100.000 u/h). The streptokinase was administered 48-72 h followed by heparin, and then by oral anticoagulants. Another 13 patiens were treated with heparin followed by oral anticoagulants.

After remission of acute signs diagnostic procedures to confirme the presence of thoracic outlet syndrome were performed.

After 14-21 days of conservative treatment patients were operated on. In all cases transaxillary 1-st rib resection was performed. There were no complication in the perioperative period, and there were no recurrence of thrombosis of subclavian vein durind follow-up (1-5 years).

In the early follow-up (up to one year there 90% good and very good results (criteria of Roos [7]), and in the late follow-up (1-5 years) there were 87% such results.

Conclusions:

- Subclavian vein effort thrombosis should be managed conservatively until anticoagulant therapy results in remission of acute clinical signs.

- Precise transaxillary 1-st rib resection with transsection of all fibrous tracts, cervical ribs, adhesions, etc. is the procedure of choice, irrespective of mechanism of compression of the vein.

References:

1.   Dale WA. Thoracic outlet compression syndrome.
     Critique in 1982
     Arch. Surg. 1982; 117:1437-45.
2.   Deskalakis E., Bouhoutsos J.
     Subclavian and axillary vein compression of musculoskeletal origin.
     Br. J. Surg. 1980;67:573-6.
3.   Gruss J.D., Bartels D., Karadedos C., Tsafandakis E., Straubel H., Ohta T.
     Unser Behandlundskonzept baim akuten Vorschlus der V subclavia.
     Phlebol. n. Proktol. 1981;10:25-32
4.   Hughes Esr: Collective review; Venous obstruction in the upper extremity (Paget - Schroetter's syndrome)
     Surg. Gynecol. Obstet (Suppl):89, 1949
5.   Riddel D. H.
     Thoracic and vascular aspect of thoracic outlet syndrome 1986 up date
     Clin. Orthop. 1986; 31-36.
6.   Ruckley C.V.
     Thoracic outlet syndrome.
     Br. J. Surg. 1983;287:447-8.
7.   Roos D. B.
     Transaxillary approach for first rib resection to relieve thoracic outlet syndrome.
     Ann. Surg. 1966;163:354-8
8.   Schubart P. J.
     Intermitted subclavian venous obstruction: utility of venous pressure gradients.
     Surgery, 1986, 365-8.

Phlebology '95, D. Negus et al. (eds.). Phlebology (1995) Suppl. 1: 1022-1024

P016

Archicture Types of the Superficial Forearm Veins

R. Jasinski[1] and M. Wozniewski[2]

[1] Departmentof Anatomy and [2] Department of Rehabilitation, Academy of Physical Education Wroclaw, Poland

INTRODUCTION

Superficial veins of the the upper limb drainage the blood by the cephalic vein and basilic vein from the skin and connective tissue. Deep veins drainage the blood from the subfascial area of the extremities. Both of these systems can complete and substitute for owing to their anastomosis (1). However the connections between the cephalic vein and basilic vein are hereditary, but they can be different. It depends on the intensity of the blood circulation (3). If the blood circulation is increased then the connection between the veins is different than the circulation is decreased. Intensity of the blood circulation increases during the physical activity. Evaluation of the connection types of the forearm veins is very important in surgery and physiotherapy.

METHODS

250 women (age from 18 to 25) were examined. 45.2 per cent of the women practised sport (increase of the physical activity).

The upper limb was compressed at the arm level and the superficial veins of the forearm were observed. M, N, Y types of the veins connections were estimated and types I for the others connections.

RESULTS

Y type of the connection between the basilic vein and cephalic vein was observed in 55.0 per cent of the women, M type in 35.0 per cent and N type in 10.0 per cent. Y type was the most frequent connection of the vein on the right forearm (60.0 per cent) , and M type on the left forearm (40.0 per cent).

Y type of the veins connections was observed the most often in the women who practised sport (76.8 per cent on the right forearm and 69.6 per cent on the left forearm). The women who did not practise sport had the most often M type of the veins connections (58.8 per cent on the both of the forearms).

DISCUSSION

Superficial veins of the upper limbs are often used in the artery occlusions operations, particularly when the legs veins are incompetent. Venous system is very important in the development of the lymphedema too. Increase of the venous pressure in the extremity results in the pressure increase in the lymphatics leading to the hemodynamic insufficiency of the lymph flow. Efficacy of the blood drainage from the extremity depends on the veins connections.

The blood circulation is increased in the physical activity and the drainage of the blood should be greater. Then the venous system must be more efficacious. Y type of the connection between the basilic vein and cephalic vein is the best connection for the drainage of the blood. Main blood stream flows by the cephalic vein which is localized more medial then usually, the medial basilic vein and the basilic vein (1, 2, 3).

Y type of the veins connections was observed the most often in the women practising sport and on the right forearm. Physical activity leads to the development of the veins connections which drainage the blood from the upper limb better than in the women who did not practise sport. It concerns the right forearm which is used more often than the left forearm too.

CONCLUSIONS

1. Y type of the connection between the basilic vein and the cephalic vein was stated the most frequent.
2. Y type, which is the best of the vein connection for the drainage of the blood was observed the most often in the women who practised sport and on the right forearm.
3. The simple examination of the vein connection types can be useful in the selection of the superficial forearm veins in the artery occlusions operations and in the physiotherapy of the patients with the lymphedema.

REFERENCES

1. Bochenek A., Reicher M., Human anatomy (in Polish). PZWL Warszawa 1993.
2. Gościcka D., Flisiński P., Superficial veins of the elbow region in the rural children (in Polish). Antrop. Rev. 1992 ; 55 : 119-23.
3. Masłowski Z., Examination of the basilic vein variation in human (in Polish) . Ann. of Medical Academy , Szczecin 1967 ; 13

Phlebology '95, D. Negus et al. (eds.). Phlebology (1995) Suppl. 1: 1025-1027

P268

A Study to Differ Oedematous Swellings in the Upper Extremities

Prof Prof h c mult Dr med Dr hc N. Klüken and Dr med A. Falk

Ladenspelderstrasse 46, 45147 Essen, Germany

The intention of this study was stimulated by an increasing number of patients, suffering from oedematous swellings in the upper extremities. In this case, it is necessary to differ between venous or lymphatic flow impairment. This differentiation is possible with the assistance of invasive methods, for example phlebography or isotope lymphography. But we wanted to examine a method that is more carefully for the patients, consequently a non invasive method. Such a method may be a variant of the photoplethysmography, like the light reflection rheography. Does this method achieve such a differentiation of oedematous swellings in upper extremities?

In this study it is necessary to stress the particularity of the venous system in the upper extremities. In contrast to the legs, in the venous system and the circulation of the upper extremities it is not possible to differ a superficial from a deep venous system. Therefore it is necessary to change the method of examination. Moreover it is important to note the peculiarities of the lymphatic and the venous system and the anatomic stenose on the crossing of the clavicle by the vena subclavia.

The measuring method in our study, as I mentioned, was the light reflection rheography, published by Wienert and Blazek. Infrared radiation from three points are given vertical in the skin. The reflected rays are measured with a Siliciumphototransistor and plotted with a printer. With this method the reflected rays in the skin within a deep of zero point three to two point three mm are registered. These reflections depend on the filling of blood in the cutaneous small vessels. In this kind of measurement the filling of blood is not only registered in the venous, but in the arterial vessels of the skin, too.

Because this blood volume in the microcirculation is always constant. During this measurement it is important that the temperature of the room does not change. It is controlled by continual measurement of the room's and skin's temperature.

We had made some examinations in different places of the arm, because the best locality for measurements is in the upper extremities. The best localisation was given in the outside of the upper arm of the patient.

First the patient is requested to let down his arm in relaxation. After a time, the arm of the patient is moved in a vertical position. In this position the cutaneous venous complexus leak out. The time from the beginning of the venous leak out to the end of the registration is called venous outflow time t_a if the curve notifies a plateau.

By contemporaneous registration of the venous pressure and the time of the venous outflow it was possible to verify this behaviour.

Kind of Vascular Disturbances	Mean Value	Standard Deviation
Controls	8.1 sec	2.8 sec
Lymphostatic oedema of the arm	13.3 sec	4.5 sec
Acute axillary veinstasis	30.1 sec	11.7 sec
Chronic axillary veinstasis	16.1 sec	11.2 sec

In our following research it was assumed that most of the patients with chronic axillary veinstasis in small partial recanalisation and in different well-marked formations of collateralisation of venous vessels among conditions of immovability have normal time of venous outflow. The reason for this is seen in bigger load of venous blood volume. This bigger volume of blood is caused by hindrance in venous vascular system, which causes a retardation of the outflow.

The measurements of the time of venous outflow in condition of rest and under load were carried out in 15 patients, who suffered from chronic axillary veinstasis, and 10 patients who suffered from lymphostatic oedema of the arm. These results were compared with 47 measurements at arm with normal blood flow in vein. 15 patients with chronic axillary veinstasis, 5 male, 10 female, with an average age of 43.8 years, were examined as described. 10 patients suffered from axillary veinstasis and chronic lymphatic oedema.

The venous outflow t_{90} amounted in condition of rest, average value in probands to 6.72 sec, in standard deviation of 3.94 sec, during passive load of 60 mm mercury back-pressure for 3 minutes the observed value increased to 15.62 sec, in standard deviation of 5.79 sec.

In patients, who suffered from lymphostatic oedema, we measured a venous outflow in condition of rest of 8.1 sec in average value, in standard deviation of 4.43 sec. During passive load of 60 mm mercury back pressure for 3 minutes the observed value increased to 16.95 sec, in standard deviation of 7.9 sec.

Patients, who suffered from chronic venous stasis, had an outflow at rest of 19.93 sec, with a standard deviation of 11.54 sec. with a passive load of 60 mm mercury back pressure for 3 minutes, the venous outflow increased to 20.03 sec, in standard deviation of 10.73 sec.

Our results were as follows:

In the controls it's to find out an unequal increase of the venous outflow-time under load, as one can see statistically. The central- (or median-) value was for controls in condition of rest 5 sec and under load of 60 mm mercury back pressure for 3 minutes 15.5 sec, in lymphostatic oedema 7.25 sec, under load 16.5 sec, in chronic axillary veinstasis 12.25 sec, under load of 60 mm mercury back pressure for 3 minutes 7.25 sec.

Our researches result using the light reflection-rheography without and with load in 231 measurements in controls, 50 in patients with lymphostatic oedema and 79 in patients with chronic axillary veinstasis are the following:

In patients with lymphostatic oedema of the arm we found nearly the same venous outflow as in controls.

In patients with chronic axillary veinstasis were measured without and with load significant longer times as from persons or both other groups.

P276

EXPERIENCE OF TREATMENT PRIMARY SUBCLAVIAN VEIN THROMBOSIS.

Saveliev V., Kirienko A., Leontiev S.

Research Vascular Laboratory State Russian Medical University, Moscow, Russia

OBJECTIVE: To develop complex and effective method of the primary subclavian vein thrombosis treatment.
DESIGN: Retrospective review of consecutive series.
PATIENTS: 26 patients with acute primary subclavian vein thrombosis(PSVT).
INTERVENTION: Local thrombolytic therapy by streptaze (100.000 units/hour) was conducted during 3-5 days. In 8 cases were used catheter aspiration thrombectomy before thrombolysis. Ballon angioplasty of tight stenosis in typical subclavian vein segment was applied in 8 cases in addition.
MEASUREMENTS: Dynamic DS-phlebography, Duplex-scanning and radionuclide phlebog-raphy were applied in 1-5 days, in 1,6,12 months after intervention.
RESULTS: 12 patients had wide patency of subclavian vein. We had three cases of rethrombosis in early period and two one after 2 and 18 months.
CONCLUSION: Complex endovascular interven-tion is effective method of desobstruction in patients with PSVT.

P278

INTERMITTENT OEDEMA:AN ALARM FOR UPPER EXTREMITIES' MAJOR VEIN THROMBOSIS

Rigopoulos J.,Thalassinos N.,Kouremenos G. Tsipas C. Rouskas A.

Department of Vascular Surgery,1st IKA Hospital Athens,Greece

Objective:Evaluation of the role of intermittent oedema in the subclavian or axillary vein throm-bosis.
Design:Retrospective review of cases with upper extremities'major vein thrombosis and intermit-tent oedema.
Patients:33 patients with upper extremities' ma-jor vein thrombosis and 20 with intermittent oe-dema.
Measurements:All patients were examined by color duplex scan and patients with intermittent oede-ma were also examined by descending phlebography
Results:In 15 patients with intermittent oedema, phlebography showed compression of the subclavi-an vein in the outlet area.14 patients with thrombosis reported intermittent oedema as first symptom.
Conclusions:In intermittent oedema,the compres-sion of the vein in the thoracic outlet area, predisposes in thrombosis of the subclavian or axillary vein and action must be taken to pre-vent this complication.

P279

IS ARM VENOUS INSUFFICIENCY PROVABLE ?

I.O. Rada, F.C. Rada, V. Santimbreanu, Domnita Rada
Timisoara Medical and Pharmaceutical University,
str.Siret no.6, 1900 Timisoara, Romania

Post-thrombotic syndrome (PTS) of the superior limb is controversial. Secondary development of edema after phlebitic processes represents the major syndrome of PTS.

We have studied 41 patients (31-64 years old, 31 female, 9 male) with superior limb PTS. These patients presented one common symptom: edema in the superior limb, whose volume increased towards the end of the day and which, in 37 of our patients, also involved the shoulder. 17 patients had a previous history of lymph-nodes ablation in the past several years, while 14 had a history of post-surgical radiotherapy. In these cases (with shoulder-axillar obstruction and ample collateral circulation on the phlebography) the cause of lymphedema might be the post-surgical or post-radio-therapy axillar fibrosis.

In none of the 41 cases haven't we met trophic disturbances of the forearm or trophic skin alterations - which represent an almost permanent complication in the similar conditions of the calves. In all the cases with upper limb PTS thrombosis occurred at the subclavii-axillar (superior humeral) level, on vessels with an integrum valvular system of the forearm and inferior half of the arm. Such phlebo-graphical aspects could explain atypical, incomplete symptoms of PTS in the upper limb. Shoulder edema is a characteristic clinical sign, differentiating between venous and lymphatic edema of the superior limb. We support the hypothesis that axillar vein thrombosis starts in one of its affluents, wherefrom it extends afterwards to the principal axillar axle.

Gynaecology, Hormones and Pelvic Disorders

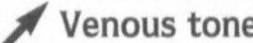
Venous tone

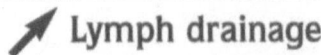
Lymph drainage

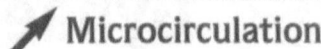
Microcirculation

daflon 500mg

Micronized, purified flavonoidic fraction

micronized

Presentation and composition: Box of 30 coated tablets. Micronized flavonoidic fraction 500 mg: diosmin 450 mg; hesperidin 50 mg. **Therapeutic properties:** Vascular protector and venotonic. Daflon 500 mg acts on the return vascular system: it reduces venous distensibility and venous stasis; in the microcirculation, it normalizes capillary permeability and reinforces capillary resistance. **Therapeutic indications:** Treatment of organic and idiopathic chronic venous insufficiency of the lower limbs with the following symptoms: heavy legs; pain; nocturnal cramps. Treatment of hemorrhoids and acute hemorrhoidal attacks. **Side effects:** Some cases of minor gastrointestinal and autonomic disorders have been reported, but these never required cessation of treatment. **Drug interactions:** None. **Precautions:** *Pregnancy:* experimental studies in animals have not demonstrated any teratogenic effects and no harmful effects have been reported in man to date. *Lactation:* in the absence of data concerning the diffusion into breast milk, breast-feeding is not recommended during treatment. **Contraindications:** None. **Dosage and administration:** *In venous disease:* 2 tablets daily. *In acute hemorrhoidal attacks:* the dosage can be increased to up to 6 tablets daily. *Refer to data sheet for complete prescribing information.* **Les Laboratoires Servier** - 45520 Gidy France. Correspondent: **Servier International** 6, Place des Pléiades - 92415 Courbevoie Cedex France.

✦ SERVIER

A *decisive therapeutic benefit* for patients with:

Chronic venous insufficiency:

2 tablets daily

Acute hemorrhoidal attacks:

up to 6 tablets daily

Phlebology '95, D. Negus et al. (eds.). Phlebology (1995) Suppl. 1: 1033-1035

V/1.10

Pelvic Varices: Evaluation by Duplex Ultrasonography - Pelvic Phlebography and Surgery: Case Report

E. Burihan[1], S. Ikeda[1], J.C.C. Baptista-Silva[1], J. Francisco Jr[1] and V. Freitas[2]

[1] *Division of Vascular Surgery, Department of Surgery* [2] *Division of Gynecology, Department of Tocogynecology, Escola Paulista de Medicina, Universidade Federal de São Paulo, São Paulo, Brazil*

INTRODUCTION

Pelvic congestion or pelvic pain syndrome is a common gynaecological symptom which presents a difficult diagnostic and treatment [1,2]. Since the last century pelvic varices are studied as a cause of genesis of chronic pelvic pain syndrome(CPPS). Recent studies have shown that pelvic varices are a common finding in women with CPPS [3].

The clinical features of CPPS include pelvic pain of variable intensity which is exacerbated by postural changes and walking. Congestive dysmenorrhea, dyspareunia, post-coital ache and urinary symptoms are common features of CPPS. This condition affects women of reproductive age; it is more common in the multiparous patient, without evidence of pelvic inflammation or other obvious pathology. The use of non-invasive method propedeutics as ultrasound techniques include colour Doppler imaging, utilizing specific anatomical windows or transvaginal approach increased the diagnostic of this affection [2].

Pelvic pain is the commonest reason for laparoscopy in the United Kingdom, but in 75% of cases, no cause is found[3]. Various imaging modalities have been employed in the diagnostic of this condition, but only selective ovarian venography provides the most anatomical information. Although an association between pelvic varices and CPPS has been known for many years[4], uncertainty regarding its etiology has resulted in different therapeutic approaches, producing variable results[2].

CASE REPORT

A 29-year-old woman was referred with a 2 year history of chronic pelvic pain principally with congestive dysmenorrehea and urinary symptoms. Her symptoms were aggravated by prolonged standing, were worse during menstruation and pos-coital ache.

She was pregnant twice, one was born by cesarean operation and the other was aborted.

During the gynecological examinations no alterations were encountered.Color Doppler fluxometry of this case showed enlargement of pelvic veins and increased venous flow.

The phlebography showed retrograde blood flow back by enlarged the left and right ovarian, and the right hypogastric veins.

The treatment in this patient was ligation of left and right ovarian and right hipogastric veins by surgical approach. During operation was noted transposition of inferior cava vein to left side. Five months later she remained asymptomatic.

DISCUSSION

In 1857, Reichet described for first time the pelvic varices, calling it tubo-ovarian varicocele [1].

Lefévre [5] suggested that the pelvic varices observed in multiparaous women were decorrent of dilated veins during the pregnancy which not did retrograde after the delivery. Giacheto et al [6] realized the phlebography of the ovarian and iliac vein in women with CPPS, observed that patients with retrograde blood flow back by large the left and right ovarian veins showing age and number of pregnants significantly increased in relation to normal women. It has been suggested recently that the primary problem is that of venous reflux in incompetent, dilated ovarian veins [1,7,8]. Anatomical studies have shown that ovarian venous valves are absent in 15% of women on the left side and 6% on the right [9]. Valvular incompetence is common and may occur on either side, in 35-43% [10]. Besides valvular incompetence, alterations primary of the venous wall and arteriovenous malformation are causes of the pelvic varices [11]. During pregnancy the capacity of ovarian veins may increase by 60 times and these changes may persist up to 6 month after delivery [12]. This may explain why CPPS is more common in multiparous women [2]. Vulval varices and atypical varicosities of the thigh or buttock may be part of the clinical presentation and are caused by reflux from the dilated pelvic veins [8]. These varices appear in the vulva and labia on inner side and of the thigh. These veins arise predominantly from the internal pudenda and obturator veins, which are tributaries of the internal iliac vein, and it may spreading down the back of the thigh and giving to rise to large veins in the popliteal area [13]. The left renal vein may be compressed between the superior mesenteric artery and the aorta (the nutcracker syndrome) and as result in a common problem as varicocele in men and ovarian vein syndrome in women[14].

The gynecological examination in general is not conclusive, but may be encountered vulval varices and pain during adnexal palpation [3]. The phlebography was considered the principal method of diagnosis of the pelvic varices, but it is invasive and may present risks. A ultrasound examination is a good method to demonstrate pelvic varices, but it is important that it is realized in erect position and Valsalva maneuver to show the filling of pelvic veins, because in a position that favours venous drainage from the pelvis and the degree of pelvic congestion is therefore underestimated [2,6]. The laparoscopy may demonstrate congestive pelvic state and venous ectasia [1], it may be used to ligate the dilated ovarian veins. Edwards [2] realized a transcatheter embolization in one case with good result. The surgical ligation and resection on the dilated ovarian veins has been performed in small series of patients. This appears to be a relatively simple, safe procedure which provides an effective cure for CPPS [1,7,8].

The hysterectomy and ooforectomy bilateral should be used only in case that the results above were not good, because these women are young and in reproductive age [3].

Finally in this case we realized the ligature of the right hypogastric and ovarian bilateral veins improved the CPPS symptoms.

REFERENCES

1. Hobbs JT. The pelvic congestion syndrome. Br J Hospital Med 1990;43:200-6.
2. Edwards RD, Robertson AB, MacLean AB, Hemigway AP. Case report: pelvic pain syndrome - successful treatment of a case by ovarian vein embolization. Clin Radiol 1993;47:429-31.
3. Beard RW, Kenndy RG, Gangar KF, Stones RW, Rogers V, Reginald PW, Anderson M. Bilateral oophorectomy and hysterectomy in treatment of intractable pelvic pain associated with pelvic congestion. Br Obstet Gynecol 1991;98:988-92.
4. Topolanski-Sierra R. Pelvic phlebography. Am J Obstet Gynecol 1958;76:44-5.
5. Lefréve H. Broad ligament varicocele. Acta Obstet Scand 1964;43:122-3.
6. Giacchetto C, Cotroneo GB, Marincolo F, Camisulu F, Caruso G, Catizone F. Ovarian Varicocele: ultrasound and plebographic evaluation. J Clin Ultrasound 1990;18:551-5.
7. Lechter A. Pelvic Varices: treatment. J Cardiovasc Surg 1985;26:111.
8. Lechter A, Alvarez A. Pelvic Varices and gonadal veins. In: Negus D, Janet G, editors. Phlebology '85. London: John Lbbey, 1986;225-8.
9. Ahlberg NE, Bartley O, Chidekel N. Circumference of the left gonadal vein. An Anatomical and statistical study. Acta Radiol 1965;3:503-12.
10. Ahlberg NE, Bartley O, Chidekel N. Right and left gonadal veins. An Anatomical and statistical study. Acta Radiol 1966;4:593-601.
11. Goren G, Yellin AE. Primary varicose veins; and hemodynamic correlations. J Cardiovasc Surg 1990;31:672-7.
12. Hodgkinson CP. Physiology of the ovarian veins during pregnancy. Obstet Gynecol 1953;1:26-37.
13. Dodd H, Cockett FB. Varicose veins in pregnancy. In: Dodd H, Cockett FB, editors. The pathology and surgery of the veins of the lower limb. Edinburgh: Churchill Livingstone, 1976:155-9.
14. Barnes RW, Fleisher HL, Redman JF, Smith JW, Harshfield DL, Ferris EJ. The nutcracker syndrome. J Vasc Surg 1988;8:415-21.

Phlebology '95, D. Negus et al. (eds.). Phlebology (1995) Suppl. 1: 1036-1038

P285

Role of Hormonal Therapy and Pregnancy on the Varicose Vein Recurrence After Stripping of the Long Saphenous Vein: Study on 630 Women

S. Sadoun[1], C. Garde[2], A. Cornu-Thénard[3] and P. Danel[4]

[1] 10 Rue Benjamin Moloïse, 94000 CRETEIL, [2] Hôpital Tenon, 4 Rue de la Chine, 75020 PARIS, [3] Hôpital St Antoine, 184 Rue du Fbg St Antoine, 75575 PARIS Cedex 12, [4] Avenue de la Redoute, 92600 ASNIERES SUR SEINE

INTRODUCTION

The treatments correctly suggested for varicose veins try to treat the lesions and to master the evolution of the disease.

The natural history of the disease may accelerate in numerous circumstances (puberty, peri-menstrual period, pregnancy, menopause, contraceptive pills, substitutive treatments), where modification of absolute and relative levels of oestrogens and of progesterone are encountered.

MATERIALS AND METHODS

This survey has compared a group of factors in patients who had stripping with ligation of the long saphenous vein 1 to 10 years previously.

The investigators have studied all the patients coming to their office during 2 randomised days each month.

The existence of one or more varicose vein(s), originating from the superior third of the antero-medial aspect of the thigh of the operated side, combined with reflux of more than 1 second by continuous wave Doppler defined a recurrence.

The data have been collected by questioning the patients, from the charts and at clinical examination.

Statistical analysis has compared the Recurrent (R) and Non Recurrent (NR) groups for the variables related to the period before and after surgical treatment.

RESULTS:

Between March 1992 and 1993, 47 angiologists included 741 patients, totalling 1142 operated lower limbs: 585 right limbs and 557 left limbs: the complete results have been published elsewhere. The patients are 15% men and 85% (630) women (p=0.45), the relative percentage of recurrence in the 2 genders is comparable. The annual recurrence rate since stripping is between 20 and 40%.

Before the stripping:
By comparison to NR, the R have an elevated weight and Body Mass Index (Weight in Kg/(Height in meters)^2), flat feet, stand more often and practice less sporting activities.

The average number of pregnancies is comparable in the 2 groups. There is no correlation between the weight before stripping and the number of pregnancies.

The recurrence rate for each 10-year-old-age-group (<30; 30-40: 40-50,...) is not different for those of more than 30 years, who total 15% of the total pregnancies whereas patients of less than 30 years have only 2.7%.

Perineal veins (PVV) are more often present before stripping on the same side of the surgery (p=0.003) on the R. PVV are associated with the pregnancies before stripping (p=0.013).

More than 75% of the patients older than 31 years do not receive any hormonal treatment (the results are the inverse for those younger than 30 years).

Patients who received hormonal treatment (HT) before stripping are more often R; but this concerns patients older than 51 years (p<0.015). The mean age of R patients receiving oestro-progestative (ROP) (40.7±9.6) is different from the age of those without HT (45.2± 10.9) (p< 0.05). The mean age of RP is of 40± 7 versus 48.9±8.2 for the NRP (p<0.05), however the RP number only 4, and this result has to be regarded cautiously.

The mean age of patients not taking any treatment is 51.3 ± 11.2 for the R and 49.4± 10.3 for the NR (p<0.05). For the patients of less than 45 years, there is no relation between HT and the absence of pregnancy (p=0.5).

Period after the LSV stripping:

Post surgical compression was prescribed for more than one month more often to R (67%) than to NR (82%) (p<0.001). The R have a higher weight and BMI, stand more often and practice less sport activities than the NR. Pregnancies before stripping are not responsible for the rise in weight after stripping (p>0.05). The average number of pregnancies is 0.2± 0.7 for the R and 0.05 ± 0.3 for the NR (p=0.001).

Hormonal treatment is comparable between R and NR: more than 75% of patient do not receive any treatment, 18% receives an Estro-Progestative Hormonal Treatment (OPHT), and 7% a Progestative one (PHT). The patients having had their first pregnancy after stripping are more R (p=0.078), but this concerns only 2 patients.

Ipsi or controlateral PVV to the stripping are associated with recurrence no matter which side was the stripping performed (p<0.001).

Study of the evolution of factors before and after the stripping:

11% of R had a weight which increases (more than 10%) against 6.5% for NR (p=0.03). There is a correlation between pregnancies before the stripping and perineal veins after the stripping (p=0.005). There is a correlation between pregnancies after stripping and perineal varicose veins after stripping (p<0.05).

Among the whole group there is no correlation between HT after stripping and a recurrence. The recurrence rate shows a tendency to a difference for patients having the same hormonal treatment before and after (no, OP or P), however, detailed study of the treatment given to each patient shows that:
- the patients having received a OPHT before and P after, a treatment P before and P after, a treatment P before and nothing after, are less often R.
- the patients having received a OPHT before and nothing after, nothing before and a OPHT after, are more often R (p=0.03).

Patients older than 61 years with HT neither before nor after, are more often R (p=0.047).

DISCUSSION

Recurrence seems ineluctable in the normal evolution of the illness for about 40% of the patients, there is no correlation between the recurrence rate and the elapsed time since the stripping.

In international literature, we find a recurrence rate of 0.66% to 45%.

The sex ratio men: women of 1.5 is the same as for functional pathology; usually the sex ratio concerning the varicose veins is less balanced.

Flat feet, standing position , particularly stamping, no sport activities, are known risk factors for venous disease and now we may add recurrence. The number of pregnancies before stripping doesn't have any influence on the recurrence, even though we know the responsibility of the pregnancies in the development of varicose veins; on the other hand, a pregnancy after stripping is associated with R.

In our study, we find the classical association between perineal varicose veins (VP) and pregnancies, the association of PVV and surgical varicose vein of the long saphenous vein (LSV), at the same side before and on either side after.

An international study in 1972 has shown the aggravating role of HT on the venous system. Recent work demonstrated that the intensity of functional signs are significantly lower with the low dose pills (mono, bi or tri-phasic) by comparison to normo-dosed monophasic pills (containing 50g of oestrogen and 500 mg of Progesterone).

Many works showed the responsibility of high doses Ethinyloestradiol, in thrombo-embolic arterial accidents and of high doses of progesterone in accidents of venous origin.

In our study, patients younger than 30 years, taking contraception are less R and this may be because pregnancy will occur in fewer of these patients.

CONCLUSION

Varicose recurrence is multifactorial and its preventive treatment is yet to be found. The initiation of comparative prospective studies over several years will be the only means of testing new treatments for varicose veins. The protocols will have to stratify according to these preliminary results. For the moment, only phlebological follow-up, is available for patients to help then live with their disease and to avoid complications.

Phlebology '95, D. Negus et al. (eds.). Phlebology (1995) Suppl. 1: 1039-1041

OP/13.2

Varices of Pelvic Origin Reappraisal of a Clinical, Radiological and Surgical Condition

A. Lechter, C.A. Franco, G. Bayona, L.G. Cadavid and D.A. Rojas

Service of Vascular Surgery and Angiology, Hospital Militar Central, Bogota D.C., Colombia, South America

INTRODUCTION

In the past, vulvar and pelvic types of varicose veins were poorly understood; hence their treatment was not rational. With the advent of vascular radiology, ascending and descending phlebography of pelvic and gonadal veins became possible. In 1.954, with publication of the classic work by Guilhem and Baux, exploration and invasion of this veins began.

From 1.965 through 1.968, reports from Ahlberg, Bartley and Chidekel of Scandinavia furnished substantial information about exploration of gonadal veins from above in a downward direction.

On September 14, 1.984, we performed the first operation of bilateral gonadal vein resection.

The evolution of concept of pelvic varices include:

1- Segmental pelvic varices without direct connection to the saphenous vein were commonly noted.

2- High-pressure escape points from the pelvis into the vulva, labia and upper thigh, constituting a true pelvic varicocele, were suspected, and positive diagnostic phlebography of gonadal veins confirmed the clinical impression.

3- Excellent surgical results obtained by bilateral resection of gonadal veins and ligation of communications to uterine veins, followed by varicectomy with sparing of the saphenous system, further confirmed the non-saphenous cause of pelvic varices.

The concept of high-back pressure as the cause of varicose veins in the legs was proposed by Trendelenburg in the first decade of the twentieth century and by Dodd and Cockett in the 1.940s, relating their work to the sapheno-femoral junction and perforating veins in the leg, respectively. There are, however, varicose veins in the leg that cannot be explanied by back pressure. The purpose of this study is to present our findings, collected during a 10 year period, of these patients in which we have been studying and operating, who had high-pressure scape points located in pelvic and abdominal veins.

1040

METHODS

A prospective and descriptive study realized between September 1984 and September 1994.
The inclusion criteria were:
1. Women with varicosities in the vulvar and pelvic area that consult to the service of vascular surgery and angiology
2. Gonadal insufficiency confirmed with invasive phlebography.

SURGICAL TREATMENT
Gonadal veins are exposed through a curved, almost transverse 6 cms incision located anterior and medial to the iliac spine . Extensive muscle splitting exposed the retroperitoneal space . The gonadal vein is usually attached to the peritoneal fat. Because the gonadal vein is large and fragile, it is dissected carefully for a few centimeters, ligated and divided . The ovarian veins is handled with utmost care through the use of atraumatic vascular forceps and ligatures are passed around and securely tightened above and below the dissected gonadal vein . A carefully search for other gonadal veins is performed since at this level the ovarian vein may be double or triple. As dissection progresses downward , the gonadal veins opens, in an umbrella-like fashion, in the front of the ovary. Instead, en bloc dissection and ligature are performed at this level. The second part of the operation consists of varicectomy of the vulvar veins and removal of leg veins through small transverse incisions done with the hemostatic technique or phlebectomy.

RESULTS

A total of 400 patients presented for treatment .All were women aged 31 to 49, with a mean age of 40 . All patients had multiple full-term pregnancies (2 to 14) , with and average of four deliveries. Their symptoms included pain and often incapacitating heaviness in the thighs and legs. Premenstrual and menstrual pelvic, vulvar and thigh pain also were present . No trophic changes were observed.Vulvar varices were present in 280 of the 400 patients. Varicose veins began at the root of the thigh at the union of the external border of the labia and the inner area of the thigh . The course of the varices did not follow the saphenous system. Tipically , it crossed the posterior or anterior area of the thigh to the lateral leg , foot and popliteal fossa. These very superficial veins were usually deep blue or violaceous. They were fragile, prone to ecchymosis and hematomas and difficult to surgical removal.

Both gonadal veins were studied in 332 of the 400 patients. The left gonadal vein was almost always catheterized . With more experience the orifice of the right gonadal vein in the vena cava was catheterized in 80% of the attempts. The classical pattern of junction of the gonadal veins to the left renal vein and vena cava was found in only 78% of the cases. The remaining cases were anatomic variations that may explain some failures in gonadal phlebography.

Bilateral gonadal vein ligation was performed in 382 patients (95.5%). Unilateral ligations were done in the remaining patients (12 right and 6 left). Of 64 patients (16%) with saphenous insufficiency , 40 patients(10%) had unilateral and 24 patients(6%) had bilateral .The operation was always completed by treating both conditions , pelvic and saphenous . Among 40 patients (10%) one or more pregnancies followed this surgery.

Complementary scleroterapy should be performed on small veins for cosmetic reasons. Most patients (90%) request this additional procedure. Of the 400 patients, 344 (86%) showed excellent results and 40 (10%) had good results. A total of 384 (96%) had very satisfactory outcomes. Ten patients had fair outcomes and two patients showed no improvement even though gonadal veins were ligated (both unilateral) and varicose veins were removed .

REFERENCES

1. Guilhem P, Baux R, La Phlebographic Pelvienne par Voies Veineuse, Osseuse et Uterine, Paris: Masson et Cie, 1.954
2. Ahlberg EN, Bartley O, Chidekel N. Right and left gonadal veins: An anatomical and statistical study. Acta Radiol 4: 593-601, 1.966
3. Ahlberg EN, Bartley O, Chidekel N. Retrograde contrast filling of the left gonadal vein. A Roetgenologic and Anatomical study. Acta Radiol 3: 385, 1.965
4. Lechter A, Pelvic Varices: Treatment. J Cardiovasc Surg. 26: 111. 1.985
5. Lechter A, Alvarez A. Pelvic varices and gonadal veins. In Negus D, Jantet G, eds. Phlebology, 1.985. London, libbey, 1.986 pp 225-228.
6. Lechter A, Alvarez A, Lopez G. Pelvic varices and gonadal veins. Phlebology 2: 181-188, 1.987
7. Lechter A, Lopez G, Martinez C, Camacho J. Anatomy of the gonadal veins: A reappraisal. Surgery 109: 735-739, 1.991
8. Hobbs JT. Treatment of vulvar and pelvic varices. In Bergan JJ, Yao JST, eds. Venous disorders. Philadelphia: WB Saunders, 1.991, pp 250-257.

Phlebology '95, D. Negus et al. (eds.). Phlebology (1995) Suppl. 1: 1042-1044

OP/13.5

Male Sexual Venous Dysfunction

A. Diaz[1] and K. Diaz[2]

Instituto de Angiologia, Cirugia Vascular e Impotencia Sexual, Av de la Republica
770 y Eloy Alfaro, Quito, Ecuador

INTRODUCTION

Male sexual dysfunction,also called some years ago as sexual impotence,is divided into:erection,eyaculation,desire and sensitive dysfunctions,these 4 types of male dysfunction recognize two main causes:Psycological Primary and organic.
  Among organic causes there are neurological,endocrinologi-cal,traumatic and vascular factors.Actually,we know highest average of male sexual dysfunction, is caused by vascular problems: arterial,venous and micro capillar.
  The not well known venous outflow,has been the first and major cause for venous origin male sexual dysfunction. On the past years it was beleived that problem was due to a loss on venous tone and valves system failure;but this concept has been changed,because it was demonstrated,the problem appears due to a lack of compression over the emissary veins,between cavernous body and albiginea, due to a loss of albuginea's rigidity and cavernous bodies eslas-ticity, which become fibrosed.
  This fact called veno-occlusive dysfunction can be demonstrated by radiological and hemodynamical methods (cavernosography and cavernosometry).

MATERIAL AND METHODS

In our institution we use the following steps: 1.A careful medical record containing: the exact date of problem's appearance, the way it appeared, the aggravating causes and evolution of simptomatology,as well as the results of a complete and specific physical examination,to determine anomalies of cavernous bodies as well as of circulatory and neurological systems. 2.We perform test to discharge psycological origin: psycosexual test, nocturnal penile tumescence test, and visual erotic stimulating test. 3.We perform test to confirm organic origin: we have divided into endocrine, metabolic, urologic, neurologic and vascular investigations.

On patients with apparently neurological problem we perform on limbs and penis nerves,electro-neuro-physiological test specially R1 and R2 reflexes answers.

To investigate arterial flow we perform the test called : penis-arm arterial index,penis thermograpy,arterial penis doppler and selective arterial angiography.

Venous flow is studied specially on those patients whom we suspected to present venous outflow (fast detumescence and inability to maintain intravaginal erection):erotic stimula- ting test is performed with and without vasodilatador drugs. Cavernosometry test which give us some information about the amount of necessary blood to obtain and maintaim a good erection. Cavernosography test has two phases:normal and vasodilating and it is necessary to confirm venous outflow.

Our experience between January 1991 and december 1992 was: 223 patients complained some kind of sexual simptomatology. In 118 cases we suspected venous outflow,but we are in a right diagnosis on 33 cases. 85 patients, were not confirmed on their diagnosis or do not have their studies completed.

We have had one 18 years old patient,with spongiosum body anomaly,and the youngest patient with venous outflow disease was 20 years old and 63 the oldest;although we have had one patient 69 years old associate with Peyronie disease. The largest incidence was found between 40 and 60 years old.

About the ethiology we have found 6 cases of diabetes,8 cases of atherosclerosis,one of congenital anomaly,3 Peyro- nie´s disease,12 patients with hormonal problems and the last three with pure venous outflow.

One patient complained about some type of spongiosum body deformity,12 not be able to otain a rigid erection,15 only be able to obtain a very brief erection,16 have very rapid lost of rigidity and 5 not be able to maintain an intrava- ginal erection.

In 19 patients fluxometry was normal and in 14 cases were not.

The visual erotic stimulation test was normal in 16 cases but it was not in 17 cases.

Cavernosography shows:spongiosum fistulae in 3 cases,degree one venous outflow 7 cases,degree two venous outflow in 2 cases,degree three venous outflow 21 cases,congenital anomaly 2 cases,peyronie disease in 3 cases,and venous occlusive dysfuntion 15 cases;of course some of these radiologic pathology were found concomitant.

RESULTS

By,these results we have divided as clinical or surgical treatement. The first was carried to correct the endocrino- metabolic and toxic problems. Five patients were treated in this way and one of them must be transferend to surgery.

We have proposed surgical correction in 13 patients;11 venous outflow procedures,1 deformity correction and one penile prosthesis implantation;but they did not accept.

On the other hand we have performed 6 single venous outflow operations,one of them with a litle problem by shortening of his penis and 3 simultaneus venous outflow surgery plus penile prosthesis implantation. All of these cases with good results except one of them with penis shortening.

Our casuistics are not so large to take conclutions.

We have used Tullii´s technique in 6 cases and Wespes technique in 3 cases.

We think decreasing of the albuginea layer compliace is necessary to get the best results.

REFERENCES

1. Lue T, First world Meeting on Impotence.Paris 1984.
2. Tullii RE, Degni M, Surgery for venous leakage in diabetic patients. Rev Bras de Ang e Circ Vas 1988;18:89-92.
3. Tullii RE, Degni M. Ligadura venosa no tratamento da Impotencia sexual masculina de origen venosa pura. Rev Bras ve Ang e Cir.Vasc.1988;18:77-79.
4. Tullii RE, Dilorio JM. Correction of venous leakage according to modified Wespes Technique. Rev.Bras de Ang e Cir.Vas.18:73-76
5. Wespes E, Schulman, C.Surgical treatement of the Organic Impotence due to a venous leak.Deparment of urology,University Clinics of Brussels,Erasm Hospital,Brussels,Belgiu.

OP/13.4

PLACEBO CONTROLLED TRIAL OF NAFTAZONE IN WOMEN WITH PRIMARY NON COMPLICATED SYMPTOMATIC VARICOSE VEINS

VAYSSAIRAT M and the French venous Naftazone trial group
Rothschild Hospital , Paris , France

Objective : The efficacy , tolerance , and best rhythm for the prescription of 30 mg/day oral Naftazone (N) in women with primary non complicated symptomatic varicose veins (PNCSVV)
Patients and methods : Two parallel multicentric randomized double blind trial comparing Naftazone and placebo in 270 women with PNCSVV. Comparison by ANOVA , at day 0 and after 14 days of treatment, of 1- clinical disability, using an analogous scale, and 2 - morning and evening leg volumes .
Results : The improvement in disability at day 14 was 32 ± 23 mm in the N group and 24 ± 20 in the placebo group (p=0.01) . Best clinical efficacy was obtained in the sub-group given 30 mg Naftazone at midday (35 ± 22mm) . Differences between morning leg volumes at days 0 and 14 were 19 ± 73 ml in the N group and 1.5 ± 57 in the placebo group (p=0.10).
Conclusion : Naftazone was more efficient than placebo for the clinical improvement of patients with PNCSVV .

P283

THE EXTERNAL PUDIC VEINS: AN ANATOMO-CLINICAL STUDY OF THEIR TREATMENT BY AMBULATORY PHLEBECTOMY (MULLER METHOD)

Dortu J A, Dortu J, Constancias-Dortu I

2 rue des Glieres, 74000, Annecy, France

41 cases of external pudic varicose veins were identified after examining 1371 patients followed up during four years and treated by ambulatory phlebectomy.
Analysis of the history, the clinical and doppler signs and the treatment by ambulatory phlebectomy of the thighs made it possible to establish an accurate anatomical description of these poorly understood venous territories.
Physiopathological investigation can establish the frequently autonomous nature of these external pudic varicose veins.
The high incidence of primary reflux, their wide distribution along the varicose axes prolonged over 1 to 3 segments of the limbs, characterize the 41 cases of major external pudic varicosis.
Therapeutic analysis reveals the inadequacy of surgery or sclerosis in severe cases and the efficacy of ambulatory phlebectomy.
Ambulatory phlebectomy presents specific characteristics of method and bandaging related to the quality of the skin and venous tissue an the external pudic site.

OP/13.1

PELVIC VARICOCELE: PHYSIOPATHOLOGICAL CLASSIFICATION AND CORRELATED LOWER LIMBS VENOUS INSUFFICIENCY.

A Vercelli, F Ghilardi, U Riba

Centro Studio Malattie Vascolari, Torino, Italia

Objective: Latest achievements in instrumental diagnostics suggest revising pelvic varicocele (FV) physiopathology and propose a new way of classification.

Patients: Study of 64 patients with PV in 3 out of these associated with venous insufficiency in lower limbs.

Measurements: Transvaginal Ecodoppler study and investigation on venous connections with lower limbs.

Results: 3 (three) types of P.V. were found
1) Hyperestomy P.V.
2) Reflux P.V.
3) Mixed P.V.
anastomotic channels between P.V. and venous circulation in lower limbs were investigated.

Conclusion: This classification allows the tracing back to P.V. pathogenesis, highlighting mutual relationships and aggravating elements in the two systems, detecting physiopathological factors of some varicose recidivous.

P286

PELVIC PAIN ASSESSMENT IN THE TREATMENT OF THE PELVIC CONGESTIVE SYNDROME

Louis Grondin, Ron Young, Lilly Wouters

The Grondin Medical Centre
3rd Floor, 1504 15 Avenue S.W.
Calgary, Alberta   T3C OX9   Canada

The pelvic congestive syndrome is a distinct clinical and vascular entity caused by venous insufficiency of the ovarian veins. It was previously described by Abraham Lecter and John Hobbs. The treatment for this condition consists of firstly ligating the ovarian vein bilaterally (Hobbs), as near its termination as possible, and removing the para-uterine varices (Lecter). Little objective data has been put forth in their respective studies.

In combination with the University of Calgary we have designed a three year prospective efficiency study for proximal ovarian vein ligation. The surgery consists of ligating the ovarian vein and removing it over a segment of 6.0 to 8.0 cm. Since it is a female duplicatum of the varicocele surgery, it is performed in our service by urologists. Prior to being placed into this study, patients must have a normal gynecological assessment, normal pelvic abdominal ultrasound, and laparoscopy. Ovarian insufficiency must be demonstrated by selective descending ovarian venography (previously described in San Francisco at the North American Society of Phlebology Meeting). Furthermore patients will undergo a psychiatric evaluation and a pelvic pain assessment score will be performed one month pre-op, one month post-op, three months post-op, six months post-op and one year post-op. Repeated ovarian venography's will be carried out to ascertain physiological interruption of the ovarian venous reflux.

The purpose of this study is to offer objective data to the effectiveness of the previously described surgical intervention.

P287

CHRONIC PHLEBOLOGICAL DISORDERS OF THE FEMALE PELVIS

Figueirôa C L S, Figueirôa E S, Soares M V

Hospital Stalzabel Escola de Medicina Salvador - Bahia, Brazil

The author makes a detailed study of pelvic phlebological disorders in women, which includes anatomical, physiological and pathological concepts, as complementary methods of diagnosis in order to obtain adequate treatment for the different pathological degrees.

The material obtained during the period from 1987 until 1992 represented a universe of 496 patients with chronic pelvic disorders related to the menstrual cycle: from this total 52.7% of the patients were multiparous with the age between 20 and years old, and nearly 70% developed varices in other areas.

The phlebographical studies, in conjunction with the clinical information and with the reproductive history of each patient, will allow us an adjustment of our material in Schaupp's therapeutic proposal (1978), which includes the simple resection of the segments of the lumbarovarian plexus until extensive procedures with the total paramaterial and pampiniphiorm dissection associated with the total hysterectomy, remaining the alternative of the tubal resection when it is involved.

P031

THE HORMONAL FACTOR IN THE GENESIS OF VARICOSE VEINS. DETECTION OF HORMONE RECEPTORS.

Salvadore Nieto, M.D., F.I.C.A.
Salvador Nieto Foundation. Av. Santa Fe 2679, 2nd. "D"; (1425) Buenos Aires, Argentina. Telefax: (541) 826-8519.
Buenos Aires Naval Hospital. Buenos Aires, Argentina.

Objective:
To display the actual presence of estrogen and progesterone receptors in varicose veins.

Material and methods:
40 patients that presented varicose veins were studied. Characteristics of the sample were:

- All of them were women.
- Greater saphenous vein stripping was performed in everyone (in one or both limbs) and immediately sent to study.
- 13 (32,5%) belonged to the premenopausal group.
- 27 (67,5%) belonged to the postmenopausal one.
- Defined techniques were used to prepared and study veins.

Results:
Positive receptor findings were significant:

- Premenopausal patients: 69,24% for both estrogen and progesterone receptors.
- Postmenopausal patients: 59,26% for estrogen receptors and 85,19% for progesterone receptors.

Conclusions:
Tissues which are positive in hormone receptors are exposed highly to the influence of the corresponding hormones. Their detection in varicose veins allow to develop an interpretation of the intimate mechanism of the activity of hormones and their effects on the vascular system involved.

Lymphoedema

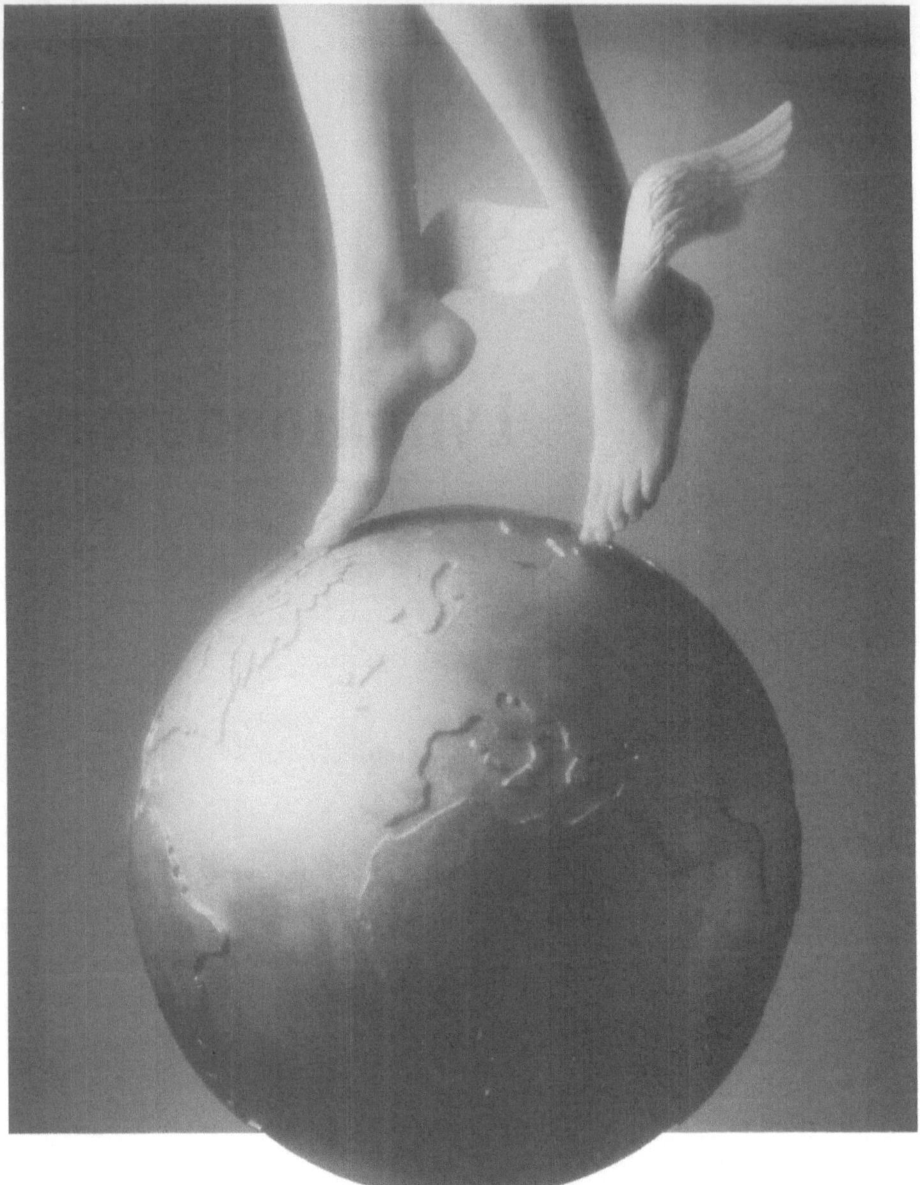

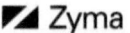

LEADER IN PHLEBOLOGY

VENORUTON®
O-(β-hydroxyethyl)-rutosides

*VENORUTON® = PAROVEN® in Australia,
New Zealand, the Republic of South Africa,
RELVÊNE® in France, VERUTIL® in Venezuela*

ANGOLA
ARGENTINA
AUSTRALIA
AUSTRIA
BAHRAIN
BELGIUM
BOLIVIA
BRAZIL
BULGARIA
CAMEROON
CHILE
CIS
COLOMBIA
CONGO
COSTA RICA
CYPRUS
CZECH REPUBLIC
DENMARK

DOMINICAN REP.
ECUADOR
EGYPT
ETHIOPIA
FRANCE
GABOON
GERMANY
GREECE
GUATEMALA
GUINEA
HONDURAS
HONG KONG
HUNGARY
IRELAND
ISRAEL

ITALY
IVORY COAST
JORDAN
KUWAIT
LEBANON
LIBYA
LUXEMBOURG

MALAYSIA
MALTA
MAURITIUS
MEXICO
MOROCCO
MOZAMBIQUE
NETHERLANDS

NETHERLANDS
ANTILLES
NEW ZEALAND
NICARAGUA
PANAMA
PARAGUAY
PERU
PHILIPPINES
POLAND
PORTUGAL
QATAR
RUMANIA
RUSSIA
SALVADOR
SAUDI ARABIA

SINGAPORE
SLOVAK REPUBLIC
SOUTH AFRICA
SOUTH KOREA
SPAIN
SRI LANKA
SWITZERLAND
SYRIA
THAILAND
TUNISIA
TURKEY
UNITED ARAB EMIRATES
UNITED KINGDOM
UKRAINA
URUGUAY
VENEZUELA
YEMEN
ZAIRE

*Full prescribing information is available on request.
Zyma SA, CH-1260 Nyon, Switzerland – A Member of the Ciba Group*

Zyma

Phlebology '95, D. Negus et al. (eds.). Phlebology (1995) Suppl. 1: 1051-1053

P080

Physiotherapy of the Patients with Lower Extremities Lymphedema

M. Wozniewski, U. Pilch and Cz. Jezierski

Department of Rehabilitation, Academy of Physical Education, Wroclaw, Poland

INTRODUCTION

The extremities lymphedema is observed in about 200-300 million of the people in the world. Pharmacological methods of the lymphedema treatment are inefficacious, and the indications to the surgical treatment are limited. Now the physiotherapy methods are essential in the treatment of the lymphedema, particularly the intermittent pneumatic compression (IPC) (1,2,3). Successful results can be obtained in 50-90 per cent of the patients with the lymphedema of upper limb owing to the IPC use. Physiotherapy of the patients with the lymphedema of the legs is more difficult than with the uuper limb lymphedema. The efficacy of the physiotherapy in the treatment of the legs lymphedema has been analyzed.

METHODS

20 patients (age from 17 to 83) treated due to the lymphedema of the legs were examined. The removal of the inguinal lymphatic nodes in the course of the radical treatment of the melanoma malignum was of the cause of the secondary lymphedema in 12 patients. 8 patients had the primary lymhedema of unknown origin (Table 1.).

Table 1. General characteristic of patients

Type of edema	Number of patients	Sex		Age	Leg	
		Women	Men		Right	Left
Primary	8	8	0	34.3 (17-68)	4	4
Secondary	12	7	5	50.7 (23-83)	7	5

The patients were treated with the intermittent pneumatic compression (IPC), exercises and the manual lymphdrainage. The procedure was performed 5 times a week for 1 hour a day during 5-12 weeks. The circumferences on the 9 levels of the both legs were measured prior and post IPC. Difference between normal and edematous legs determined the size of the edema. Decrease of the edema size was calculated in per cent according to the formula :

$$\% \downarrow = \text{I-II/I} \times 100\%,$$

I - difference between normal and edematous legs prior the physiotherapy,
II- difference between normal and edemayous legs post the physiotherapy.

RESULTS

The highest size of the edema was 15.5 cm in the patients with the secondary lymphedema (average from 1.1 to 4.1 cm) and 13.0 cm with the primary lymphedema (average from 1.4 to 3.9 cm). The highest difference of circumferences was 4.1 cm at the 1/2 thigh level in the patients with the secondary lymphedema and 3.9 cm at the ankle level with the primary lymphedema. Average the edema decreased varied from 3.8 to 54.5 per cent in the patients after the lymphangectomy and from -6.9 (increase of the edema) to 33.3 per cent in the patients with the primary lymphedema (Table 2).

Table 2. Results of the physiotherapy

Level of measurement	Primary lymphedema Difference of circumference		%↓	Secondary lymphedema Difference of circumference		%↓
	I (cm)	II (cm)		I (cm)	II (cm)	
1.Thigh at inguinal level	2.7	1.8	33.3	2.4	1.9	20.8
2. 1/2 of the thigh	3.1	2.3	25.8	4.1	3.2	22.0
3. Above the knee	3.6	2.8	22.2	4.0	3.2	20.0
4. The knee	3.3	2.7	18.2	2.9	2.0	31.0
5. Below the knee	2.9	3.1	-6.9	2.6	2.5	3.8
6. 1/2 of the calf	3.3	3.4	-3.0	3.7	3.0	18.9
7. Above the ankle	3.9	3.7	5.1	3.5	2.8	20.0
8. The ankle	2.5	2.1	16.0	2.6	2.0	23.1
9. The metatarsus	1.4	1.3	7.1	1.1	0.5	54.5

I - prior physiotherapy ;
II - post physiotherapy ;
%↓ - decrease of the edema size

DISCUSSION

The IPC increases the hydrostatic pressure in the tissue of the legs, which was decreased under the influence of the edema. The natural muscular pump and the lymphatic drainage from the legs are helped by the physiotherapy. That leads to the improvment of the efficiency of the lymphatics remaining after the lymphangectomy. The development of the lymphatic collateral anastomosises is facilitated too. The decrease of the size of the edema and the restitution of the equilibrium of the lymphatic circulation of the legs are results of the physiotherapy (2).

The efficacy of the IPC depends on the type of the edema. The best results of the treatment were obtained in the patients with the secondary lymphedema. Reduction in lymphedema of the patients with the secondary lymphedema was greater than that of the primary. Reduction in the degree of the lymphedema at the thigh and calf level were comparable in the patients with the secondary lymphedema. The worst results of the treatment were obtained at the calf level in patients with the primary lymhedema.

We used less pressure than the others authors (3) (about 40-70 mm Hg), because the lymphatics are very fragile. Even a light touch can tear them. Casley-Smith (1) estimated that a safe, non-injurious pressure , would be up to 100 g/cm^2 (75 mm Hg). The lymphatics are closed by applied pressures of above about 80 g/cm^2 (60 mm Hg). At least, 60 mm Hg is well below that likely to cause injury. It was found that the optimal pressure was the maximum which would not cause lymphatic collapse : 60 g/cm^2 (45 mm Hg).

CONCLUSIONS

1. The physiotherapy (IPC, exercises, manual lymphdrainage) is the efficacious method of the conservative treatment of the lymphedema of the legs, particularly in the patients with the secondary lymphedema.
2. The reduction of the lymphedema depends on the type of the lymphedema and part of the leg.

REFERENCES

1. Casley-Smith J.R., Other techniques : compression pumps and devices, and heating.Proceedings of the Conference " The lymphatic system, lymhedema and its physical therapy ", Australia 21 Jan- 2 Feb 1990: 132-9.
2. Raines J.K., O' Donnell T.F., Kalisher L., Darling R.C. ,Selection of patients with lymphedema for compression therapy. The Am. J. of Surg. 1977; 133 : 430-7.
3. Richmand D.M., O' Donnell T.F., Zelikowski A., Sequential pneumatic compression for lymphedema. Arch. Surg. 1985 ; 120 : 1116-19

Phlebology '95, D. Negus et al. (eds.). Phlebology (1995) Suppl. 1: 1054-1057

P038

Thermotherapy for Primary Lymphedema

A. Misuri

Cattedra di Chirurgia Vascolare, Università degli Studi di Genova, Genova

INTRODUCTION

An increasing interest in lymphatic pathology has brought real progress in pathophysiological, diagnostic and therapeutic fields about over the last thirty years.

It's important to remember that, with regard to conservative therapy, normal hygienic measures such as elevation of the limb, manual lymphatic drainage, elastic and rigid compression and drugs are all of sure effectiveness.[1, 2, 3]

The aim of conservative therapy is :
-reduction of edema;
-improvement of skin condition;
-prevention of complications (lymphangitis).

Recently, among the various forms of treatment, positive results have been obtained by thermotherapy.

In 1964 Zhang and collaborators [4] started to treat primary and secondary lymphedemas in a chamber heated by infrared rays and obtained satisfactory results. According to the authors, advantages of this method are: nonivasive, simple to perform, highly effective and inexpensive.

In 1988 Fox and collaborators [5] developed an apparatus using microwaves.

More recently Ohkuma, Liu and Misuri [6, 7, 8] have obtained a significant reduction of edema and a decrease of infection of lower limbs using microwave hypertermia.

The heat breaks down the protein of different molecular weight, thereby obtaining others of a lighter molecular weight [9].This breakdown favours reabsorption into the circulation and consequently reduces the accumulation of protein macromolecules with less subcutaneous fibrosis, therefore reducing the volume of the limb. On this basis, we feel that examination of the effects of heat therapy on primary lymphedema of the limbs could be of interest.

MATERIAL AND METHODS

Thirty-five patients (44 lower limbs) of which 5 males and 30 females affected by primary lymphedema (26 unilateral and 9 bilateral) were subjected to thermotherapy.Their ages ranged from 11 to 78.

All patients were given a clinical examination, Doppler C.W. and lymphoscintigraphy of the lower limbs. The apparatus used for the treatment consisted of a chamber using electromagnetic waves, called "Lymphotherm 24" (patent 209407).This chamber consists of 3 generators, "Magnetrons", 2,4 GHz, whose outlets differentiate between foot, knee and thigh.

Each "Magnetron" has a power regulator (0-900 WRF) and has visual controls and acoustic alarms. A digital electronic thermoregulator showing the temperature of the patient's limb automatically blocks the amount of heat when the maximum temperature required is reached in this first experimental stage.

The therapy consists of a cycle of 15 sessions of 45 minutes each, once a day, 5 days a week for 3 weeks, according to the method elaborated by Fox and collaborators [5]. The power of the "Magnetrons" is regulated so that the inner temperature of the limb is about 41.0-42.0 C°. After each session patients wore an elastic stocking and continued normal activities.

The evaluation criteria of the results was the circumference reduction of the limb and of lymphangitis.

Measurements were taken half way across the foot, at the malleolus and at 10, 20 and 30 cm. above and below the knee. The edema reduction in patients affected by unilateral lymphedema was calculated according to the formula used by Zhang and collaborators [4] and Richmand and collaborators [10]:

Amount of reduction of edema =

(Sum of the circumferences before therapy - Sum of the circumferences after therapy):
(Sum of the circumferences before therapy - Sum of the circumferences of the healthy limb) x 100%.

The results were clessified in four categories:
- excellent: the treated limb equals the healthy one, a reduction of 100%;
- good: a reduction of 50% or more;
- fair: a reduction less than 50%;
- poor: no reduction of the edema.

In bilateral lymphedema patients, for whom it was impossible to check against a healthy limb, average circumferences of each limb before and after therapy were compared. The results are defined by the average circumference reduction .

These results were classified in four categories:
- excellent: 3 or more cm of reduction in the average circumference;
- good: 1-2.9 cm of reduction in the average circumference;
- fair: 1 cm of reduction;
- poor: no reduction.

RESULTS

In the case of unilateral lymphedema, results classifiable as excellent were obtained in 6 cases out of 26 (24%), good in 10 out of 26 (38%) and fair in 10 cases out of 26 (38%). In cases of bilateral lymphedema results were excellent in 4 cases out of 9 (44%), good in 4 out of 9 (44%) and fair in 1 out of 9 (12%).

Finally, in 26 limbs with previous episodes of lymphangitis, these episodes were not repeated in the 36 month follow-up to which all patients were subjected.

1056

DISCUSSION

There are different methods of conservative treatment of lymphedema of the lower limbs.

To establish some order, the basic principles of applied therapy were classified at the Congress in Adelaide in 1985 [11]. These aim to improve skin quality and reduce limb dimension.

Regarding the techniques used to reduce limb volume, there are various external mechanical methods of compression.

In 1974 van der Molen and Toth [12]proposed a method by which soft rubber tubes ("tuyautage") were wrapped around the limb and pressure up to 500 mmHg was applied. The authors reported a reduction of nearly 3 cm in the circumference of the treated limbs in 70% of the patients with a follow-up of more than 5 years. Other methods adopt external, intermittent pneumatic compression. In 1974 Raines and co-workers [13] developed a method using an apparatus which applies slight pressure (60 mmHg) intermittently (at 30 second intervals) for 4 hours. Limb volume reduction by this method was between 33% and 52%.

In 1985 Richmand and collaborators [10] used an apparatus which applied a short period of compression at high pressure (130 mmHg) 6 to 8 hours daily. There were positive results in 45% of cases.

In 1990 Orhan and Lavavasseur [14] obtained 65% positive results using 80 mmHg, 2 hours per day for 6 days.

A new method can be added to these principles: thermotherapy.

Over the last 20 years Zhang and collaborators [4] have treated more than 1,000 cases and have demonstrated that infrared heat treatment produces significant volume reduction, using various mechanisms such as lymphatic neoangiogenesis near the damaged lymphatic channels. Another mechanism improves the clearance from tissue of serum labelled albumin, showing that treatment by means of heat stimulates the metabolism and local blood circulation so that absorption of composite molecules broken down and trasformed by heat is more readly effected by the blood stream.

As we said before, in 1988 Fox and collaborators [5] together with bioengineers perfected a microwave apparatus. The results obtained by the authors are encouraging.(51% positive).

In 1993 Liu and Olszewski [7] demonstrated, by immunohistological data, a decrease and sometimes disappearance of inflammatory infiltrates in lymphedematous skin. Moreover, immunohistochemical evaluation showed increased immunological activity. As a result, the effect of hyperthermia may be the production of an anti-inflammatory effect.

With regard to our experience, although limited to a single cycle of therapy, the results are positive as far as reduction of limb girth, subcutaneous tissue and episides of lymphangitis are concerned.

REFERENCES

1. Lucertini G,Misuri A,Viacava,Alonzo A. La terapia del linfedema dell'arto inferiore: attualità e prospettive. In: Nuzzaci G, a cura di. Atti del 7° Congresso Nazionale della Società Italiana di Flebologia Clinica e Sperimentale. Firenze, 10-12 dicembre 1990. Bologna: Monduzzi Editore, 1990: 369-80.
2. O'Donnell F Jr,Yeager A. Diagnosis and management of lymphedema. In: Haimovici H, Callow AD, DePalma RG, Ernst CB, Hollier LH, eds.Haimovici's Vascular Surgery. Principles and techniques. 3rd ed. Norwalk: Appleton and Lange, 1989: 1005-17.

3. Clodius L,Foldi E, Foldi M. On nonoperative management of chronic lymphedema. Lymphology 1990; 23: 2-3.

4. Zhang TS, Huang WY, Han LV, Liu WY. Heat and bandage treatment for chronic lymphedema of extremities.Chin Med J 1984; 97: 567-77.

5. Fox U, Romagnoli G, Ribaldone G. Assotiation of microsurgery and thermotherapy in the treatment of limb lymphedemas: preliminary experience.In:Partsch H, ed. Progress in Lymphology-XI.Amsterdam:Elsevier Science Publishers BV (Biomedical Division), 1988:437-43.

6. Ohkuma M. The treatment of lymphedema by microwave and elastic dressing-The second report. In: Cluzan RV, Pecking AP, Lokiec FM ed. Progress in Lymphology-XIII.Elsevier Science Publishers BV (Biomedical Division). Excerpta Medica 1992, 493-496.

7. Liu NF, Olszewski W. The infuence of local hyperthermia on lymphedema and lymphedematous skin of the human leg. Lymphology .1993; 26: 28-37.

8. Misuri A, Grana A, Lucertini G, Belardi P. Thermotherapy for lymphedema of lower extremity:preliminary experience. Proceedings of the European Congress of The International Union of Phlebology. Budapest 6-10 september 1993: 287-289.

9. Frazer JW. Biophysical chemical basis of RF field interactions. In: Osepchuk JM, ed. Biological effects of electromagnetic radiation. NewYork: IEEE Press, 1983: 101-7.

10. Richmand DM, O'Donnell TF Jr, Zelikovski A.sequential pneumatic compression for lymphedema.A controlled trial. Arch Surg 1985; 120: 1116-9.

11. Casley-Smith JR, Foldi M, Ryan TJ, Witte MH, Witte CL, Cluzan R, Partsch H, Jamal S,O'Brien B. Summary of the 10th International Congress of Lymphology Working Group Discussions and Recommendations, Adelaide, Australia, August 10-17,1985. Lymphology 1985; 18: 175-80.

12. van der Molen JR, Toth LM. The conservative treatment of lymphedema of the extremities. Angiology 1974; 25: 470-83.

13. Raines JK, O'Donnell TF Jr, Kalisher L, Darling RC. Selection of patients with lymphedema for compression therapy. Am J Surg 1977; 133: 430-7.

14. Orhan J, Lavavasseur O. Approche de la pressothérapie pneumatique des lymphoedèmes des membres inférieurs. Phlébologie 1990; 2: 243-51.

Phlebology '95, D. Negus et al. (eds.). Phlebology (1995) Suppl. 1: 1058-1060

P295

Effect of 0 (Beta-Hydroxyethyl)-Rutosides (Venoruton) in the Treatment of Primary and Secondary Lymphoedema

D. Kalas, M. Redling, K. Prodán and J. Daróczy

Department Dermatol, St Stephen Hospital of Kun Hospital, Budapest, Hungary

Introduction

Lymphoedema is caused by functional impairment of the lymphatic and tissue systems (1). It has been shown that alterations occur not only in the lymphatics themselves, but also in the adventitia of the large lymphatics, in the surrounding tissues in general and in the blood vessels (2) (Beta-hydroxyethyl) rutosides (Venoruton) has been known for decades as a drug which acts by influencing the microcirculation. It decreases inflammation by blocking cyclo-oxygenase, increases the endothel resistance by reducing intercellular permeability and increases venous pressure (3,4) It also blocks thrombocyte aggregation, reduces capillary permeability and filtration (5). Venoruton may decrease the protein content of intercellular space and may reduce lymphoedema. The aim of the present study was to measure the additional effect of Venoruton treatment in the complex oedema-reducing therapy of lymphoedema. We also compared the effect of Venoruton in primary and secondary lymphoedema.

Methods
Forty patients of grade II-III lymphoedema of primary or secondary origin were involved in the study. They received no treatment for one month prior to entering the study. There were 38 women and 2 men with a mean age of 49 ± 6 years range 37-68). Patients with acute venous or arterial insufficiency, those with systemic disease such as cardiac oedema, renal failure, diabetes, pregnancy or liver disease and those immobilised were excluded from the study. All studies were performed in accordance with the declaration of Helsinki. Past history (individual and family) and complete physical and laboratory examination was performed. Laboratory parameters such as total protein, serum cholesterol and triglycerides, serum potassium and sodium were evaluated. Total volume of leg was estimated by measuring the circumference of legs every 4 cm (20 measurements). Volume was calculated by the equation

$$V^2{}_1 + V^2{}_2 + \ldots V^2{}_{20} = V$$

Patients' complaints such as heavy leg syndrome, paraesthesia, burning skin, decreased activity, restless leg, muscle cramps, general ill health were scored on a quantitative 2 point scale every two weeks. Complaints judged serious were 2, mild were 1.5 or 1.0, marginal 0.5 and no complaint 0. All patients received complex physiotherapy such as manual lymph drainage, compression bandaging, special lymph-exercise for two weeks and elastic stockings for an additional four weeks. All patients were on low cholesterol diet for six weeks. Ten patients with primary and ten with secondary lymphoedema received Venoruton (3 x 500 mg/day for six weeks. Statistical analysis was done by a NWA Statpack computer package.

Results
Total volume of the legs decreased significantly in each group after two weeks with complex therapy. There was no difference in the decrease in volume between those receiving Venoruton treatment as compared to those without the drug (Fig.1). At four and six weeks, however, a further decrease of total leg volume was observed only in the Venoruton-treated group. When the primary and secondarily lymphoedema groups were compared, a more pronounced decrease in volume was observed in the primary lymphoedema group with Venoruton treatment. Complaints of patients decreased significantly in each group (Fig.2). Unexpectedly, there was an increase in plasma total protein after 6 weeks in all groups irrespective of Venoruton treatment. No side effects of Venoruton treatment were observed.

Fig 1.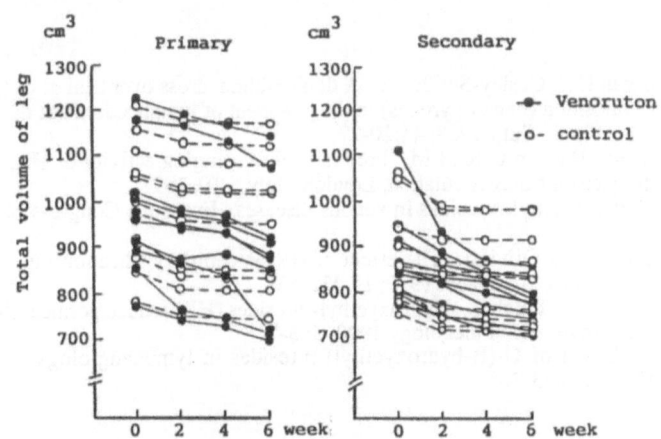

Fig. 2   Decrease in patient complaints during Venoruton treatment
quantitativ score

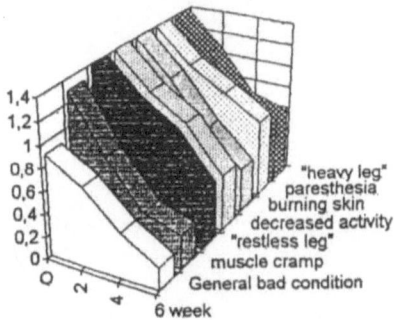

Discussion

0-(B-hydroxyethyl) - rutosides (Venoruton) is a well known flavonoid with pronounced anti-inflammatory, anti-oxidant and endothelial sealing effects. Previous double blind clinical studies have proved the efficacy of the drug in the treatment of post-mastectomy lymphoedema of the limb was reduced significantly by 3000 mg/day for 6 months [1]. The drug reduced extravasation of contrast material in men on lymphangiography [6]. Clinical studies evaluating the effect of Venoruton in primary and secondary lymphoedema have not yet been published.

We found a significant reduction of total leg volume following 6 weeks Venoruton treatment. There was a considerable relief of patients symptoms as scored by a quantitative scale. No patient withdrew from the study, showing the safety of the drug and patient compliance. In addition, no side effect was reported.

We also measured the total protein concentration in the blood prior and after the treatment. Interestingly, there was an increase in the plasma total protein after 6 weeks of the treatment. This finding does not directly prove the reduction of protein content in the oedematous leg, but may indirectly suggest the mechanism of oedema-reducing activity of Venoruton (the increased osmotic pressure of blood, and reduction in permeability of capillaries).

Venoruton can be considered effective in the treatment of both primary and secondary lymphoedema of the legs. The fact that there was no difference between primary and secondary lymphoedema suggests that the mechanism of oedema reduction is independent of the aetiology of lymphoedema.

References
1. Piller N B, Morgan R G, Casley-Smith J R. A double-blind, cross over trial of O-(Beta-hydroxyethyl) - rutosidon (benzo-pyrones) in the treatment of lymphoedema of the arms and legs. British J Plastic Surg 1988; 41:20-27.
2. Bast A, Jansen F P, Haeuen G R M M. Free radical scavenging activity of HR. 17th European Conference on Microcirculation, London, July 5-10, 1992.
3. Thukesins O. Hydroxyethyl rutosides in venous diseases. European Congress of IVP. Budapest, 6-10, 1993.
4. Roztocil K, Prerovsky I, Olivia I. The effect of HR on capillary filtration rate in the lower limb of man. Eur J Pharmacol 1977; 11:435-438.
5. Michel C, Blumberg S, Clough G. Hydroxyethyl-rutosides (HR) reduce permeability of frog mesenteric microvessels. Phlebology 1990; 5: 3-7.
6. Brocks P D C. Effect of O-(B-hydroxyethyl) rutosides in lymphangiology. Am J Roentgenol 1977; 128: 263-265.

P047

GRADE OF NODAL FIBROSIS AND VERRUCOSIS LYMPHOSTATICA OF PRIMARY LYMPHOEDEMA

Bechyně M.
Dermat. clinic , Charles University

Praha, Czech republic

Seventy five patients with primary lymphoedema of the lower limb have been studied,twelve of them with familial congenital ones.Because it seems as from the literature so from our studies, that biopsies did not increase them,therefore they were done.The pericortical fibrosis have been found in control group of 25 patients with a history of the inflamation but an extensive fibrosis at the primary lymphoedema.At patients with Milroy's disease/congenital familial lymphoedema/ the nodes were small and lightly fibrosed.The degree of the fibrosis was lesser with a bilateral mild lymphoedema which did not progressed to the knee. When there was the history with the erysipel, the fibrosis was much more greater in accordance to the extensibility of the oedema.At the distal hypoplasia or at the subcutaneous changes with the distal lymphoedema was the fibrosis very slight when the history of the lymphoedema was over ten years.As, an agravationable complication is the verrucosis lymphostatica between the toes, on the genital organs or in the anal area.The highest fibrosis and the extent verrucosis after the contrast lymphography or phlebography was at all ten patients.
Conclusions:history, inspection, palpation,lymphoscintigraphy and the grade of nodal fibrosis with verrucosis lymphostatica as the worst change of the skin are indicator for the patient's state of the lymphoedema.

P012

VENOUS LESIONS IN BEHÇETS DISEASE

Saba D., Özer Z.G., Sagdiç K., Cengiz M.

Uludag University, School of Medicine, Department of Thoracic and Cardiovascular Surgery, Bursa, Turkey.

Behçet's disease was first described as a triad (oral and genital ulcerations with iridocyclitis) in 1937 by Hulusi Behçet. Soon it was though tht this disease was a systemic vasculitis and had an autoimmune aetiology. The prognosis is related to the cardiovascular, gastrointestinal and central nervous system complications.

The percentage of vascular lesions is 7.7-60% with the mean of 25% in Behçet's disease. Despite the fact that venous system involvement takes an important place with the frequency of 18-24%, reports about venous lesions in the literature are quite rare. For this reason we decided to present 39 (72.2%) venous lesions in 52 patients with Behçet's disease having 54 vascular lesions that we have treated in our department for the past 10 years. The youngest patient was 18 years old and the oldest patient was 57 years old with the mean age of 36. Male/Female ratio was 3.7/1.

Although venous lesions are not rare and affect prognosis in Behçet's disease, it is not easy to recognize if it is the first system involved in the nature of the disease.

Miscellaneous Topics

Miscellaneous Topics

Phlebology '95, D. Negus et al. (eds.). Phlebology (1995) Suppl. 1: 1065-1067

P001

Effect and Morphologic Evolution of Autogenous Jugular Vein and Glutaraldehyde-Stabilized Human Umbilical Cord Vein Grafting in Dog

Chen Weipei, Xu Ko and Chen Xiwei

Departmentof Applied Surgical Anatomy and Operative Surgery, Third Military Medical College, Chongqing, China

INTRODUCTION

The modified human umbilical cord vein graft for peripheral vascular reconstructions has been extensively used clinically, because of its favorable biological. physical and chemical characteristics since it was first reported by Dardik, et al[1]. Giodano and keshishiaw reported three cases of aneurysm formation in implanted human umbilical vein grafts[2]. Animal investigation give useful and analogous information, which can be applied to clinical treatment[3].

The purpose of this paper. therefore. is to provide interesting data on the ultimate fate of an implanted human umbilical cord vein (HUV) graft and morphologic evolution of HUV grafting in dog. compared with autogenous jugular vein.

METHODS

The glutaraldehyde-stabilized human unbilical cord vein

was used in the experiment. A 3cm segment of the
infraabdominal aorta of an adult dog was resected and
was replaced with a HUV. using autogenous jugular vein
(AJV) as control. The healing mechanism was revealed by
gross finding. angiogram. radioistope scanning of blood.
Doppler ultrasonic. LM. SEM and TEM. with 6 experimants
carried out at 1 day, 1 week. 2 weeks. 1 month. 3 months,
6 months. in order to find the highest patency rate as
the scientific foundation for clinical using.

RESULTS

This study shows:
1.The patency rate in 6 months is 95.2% in AJV. 87.5% in
HUV. It is no significant difference between two venous
mateials (P>0.05).(Table 1)
Table 1 Comparison of the implanted result of AJV and HUV
grafts

groups	number of dogs	graft patency	graft thrombosis	cpok
AJV	21	20 (95.2%)	1 (4.8%)	1~180 days
HUV	24	24 (87.5%)	3 (12.5%)	1~180 days

2.The wall of umbilical vein grossly is intact. in which
there are no dilatation and rupture. In the early phase.
there is some yellow gray membranous material attaching
on the inner wall. In the late phase. the inner wall is
smooth covered with a white gray membrane. which grows
into the graft from the anastomotic site.
3. The pathologic histology of the AJV and HUV after
implantation showed three stages: acute tramatic. acute
inflammatory reaction and hyperplastic repairing of
tissue. The endothelium degenerated and shed during the
process of preparation and implant of HUV; and the
subendothelial fibrous tissue could be observed. The new
endothelial cells which grow from the remainder of the

endothelial cells of AJV cover the intima gradually. The new endothelial cells of AJV grow earlier and faster than those of HUV. But. both the veins were endothelialized 6 months postoperatively. the subendothelium of new intima consisted of fibroblasts and collegen fiber; the myointimal cells derived from smooth muscle cells in media were less; the media and the adventitia were replaced by fibrous connective tissue.

4. HUV stabilized with 0.5% glutaraldehyde and used in grafting didn't cause immunologic rejection. but possessed the structure of the wall of the vein. and showed antithrombotic function and kept the patency of the grafts.

DISCUSSION

The correct technique of suture. decreasing the endothelial lesion and the using of antiplatelet drugs early post operately are the key to raise the early patency of the grafts.

The morphologic and histologic evolution of stabilized HUV after implanting is similar to that of AJV. HUV is easy to get, simple to prepare. with mild reaciton. good patency rate and great flexibility and toughess so that it is convenient to use a middle or small caliber arterial graft clinically.

REFERENCES

1. Dardik H, Dardik I. Successful arterial substitution with modified human umbilical veiw. Ann Surg 1976;183:252-8.

2. Gioradano JM. Keshishian JM. Aneurysm formation in human umbilical vein graft. Surgery 1982;91:343-5.

3. Heynen YG. Immediate and longterm evolution of the blood-venous graft interface. Eur Surg Res. 1983;15:230-5.

Phlebology '95, D. Negus et al. (eds.). Phlebology (1995) Suppl. 1: 1068-1070

P053

Proposal of a Mnemonic and Complete Description of the Superficial Venous Disease "PRSTUVWX"

S. Sadoun

10 rue Benjamin Moloïse, 94000 Créteil, France

INTRODUCTION :

There are many classifications of the superficial venous disease.

The proposed stages, which are correct of course, are mutually exclusive or inclusive and describe with variable and non exhaustive precision the patients' phlebological symptoms, or consider only one aspect of the disease at a time[1,2,3,4].

Even though the classifications are of great value, there are imprecisions : a patient operated of a stripping of the long saphenous vein (LSV), has «no more» any LSV varicose vein on the medial aspect of the limb, but in any case this patient can be considered as being at the same evolutive stage as a patient who has never had varicose vein(s) of the LSV, even if the two of them do not have LSV varicose veins.

Objective :

1) to propose a symptomatic and very precise description of the superficial venous disease to be used for the characterization of 7 symptoms and one antecedent of the disease.

2) to produce a very precise and very clear stratification of patients in clinical and epidemiological studies.

3) the classification proposed is very simple with no arbitrary grades or stages.

Examples :

1) Patients unscathed are :

$$P_\emptyset \, R_\emptyset \, S_\emptyset \, T_\emptyset \, U_\emptyset \, V_\emptyset \, W_\emptyset \, X_\emptyset .$$

2) Patients with 4 symptoms and nothing else are :

$$P_\emptyset \, R_\emptyset \, S_4 T_\emptyset \, U_\emptyset \, V_\emptyset \, W_\emptyset \, X_\emptyset \qquad \text{or} \qquad S_4$$

3) Patients with a reflux from the perforators in the LSVt and SSVt (P_LP_S), a reflux of the LSV (R_L), 3 symptoms (S3), panniculitis (T1), 1 ulcer in the LSVt (U_L), 1 ulcer in the SSVt (U_S), varicose veins in the LSVt (V_L), non systematized telangiectatic veins (W_O), and a ligation/section of one LSV (X_L) are :

$$P_L\,P_S\,R_L\,S3\,T1\,U_L\,U_S\,V_L\,W_{\emptyset}\,X_L$$

or

$$P_{LS}\,R_L\,S3\,T1\,U_{LS}\,V_L\,W_{\emptyset}\,X_L.$$

It is desirable to put an apostrophe (')for the symptoms originating from the left side (A',n'):

4) Patients with a reflux of the perforators in the left LSVt (P'_L or P_L'), a LSV reflux on the right (R_L), left SSV reflux (R'_S or R_S'), 3 symptoms (S3), a panniculitis in the right LSVt (T_L), a circonferencial stasis pigmentation and eczema on the left side (T'_{2O} or T_{2O}'), 1 ulcer at the right medial malleolus (e.g. LSVt = U_L), 2 ulcers at the left lateral malleolus. (e.g. SSVt) ($2U'_S$ or U_{2S}'), varicose veins in the right LSVt (V_L) and non systematized on the left side (V'_O or V_O'), telangiectatic varicose veins in the right and left LSVt (W_L & W'_L or W_{LL}') and a ligation/section of the left LSV (X_L') are :

$$P'_L\,R_L\,R'_S\,S3\,T_L\,T'_{2O}\,U_L\,U'_{2s}\,V_L\,V'_O\,W_L\,W_L'\,X_L'$$

or

$$P_L'\,R_{LS}'\,S3\,T_L\,2O'\,U_L\,2s'\,V_L O'\,W_L'\,X_L'\,.$$

<u>Conclusion :</u> the use of such a summarized identification will lead to more accurate population selection, and a less dispatched patients' population phlebological symptoms.

<u>Design :</u>　　the classification is based on 7 symptoms and one antecedent.
　　　　　　　it is named PRSTUVWX :

P =	incompetence of the Perforators
R =	Reflux
S =	Symptoms
T =	Trophic cutaneous disorders
U =	Ulcer (s)
V =	Varicose veins
W =	small telangiectatic VVeins
X =	ligation/sections.

BY CONVENTION :
♦ the suffixes are
"∅" = absence of the element
"L" = territory of the Long Saphenous Vein [LSVt]
"S" = territory of the Short Saphenous Vein [SSVt]
"O" = other territory.
♦ Figures in suffixes indicate the number of elements.

PRSTUVWX CLASSIFICATION BOARD :

	Right : X Left : X'	Right LSV	Left LSV	Right SSV	Left SSV	OTHER Right	OTHER Left	NUMBER = figure in suffix (n) LOCALISATION=letter in suffix (x)
Reflux Perforators	P	L	L'	S	S'	O	O'	P_{xn}
Superficial Reflux	R	L	L'	S	S'	O	O'	R_x
Symptoms	S							S_n
Trophic cutaneous disorders	T	L	L'	S	S'	O	O'	T_{nx}
Ulcer	U	L	L'	S	S'	O	O'	U_{nx}
Varicose Vein	V	L	L'	S	S'	O	O'	V_x
Telangiectatic varicose veins	W	L	L'	S	S'	O	O'	W_x
Ligation/ section	X	L	L'	S	S'			X_{nx}

Bibliography :

1. Griton P., Widmer L-K. Classification des varices et de l'insuffisance veineuse.J.Mal.Vasc.,1992, 17, 102-108.
2. Hach W. : Neue aspekte zum spontanverlauf einer stammvarikose der V. saphena magna.Phlebol.Proktol.1988,17, 79-82.
3. Porter & al. : Reporting standards in venous disease.J Vasc.Surg.1988; 8:172-181.
4. In Vin F, Schadeck M : La maladie veineuse superficielle, Ed. Masson, Nov.90.

Phlebology '95, D. Negus et al. (eds.). Phlebology (1995) Suppl. 1: 1071-1072

P155

A Comparison of a Hydrocolloid and a Knitted Viscose Dressing in the Treatment of Arterial Leg Ulcers

B. Gibson[1], D.R. Harper[1], E.A. Nelson[2], R.J. Prescott[3] and C.V. Ruckley[2,3]

Lothian and Forth Valley Leg Ulcer Study, [1] Falkirk and District Royal Infirmary,
[2] Royal Infirmary Edinburgh, [3] University of Edinburgh

INTRODUCTION

There is little evidence on the most effective dressing for ischaemic leg ulcers. Since compression cannot safely be offered, the choice of dressing may be more important [1]. Acute pain is often associated with this type of ulceration and a dressing which reduces patient discomfort is preferable [2].

STUDY DESIGN

As part of a multi-arm trial of dressing type, compression (venous ulcers) and oxpentifylline vs placebo, patients with arterial impairment (ABPI <0.8) were randomised to either hydrocolloid (Improved Formulation Granuflex - Convatec) or N-A (Johnson & Johnson) dressings.

PATIENTS

Twenty two patients with ischaemic leg ulcers were randomised to either H or N-A dressings and crepe bandage in the arterial arm of a larger study of 286 ulcer patients. Written informed consent was obtained.

INTERVENTION

Dressings were changed regularly by specialist nurses and the pain score was recorded at every dressing change according to protocol.

RESULTS

The study was stopped after 22 patients were entered. 100% withdrawal from the N-A group because of pain (after mean of 7 days). 33% withdrawal from H group because of skin maceration, cellulitis or ulcer deterioration. P<0.05.

CONCLUSIONS

Hydrocolloid dressing was superior to N-A dressing in the treatment of chronic leg ulcers in patients with arterial impairment.

REFERENCES

1.   Callam MJ, Ruckley CV, Dale JJ, Harper DR. Hazards of compression treatment of the leg: an estimate from Scottish surgeons. BMJ 1987; 295:1382.

2.   Dale JJ, Gibson B. Treatment of leg ulcers. The Professional Nurse 1986; 9:321-324.

Phlebology '95, D. Negus et al. (eds.). Phlebology (1995) Suppl. 1: 1073-1075

P008

A Rat Cortical Vein Occlusion Model Using Photochemical Dye: A New Technique

H. Nakase, A. Heimann and O. Kempski

Institute for Neurosurgical Pathophysiology, Johannes-Gutenberg University Mainz, Mainz, Germany

INTRODUCTION

The pathophysiological mechanisms responsible for the high variability of symptoms following sinus-vein occlusion observed in patients and experimental animals still remain unclear. Recent experiments on SVT have demonstrated that occlusion of the superior sagittal sinus (SSS) alone is not sufficient to block venous outflow, and that a cerebral venous thrombosis becomes critical for the parenchymal blood supply only if draining cortical veins are occluded [1-6]. These reports, however, could not satisfactorily explain the mechanisms of the inconsistency of symptoms after venous occlusion.

To elucidate these mechanisms, we examined changes of the cerebral venous flow pattern by fluorescence angiography, regional cerebral blood flow (rCBF) and cerebral blood volume fraction (CBVF) assessed by a modern laser Doppler "scanning" technique, and brain damage histologically in a rat cortical vein occlusion model using a photochemical thrombotic technique.

METHODS

Twenty-two male Wistar rats (260-360g) were used. Cortical vein occlusion was induced photochemically by rose bengal and local fiberoptic illumination at 540nm. The procedure of cortical vein occlusion using photochemical dye has been previously reported [7]. rCBF and CBVF were measured by laser Doppler in 15 min intervals for 90 min after occlusion at 48 (8x6) locations using a computer-controlled micromanipulator. Fluorescence angiography was carried out before, 30 and 90 min after venous occlusion. After 48 hours, the rats were submitted to perfusion fixation and examined histologically.

RESULT

Fluorescence angiographic findings could classify animals into 3 groups: (1) Group A, with a changed venous flow pattern after occlusion (n=12); (2) Group B, with an interruption of blood flow and/or a growing venous thrombus (n=5); (3) Group C: sham-operated animals (N=5). Extravasation of fluorescein, a massive decrease of rCBF (after 60, 75 and 90 minutes, P<0.05), a short-lasting increase of CBVF (after 30 minutes, P<0.05) and regional brain damage were typical for group B.

Cortical CBF mapping revealed a transient hyperperfusion zone with hyperemia surrounding a hypoperfused ischemic core in group B (Fig.1).

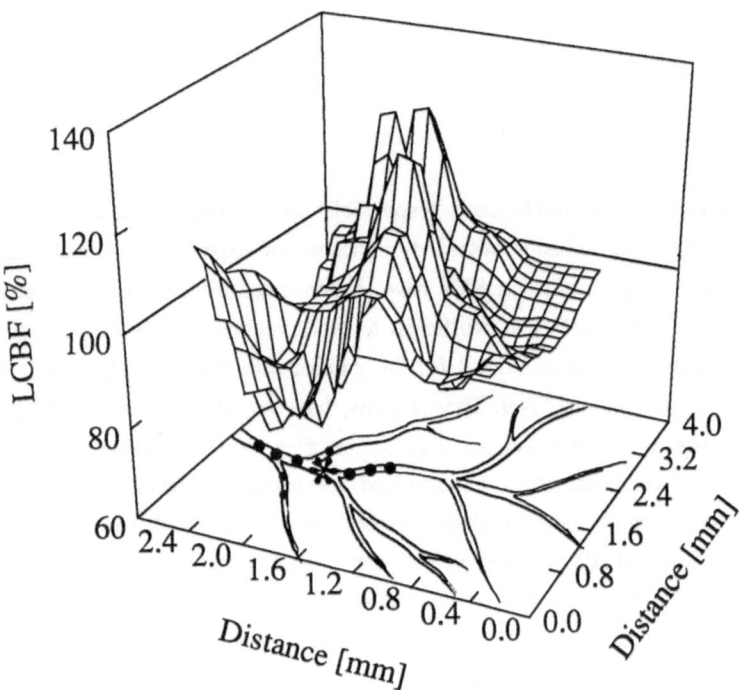

Fig. 1. Graph showing cortical CBF mapping of 30 min after thrombosis induction in a typical experiment (No.6). Data are expressed as percentage change from baseline. The location of the inducted thrombus photochemically is indicated by asterisk. The growing thrombus is indicated by black dots. The mapping reveals a hyperperfusion zone around an area of hypoperfusion. Ninety min after thrombosis induction the thrombus had grown and rCBF had decreased massively below control level in the whole tissue section study (data not shown).

CONCLUSION

The circulation perturbation appears adjacent to cerebral veins without sufficient collateral flow even in the very early period following venous occlusion and results in the further growth of the venous thrombus, local ischemia, and severe brain damage.

This new experimental approach provides a useful tool to examine injury after venous compromise in brain but also in other organs.

REFERENCES

1. Cervos-Navarro J, Kannuki S. Neuropathological findings in the thrombosis of cerebral veins and sinuses - vascular aspects. In: Einhäupl K, Kempski O, Baethmann A, editor. Cerebral Sinus Thrombosis: Experimental and Clinical aspects. New York: Plenum Press,1990:15-26.

2. Frerichs KU, Deckert M, Kempski O, Schurer L, Einhäupl K, Baethmann A. Cerebral sinus and venous thrombosis in rats induces long-term deficits in brain function and morphology - Evidence for a cytotoxic genesis. J Cereb Blood Flow Metab 1994;14:289-300.

3. Fries G, Wallenfang T, Hennen J, Velthaus M, Heimann A, Schild H, et al. Occlusion of the pig superior sagittal sinus, bridging and cortical veins; multistep evolution of sinus-vein thrombosis. J Neurosurg 1992; 77:127-133.

4. Gotoh M, Ohmoto T, Kuyama H. Experimental study of venous circulatory disturbance by dural sinus occlusion. Acta Neurochir (Wien) 1993;124:120-126.

5. Takeshima T, Miyamoto K, Okumura Y, Tominaga M, Tsujimoto S, Sakaki T. Experimental study of local cerebral blood flow in cerebral venous occlusion, In: Tomita M, Mchedlishvili G, Rosenblum WI, Heiss W-D, Fukuuchi Y, editor. Microcirculatory Stasis in the Brain. Amsterdam: Elsevier Science Publishers B.V., 1993, 441-444.

6. Ungersböck K, Heimann A, Kempski O. Cerebral blood flow alterations in a rat model of cerebral sinus thrombosis. Stroke 1993;24:563-570.

7. Nakase H, Kakizaki T, Miyamoto K, Hiramatsu K, Sakaki T. Prediction of brain damage subsequent to venous circulation disturbance by local cerebral blood flow monitoring - Cortical vein occlusion model by photochemical dye. Neurosurgery 1995 (in press)

Phlebology '95, D. Negus et al. (eds.). Phlebology (1995) Suppl. 1: 1076-1078

P009

Cerebral Blood Flow and Tissue Oxygen Saturation Alteration after Sinus-Vein Thrombosis

H. Nakase, A. Heimann and O. Kempski

Institute for Neurosurgical Pathophysiology, Johannes-Gutenberg University Mainz, Mainz, Germany

INTRODUCTION

Sinus-vein thrombosis (SVT) is increasingly recognized as a much more frequent neurological disorder than anticipated before, because it is often overlooked due to the wide spectrum of clinical manifestations: namely the clinical symptoms and prognosis of SVT observed in patients and animal experiments are quite variable, ranging from no symptom to severe venous infarction [2]. However, the mechanisms underlying the high inconsistency of clinical symptoms and prognosis after SVT observed in patients and experiments are currently still unclear and one of the main foci of attention in this field. Recent publications on SVT [1,3-5] demonstrated that the occlusion of the SSS alone doesn't cause brain tissue damage, and that cerebral venous thrombus becomes critical for the parenchymal blood supply only if draining cortical veins are occluded, and still more that increase of CBV and cerebral edema by venous flow obstruction results in intracranial hypertension and decrease rCBF. However, the relationship between the occurrence of ischemia and brain damage after SVT is still poorly defined.

This present investigation was designed to examine the pathophysiological mechanisms after SVT, especially the relationship between ischemia and brain function after SVT. Regional cerebral blood flow (rCBF) were studied by laser Doppler flowmetry and tissue hemoglobin oxygen saturation (Hb SO2) of the brain by a microphotometric scanning technique, the venous flow by fluorescence angiography, and brain damage histologically using a rat SVT model.

METHODS

Twenty-three male Wistar rats (260-370g) were used. SVT was induced by a technique combining sinus ligation and thrombosis induction in the superior sagittal sinus (SSS). We examined the local cerebral blood flow (LCBF) using a laser doppler scanning technique, tissue Hb SO_2 by a microphotometric technique (EMPHO), the venous flow by fluorescence angiography, and brain damage histologically. LCBF and tissue Hb SO_2 were measured at 48 (8x6) identical locations in the right fronto-parietal cortex in a scanning procedure by means of a computer-controlled micromanipulator in 15 minutes intervals for 90 minutes after occlusion. Fluorescence angiography was performed before, 30 and 90 minutes after induction. After operation the rats were returned to individual cages for 48 hours, and they were sacrificed for histology.

RESULT

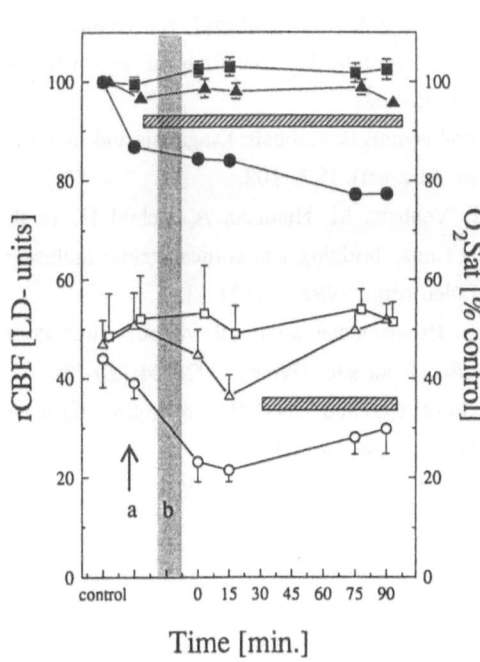

Time [min.]

Fig. 1. Upper: Sequential changes in tissue Hb O_2 saturation (O_2 Sat), expressed in % control (right ordinate, mean ± SEM), in each group. Tissue O_2 Sat of group B significantly decreased from the ligation of SSS to 90 min after injection compared with that of group A (ANOVA for multiple comparison, hatched box: P<0.001). a: Ligation of SSS, b (gray bar): Injection of kaolin-cephalin suspension, ▲ : Group A, ●: Group B, ■: Group C. Lower: Sequential changes in rCBF, expressed in LD-units (left ordinate, mean ± SEM), in each group. In group B, rCBF significantly decreased from 30 min to 90 min after injection compared with that in group A (ANOVA for multiple comparison, hatched box: P<0.01). △: Group A, ○:Group B, □: Group C

According to the pattern of the fluorescence angiographic findings, animals could be divided into 3 groups: (1) Group A, in which the SSS was thrombosed without cortical vein thrombosis (n=8); (2) Group B, which showed a thrombosis of SSS and cortical veins. (n=10); (3) Group C, which is a sham-operated group (n=5).

A massive decrease of LCBF, a decrease of tissue Hb SO2 and severe brain damage were seen in group B. Interestingly, tissue SO2 monitoring was more sensitive to predict the outcome. Animals with thrombosis in cortical veins suffered from a significantly reduced tissue Hb SO2 already after sinus ligation when rCBF reduced only slightly (Fig.1).

CONCLUSION

The venous system of the brain becomes critical for the parenchymal blood supply only if bridging and cortical veins are involved, and brain metabolism disturbance due to severe ischemia mainly causes brain damage after SVT. Also, CBF and tissue Hb SO2 can be helpful monitors for the early detection of critical flow reductions after SVT.

REFERENCES

1. Cervos-Navarro J, Kannuki S. Neuropathological findings in the thrombosis of cerebral veins and sinuses - vascular aspects. In: Einhäupl K, Kempski O, Baethmann A, editor. Cerebral Sinus Thrombosis: Experimental and Clinical aspects. New York: Plenum Press,1990:15-26.
2. Einhäupl KM and Villringer A. Cerebral venous thrombosis: Diagnosis and therapy. In: Microcirculatory stasis in the brain (Abstract). 1993:102.
3. Fries G, Wallenfang T, Hennen J, Velthaus M, Heimann A, Schild H, et al. Occlusion of the pig superior sagittal sinus, bridging and cortical veins; multistep evolution of sinus-vein thrombosis. J Neurosurg 1992; 77:127-133.
4. Gotoh M, Ohmoto T, Kuyama H. Experimental study of venous circulatory disturbance by dural sinus occlusion. Acta Neurochir (Wien) 1993;124:120-126.
5. Ungersböck K, Heimann A, Kempski O. Cerebral blood flow alterations in a rat model of cerebral sinus thrombosis. Stroke 1993;24:563-570.

Phlebology '95, D. Negus et al. (eds.). Phlebology (1995) Suppl. 1: 1079-1081

P015

Tennis Leg Syndrome: Is it an Appropriate Definition?

E. Melillo, M.L. Iabichella, R. Berchiolli, F. Porcelli and M. Ferrari

Medicina Interna, Instituto di Chirurgia Generale e Sperimentale, Azienda Ospedaliera Pisana e Università di Pisa, Pisa, Italy

INTRODUCTION

The Tennis Leg Syndrome (TLS), first described by Martorell[1] in 1955 and defined as "Pedrada" syndrome, is an acute affection characterized by a muscolo-tendinous strain and by the laceration of muscolar veins, sometimes associated with deep vein thrombosis[2].This relatively rare syndrome usually affects apparently healthy young subjects who practice sports like, for istance, tennis (that is why this syndrome has been called TLS) implying springs and sudden stops[3]. The patient usually complains of sudden and acute calf pain followed by a poor leg functionality which may be totally disabling. Its clinical aspect is a swelling calf with edema and hematoma extending to the lower malleolar area.
Although Martorell has stressed an high frequency of deep vein thrombosis associated with TLS, this syndrome usually is a benign one and fully clinical recovery occurs in few weeks.
Aim of this study is the evaluation of the prevalence of TLS among patients suspected to be affected by venous disease; its relationship with patient's lifestyle; the frequency of venous thrombosis complications and the duration of any clinical and or instrumental signs of TLS.

PATIENTS

Between January and December 1993 three male patients aged 38, 58 and 66 were referred to us with suspected leg deep venous thrombosis (1,2% of the total instrumental investigations for suspected venous diseases). All patients complained of a sudden violent monolateral medial calf pain occurred one month before, during daily activities, such as lifting of an heavy item, in the first case, or crossing a road, in the others, followed by swelling and muscolar tension of the calf and, after few days, by malleolar hematoma. All the patients underwent clinical and instrumental evaluation by ultrasound (doppler c. w. and duplex scanner) and pletismography (Light Reflection Reography)
During clinical examination an increased size of the symptomatic calf was observed (compared to the controlateral leg), together with acute palpatory pain and residual malleolar bluish areas.

The patients were treated with prophylactic subcutaneous calcium heparin (15.000 U/a day) for two weeks and bound up with gradient elastic compression for the following (3 to 6) months.

RESULTS

The CW doppler ultrasounds and plethysmographyc investigations did not show any thrombosis nor shortened venous refill time, while the Echo-Doppler demonstrated in all cases a wide medial gemellus hematoma, which did not cause any hemodynamic compression of the main vein trunks (fig. n°1: hematoma pointed by arrow).

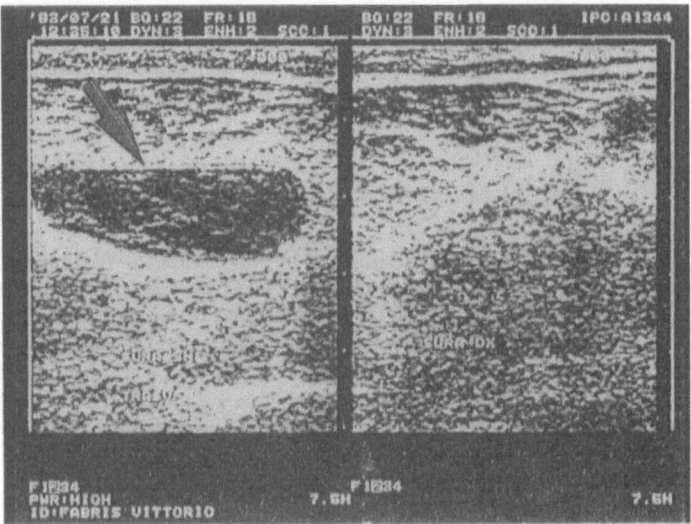

All the patients had a rapid clinical remission, while an echographic follow-up, on the contrary, showed, in two cases, a persistent small hematomas even three months later (fig. n°2: hematoma pointed by arrow).

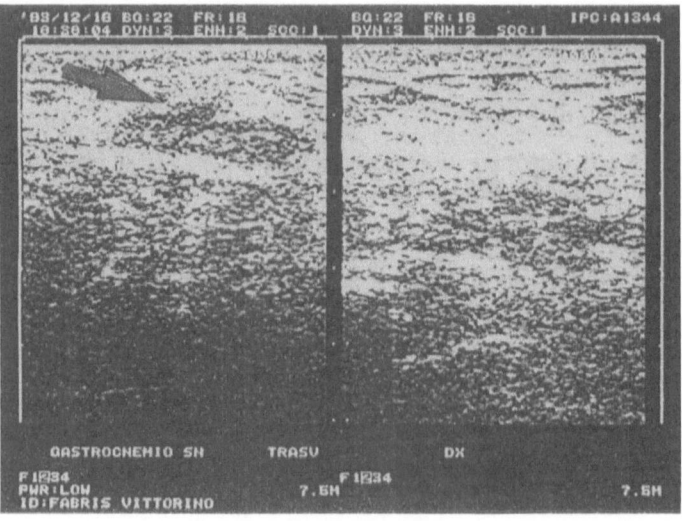

CONCLUSIONS

Our limited experience suggests that, in case of a suspected TLS, only an echographic investigation can confirm this diagnosis and, since this syndrome affects subjects during the perfomance of routine activities, it is rarely diagnosed and its real incidence is probably underestimated. However, since Tennis Leg Syndrome is not only related to young subjects who usually practice sports, we think that it is more appropriate to define it as "Pedrada" syndrome, like Martorell did in his report.

REFERENCES

1) Martorell F.: El sindrome de la pedrada. Angiologia 7, 245-251

2) Lacoste J.: Le coup fe fouet. In Olivier C., Merlen J. F.. Paris 1983: 377-379

3) Goldberg M.J.: A syndrome that is already a syndrome "coup fe fouet" is "tennis leg"?. Angiology 21: 260-264, 1970

Phlebology '95, D. Negus et al. (eds.). Phlebology (1995) Suppl. 1: 1082-1084

P018

Histological Changes in the Kidneys, Testes and Adrenal Glands after Total Ligation of the Left Renal Vein in EPM1-Wistar Rats

J.C.C. Baptista-Silva[1], J.O.P. Medina[2], J.G.H. Vieira[3], M.S. Dolnikoff[4], L.A.R. Moura[5], F. Miranda Jr[1] and E. Burihan[1]

[1] Division of Vascular Surgery, Department of Surgery, [2] Division of Nephrology, [3] Division of Endocrinology, [4] Department of Medicine, Department of Physiology and [5] Department of Pathology, Escola Paulista de Medicina, Universidade Federal de São Paulo, São Paulo, Brazil

INTRODUCTION

Total left renal vein ligation (TLRVL) has been applied during some surgical procedures, as in abdominal aortic aneurysm repair, and there is some controversy about its safety in the renal function[1,2,3,4,5,6]. Perirenal aortic exposure and control can be facilitated by division of the left renal vein (LRV), but only if adequate collateral venous drainage is present. When incremental elevations in LRV pressure were produced in nine dogs, we noted that the left renal glomerular and tubular function (creatinine clearance, sodium retention, urine osmolarity, and urine output) were virtually lost if the pressures is more than 50 to 60 cm water [7]. But the repercussion of the total left renal vein ligation in the testes and adrenal glands in human was not previously described [8].

METHODS

Sixty four mature, male EPM1-WISTAR rats, weighing 264 to 369 g were used, divided into eight groups, eight animals each. Four groups underwent a total left renal vein ligation close to inferior vena cava (ligature groups) and the other four were control groups. The control groups were submitted to the same surgical procedure without TLRVL. The animals were sacrificed at the seventh, 15 th, 30 th, 60 th day after the initial operation. Samples of urine from each animal for proteinuria over 24 h were collected before decapitation. The trunk blood was collected for determination of creatinine, testosterone and corticosterone. The kidneys, testes, and adrenal glands were extracted; weighed, and formalin fixed for histological examination. Changes in renal, testicular, and adrenal glands function as result of total left renal vein ligation were assessed by multiple comparisons of laboratory data (proteinuria; and creatinine, testosterone, corticosterone in serum) of ligature and control groups, and by multivariate analysis of variance. Changes in histological examination were assessed by the Fisher test. In all statistical analysis the level of significance was set to $p < 0.05$.

RESULTS

Histological changes by light microscopy

Ligature groups: *the kidneys* showed severe lesions as tubular atrophy, thickening of the tubular basement membrane, focal and / or diffuse necrosis; *the testes* showed severe lesions as atrophy, fibrosis widening and necrosis with calcification; *the adrenal glands* also showed severe lesions such as atrophy, fibrosis widening, medullar and cortical necrosis. All lesions found in the kidneys, the testes, and the adrenal glands were interpreted as the resulty from a ischemic process, being more intense on the left side.

Control groups: there are no histological lesions.

Only the lesions in the kidneys and testes from the ligature groups were statistically significant by means of the FISHER exact test.(p <0.05).

Biochemical results

The proteinuria; and creatinine, testosterone, corticosterone in serum had theirs values in ligature groups different from control groups, but not above of the normal levels for rats.

DISCUSSION

We have found damage in the kidneys, testes, and adrenal glands only in hystological analysis after the total left renal vein ligation, but the results of biochemical analysis data (proteinuria; and creatinine, testosterone, corticosterone in serum) were not above the normal levels for rats. These findings were discussed elsewhere by other authors [9,10,11,12,13,14], and it proves that only biochemical analysis was not sufficient to demonstrate injury in the kidneys, testes, and adrenal glands [8]. According to some authors the damage in the left kidney by the TLRVL may induce injury in the right kidney mediated by immune-complex deposit [9,12].

For a better approach to the abdominal aorta a mobilization of the left renal vein may be used by the ligation of its tributaries as the renal lumbar, and the gonadal, and the adrenal veins, this technique allows mobilization of the left renal vein 6 to 7 cm cephalad [15]; or the retroperitoneal incision and retracts upward to the right of the left kidney [16]; or partial extraperitoneal mobilization of left-sided viscera including kidney, or aortic exposure afforded by a medial rotation including the left kidney, or aortic exposure achieved by medial rotation in plane between pancreas and kidney [17]. When these techniques above were impossible and had to divide the left renal vein, it must be reanastomosed after the end of the aortic operations to prevent injury in the left kidney(18).

CONCLUSION

We concluded that the ligation of the left renal vein in EPM1-WISTAR rats is a procedure of high risk to the kidneys, the testes and the adrenal glands, and by analogy it should be avoided in human.

1084

REFERENCES

1.   Brener BJ, Darling RC, Frederick PL, Linton RR. Major venous anomalies complicating abdominal aortic surgery. Arch Surg 1974;108:159-65.
2.   James EC, Fedde CW, Khuri NT, Gillespie JT. Division of the left renal vein: A safe surgical adjunct. Surgery 1978;83:151-4.
3.   Devine TJ, Scott DF, Myers KA, King RB. Massive hemorrhage caused by left renal vein ligation. Br J Surg 1980;67:594-5.
4.   Johnston KW. Basis for technically difficult decisions in abdominal aortic aneurysm repair. In: Veith FJ, editor. Current critical problems in vascular surgery. Saint Louis, Quality Medical Publishing, 1989:281-3.
5.   Dearing PD, James EC, Siegel MB, Swenson WM, Slotnick HB, Schmidt MJ. Further experience with division of the left renal vein. Surgery 1990;107:105-9.
6.   Aburahma AF, Robinson PA, Boland JP, Lucente FC. The risk of ligation of the left renal vein in resection of the abdominal aortic aneurysm. Surg Gynecol Obstet 1991;173:33-6.
7.   Calligaro KD, Savarese RP, McCombs PR, DeLaurentis DA. Division of the left renal vein during aortic surgery. Am J Surg 1990;160:192-6.
8.   Baptista-Silva JCC. Ligadura da veia renal esquerda em ratos EPM1-Wistar: complicações renais, testiculares e das glândulas supra-renais. Tese de doutoramento. Escola Paulista de Medicina, Universidade Federal de São Paulo, 1994.
9.   Omae T, Masson MC, Corcoran AC. Experimental production of nephrotic syndrome following renal vein constriction in rats. Proc Soc Exper Biol Med 1958;97:821-5..
10. Siderys H, Kilman J W. The effects of acute occlusion of the renal vein in dogs. Surgery 1966;59:282-5.
11. Fisher ER., Sharkey D, Pardo V, Vuzevski V. Experimental renal vein constriction. Lab Invest 1968;18(6):689-99..
12. Harris JD, Ehrenfeld WK, Lee JC, Wylie EJ. Experimental renal vein occlusion. Surg Gynecol Obstet 1968;126:555-62.
13. González-Avila G, Vadillo-Ortega F, Perez-Tamayo R. Experimental diffuse interstitial renal fibrosis. A biochemical approach. Lab Invest 1988;59(2):245-52.
14. Stanley JC. Renal revascularization: Errors in patient selection and complications of operation. In: Bernhard VM, Towne JB, editors. Complications in vascular surgery. Saint Louis, Quality Medical Publishing, 1991:180-203.
15. Cooley DA, Wukasch DC. Aneurysms of the abdominal aorta. In: Cooley DA, Wukasch DC, editors. Techniques in vascular surgery. Philadelphia, Saunders, 1979:54-68.
16. Crawford ES, Crawford JL. Aneurysms of Degenerative Origin. In: Crawford ES, Crawford JL, editors. Diseases of the aorta. Baltimore, Williams & Wilkins, 1984:1-166.
17. Stoney RJ, Matsumoto K. Transabdominal exposures of the upper abdominal aorta: techniques and strategies. In: Veith FJ, editor. Current critical problems in vascular surgery. Saint Louis, Quality Medical Publishing, 1989:275-80.
18. Ristow A, Abreu RC, Bonamigo TP, Burihan E, Cinelli Jr, M. Complicações precoces e tardias das restaurações arteriais aorto-ilíacas. In: Bonamigo TP, Burihan E, Cinelli Jr M, Von Ristow A, editors. Doenças da aorta e seus ramos. São Paulo, Fundo Editorial Byk, 1993:362-82.

Phlebology '95, D. Negus et al. (eds.). Phlebology (1995) Suppl. 1: 1085-1087

P019

Anatomical Study of the Renal Veins and Its Variations Observed During Living Donor Nephrectomy

J.C.C. Baptista-Silva[1,2,3], J.O.P. Medina[1,3] and E. Burihan[3]

[1] Centro Hospitalar Dom Silvério Gomes Pimenta, [2] Beneficência Portuguesa, and [3], Escola Paulista de Medicina, Universidade Federal de São Paulo, São Paulo, Brazil

INTRODUCTION

It is very important to know the anatomy of the renal vessels during retroperitoneal approach to prevent bleeding by accidental tearing [1,2,3]. Comparably, the renal venous pattern of the right side bears little resemblance to that of the left. In its relatively short course from the kidney to the inferior vena cava, the right vein rarely receives a tributary vein. The longer left renal vein (LRV), on the contrary, regularly receives the following tributaries: adrenal and inferior phrenic, from above, frequently by a common; gonadal (testicular or ovarian) below; and lumbar renal vein posteriorly, often by confluent with the gonadal vein [4,5,6]. During the nephrectomy in a living donor the left kidney is more used as a donor organ due that its vein is longer than the right renal vein.

Usually the LRV crosses anteriorly the aorta before reaching the vena cava.

METHODS

Throughout the last four years, 219 living donor nephrectomies (197 were on the left side) have been performed at Dom Silvério Gomes Pimenta and Beneficência Portuguesa Hospitals. The 136 cases were female and 83 male, white were 83%. The mean age was 40,3 years. We have studied preoperative renal angiography and intraoperative observation of all cases.

RESULTS

On the left side

We encountered in 197 cases which were submitted to the left nephrectomy: *a:* 122 left renal veins (61,92%) had three or more major tributaries as one adrenal, one gonadal and one or more lumbar renal veins; but three cases had the retroaortic renal vein; *b:* 75 left renal veins (38,07%) had only two tributaries as one adrenal and one gonadal veins; but two cases had the duplication of inferior vena cava (DIVC) (Table 1).

On the right side

We encountered in 22 cases which were submitted to the right nephrectomy: *a:* 12 cases had only one renal vein ; *b:* 10 cases had with two renal veins (Table 1).

Table 1. Results of the 219 living donor nephrectomies showed the variations of the renal veins and its tributaries. (G= gonadal vein, A= adrenal vein, L= lumbar renal vein, DIVC= duplication of the inferior vena cava, RLRV= retroaortic left renal vein)

VEINS		RIGTH SIDE	LEFT SIDE
One renal vein		12	197
Two renal veins		10	0
Tributaries of renal vein	two (G+A)	0	75
	three or more (G+A+L)	0	122
RLRV		0	3
DIVC		0	02

DISCUSSION

We have found that the left renal vein receives always two tributaries as the adrenal vein cranially and the gonadal vein (testicular or ovarian veins) caudally; and usually one or more lumbar renal veins in 61,92 per cent of cases, Lejars [7] encountered it in 88 per cent and Yang et al [2] in 60.8 per cent.

We have observed that the lumbar renal vein may be one or multiple and has many variations in its diameter and the local that reaches the left renal vein. Usually it reaches the LRV close to the gonadal vein, also observed by other autors [2,4,5,6].

We observed on the left side when there is more than one renal artery in angiography it is more common to find in surgery more than one renal vein on the right side. It is clear that the left renal vein curving caudally in preoperative angiography, strongly suggests that its course is retroaortic [2].

CONCLUSION

We conclude that there are many anatomical variations in the renal veins, and these must be aware in our mind to prevent bleeding by accidental lesion of them when operating on these particular regions.

REFERENCES

1. Wylie EJ. Discussion. In: Najarian JS, Delaney JP. Vascular surgery. Chicago, Symposia Specialists, 1978:405-14.
2. Yang SC, Suh DH, Kim YS, Park K. Anatomical study of left renal vein and its draining veins, as encountered during living donor nephrectomy. Transplant Proc 1992;24(4):1333-4.
3. Cooley DA, Wukaschi DC. Aneurysms of the abdominal aorta. In: Cooley DA, Wukaschi DC, editors. Tecniques in vascular surgery. Philadelphia: Saunders, 1979:54-68.
4. Anson BJ, Cauldwell EW, Pick JW, Beaton LE. The anatomy of the pararenal system of veins, with comments on the renal arteries. J Urol, 1948;60:714-37.
5. Latorre J. Embriología. In: Villallonga JT, editor. Sector iliocava. Barcelona: Uriach, 1993:17-23.
6. Latorre J. Anatomía Y Fisiología. In: Villallonga JT, editor. Sector Iliocava. Barcelona: Uriach, 1993:37-66.
7. Lejars F. Les voies de surete de la veine renale. Bull Soc Anat (Paris) 1888;63:504-11.

Phlebology '95, D. Negus et al. (eds.). Phlebology (1995) Suppl. 1: 1088-1090

P026

Is Chronic Pancreatitis Source of Portal Hypertension

M. Ruzicka, P. Dite, L. Veverkova and D. Konecna

Surgical Clinic, University Hospital, Brno - Bohunice
3rd Med./Gastroenterol. Dept., University Hospital, Brno - Bohunice
1st Surgical Clinic, University Hospital, Brno, Pekarska 53

INTRODUCTION

The portal vein (PV) is formed from the union of two main tributaries - splenic vein (SV) and superior mesenteric vein (SMV). The place of the union lies on the posterior surface of the body of the pancreas, where both veins make a 90-degree angle to form the portal vein.

Close proximity of the PV, SMV and SV to the pancreas leads to entrapment of the veins by the pancreatic and peripancreatic fibrosis which is characteristic for all four types of chronic pancreatitis. Rarely this inflammation process may extend into the venous wall and cause secondary thrombosis, mostly of the splenic vein.

In the treatment of chronic pancreatitis we prefare duodenum sparing resection of the head of the pancreas. The result of this procedure is releasing of the stenosis of the common bile duct, duodenum and portal vein from adjacent inflammatory process and thus from compression.

The goal of our investigation was to discover if venous involvement by inflammatory process is so severe that can cause portal hypertension.

MATERIAL AND METHODES

70 patients were operated on by our team since 1985 because of CHP.

Following procedures were done:

Duodenum sparing resection of the pancreatic head   37
Hemipancreatoduodenectomy   18
80% distal pancreatectomy   2
Resection of the middle segment of the pancreas   2
Pancreaticojejunoanastomosis (Partington-Rochelle)   10
Pancreaticoduodenoanastomosis   1

The measurement of pressure in the superior mesenteric vein (SMV) was done in last 10 patients. Plastic needle was inserted into the vein before and after resection of the pancreatic head and direct measurement of the venous preassure was done.

Fig. 1
The arrow showes the point where the needle was introduced

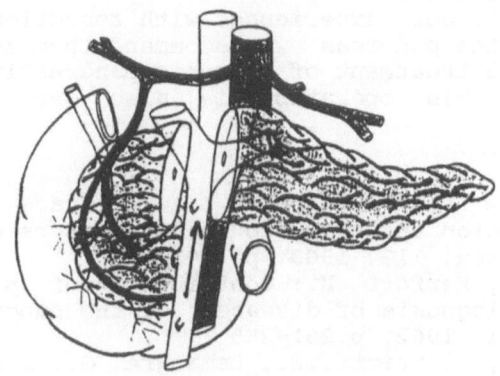

Table 1. Comparison of the pressures in the SMV before and after the resection of the pancreatic head

	mm Hg	mm Hg
1.	5	1
2.	12	5
3.	9	7
4.	22	10
5.	23	7
6.	12	8
7.	15	7
8.	10	6
9.	21	10
10.	20	10

Normal value of the pressure in the portal vein is aproximately 6 mm Hg.
The venous pressure was lower after resection of the head of the pancreas in all 10 patients but in some of them remains higher then normal value. It can be caused by cirrhosis of the liver.

RESULTS
Indications to the resection of the head of the pancreas in patients suffering of CHP are usually:
- intractable abdominal pain
- stenosis of the duodenum
- stenosis of the common bile duct
Resection procedures of the head of the pancreas have very good results and all patients lost the pain. Problems with digestion caused by exocrine pancreatic insufficiency are managed by oral enzyme substitution.

DISCUSSION

It seems that high pressure in the portal vein and superior mesenteric vein is another symptom related to the chronic pancreatitis causing subjective problems of the patient.

It's in accordance with comparison of results of decompression pancreaticojejunoanastomosis and resection procedures of the pancreatic head. Good long termed results of the first one are in 40-60%, of the second in 90-95% of operated patients.

On the base of our experiences with resection procedures of the head of the pancreas we recommend them as procedures of choice in the treatment of chronic pancreatitis. One of the results of this operation is also decompression of the portal vein.

REFERENCES

1. Varriale P., Bonnano C,A., Grace W.J.: Portal hypertension secondary to pancreatic pseudocysts. Arch. Intern. Med. 112, 1963, p. 191-198.
2. Rosch J., Herfort K.: Contribution of splenoportography of the diagnosis of diseases of the pancreas. Acta Med. Scand.171, 1962, p.251-255
3. Leger L., lenriot J.P., Lemaigre G.: L'hypertension et la stase portales segmentaires dans les pancreatites chroniques: A propos de 126 cas examines par splenoportographe et spleno-manometrie. J.Chir.(Paris) 95, 1968, p.599-608.
4. Rignault D., Mire J., Moine D.: Splenoportograhpic changes in chronic pancreatitis. Surgery 63, 1968, p.571-575.
5. McDermott W.V.: Portal hypertension secondary to pancreatic disease. Ann. Surg.1525, 1960, p. 147-149.
6. Burbige E.J., Tarder G., Carson S. et al: A complication of pancreatitis with splenic vein thrombosis. Am. J. Digest. Dis. 23, 1978, p.752-755.
7. Bradley E.L.: The natural history of splenic vein thrombosis due to chronic pancreatitis: Indications for surgery. Int. J. Pancreatol. 2, 1987, p.87-92.
8. Little A.G., Moossa A.R.: Gastrointestinal hemorrhage from leftsided portal hypertension: An unappreciated complication of pancreatitis. Am. J. Surg. 141, 1981, p.153-158.
9. Warshaw A.L., Jin G., Ottinger L.W.: Recognition and clinical implications of mesenteric and portal vein obstruction in chronic pancreatitis. Arch. Surg. 122, 1987, p. 410-415.
10. McElroy R., Christiansen P.A.: Hereditary pancreatitis in a kinship with portal vein thrombosis. Am.J.Med. 52, 1972, p.228-241.
11. Alwmark K., Gullstrand P., Ihse I. et al: Regional portal hypertension in chronic pancreatitis. Acta Chir.Scand. 147, 1981, p.155-157.

P275

CLIVILIAN INFERIOR VENA CAVA INJURIES

Naga R, Molokhia F, Hamza M

Department of Vascular Surgery, Faculty of Medicine Alexandria University Eygpt

Objective: To evaluate the outcome of the different methods of management of inferior vena cava injury
Design: Retrospective review of a consecutive series.
Patients: 39 case of major inferior vena cava injuries. 22 iatrogenic and 17 due to abdominal trauma. In 17 cases there was an associated organ injury.
Intervention: All cases were explored for surgical repair of the IVC. Different manoeuvres were used for control of IVC blood flow.
Measurements: Early and late morbidity were clinically evaluated in terms of manifestations of venous outflow impairment from the lower limbs.
Results: Lateral caval sutures gave excellent results. Caval ligation was followed by accepted morbidity.
Conclusions: Trial for IVC reconstruction is mandatory after iatrogenic injury. IVC exploration should be a part of exploratory laparotomy after blunt abdominal trauma.

Satellite Symposia

Satellite Symposia

SERVIER
Medical and socio-economic impact of venolymphatic disease: benefit of Daflon 500 mg

Phlebology '95, D. Negus et al. (eds.). Phlebology (1995) Suppl. 1: 1095-1097

Chronic Venous Insufficiency - Well Known Disorder(s) With Many Questionmarks!

Lars Norgren

Professor of Vascular Surgery, Lund University, S 221 85 Lund, Sweden

By definition chronic venous insufficiency of the legs (CVI) is a condition with an ambulatory venous hypertension, involving either the superficial vein system alone or the deep and the superficial systems together. The definition of CVI claims that skin changes should be present. It has, however been advocated to classify all non-acute venous pathology of the lower limb as CVI, also including all kinds of symptomatic varicose veins, not only those with skin changes, excluding only the cosmetic ones. For several reasons this seems relevant, as it reduces the problem to find a cut off point between "advanced" varicose veins and chronic venous insufficiency.

CVI is a common condition in great parts of the world, with a prevalence of 30 - 50 % if varicose veins are counted (1). Advancing age and female sex increase the prevalence.

One may ask why CVI is that common, and despite a lot of theories many questions still remain open. One important point may be mankind's upright position, which makes the resting venous pressure high in the target part of the body, the lower leg and the foot.

Many predisposing factors have been proposed, such as heredity, previous pregnancies, standing work, obesity, however few of them have been proven (2).

Also pathophysiology is partly unclear. It seems evident that a continuous venous hypertension may distend the veins, which prevents the valves from closing efficiently. Thereby a reflux occurs, which in turn increases the distension of the veins. If a deep vein thrombosis is present it is understandable that the venous return is prevented, which influences both perforating and superficial veins. After recanalization the valvular function is destroyed, which causes reflux. About 15 % of all cases suffering from deep vein disease do not have a postthrombotic, but a primary deep vein incompetence, the pathophysiology being unexplained.

The question how varicose veins develop is not sufficiently explained either. Apparently not all saphenous varicose veins start from the sapheno-femoral junction, some might develop from vein wall weakness and valvular dysfunction in other parts of the main stems.

The muscle pumps are of the greatest importance, as weakness may precipitate valvular dysfunction, while good muscle forces may compensate and prevent from symptoms of reflux. Another less well understood fact is the finding of incompetent perforating veins in cases with exclusively superficial venous insufficiency, which should imply that the superficial venous hypertension is transmitted to the perforators, dilating them to a level where the valves start to leak. The role of perforator incompetence in case of deep vein disease has been studied, and there is some evidence that surgical treatment of the perforators may not be necessary. When there is little relief of the ambulatory venous hypertension, the microcirculation is severely afficiated, and skin changes and ulcers may occur. Formerly it was understood that a deep vein incompetence necessarily had to be present before an ulcer could develop. Recent studies have, however, shown that a superficial venous hypertension may cause up to 30 - 40 % of all venous ulcers (3).

Symptoms and signs

Varicose veins should be a common denominator in CVI, and if accepting all from telangiectasiae and reticular veins as varicose veins it may be so, but evident varicose veins are not present in a considerable number of patients seeking advice for swelling, leg tiredness and other, less well defined sensations in the legs.

More severe signs, such as skin changes and ulcers are often simple to diagnose, but there is evidence that many patients with these severe problems do not consult the medical profession. There may also be problems in differentiating between various ulcer etiologies, and care must particularly be taken not to misjudge an ischemic, arterial ulcer.

Diagnosis

Details of the diagnostic procedures fall outside this topic, but it has to be stated that a clinical examination alone is insufficient in most cases of CVI, as it does not reveal the functional status of the venous system or of the muscle pumps. A simple Doppler examination, performed as part of the clinical examination helps considerably. More detailed investigations with duplex scanning and plethysmographic examinations are advised in most cases with CVI. A careful examination is the only way to give an appropriate and individualized treatment to each patient.

Treatment

It is disappointing to find that such a common disorder as CVI is stepmotherly treated. One reason may be that the pathophysiology is not well understood, another that the disorder is not linked with mortality, and simpler cases not even with disability. However, prevention of disabling symptoms such as severe swelling and ulcer development by an adequate treatment is naturally as desirable as treatment of the obvious signs, varicose veins and ulcers.

Too much varicose vein surgery has been performed during the years! Removal of a competent long saphenous vein in a case of local varicose veins is not acceptable, as the vein may be of great importance as an arterial conduit in the future. Partial removal of incompetent parts of saphenous veins are possible after careful instrumental investigation.

Also a graduated compression treatment can be almost as helpful and as effective as surgery in some cases.

Compression treatment in case of deep vein incompetence is a must, but still this is not very well performed.

Surgical correction of deep vein incompetence and obstruction is still under development, despite years of trial and error, the results are far from those achieved in arterial surgery. Drugs to treat symptoms of CVI are used with great variations over the world. There are presently too few studies to clearly validate the efficacy of drugs for healing of ulcers, while some studies point at beneficial effects on symptoms such as edema.

Comments

There are more areas to explore than there is full evidence concerning both pathophysiology and treatments in chronic venous insufficiency.

From a surgical point of view the role of the incompetent perforators has to be studied, as well as new ways have to be tried to handle the deep vein incompetence.

The place for pharmacotherapy has to be established, which is only possible if controlled randomised studies with strict protocols are used with a sufficient number of patients included. Training of the medical profession to use compression adequately, to give appropriate advice concerning physical activity etc. are also goals which have to be reached.

References

1. Widmer LK (ed.). Peripheral venous disorders - prevalence and sociomedical importance. Hans Huber, Bern 1978;1-90.
2. Evans CJ, Fowkes FGR, Hajivassiliou CA, Harper DR, Ruckley CV. Epidemiology of varicose veins. Inter Angio 1994;13:263-270.
3. Nelzén O, Bergqvist D, Lindhagen A. Prevalence of leg ulcers in a population of industry workers. Abstract at Eur Congr Int Union Phlebology, Budapest 1993. Abstract Book p. 29.

Phlebology '95, D. Negus et al. (eds.). Phlebology (1995) Suppl. 1: 1098-1100

Microcirculation Changes in Venous Disease: An Update

A. Bollinger, A.J. Leu and U.K. Franzeck

Department of Internal Medicine, Angiology Division, University Hospital, CH-8091 Zürich, Switzerland

Microangiopathy of blood capillaries in the skin of patients with chronic venous insufficiency (CVI) may be assessed by intravital capillaroscopy (6) and in a more sophisticated way by fluorescence videomicroscopy (2,4,8). Meandering capillary convolutes at the lower leg in regions with trophic changes are detected by conventional capillary microscopy without the use of fluorescent dyes. After intravital bolus injection of Na-fluorescein non-perfused capillaries (microvascular thrombosis) are identified and the perivascular compartments ("halos") visualized (2,9,10).

Typically there is a patchy distribution of microvascular changes. Areas with normal numbers of perfused microvessels may be adjacent to regions with a markedly reduced capillary number (4,7). In the extreme situation (atrophie blanche) there are areas without perfused capillaries.

The enlarged and tortuous microvessels are embedded in pericapillary halos of increased size (8). In severe CVI mean halo diameters were 146 ± 47 µm, in healthy controls 81 ± 15 µm ($p < 0.001$). The distances between the halo borders are decreased in CVI causing a "cobble stone" aspect. Micropuncture of halos (6) results in evacuation of pericapillary edema. Transcapillary diffusion which is measured by fluorescence videomicroscopy and densitometry, is increased in patients with CVI, provided that there is no rarefaction of capillary loops (2).

Normally, the superficial lymphatic capillary network of the skin is regular. In severe CVI some regions of the network are interrupted by obliterations (3). There may even be areas without lymphatic capillaries which are visualized by almost atraumatic fluorescence microlymphography (subepidermal injection of 0.01 - 0.05 ml FITC-dextran 150'000). The **lymphatic microangiopathy** just described may result from repeated infections (ulcers), but is also observed in other skin regions. Enhanced permeability of microlymphatics often develops with increased amounts of the fluorescent dye leaving the intravascular compartment and re-entering the interstitial space.

Skin blood flow may be evaluated by **laser Doppler fluxmetry** in arbitrary units. Hyperperfusion is found in skin sites with CVI changes (1,9,10). In contrast to these findings **transcutaneous oxygen tension** (tc PO_2) is reduced in CVI (7,12,13). The decrease is correlated to the number of perfused capillaries. The lower the number becomes the lower are the tc PO_2 values. With a special window probe allowing combination of capillaroscopy and tc PO_2 measurements it was found that tc PO_2 approaches zero values in atrophie blanche spots (7). The reduced number of perfused capillaries is probably due to microvascular thrombosis which may be promoted by leucocyte plugging (5,14).

The apparent paradox of increased laser Doppler flux and decreased tc PO_2 is probably due to the different sampling areas of the two techniques of measurement. Whereas flux is determined mainly in deeper skin layers, oxygen diffuses through the skin mainly from the superficial nutritive capillaries. Hyperperfusion in deeper skin which may be due to shunt flow, does not exclude ischemia in the most superficial parts. Indeed, it may be postulated on the basis of the objective findings reviewed that patchy microvascular ischemia resulting from reduced capillary numbers is the main cause for venous ulcer formation (2,10,11).

REFERENCES

1. Belcaro G, Christopoulos D, Nicolaides AN. Skin flow and swelling in post-phlebitic limbs. Vasa 1989;18:136-9.
2. Bollinger A, Fagrell B. Clinical capillaroscopy. A guide to its use in clinical research and practice. Toronto, Lewiston NY, Bern, Göttingen, Stuttgart: Hogrefe and Huber, 1990.
3. Bollinger A, Isenring G, Franzeck UK. Lymphatic microangiopathy: a complication of severe chronic venous incompetence (CVI). Lymphology 1982;15(2):60-5.
4. Bollinger A, Jäger K, Geser A, Sgier F, Seglias J. Transcapillary and interstitial diffusion of Na-fluorescein in chronic venous insufficiency with white atrophy. Int J Microcirc: Clin Exp 1982;1:5-17.
5. Cheatle TR, Sarin S, Coleridge Smith PD, Scurr JH. The pathogenesis of skin damage in venous disease: a review. Eur J Vasc Surg 1991;5:115-23.
6. Fagrell B. Microcirculatory disturbances - the final cause for venous leg ulcers? Vasa 1982;11:101-3.
7. Franzeck UK, Bollinger A, Huch R, Huch A. Transcutaneous oxygen tension and capillary morphologic characteristics and density in patients with chronic venous incompetence (CVI). Circulation 1984;70:806-11.
8. Haselbach P, Vollenweider U, Moneta G, Bollinger A. Microangiopathy in severe chronic venous insufficiency evaluated by fluorescence videomicroscopy. Phlebology 1986;1:159-69.
9. Leu AJ, Yanar A, Geiger M, Pfister G, Franzeck UK, Bollinger A. Mikroangiopathie bei chronischer venöser Insuffizienz. Dtsch Med Wschr 1991;116:447-51.
10. Leu AJ, Yanar A, Geiger M, Franzeck UK, Bollinger A. Microangiopathy in chronic venous insufficiency before and after sclerotherapy and compression treatment: Results of a one-year follow-up study. Phlebology 1993;8:99-106.
11. Leu HJ. Morphology of chronic venous insufficiency - light and electron microscopic examinations. Vasa 1991;20:330-41.

12. Mannarino E, Pasqualini L, Maragoni G, Sanchini R, Regni O, Innocente S. Chronic venous incompetence and transcutaneous oxygen pressure: a controlled study. Vasa 1988;17(3):59-62.
13. Neumann HAM, van Leeuwen M, van den Broek MJTB, Berretty PJM. Transcutaneous oxygen tension in chronic venous insufficiency syndrome. Vasa 1984;13:213-9.
14. Scott HJ, Coleridge Smith PD, Scurr JH. Histological study of white blood cells and their association with lipodermatosclerosis and venous ulceration. Br J Surg 1991;78:210-11.

Phlebology '95, D. Negus et al. (eds.). Phlebology (1995) Suppl. 1: 1101-1103

Microvascular Reactivity after Ischemia/Reperfusion in the Hamster Cheek Pouch. Beneficial Effects of Different Oral Doses of S 5682 (Daflon 500 mg)

E. Bouskela

Laboratório de Pesquisas em Microcirculação, Universidade do Estado do Rio de Janeiro, Rua São Francisco Xavier, 524, 20550-013 Rio de Janeiro RJ, Brazil

INTRODUCTION

Ischemia followed by reperfusion is characterized by sequestration of leukocytes within the microvasculature of ischemic tissues and organs where they interact with the microvascular endothelium and aggravate the extent of the reperfusion injury. This phenomenon has been demonstrated in various tissues and organs including the hamster cheek pouch.

Previous experiments in our laboratory, using the hamster cheek pouch preparation, have shown that in animals treated orally for 10 days with S 5682, 20 mg/kg body weight/day, the permeability increase (measured as number of leaks per cm^2) and the number of adhering leukocytes (measured per 6 mm^2), after reperfusion after 30 min total ischemia, are significantly reduced compared to placebo-treated animals.

The objectives of this study were to determine if (1) S 5682 also improved the microvascular reactivity and functional capillary density during reperfusion after 90 min total ischemia compared to placebo-treated animals and (2) there is a dose-dependent relationship.

MATERIAL AND METHODS

Male hamsters (Mesocricetus auratus, Engle Labs Farmersburg, Indianapolis, USA) were treated for 10 days, twice a day, with different doses (5, 20, 80 and 160 mg/kg body weight/day) of S 5682, suspended in 0.2 ml of 10% lactose solution. Placebo-treated animals were also tested and handled in the same way.

Microvascular reactivity

Experiments were performed on arterioles and venules of the cheek pouch of 7 to 10 weeks old hamsters. Anesthesia of the animals was induced by an intraperitoneal injection of 0.1-0.2 ml of sodium pentobarbital, 60 mg/ml and maintained with α-chloralose administered through the femoral vein. The femoral artery was also cannulated for pressure measurements. Throughout the surgery and subsequent experiment, the temperature of the animals was kept at 37.5°C with a heating pad controlled by a rectal thermistor. A tracheal tube was inserted to facilitate spontaneous breathing. The preparations were dissected by the method of Duling (1) modified by Bouskela and Grampp (2) and mounted in the experimental chamber where they continuously superfused with a HEPES-supported HCO_3^--buffered saline solution at 36.5°C, pH set to 7.40 by bubbling the solution continuously with 5% CO_2-95% N_2. Local ischemia was obtained by a cuff which was mounted around the neck of the everted pouch where it leaves the mouth of the hamster (3). For measurements of arteriolar and venular internal diameters with an image shearing monitor, IPM model 907, the preparations were placed under an intravital microscope coupled to a close circuit TV system. Red blood cell (RBC) velocity was measured continuously by the dual-slit photometric technique (4). Microvessel volume flow was calculated from the recorded diameters and RBC velocities using an analog circuit. These variables were recorded at the onset of reperfusion, 10, 20, 30, 45 and 60 min thereafter in a six-channel stripchart recorder (Grass polygraph model RCS7C8).

Functional capillary density (FCD)

Defined as the length of the red blood cell-perfused capillaries per observation field (5), it was assessed in one to three different sites (each site = 1 mm²) within the observation area and determined in control conditions, at the onset of reperfusion, 10, 20, 30, 45 and 60 min thereafter.

RESULTS

No significant changes in mean arterial pressure could be detected in any of the groups studied.

During reperfusion, placebo-treated animals showed (1) an increase in venular (30%) and arteriolar (45%) diameters; (2) a decrease in venular (45%) and arteriolar (40%) flows and (3) a decrease in FCD (50%) throughout the observation period. In animals treated with 5 mg/kg body weight/day S 5682 we observed (1) an increase in venular (20%) and arteriolar (30%) diameters which lasted for 30 min; (2) a decrease in venular (30%) and arteriolar (30%) flows and (3) a reduction in FCD (30%) throughout the observation period. In animals treated with 20 mg/kg body weight/day S 5682 we observed (1) no change in venular and arteriolar diameters; (2) a reduction in venular (30%) and arteriolar (30%) flows and (3) a reduction in FCD (25%) throughout the observation period. In animals treated with 80 mg/kg body weight/day we observed (1) no change in venular and arteriolar diameters; (2) a decrease in venular (20%) and arteriolar (15%) flows and (3) a reduction in FCD (20%) throughout the observation period. In animals treated with 160 mg/kg body weight/day we observed (1) no change in venular and arteriolar diameters; (2) a decrease in venular (20%) and arteriolar (15%) flows and (3) a reduction in FCD (20%) throughout the observation period.

CONCLUSION

During reperfusion, placebo-treated animals showed a vasodilation and a significant decrease in blood flow and FCD compared with pre-ischemic values, with an impairment of the myogenic response. S 5682 improved, in a dose-dependent fashion, all the parameters measured including the myogenic tonus.

REFERENCES

1. Duling BR. The preparation and use of the hamster cheek pouch for studies of the microcirculation. Microvasc Res 1973;5(3):423-429.
2. Bouskela E and Grampp W. Spontaneous vasomotion in hamster cheek pouch arterioles in varying experimental conditions. Am J Physiol 1992;262(Heart Circ Physiol 31):H478-H485.
3. Persson NH, Erlansson M, Svensjö E, Takolander R and Berqvist D. The hamster cheek pouch - an experimental model to study postischemic macromolecular permeability. Int J Microcirc: Clin Exp 1985;4:257-263.
4. Wayland H and Johnson PC. Erythrocyte velocity measurement in microvessel by a two-slit photometric method. J Appl Physiol 1967;22:333-337.
5. Nolte D, Lehr H-A, Sack F-U and Meßmer K. Reduction of postischemic reperfusion injury by the vasoactive drug buflomedil. Blood Vessel 1991;28:8-14.

Phlebology '95, D. Negus et al. (eds.). Phlebology (1995) Suppl. 1: 1104-1106

Assessing Quality of Life (QOL) in Venous Diseases of the Lower Limbs

D. L. Lamping

Health Services Research Unit, London School of Hygine & Tropical Medicine, London, UK

INTRODUCTION

This paper reviews methods for assessing quality of life (QOL) in venous diseases of the lower limbs and summarizes research findings regarding venous disease-related QOL.

QOL IN VENOUS DISEASE: ASSESSMENT METHODS

Comprehensive assessment of QOL in venous diseases of the lower limbs includes an evaluation of clinical (objective symptoms and functional signs) and psychosocial (interference with activities of daily living, functional limitations, psychological impact, social consequences) outcomes. QOL in venous disease has been evaluated using standardized generic measures developed for use across different patient populations and applied to patients with venous disease, and disease-specific measures, developed specifically for use in venous disease. One generic measure, the SF-36, and three disease-specific measures have been used to assess QOL in venous disease.

Generic QOL Measures

The SF-36 has been used to assess quality of life in venous disease in two studies in the UK, both for use with patients with varicose veins [1,2]. The SF-36 satisfied rigorous psychometric criteria for validity and internal consistency [2]. SF-36 scores lower in referred patients than in patients not referred and were closely related to general practitioners' perceptions of severity [2].

Disease-Specific QOL Measures

Three disease-specific measures have been developed to assess quality of life in venous disease. Two of these instruments were developed in the UK; one was developed initially for use with patients with venous disease [3] and then adapted for use with patients with ulcers [4], and the second was developed for use with patients with varicose veins [1]. A third instrument was developed in France for use with patients with chronic venous insufficiency [5].

Questionnaire to measure quality of life in venous disease [3]

This is a 36-item questionnaire designed to measure QOL (symptoms, psychiatric morbidity), risk factors, costs, symptoms in patients with venous disease. Symptoms assessed include: swelling of one leg, swelling of both legs, night cramps, itching, restless legs at night, pain in legs, heaviness of legs. Psychiatric morbidity is assessed by the Symptom Rating Test, with subscale scores for depression, anxiety, hostility, subjective cognitive function, somatic symptoms of psychological distress. Costs (use of medical and social services) and risk factors are also assessed. The reliability, validity and responsiveness of the questionnaire have not been evaluated.

Questionnaire adapted from above to measure quality of life in leg ulcer treatment [4]

This questionnaire, designed to assess QOL with ulcer patients, was adapted from the questionnaire described above [3]. It measures psychiatric morbidity using the Symptom Rating Test, with subscale scores for depression, anxiety, hostility, cognition, somatic well-being, and includes questions about interference in daily activities, pain and feelings about the ulcer. The reliability and validity of the measure have not been assessed. However, it has been shown to be responsive to changes in QOL following 12 weeks of ulcer treatment.

Questionnaire to measure quality of life in patients with varicose veins [1]

This is a 15-item questionnaire containing questions commonly used in the clinical assessment of patients with varicose veins, e.g. distribution of veins, duration of pain, time of day with worst pain, duration of analgesia, degree of ankle swelling, use of support stockings, use of diuretics, extent of itching, discolouration, rash or eczema, skin ulcer, degree of concern at appearance, influence on choice of clothes, interference with work, interference with leisure. There is some evidence for the reliability and validity of the questionnaire. It shows good internal consistency as measured by item-total correlations. Factor analysis identified four important health factors: pain and dysfunction, cosmetic appearance, extent of varicosity, complications. The validity of the questionnaire has been demonstrated by a high correlation with the SF-36.

Questionnaire to measure quality of life in chronic venous insufficiency [5]

This is a 20-item questionnaire to measure QOL in chronic venous insufficiency. It is based on an earlier 18-item version [6] with the addition of two new items. The questionnaire assesses psychological consequences, physical consequences, pain, and social consequences. The Launois et al. measure was tested in a large sample of patients and is simple, practical and easy to administer. There is some evidence for the reliability and validity of the questionnaire [7]. It has good internal consistency and has been shown to differentiate CVI patients from non-CVI patient controls. Evidence for test-retest reliability, convergent/discriminant validity, and responsiveness has not yet been reported, but further studies on the reliability and validity of the measure are currently in progress.

QOL IN VENOUS DISEASE: RESEARCH FINDINGS

Findings based on the SF-36 show that QOL is: i) lower in varicose vein patients compared to the general population but higher than in patients with low back pain, menorrhagia, and suspected peptic ulcer [2]; ii) related to general practitioners' perceptions of severity [2].

Findings based on disease-specific measures show that: i) venous disease patients report more symptoms but do not differ on psychiatric morbidity compared to controls [3]; ii) ulcer patients show improved QOL following treatment, in terms of reductions in symptoms, depression, hostility, pain and interference with daily activities [4]; iii) chronic venous insufficiency patients report poorer QOL than non-CVI patient controls [5].

CONCLUSIONS

Comprehensive assessment of QOL in venous diseases of the lower limbs should include both generic and disease-specific measures which are known to be reliable, valid and responsive. The SF-36 has proven to be a useful measure of QOL in venous diseases of the lower limbs but must be supplemented with a venous disease-specific measure in order to comprehensively assess QOL. Few of the disease-specific measures have been evaluated in terms of rigorous scientific criteria of reliability, validity and responsiveness. What is needed is a venous disease-specific measure which is both scientifically sound and practical to administer on a routine basis to monitor outcomes. In conjunction with the Task Force on Venous Diseases of the Lower Limbs, we are currently developing and validating a venous disease-specific QOL measure.

REFERENCES

1. Garratt AM, MacDonald LM, Ruta DA, Russell IT, Buckingham JK, Krukowski ZH. Towards measurement of outcome for patients with varicose veins. Quality in Health Care 1993;2:5-10.
2. Garratt AM, Ruta DA, Abdalla MI, Buckingham JK, Russell IT. The SF-36 health survey questionnaire: An outcome measure suitable for routine use within the NHS? Br Med J 1993;306:1440-4.
3. Franks PJ, Wright DDI, Fletcher AE, Moffatt CJ, Stirling J, Bulpitt CJ, McCollum CN. A questionnaire to assess risk factors, quality of life, and use of health resources in patients with venous disease. Europ J Surg 1992;158:149-55.
4. Franks PJ, Moffatt CJ, Connolly M, Bosanquet N, Oldroyd M, Greenhalgh RM, McCollum CN. Community leg ulcer clinics: Effect on quality of life. Phlebology 1994;9:83-6.
5. Launois R. At the crossroads of venous insufficiency and hemorrhoidal disease: Daflon 500 mg - Repercussions of venous insufficiency on everyday life. Angiology 1994;45:495-504.
6. Launois R, Reboul-Marty J, Henry-Launois B. Les manifestations de l'insuffisance veineuse: Retentissement sur la qualité de vie - Résultats de la 1ère phase de recherches: Identification et sélection des dimensions spécifiques. Report to Servier, March 1992.
7. Launois R, Reboul-Marty J, Henry-Launois B. Les manifestations de l'insuffisance veineuse: Retentissement sur la qualité de vie - Résultats de la 2ème phase de recherches: Mesure quantitative de l'impact sur un échantillon national de patients. Report to Servier, May 1993.

Phlebology '95, D. Negus et al. (eds.). Phlebology (1995) Suppl. 1: 1107-1109

Socio-Economic Impact of Chronic Venous Insufficiency and Leg Ulcers

C.V. Ruckley

Edinburgh Royal Infirmary and University of Edinburgh

In industrial countries where population surveys have been carried out chronic venous insufficiency and leg ulceration are major health care problems. In non-industrialised countries the scale of the problem is not known. Roughly 5% of the adult population suffer from chronic venous insufficiency and 1% from leg ulcer disease (1-8). The socio-economic aspects will be considered first in terms of quality of life and second in terms of health care costs. It has to be said however that reliable socio-economic data in this field are scanty.

It is probably true to say that leg ulcer disease is not sufficiently recognised as a problem, either by the population at large or by the medical community. There are several reasons. Leg ulcers are often concealed, not only physically by clothing, but also concealed from medical attendants by patients who prefer, because of diffidence, social stigma, fear, embarrassment or potential cost not to consult a doctor. Because leg ulcers are dealt with by many different specialists: general, plastic and vascular surgeons, phlebologists, angiologists, dermatologists, rheumatologists, geriatricians, physiotherapists, nurse specialists etc, it is often the case that no single specialist acquires a proper perspective on the scale of the problem nor of the true disease spectrum. Furthermore the majority of patients with chronic leg ulcer are managed in the community. For all these reasons ignorance as to the importance of chronic leg ulcer as a health care problem and consumer of resources is also shared by health care authorities and funding bodies.

It is only recently that socio-economic and quality of life evaluation has been recognised to be an important part of clinical research. However Widmer and colleagues in their pioneering Basle studies drew attention to the serious effects of leg ulcer on the subjects' health and working practices (2).

Considering first quality of life: Phillips et al collected data by standardised personal interviews from 73 patients with chronic leg ulcer. A significant number had moderate to severe symptoms, principally pain, related to the ulcer. Eighty-one percent reported that their mobility was impaired. Leg ulceration was significantly correlated with time lost from work, job loss, and adverse effects on finances. There was a strong correlation between time spent on ulcer care and feelings of anger and resentment. The authors concluded that leg ulcers pose a substantial threat to a variety of dimensions of the patients' quality of life (9).

The next step was to examine the effects of ulcer therapy on quality of life scores. Franks et al used a Symptom Rating Test in 185 patients presenting to Community Leg Ulcer Clinics in the Riverside Health District (10). Anxiety, depression, hostility and cognition impairment were found to be common and to be significantly reduced after 12 weeks of therapy during which time 52% of the ulcers were healed. Other quality of life assessments were also documented. Pain was present in 78%, falling to 22% after 12 weeks of treatment. Worry about the ulcer fell from 15% to 1% and interference with leisure and/or social activities fell from 42% to 30%. Thus the authors were able to demonstrate clear improvements in a range of parameters of quality of life in response to treatment in a community clinic.

Turning next to the economic aspects. Social class has not been shown to influence predisposition to ulceration. But the duration of the ulcer diathesis has been shown to be longer and the numbers of episodes of ulceration to be greater in the lower social strata (11). In the same study almost 50% of the ulcer population of 600 patients were of working age and 21% had severe limitations of work or were unable to work.

The cost of ulcer care in the UK has been estimated at between £230-£400 million at 1990-91 prices (12). There is no doubt that ulcer care consumes a substantial proportion of the health care budget. Estimates based on national statistics suffer from the lack of precision of classifications. Utilising ICD9 numbers 454 (varicose veins of the lower extremities), 459 (venous insufficiency and post-phlebitic syndrome) and 451 (phlebitis and thrombophlebitis) Laing has estimated using 1986-89 costings, for the European countries for whom the data were available (UK, France, West Germany) utilised 1.5-2% of the total health care budget, giving a range, at 1992 currency exchange rate, of 418 to 1135 million ECUs per annum (13).

REFERENCES

1. Bobek et al. Etude de la fréquence des maladies phlébologiques et de l'influence de quelques facteurs étiologiques. Phlebology 1966;19:217-30.
2. Widmer et al. (1978) Peripheral Venous Disorders. Basle Study 111. Hans Huber (Berne, Stuttgart, Vienna).
3. Callam MJ. Chronic ulcer of the leg: extent of the problem and provision of care. Brit Med J 1985;294:1389-91.
4. Cornwall JV. Leg Ulcers: epidemiology and aetiology. Brit J Surg 1986;73:693-6.
5. Henry M. Incidence of Varicose Ulcers in Ireland. Irish Medical Journal 1986;79(3):65-7.
6. Hannsson C, Andersson E, Swanbeck G. Leg ulcer epidemiology in Gothenburg. Acta Chir Scand (Suppl) 1988;544:12-6.
7. Baker SR, Stacey MC, Jopp-Mckay AG, Hoskin SE, Thomson PJ. Epidemiology of chronic venous ulcers. Br J Surg 1991;78:864-7.
8. Nelzen O, Berqvist D, Lindhagen A, Halbook T. Chronic leg ulcers: an underestimated problem in the primary health care among elderly patients. J Epid and Com Health 1991;45:184-7.
9. Phillips T, Stanton B, Provan A, Law R. A study of the impact of leg ulcers on quality of life: financial, social and psychological implications. Journal of the American Academy of Dermatology 1994;31(1):49-53.
10. Franks et al. Community leg ulcer clinics. Phlebology 1994;83-6.
11. Callam MJ, Harper DR, Dale JJ, Ruckley CV. Chronic leg ulceration: socio-economic aspects. Scottish Medical Journal 1988;33:358-60.

12. Bosanquet N. Cost of venous ulcers: from maintenance therapy to investment programmes. Phlebology Suppl 1: 1992;44-6.
13. Laing W. Chronic venous disease of the legs. Office of Health Economics. 1992.

Phlebology '95, D. Negus et al. (eds.). Phlebology (1995) Suppl. 1: 1110-1112

Pathophysiology of Leg Ulceration - Update and Prospectives

Professor John A. Dormandy D.Sc. FRCS

St George's Hospital Medical School, University of London

A number of theories have been advanced to explain the primary abnormality in the veins which gives rise to primary varicose veins, including some biochemical abnormalities in the vein wall altering its physical properties. There is however no general agreement on the sequence of events leading to primary varicosities in the leg veins. Much more is known about the causes of secondary varicose veins, the aetiology of venous thrombosis and chronic venous insufficiency. All these disorders of the macrocirculation lead to a common haemodynamic abnormality characterised by a raised ambulatory venous pressure. Increased pressure at the venous end of the microcirculation would tend to decrease the capillary perfusion pressure and increase in the intra-capillary pressure. In older patients, with concomitant arterial disease, the pressure gradient along the capillary would be further decreased. The concept of venous stasis was first suggested by Homans in 1917 and he postulated the hypothesis of tissue anoxia due to poor capillary flow [1]. Although this seemed a plausible theory it has now been largely discredited by measurements of oxygen content in the venous and capillary blood. Despite continuing controversy the balance of evidence seems to suggest that the oxygen content of venous blood in patients with raised venous pressure is not decreased. The alternative, current and more complicated, hypothesis is that there is an abnormality in microcirculatory function resulting in maldistribution of the blood flow and hence areas of relative ischaemia. Using positron emission tomography Hopkins was the first to confirm this by direct measurements in 1983 [2]. This has been confirmed by several subsequent studies using different methodologies suggesting a complex series of abnormalities in the microcirculation of patients with venous hypertension.

A number of observations in the microcirculation of patients with venous hypertension have to be reconciled with any hypothesis on the aetiology of the symptoms and complications of venous diseases. In the area of the leg most severely affected, around the ankles, it is now accepted that there is a decrease in the total number of capillaries associated with an increase in their tortuosity [3]. At a more advanced stage of disease microcirculatory thrombosis [4], as well as pericapillary fibrin cuffs have also been observed [5]. More recently, it has been suggested that the pericapillary fibrin cuff is a secondary response to inflammation rather than an important primary cause of tissue ischaemia. Of at least equal importance are the functional abnormalities which have been observed in the microcirculation. Direct measurement of tissue oxygen tension would be particularly relevant, but is technically difficult and no such studies have yet been reported. Indirect measurements of transcutaneous oxygen tension have been difficult to interpret, particularly because the probes used or its measurement are usually at the unphysiological temperature of 42°C. Transcutaneous oxygen tensions are influenced by a number of factors other than cutaneous capillary oxygenation making interpretation of these indirect measurements very difficult. Xenon clearance techniques suggest that the delivery of oxygen to the tissues of patients with chronic venous insufficiency is not impaired [6]. Physiological abnormalities which are generally accepted as present in patients with raised venous pressure include abnormal vasomotion, increased capillary permeability, tissue oedema, dampened veno-arterial reflex and decreased fibrinolytic potential of the endothelium. Rheological abnormalities described included increased whole blood viscosity associated with a raised plasma fibrinogen and increased red cell aggregation. But possibly one of the most important recent findings relate to white cell rheology and white cell activation.

The white cell trapping hypothesis is based on a series of experiments carried out at St George's Hospital in the late 1980s. The results showed a 5% loss of white cells in the lower leg of normal subjects and a similar change in patients with simple varicose veins when the leg was dependent. However in patients with chronic venous insufficiency there was a mean 28.6% loss of white cells after one hour of dependency. Thus, in patients with venous insufficiency lowering the leg for an hour caused an increase in the concentration of red cells but a decrease in relative number of white cells leaving the foot [7]. In a parallel set of experiments similar measurements were carried out counting platelets. This showed a significant correlation between the number of white cells and the number of platelets trapped in the microcirculation of patients with chronic venous insufficiency during dependency. Finally, the effect of graduated external compression on white cell trapping was investigated. The results showed that such external compression significantly reduced the number of white cells 'lost' during dependency. This gave supportive evidence to the role of white cells in the pathophysiology of chronic venous insufficiency and offered another explanation for the beneficial effect of external compression [8].

The next piece of experimental evidence supporting this hypothesis came from the Middlesex Hospital. Skin biopsies of the ankle region were taken in patients undergoing varicose vein surgery. The results showed that there were eight times as many white cells in the skin of patients with trophic skin changes compared to those with normal skin and forty times more in patients who had a history of ulceration in the past [8]. The most recent evidence comes from the work of Vanscheidt and colleagues [9], who studied 30 patients with chronic venous insufficiency and 30 matched controlled studies. They produced venous hypertension in the arms using a cuff and showed that white cell trapping was significantly more in the arms of patients who had chronic venous hypertension in the legs. This interesting experiment suggests that patients with chronic venous insufficiency have circulating white cells which are primed and therefore more susceptible to activation and trapping in the microcirculation during even a short period of induced hypertension in the arm.

The details of the processes occurring at the cellular and molecular level leading to tissue damage is still largely theoretical. The essential first step is the juxtaposition of the white cell to the endothelium. The next stage of adhesion can be brought about by stimulants acting either on the endothelium, the white cell or both. The initial stimulus causes expression of the adhesion molecules. The major adhesion molecules on the endothelium are selectins and immunoglobulins while on the leucocyte they are selectins and integrins. Expression of these molecules leads to adhesion between the leucocyte and endothelium. In the circulation, adhesion depends on the balance of the binding affinities and the shear stresses, which in turn depends on the perfusion pressure gradient. Adhesion is followed by activation with migration of the white cell and degranulation. The so-called oxidative burst from the activated neutrophil can cause damage to local tissues by a number of mechanisms, which include the release of reactive oxygen metabolism, cytokines such as interleukin 1 and tumour necrosis factor.

Experimental evidence that at least some of these manifestations of the white cell oxidative burst in fact occurs in patients with chronic venous insufficiency comes from the recent work of Whiston and colleagues. The results suggest that neutrophil free radical production is indeed increased in the legs of patients with venous hypertension [10]. In subsequent studies they also showed increased release of calcium from neutrophils coming from the leg compared to those from the arm [11].

REFERENCES

[1] Homans J. The aetiology and treatment of varicose ulcer of the leg. Surg Gynaec Obstet 1917;24:300.

[2] Hopkins NFG, Spinks TJ, Rhodes CG et al. Positron emission tomography in venous ulceration and liposclerosis: a study of regional tissue function. Br Med J 1983;286-333.

[3] Franzeck UK, Bollinger A, Huch R et al. Transcutaneous oxygen tension and capillary morphological characteristics and density in patients with chronic venous incompetence. Circulation 1984;70:806-11.

[4] Bollinger A, Leu AJ. Evidence for microvascular thrombosis obtained by intravital fluorescence videomicroscopy. Vasa 1991;20:252-5.

[5] Burnand KG, Whimster I, Naidoo A et al. Pericapillary fibrin in the ulcer-bearing skin of the leg: the cause of lipodermatosclerosis and venous ulceration. Br Med J 1982;285:1071-2.

[6] Stibe ECL, Cheatle TR, Coleridge Smith PD et al. Liposclerotic skin: a diffusion block or a perfusion problem? Phlebology 1990;5:231-236.

[7] Thomas PRS, Nash GB, Dormandy JA. White cell accumulation in dependent legs of patients with venous hypertension: a possible mechanism for trophic changes in the skin. Br Med J 1988;296:1693-1695.

[8] Scott HJ, McMullin GM, Coleridge Smith PD et al. A histological study into white blood cells and their association with lipodermatosclerosis and ulceration. Brit J Surg 1990;78:210-211.

[9] Vanscheidt W, Kresse O, Hach-Wunderle V et al. Leg ulcer patients: No decreased fibrinolytic response but white cell trapping after venous occlusion of the upper limb. Phlebology 1992;7:92-96.

[10] Whiston RJ, Hallett MB, Lane IF et al. Lower limb neutrophil oxygen radical production is increased in venous hypertension. Phlebology 1993;8:151-154.

[11] Whiston RJ, Hallett MB, Davies EV et al. Inappropriate neutrophil activation in venous disease. Br J Surg 1994;81:695-698.

Phlebology '95, D. Negus et al. (eds.). Phlebology (1995) Suppl. 1: 1113-1115

Leg Ulcer Healing with Daflon 500 mg Treatment

O. Dereure*, J.J. Guilhou, L. Marzin, P. Ouvry, F. Zuccarelli, C. Debure,
H. Van Landuyt, M.N. Gilles-Terver, B. Guillot, H. Levesque, J. Mignot, G. Pillion,
B. Février and D. Dubeaux

*Department of Dermatology-Phlebology CHRU Montpellier, France

INTRODUCTION

Venous leg ulcers, the ultimate and most severe complication of chronic venous insufficiency, remains a therapeutic challenge. Although the cornerstone of the treatment is compression therapy, drug therapy has also to be considered in case of intolerance, contraindication, lack of compliance or as an adjunct to accelerate the healing process. So far, few drugs have proven to be of benefit in the treatment of venous ulcers [1]. The main objectives of the study were to investigate the clinical efficacy of a 2 month treatment with a micronized, purified flavonoidic fraction (Daflon 500 mg)* in addition to compression therapy and standardized local care, on patients suffering from venous ulcers.

PATIENTS AND METHODS

This trial was conducted according to the criteria recently released by the Alexander House group for ulcer treatments trials [2] and according to good clinical practice guidelines. The design was a double blind, randomized, controlled versus placebo (P) trial conducted in 9 French centres. Patients were male or female, aged 18 to 85 years, with a systolic pressure index (ankle/arm) > 0.8. They had to accept to wear elastic compression therapy, and could not have skin grafting during the duration of the treatment. Diabetic patients were not excluded. Concomitant treatment excluded phlebotropic or other venoactive drugs. Patients were randomly allocated to receive either the active drug or a placebo (2 tablets/day) during a maximum 2 month duration, or less in case of complete ulcer healing before the end of the 2 month treatment period. Ulcers had to be of venous origin only, whithout infection and had to be active for at least 3 months despite proper therapy. Standardized local care was given during the trial. In case of multiple ulcers, the largest ulcer was chosen as the reference ulcer. Large circumferential ulcers were excluded. Randomisation of treatment was stratified according to the diameter of ulcer ($\leq$ 10 cm, or > 10 cm). Patients were monitored every 2 weeks. The 2 primary criteria of activity of the drug were the percentage of patients with complete ulcer healing (i.e complete reepithelialisation) and time duration of complete healing. Secondary criteria were the following : percentage of ulcer surface area healed (as assessed by serial drawing of ulcer border allowing a surface area computerized calculation, blindly performed in one centre), total number of healed ulcers in case of multiple ulcers, aspect of ulcer and periulcerous skin, evolution of symptoms and socioeconomic incidence.

Descriptive statistics were used to describe baseline characteristics of patients, and otherwise statistical analysis including chi-square test or a Fisher's exact test where appropriate for comparison of percentage, bilateral Student's t test for comparison of means and standard deviation and the logrank test for comparison of complete ulcer healing of ulcers between the 2 groups.

RESULTS

One hundred and seven (107) patients were included ; two had no data available while under treatment, thus leaving a total number of 105 patients. Two main analyses were performed, stratified according to the diameter of ulcer :

1 - An intention to treat (ITT) analysis for the 105 patients included who received at least one dose of treatment (D = 53, P = 52). Baseline characteristics of patients, including prognostic factors likely to influence ulcer outcome were not statistically different between the 2 groups.

2 - A "per protocol" (PP) analysis for the 99 patients who completed the protocol (D = 51, P = 48) since six patients dropped out for other reasons than ulcer healing : two patients in the D group because of phlebitis (n = 1) and non compliance (n = 1) and four in the placebo group because of mild cutaneous adverse events (n = 3) and personal reasons (n = 1).

Ulcer diameter was less than, or equal to 10 cm in 91 patients, (D = 44, P = 47), thus subjected to a statistical analysis, and more than 10 cm in 14 patients (D = 9, P = 5), thus subjected to a descriptive analysis only.

The study demonstrated a clear cut superiority of the micronized purified flavonoidic fraction in comparison to the placebo for the 2 primary criteria of activity among the patients whose ulcer diameter was ≤ 10 cm.

1 - A complete ulcer healing occured after 2 months in 14 patients in the D group and in 6 patients in the placebo group. The difference is significant after intention to treat analysis (32 % versus 13 %, p = 0.028) and after per protocol analysis (32 % versus 14 %, p = 0.048).

2 - Healing process was significantly shortened in the D group as demonstrated by the actuarial survival curves (p = 0.037).

When calculating odd ratios, the chance of having a complete healing is almost threefold in the D group in comparison to the placebo group, whether factors known to adversely affect the healing process were present (16.1 % versus 8.1 %) or absent (47.1 % versus 20 %). On the other hand, no ulcer healing occured in the 14 patients whose ulcer diameter was > 10 cm.

Since one of the centres recruited 41 % (44/107) of patients, it was a posteriori showed that no center effect jeopardized the results concerning the percentage of patients with complete ulcer healing (p = 0.905 for odds ratio homogeneity) and delay for ulcer to achieve complete healing (p = 0.018 for ulcer with diameter ≤ 10 cm ; p = 0.036 for all ulcers).

On the other hand, this study showed no significant differences between the 2 groups for any secondary criteria (including ulcer surface area), except two which were favourably influenced by the D treatment : heaviness, sensation severity (qualitative data, p = 0.039) and frequency of atone aspect of ulcer at the last visit (4 % versus 17.3 %, p = 0.030).

The acceptability of treatment appeared to be quite satisfactory. In the D group, 6 adverse events occured : four were minor and two were thromboses but without any obvious relationship with the treatment. In the placebo group, 5 minor adverse events occured.

CONCLUSION

Despite the short duration of the study, Daflon 500 mg at a daily dose of 2 tablets appeared to be of benefit in accelerating the healing of venous leg ulcer, in addition to conventional compression treatment and standardized local care, at least for the ulcers of size less than or equal to 10 cm diameter. The mechanisms underlying this therapeutic activity are not fully understood. However, reduction of white blood cells sticking to endothelial cells [3] and subsequent reduction of capillary hyperpermeability [4] is an attractive hypothesis.

REFERENCES

1. Colgan MP, Moore DJ, Shanik DG. Drug therapy for venous ulcers : new methods of treatment. Phlebology 1992;(suppl 1):41-43.
2. The Alexander House Group. Consensus paper on venous leg ulcers. Phlebology 1992;7:48-58.
3. Friesenecker B, Tsai AG, Allegra C, Intaglietta M. Oral administration of purified micronized flavonoid fraction suppresses leucocyte adhesion in ischemia reperfusion injury : in vivo observations in the hamster skin fold. Int J Microcirc 1994;14:50-55.
4. Bouskela E, Verbeuren TJ, Donyo KA. Effects of diosmin-hesperidin on increased microvascular permeability in the hamster cheek pouch. Int J Microcirc 1994;14(suppl1):79.

* Also registered as Arvenum 500 mg®, Capiven® and Detralex®.

Phlebology '95, D. Negus et al. (eds.). Phlebology (1995) Suppl. 1: 1116-1118

Therapy Approaches for Lymphoedema

P.S. Mortimer

St George's and Royal Marsden Hospitals, London, UK

INTRODUCTION

Lymphoedema regardless of aetiology is essentially incurable but different therapy approaches exist which serve to contain swelling. Therapy will need to be tailored to suit the needs of the patient and the medical circumstances. For example, treatment for a growing child with lymphoedema may be quite different from a patient with lymphoedema from advanced cancer.

TUMOUR EXCLUSION

Tumour rarely presents as lymphoedema except in circumstances of advanced cancer because lymph flow is maintained remarkably well through malignant nodes. More commonly, lymphoedema is a manifestation of recurrent cancer when lymph transport capacity has already been compromised through initial cancer therapy.

In any patient who has developed lymphoedema secondary to cancer therapy it is therefore always of paramount importance to exclude recurrent tumour. This may not be as easy as it sounds. Breast cancer may lie hidden within fibrotic irradiated tissue deep in the axilla and not be evident clinically or show up on soft tissue scans (CT or MRI). Clinical features which suggest tumour are pain (lymphoedema per se will cause symptoms of aching or tightness but not pain) and tense swelling concentrated around the shoulder and proximal limb. Rapidly progressive neurology is also suspicious. Pelvic tumour particularly from prostate will produce a firm brawny oedema which may produce little tissue swelling. Venous obstruction can frequently co-exist.

MIXED OEDEMA

Any oedema rises from an imbalance between capillary filtration and lymph drainage. Lymphoedema means strictly impaired lymph drainage in the face of a normal load capillary filtration, but in reality many cases of lymphoedema may be complicated by an increased lymph load e.g. co-existent venous hypertension, hypoproteinaemia, heart failure. In these circumstances the associated abnormalities need correcting before the lymphoedema.

THERAPY

The objectives of treatment are to reduce swelling, to restore shape and to prevent inflammatory episodes e.g. recurrent cellulitis. Of prime importance is to prevent inflammatory episodes otherwise all other efforts are in vain. Recurrent cellulitis is a frequent and debilitating consequence of a compromised lymph drainage which can make swelling deteriorate rapidly. Antibiotics started at the peak of an attack are probably of little use and the emphasis is on prevention. Daily low dose phenoxymethyl penicillin is recommended as prophylaxis. Care of the skin as practised in Diabetes is recommended to reduce the risk of infection.

There are essentially three main approaches in order to reduce swelling and restore shape: physical therapy, drug therapy and surgery.

a) Physical therapy

This is accepted as first line treatment. The principle of such treatment is to improve drainage of interstitial fluid and macromolecules from congested regions to normally draining lymphatic regions. This is achieved through a combination of compression, exercise and massage which serve to stimulate what lymph drainage does exist as well as move fluid and materials along tissue planes. It is believed that by reducing swelling through intensive treatment including bandages, lymphatics will be given more chance to cope in much the same way as the heart pumps more efficiently when end diastolic pressure is reduced. This of course assumes some lymph drainage still exists - a reasonable assumption otherwise swelling would tend to increase inexorably.

b) Drug therapy

In isolation drug therapy from lymphoedema is disappointing. Diuretics achieve little more than relieve symptoms such as tightness and do not improve swelling. Nevertheless their indication may be justified in the palliation of symptoms in patients with advanced cancer where venous hypertension co-exists.

A number of drugs all possessing a central benzopyrone ring e.g. coumarin, hydroxy-ethylrutoside and diosmin have been evaluated for the treatment of lymphoedema. The pharmacology of these drugs is complicated because of the inclusion of a number of active ingredients within each product and the differing pharmacodynamic effects.

Hydroxyethylrutosides (HR) have been shown to be vasoactive by reversing the increase in permeability induced in single microvessels by protein free solutions.[1] In a double-blind clinical trial in postmastectomy oedema HR reduced arm volume by statistically significant but clinically unimportant amounts when used in association with physical treatment.[2]

Other flavonoid derivatives such as a mixture of micronized diosmin and hesperidin (DAFLON 500) have also been investigated. In vitro Daflon 500 increased the frequency of spontaneous contractions in isolated rings of sheep mesenteric lymphatics. In vivo the drug increased lymph flow when compared with pre-drug levels.[3] Ten patients with upper limb lymphoedema following breast cancer treatment experienced improved lymph drainage as judged by qualitative radionuclide lymphoscintigraphy when treated with Daflon 500.[4]

Clinical trials employing coumarin (5,6 benzo-α-pyrone) a drug with anticoagulant properties have shown clinical benefit in a wide range of lymphoedemas.[5,6] Claims that the drug works through enhancement of tissue protein phagocytosis, increasing lymph flow, a reduction of blood capillary filtration or a combination of all three need further substantiation.

c) Surgery

Surgery is essentially of three types:

i) Reducing operations which serve simply to debulk tissues and tighten surrounding skin. Surgery of this type may be the treatment of choice in genital lymphoedema and where eyelid oedema is compromising vision.

ii) bridging operations where new tissue containing lymphatics e.g. omentum is transplanted to 'bridge' a gap devoid of functioning lymphatics.

iii) lymphatic microsurgery involving either a) anastomoses between existing structures e.g. lympho-venous shunts or b) reconstruction e.g. autologous vessel transplantation.

CONCLUSION

Lymphoedema may not be curable but is treatable. Patients need to understand their condition and be fully informed regarding treatment so that they can assume more and more responsibility for self management. Psychological as well as physical support is often necessary. Ongoing advice and careful (objective) monitoring from professionals experienced in lymphoedema is vital for the best results.

REFERENCES

1.   Michel CC, Kendall S.   β-Hydroxyethyl rutosides reverse the increased permeability induced in frog microvessels by protein free perfusions. Phlebology 1993;8(Suppl 1):18-21.
2.   Taylor HM, Rose KE, Twycross RG. A double-blind clinical trial of hydroxyethyl rutosides in obstructive arm lymphoedema. Phlebology 1993;8(Suppl 1):22-28.
3.   McHale NG, Hollywood MA. Control of lymphatic pumping: Interest of Daflon 500 mg. Phlebology 1994;9(Suppl 1):23-25.
4.   Pecking AP, Rambert P. Current evaluation of lymphoedema and assessment by lymphoscintigraphy of the effect of a micronized flavonoid fraction (Daflon 500) in the treatment of upper limb lymphoedema. Phlebology 1994;9(Suppl 1):26-29.
5.   Casley-Smith JR, Morgan RG, Piller NB. Treatment of lymphoedema of the arms and legs with 5,6-Benzo-[α]-pyrone. N. Eng J Med 1993;329:1158-1163.
6.   Casley-Smith JR, Wang CT, Casley-Smith JR, Cui Zi Hai. Treatment of filarial lymphoedema and elephantiasis with 5,6-Benzo-[α]-pyrone.   B Med J 1993;30:1037-1041.

Phlebology '95, D. Negus et al. (eds.). Phlebology (1995) Suppl. 1: 1119-1121

Efficacy of Daflon 500 mg* in the Treatment of Lymphoedema (Secondary to Breast Cancer Conventional Therapy)

A.P. Pecking, B. Février*, C. Wargon*, G. Pillion*

Department of Nuclear Medicine, Centre René Hugenin, Saint Cloud, France
* IRIS, Courbevoie, France

INTRODUCTION

Upper limb lymphoedema secondary to breast cancer conventional therapy occurs in about 20% of all treated cases (1). Several therapeutic approaches are available such as contention, lymphatic drainage, bandaging or surgery. Drug treatment that could interfer with the lymphatic alterations observed in high protein oedema are of interest in the treatment of lymphoedema.

The lymphagogue activity of Daflon 500 mg, a purified and micronized flavonoid fraction comprising 450 mg diosmin and 50 mg hesperidin, has been demonstrated (2). To confirm the preliminary results established in a pilot study (3) a comparative controlled versus placebo study was performed.

METHODOLOGY

To assess the activity of Daflon 500 mg (D) on lymphoedema of upper limb occuring after breast cancer therapy a monocentre randomized, parallel groups, double blind, placebo (P) controlled clinical trial was carried out.

PATIENTS

One hundred and three ambulatory women, 30 to 80 years old, affected with mild to severe lymphoedema secondary to breast cancer (remission) were involved in the study. Ninety four of whom completed the study (46 D, 48 P). A subset of 24 patients (14 P, 10 D) with more severe lymphoedema (difference between perimetric measurements of the two arms ≥ 2 cm) was subjected to a separate analysis.

---

* Also registered as Arvenum 500 mg, Capiven and Detralex

TREATMENTS

Treatments, consisting on Daflon 500 mg or placebo, were given at the daily dose of 2 tablets over a six month period.

INVESTIGATIONS/MEASUREMENTS

Radionuclide lymphoscintigraphy using technetium-99m was performed at inclusion (M0) and after a six month treatment period (M6). The lymphoscintigraphic colloidal parameters were the following : lymphatic migration speed, clearance and half life. Serial perimetric measurements, performed every 5 cm, allowed the evaluation of the upper limb volume. The integration of the measurements yieled an estimation of the volume of the arm. A volumetric index was calculated as follows = (volume of the affected arm at Mx - volume of the affected arm at M0) / (volume of the affected arm at M0 - volume of non affected arm at M0). Discomfort was assessed by the patient on a visual analogic scale and heaviness assessed by a 4 points score (absent, inconstant, constant, invalidant). Evaluations took place at M0, M2, M4, M6.

RESULTS

The two groups were comparable at the inclusion for all parameters except for age (mean ± one standard deviation): 61.5 ± 10.8 years in D group versus 57.3 ± 9.8 years in P group (p = 0.039). The duration of lymphoedema was 46.8 ± 59.9 months in D group and 31.1 ± 36.5 months in P group (p = 0.113).

In the overall population, no significant difference between D and P groups were found for lymphoscintigraphic parameters and volumetric measurements. However, when each group was considered separately, the change over time analyses showed a significant improvement in each of the two groups for discomfort (p < 0.001 in D group, p = 0.002 in P group), and a significant improvement in D group for heaviness (p = 0.035).

In the 24 patients affected with a more severe lymphoedema, the evolution of the evolutions of the colloidal parameters were as follows. D, in comparison with P, significantly improved lymphatic migration speed (Δ Speed , m ± sd : 0.84 ± 0.6 cm/min versus 0.14 ± 0.26 cm/min, p = 0.005). The half life improvement was significant over time for D (Δ half life : -10.3 ± 13.07 min, p = 0.034), but not for P (Δ half life : 0.53 ± 15.51 min, NS) and the improvement tendancy was in favour of D (p = 0.086). The clearance improvement tendancy was in favour of D comparatively to P (p = 0.072) and the change over time improvement was close to significativity with D (Δ Clearance: 2.18 ± 3.10 µl/min, p = 0.054 versus 0.11 ± 2.26 µl/min, p = 0.86).

Evolutions of functional discomfort, heaviness and volumetric index were not significantly different between the two groups.

DISCUSSION

In this population of women affected with lymphoedema of the upper limb, secondary to breast cancer treatment, the more significant and clinically relevant results where observed in the subpopulation of the more severely affected patients. This is consistent with the fact that an important lymphoedema is more likely to be improved than a mild one. Colloidal migration speed was clearly improved by Daflon 500 mg. This must be related to its known lymphagogue activity, since this parameter is an indirect evaluation of lymphatic pumping. The other two parameters (ie : colloidal clearance and half life) are a more global reflect of diffusion of locally injected macromolecules. However, for this two parameters, a consistent tendancy was observed for a better improvement with Daflon 500 mg in comparaison to Placebo.

The wide variability of volume index did not allow to show any significant difference on tendancy between the two groups, although the decrease of volume was consistantly more marked for Daflon 500 mg at each evaluation.

These results are nevertheless promising, since they could be improved with a higher number of more severely affected patients. Another important point is the dosage of the drug. The two tablets dosage (ie 900 mg of micronized diosmin) is a standard dosage for signs and symptoms of CVI. Since it has been demonstrated that high dosages of flavonoid compounds are usually required to obtain a clear clinical benefit on lymphoedema (4), it could be interesting to switch to higher doses of Daflon 500 mg to demonstrate a more clear-cut efficacy.

CONCLUSION

The efficacy of Daflon 500 mg at the usual dose of 2 tablets daily was highly suggested in patients affected with severe lymphoedema although no statististical difference could be shown in the general population. The clear improvement of the colloidal lymphatic speed is to be related with the known favorable lymphokinetic activity of Daflon 500 mg .
Further studies with higher dosage could confirm the benefical activity of Daflon 500 mg in secondary lymphoedema.

REFERENCES

1. Casley-Smith JR, Casley-Smith JR. High-protein oedemas and the benzo-pyrones. Sydney and Baltimore: Lippincott, 1986.
2. Cotonat A, Cotonat J. Lymphagogue and pulsatile activities of Daflon 500 mg on canine thoracic lymph duct. Inter. Angio. 1989;8:(suppl 4):15.
3. Pecking AP, Rambert P. Current evaluation of lymphoedema and assessement by lymphoscintigraphy of the effect of a micronized flavonoid fraction (Daflon 500 mg) in the treatement of upper limb lymphoedema. Phlebology 1994;9:(Suppl1):26-29.
4. Casley-Smith JR, Morgan RG, Piller NB. Treatment of lymphoedema of the arms and legs with 5,6-benzo-[α]-pyrone. New England J.Med.1993;326 (16):1158-1163.

ANTIOXIDANT EFFECT OF FLAVONOIDS

CATAPANO A.L.
Institute of Pharmacological Sciences, and Centro per lo studio Aterosclerosi University of Milan, Milan Italy.

Inflammatory processes are often related to a sequelae of oxidative stresses. Many pathological conditions are believed to be initiated and sustained by inflammatory responses; among them atherosclerosis and vascular diseases.

Recent in vitro and in vivo evidences support the concept that antioxidants, both of natural origin or synthetic, may retard the onset of inflammation by modulating several processes in the vascular bed.

Antioxidants modulate in vitro and in vivo the adhesion to the endothelium and the extravasation of blood white cells following appropriate stimuli, including lipopolysaccharide (LPS) or interleukin thus reducing the overall inflammatory response. Furthermore antioxidants reduce the production of inflammatory mediators, including interleukins and lipooxygenase products (leukotrienes). Finally they may protect the vascular bed from endothelial damage by directly sparing the endothelium from oxidative stresses.

A large body of evidence is also accumulating that antioxidants may reduce the formation of atherogenic low density lipoproteins (LDL) by reducing the LDL oxidative susceptibility. This has been shown with several antioxidants. We have recently obtained preliminary data with Daflon® 500 mg, purified micronized flavonoid fraction (90 % diosmin and 10 % hesperidin) indicating that administration of the drug results in an increased resistance of LDL to oxidative stress suggesting a potential role for these compounds in vascular diseases.

VENOUS ELASTICITY AFTER TREATMENT WITH DAFLON 500 MG

Ibegbuna V, Nicolaides AN, Sowade O, Leon M, Geroulakos G, Irvine Laboratory, Academic Surgical Unit, St. Mary's Hospital Medical School, Imperial College of Science, Technology and Medicine, London, UK

Objective: To assess the activity of Daflon 500 mg on elastic modulus in patients with abnormal venous elasticity.

Design: Open, randomly allocated treatment (Daflon 500 mg versus control group without treatment).

Patients: 25 healthy females volunteers (age 18-35) with symptomatic varicose veins in one leg and/or abnormal elastic modulus without varicosities in the opposite leg.

Intervention: 4 week treatment with Daflon 500 mg 2 tab/d (n = 12) or no treatment (n = 13).

Measurements: Elastic modulus (K) determined using air plethysmography before and after a 4 week period with or without treatment. Simultaneous measurements of calf volume changes were made in response to different venous pressures produced by a thigh pneumatic cuff. Statistics : Wilcoxon rank sum test.

Results: In the control group K (mean ± sd) was $10.8 \times 10^3 \pm 4.1 \times 10^3$ N/m^2 at the beginning and $10.2 \times 10^3 \pm 3.1 \times 10^3$ N/m^2 at the end of the study (p > 0.1). In the group treated with Daflon 500 mg the initial K was $10.2 \times 10^3 \pm 3.9 \times 10^3$ N/m^2 and $14.2 \times 10^3 \pm 5.1 \times 10^3$ N/m^2 at the end of the study (p < 0.02).

Conclusion: The results indicate that a 4 week therapy with Daflon 500 mg is effective in improving venous tone. Further studies are required to elucidate whether the relief of symptoms shown by large studies is the result of changes in venous tone or reduction in oedema.

Satellite Symposia

BEIERSDORF
Evaluations of Compression Effects

PRESSURE MEASUREMENTS DIRECTLY UNDERNEATH COMPRESSION THERAPY

Prof. Dr. H. A. M. Neumann, J. C. J. M. Veraart
Department of Dermatology
Academisch Ziekenhuis Maastricht, The Netherlands

Ambulatory compression is the cornerstone of phlebology, either as part and support of sclerotherapy or surgical treatment. If applied by experienced people there is no doubt about its' effectiveness. Some aspects concerning the effects of compression therapy have up to now been studied. It could be demonstrated that 1) valves with a secondary insufficiency due to dilated veins close again, 2) extra pressure over pelottes even occlude perforating veins, 3) the flow increases and the function of the microcirculation improves.

A major question that still exists is whether one should use elastic or non-elastic bandages in the treatment of phlebological disorders. Especially in the Anglo-Saxon countries elastic bandages are in favour, whereas in the Germanic countries one prefers non-elastic bandages in the treatment of venous leg ulcers. We therefore performed interface pressure measurements in patients with venous diseases and normal volunteers with a non elastic bandage (Comprilan, Beiersdorf) and elastic bandage (Elodur, Beiersdorf). Recordings were made with the Oxford Pressure Monitor MKII. Pressure recordings were made on twelve different points of the lower leg. The average measuring fault is approximately 5mmHg. The measurements were taken in lying position, standing and standing on the toes with active muscle movement of the calf.

Bandages were applied by one and the same well trained nurse. Care was taken to apply each bandage with approximately the same pressure. Recordings were made in the Comprilan group directly after the bandage had been applied, after 1 and 3 hours and after 1, 3 and 7 days. Since the elastic Elodur bandage is normally worn for only 1 day, measurements were taken directly, after 1 and 3 hours. Furthermore the patients were asked to put on these bandages themselves since this is often advised by doctors.

The results show a rapid decline of pressure in the Comprilan group after already 1 and 3 hours. The pressure in the Elodur group persisted throughout the measuring time. There was not much difference between standing and lying. When applied by patients themselves, the pressure is far less than it should be. On the basis of these results we advise the use of non-elastic bandages in the treatment of venous leg ulcers. The different advantages and disadvantages of non-elastic and elastic bandages will be discussed.

INVASIVE VENOUS PRESSURE MEASUREMENTS DURING COMPRESSION THERAPY

J. C. J. M. Veraart, Prof. Dr. H. A. M. Neumann
Academisch Ziekenhuis Maastricht, The Netherlands

Ambulatory compression is the cornerstone of phlebology, either as monotherapy or as part and support of sclerotherapy or surgical treatment. If applied by experienced people, there is no doubt about its' effectiveness. Some aspects concerning the effects of compression therapy have up to now been studied. It could be demonstrated that 1) valves with a secondary insufficiency due to dilated veins close again; 2) extra pressure over pelottes even occlude perforating veins; 3) the flow increases and the function of the microcirculation improves.

In the past there have been performed pressure recordings underneath bandages and stockings. Also there have been done pressure recordings in the superficial venous system during compression therapy. Up to now no data exists on the effect of different forms of compression therapy on the pressure in the deep venous system of the leg.

For this reason we set up a study in which we brought a small catheter under ultrasound guidance in the popliteal vein and gently moved it into one of the deep calf veins. All this was done under local anaesthesia. The pressure measurements were performed in lying and standing position and when performing ten top-to-toe movements. After this the same measurements were made after applying a non-elastic bandage (Comprilan, Beiersdorf) and elastic bandages (Eldour, Beiersdorf. The 5 different compression stockings were put on the leg (Comprinet, Compriform, Elvarex2, Elvarex3, and Elvarex3 Forte; all Beiersdorf) and even so were the pressure recordings been made. We will discuss the results and consequences for the daily phlebological practice.

LONG TERM EFFICACY OF COMPRESSION STOCKINGS IN PATIENTS WITH CHRONIC VENOUS INSUFFICIENCY - a preliminary report.

Christel Austrell, Ingrid Thulin, Cecilia Darenheim and Lars Norgren
Department of Surgery, Lund University, Sweden

The effect of graduated compression stockings in venous disease is usually reported as the patient's opinion on comfort and relief of symptoms. An objective evaluation of the effect on venous functional parameters is useful to judge whether different compression classes also mean variations in venous emptying and refilling.

The present study aims at including 40 patients with venous disease stage II according to Widmer, allocating half of them to treatment with graduated compression stockings class I and half to class II. Venous function is investigated by foot volumetry with calculation of expelled volume and refilling at two occasions, at inclusion and after eight weeks of treatment.

Patients and methods

At present ten patients are included in each group, all except one in each group suffer from the same grade of venous disease in both legs. Therefore the study is based on 19 legs in each group. During the two examinations foot volumetry is performed both without and with the stockings. Expelled venous volume (EV_{ml}) is calculated during 20 knee bendings, performed during 40 sec. The refilling rate during immediate quiet standing is recorded ($Q_{ml/min \times 100ml}$). The basic foot volume (FV_{ml}) is also registered. Finally the quotient Q/EV_{rel}, (EV related to FV), is calculated.

The stockings are used daily during the eight weeks.

For statistical analysis, Wilcoxon signed ranks test is used, and $p<0.05$ is regarded significant.

Preliminary results

Few differences were seen between the two groups at this stage, including only 19 legs in each.

Therefore the groups were put together with the following findings:

At the first examination, expelled volume increased significantly when stockings were applied ($p=0.02$); the refilling rate was constant while the calculated quotient Q/EV_{rel} was significantly reduced ($p<0.001$).

At the second examination there was no significant difference between the expelled volumes without and with stockings applied. Numerically, however, EV had increased from the first examination (11.3 ± 0.6ml to 11.9 ± 0.8ml) (median $\pm$ SEM) /$p=0.08$/.

Comments

As expected, stockings increased the expelled volume at the first examination, and this difference was not seen at the second examination, when the expelled volume had increased slightly from the first examination.

Reductions of refilling rates were not seen, in general the explanation might be that the average refilling rates were close to normal, only slight refluxes were recorded.

At the present stage it is not possible to conclude any differences between compression classes I and II. Whether this may be interpreted that lower compression (class I) is as good as higher (class II) to improve venous function remains to be proven.

IMPROVEMENT OF SKIN MICROCIRCULATION BY COMPRESSION THERAPY IN CHRONIC VENOUS INSUFFICIENCY.

Junger M., Galler S., Klyscz T., Jung M. F., Steins A., Hahn M.
Department of Dermatology, University Hospital, Liebermeisterstr. 25, D-72072 Tübingen

Does compression therapy improve the impaired skin microcirculation and thereby contribute to the healing process in patients with chronic venous insufficiency (CVI)? 20 patients with chronic venous insufficiency stage 1 (n=7) and stage 2 (n=13) were included into the study. All patients had palpable peripheral pulses and an ankle/brachial index of >1.0. Examination by means of Doppler ultrasound revealed venous valve incompetence of deep veins in 7, of extrafascial veins in 12 and of perforator veins in 6 patients.

The 4 week lasting compression therapy consisted of 2 consecutive parts: during the first 2 weeks elastic bandages (Comprilan, Jobst) were used; next 2 weeks patients wore made-to-measure compression stockings (Jobst). At the beginning, between period one and two and at the end of period 2 the clinical symptoms were assessed by several visual analogue scales (0 to 3 units), volume of lower leg was measured, and proximal the medial ankle region laser Doppler flux was measured both under resting conditions and after a 3 minutes lasting arterial occlusion test to determine the cutaneous vascular reserve.

Results: The following changes were observed: Clinical symptoms as pain, tautness, swelling and itching decreased significantly. The volume of lower leg had been reduced ($p<0.05$). During the study period LDF decreased in the inner ankle area from 29 AU to 22.5 AU and finally to 20 AU. At the same time the cutaneous vascular reserve increased from 117% to 233% and after 4 weeks of treatment to 154%.

Conclusion: Compression bandages and the here used made-to-measure compression stockings improved patients' complaints impressively. This clinical benefit seems to be caused by various positive effects to the skin microcirculation of the lower leg. Especially the luxus hyperperfusion of the skin, which often is found in CVI, decreased and a vascular reserve could be observed again after successful treatment with compressing bandages and stockings.

RANDOMISED COMPARATIVE STUDY OF CUTINOVA™ FOAM AND ALLEVYN™ WITH JOBST ULCERCARE™ STOCKINGS FOR THE TREATMENT OF VENOUS STASIS ULCERS.

Weiss RA, Weiss MA, Ford RW
Johns Hopkins University School of Medicine, Baltimore, MD

Seventeen patients with confirmed venous ulcers were randomly assigned to receive adhesive hydrocolloid foam (Cutinova™ foam, N=8) or non-adhesive absorptive foam dressing (Allevyn™, N=9) along with external compression therapy consisting of Jobst UlcerCare™ stockings. This compression regimen consisted of an inner graduated compression stocking of 10mmHg to be worn 24 hours per day and an additional graduated compression zippered stocking of 20-30mmHg to be worn only during waking hours. The ulcers had been present for at least 2 months in both groups and were between 1 and 4cm^2 in size; approximately 20% of patients had recurrent ulcers and approximately 20% had multiple ulcers. All of the ulcers enrolled in the protocol demonstrated a minimum of 50% improvement over the 16 week study duration. Complete re-epithelialization occurred in 6 out of 8 (75%) in the Cutinova™ group and in 4 out of 9 (44%) of the Allevyn™ group. One patient developed a contact dermatitis to Allevyn™ during the study and had to be discontinued. Mean time to complete healing was approximately 8 weeks for both groups. All ulcers were less painful at final evaluation. Most patients preferred the ease of application of the Cutinova™ foam since the adhesive allowed more rapid application of the inner liner compression; the Allevyn™ was difficult to hold in place. In both groups percent reduction in ulcer area after 2 weeks correlated with treatment outcome and shorter time to healing. Both dressings appeared equal in initiating healing. In this ongoing study, however, our initial conclusions were that Cutinova™ foam was better tolerated and yielded a trend towards higher total cure rate.

ASSESSMENT OF THE DYNAMICAL EFFICIENCY OF COMPRESSION STOCKINGS WITH QUANTITATIVE DIGITAL PHOTOPLETHYSMOGRAPHY (D-PPG)

Ulrich Schultz-Ehrenburg & Anneliese Ott, Berlin, Germany

A prospective study for determining the dynamic effects of compression stockings on venous calf pump by digital photoplethysmography is reported. The correlation of the measurable effects with the clinical stages of CVI (according to Widmer) and the stages of PPG insufficiency is analysed. The study comprises the following clinical and PPG groups (overlapping classification).

	planned/reached		planned/reached
1) healthy legs	8/8	a) legs with PPG insufficiency stage I	8/6
2) legs with CVI stage I	8/9	b) " with PPG insufficiency stage II, improvable	8/9
3) legs with CVI stage II	8/9	c) " ditto, nonimprovable tourniquet test	8/9
4) legs with CVI stage III	8/13	d) " PPG insufficiency stage III, improvable	8/1
		e) " ditto, nonimprovable tourniquet test	8/6

Calf length stockings, 20-30 mmHg and 30-40 mmHg (Jobst GmbH, Germany), were used. Out of all measuring parameters (venous refilling times To, venous drainage Vo, efficiency of calf pump Mo and initial plateau of refilling phase) the refilling time To proved to be as the best reproducible one. The compression stockings did not show any significant changes with the healthy legs. With the venous patients the following mean To values were found in the different groups.

	Without	20-30mmHg	30-40mmHg
CVI I	16.4s	28.4s	18.5s
CVI II	14.7s	21.0s	22.2s
CVI III	9.4s	16.7s	17.7s
D-PPG I	19.3s	29.1s	20.4s
D-PPG II	13.6s	22.1s	21.4s
D-PPG III	6.1s	12.8s	21.1s

The CVI I group showed in all cases with 20-30 mmHg stockings a prolongation of To whereas this outcome was found only in about half of the cases with 30-40 mmHg stockings. Moreover, about 90% of the legs showed a deterioration with the 30-40 mmHg stockings compared with the 20-30 mmHg ones. The CVI II group also showed in all cases with 20-30 mmHg stockings a prolongation of To whereas this outcome was found only in 3/4 of the cases with 30-40 mmHg stockings, and about half of the legs showed a deterioration with the later stockings compared with the 20-30 mmHg ones. In the CVI III group the venous refilling time could be improved in more than 90% of the legs with 30-40 mmHg stockings but only in 3/4 of the cases with 20-30 mmHg stockings.

In conclusion, it can be stated that in the CVI groups I and II 20-30 mmHg stockings were always efficient, but in 30-40 mmHg stockings only in individual legs requiring an individual testing. Contrary, in the CVI III group the 30-40 mmHg stockings were efficient in almost all of the cases.

COMPRESSION THERAPY AND MICROCIRCULATION

R. Klopp
Institute of microcirculation, Berlin, Germany

After previous bandaging, 12 female subjects aged about 60 years and suffering from chronic venous insufficiency of stage II were subjected to compression therapy using thigh-length elastic stockings on both legs. Under defined marginal conditions and the usual clinical measurements, various geometric and dynamic characteristics were measured daily in complete microvascular networks of the *cutis* and *subcutis* of the left shank. After starting the therapy, these measurements were made up to the 40th day by means of a special intravital-microscopic investigation unit (combined reflected and transmitted light method).

In addition to the well-known macrocirculatory effects of compression therapy, direct responses of the local regulatory mechanisms of microcirculation were registered and interpreted in so far inaccessible target tissue; Up to the 30th day of adequate compression therapy, the venular blood flow increased by more than 20 percent as compared with initial values. Within the same period of time, the number of bloodcell-perfused junctions in the microflow increased by more than 15 percent (Wilcoxon-test significance level $\alpha = 5\%$).

The considerable improvement of venular backflow due to a more effective pressure gradient (in terms of flow mechanics) between arterioles and venules in the networks is an expression of conditioning local regulatory mechanisms of microcirculation in target tissue.

Any inappropriate compression therapy will have contrary effects on microcirculation.

Satellite Symposia

NEGMA
Normal and Insufficient Blood Supply to the Venous Wall: New Approaches

VASA VASORUM BLOOD SUPPLY TO THE OUTER LONG SAPHENOUS WALL

F. LESCALIE
Clinique St Augustin, Nantes, France

Objective : To study the vasa vasorum network (origin, course, anastomosis) of the long saphenous veins.

Material : 20 long saphenous veins from bodies.

Methods : Post-mortem latex injection then dissection from the groin to ankle followed by diaphanisation and examination after X-ray injection.

Results : The outer blood supply of the long saphenous vein by vasa vasorum depends on staged arterial branches originated from external puddendal artery, superficial femoral artery, arteria anastomotica magna, posterior tibial artery.

Conclusion : The role of vasa vasorum in the outcome of a long saphenous by-pass has to be evaluated. From a theorical point of view the in situ technique preserving vasa vasorum supply appears more relevant than the inversed saphenous vein graft.

PRINCIPLES DETERMINING THE TRANSPORT OF OXYGEN THROUGH THE WALLS OF VEINS

Michel C C
Department of Physiology & Biophysics, St Mary's Hospital Medical School, Imperial College of Science, Technology & Medicine, Norfolk Place, London, W2 1PG

Objective: To review the mechanisms of oxygen transport in the walls of arteries and veins and to consider whether oxygen transport might limit oxygen consumption in the venous wall.

Method: (i) To review evidence for the contributions of transport from the vascular lumen and transport from the vasa vasorum to the supply of oxygen to the walls of arteries.

(ii) To use the general principles of oxygen diffusion through tissues to extrapolate the findings of investigations of oxygen transport into arterial walls to transport into the walls of the larger veins.

Results and Discussion: The magnitude of oxygen transport from the vessel lumen into the vessel wall is dependent on the partial pressure of oxygen (Po_2) in the vessel lumen. While luminal Po_2 is constant and high in arteries, it is a physiological variable in veins of healthy people. In larger veins, there is evidence that flow in the vasa vasorum increases as Po_2 in the vessel lumen falls. The extent to which this regulatory action of the vasa vasorum may be comprised by raised venous pressure and venous distension has not been defined.

1130

ANATOMICAL DISTRIBUTION OF VASA VASORUM ON THE WALL OF SUPERFICIAL VEINS, WITH PARTICULAR REGARDS TO THE SHORT SAPHENOUS VEIN

D. LEFEBVRE, P. ROUX
Laboratoire d'Anatomie Purpan, Faculté de Médecine de Toulouse, France

Objective : To evaluate the vasa vasorum network of superficial veins and especially their distribution in short saphenous veins.

Design : Post mortem injection of Baryum in the arterial femoral tree using dissection and X-ray selective injections and lens magnifying dissections

Material : 5 bodies allowing the study of twenty superficial veins (10 long saphenous veins and 10 short saphenous veins).

Results : The distribution of vasa vasorum in the short saphenous vein is made by longitudinal links provided by perforating arteries coming from the tributaries of mains axles. Vascular and nervous distribution have the same pattern. When a level is lacking, the vascularisation is provided by one of the perforating arteries coming from the upper or lower stage.

Conclusion : The vasa vasorum of superficial veins are constant structures, coming from the depth, and disposed as metameric vessels.

THE DISTRIBUTION OF VASA VASORUM CAPILLARIES IN THE LONG SAPHENOUS VEIN WALL

P. BIGEL
Laboratoire ACP, Paris, France

Objective : To review data about the distribution and morphology of the capillaries network in the wall of the normal and varicose saphenous veins.

Methods : Long saphenous vein sections were obtained from patients undergoing surgical resection for varicose or saphenous graft for arterial by-pass. Histological sections of the wall were examined by different techniques. Overall structure of the muscular layers of the sampled vein as well as the density and distribution of the saphenous wall vasa vasorum capillaries are described and compared with the data from litterature.

Results : The microvascular network is included in a wider part of the vein wall than previously described and depends on the thickness of the wall.

Conclusion : These findings point out the importance of the vasa vasorum capillaries for supplying the vein wall and their possible involvement in the pathogeny of varicose veins.

STRUCTURE AND FUNCTION OF ARTERIAL VASA VASORUM

J. Koudy WILLIAMS* , Donald D. HEISTAD**

* Bowman Gray School of Medicine of Wake Forest University, Winston-Salem, NC USA
** University of Iowa College of Medicine, Iowa City, IA, USA

Nourishment of arteries is accomplished by diffusion from the lumen of the vessel and from vasa vasorum. Most normal arteries have an extensive network of vasa in the adventitia that arise from branch points of parent arteries. When the thickness of arteries exceeds the ability of simple diffusion of nutrients from the lumen (larger muscular or atherosclerotic arteries), vasa extend into the media and intima. Vasa in the intima-media arise predominantely from adventitial vasa, but can arise from the lumen in vascular grafts and recanalized arteries after thrombosis. Vasa respond to vasoactive stimuli, and can regress after they vascularize arterial grafts and in response to regression of the atherosclerotic lesions. Therefore, vasa can increase blood flow to the artery wall by dilation of existing arteries or by formation of new vessels (neovascularization). Conversely, vasa can reduce blood flow to the artery wall by active constriction or by regression (involution) of existing vasa.

The pathophysiologic significance of vasa vasorum in normal and diseased arteries is related to their structure. Vasa in the intima-media are thin-walled endothelial cell tubes with thin or absent medial smooth muscle cells. Therefore, they are prone to collapse and rupture in response to arterial pressure, mechanical forces in the artery, necrotic substances found in diseased arteries, and vasospasm. Vasa also provide the artery with a vast absorptive endothelial surface that may have important implications for arterial lipid kinetics, and delivery and removal of neurohumoral agents from the artery wall. These properties have lead to speculation about their role in the pathogenesis of atherosclerosis, plaque rupture and thrombosis, medial ischemia leading to arterial dissection and aneurism, restenosis after angioplasty, and post-stenotic dilatation.

Finally, larger veins also have an extensive network of vasa that have been implicated in the pathogenesis of venous thrombosis and varicose veins.

LASERDOPPLER FLUX IN NORMAL AND VARICOSE VEINS WALL

G. BELCARO*, A. TACCOEN**

* Microcirculation Laboratory, CHIETI University, Italy, Irvine Laboratory, St Mary's Hospital, London, U.K.
** Laboratoires Negma , Toussu-Le-Noble, France

Venous wall flux was measured using laser-Doppler flowmetry on the external surface of 24 normal veins, partially dissected during the preparation of the vein for aortocoronary bypass grafting. Measurements were performed before the final dissection of the vein when at least 3/4 of the adventitia and periadventitia tissue was still intact for a lenght of 3 cm. The segment of vein (10 cm) proximal to the sapheno-femoral junction was studied. Measurements were repeated on 22 varicose veins before stripping or ligation of the sapheno-femoral junction.

Flux was measured with a Laserflo (Vasamedics) flowmeter. A Delrin (polycarbonate) spacer was placed between the probe and the vein wall surface. Measurements shown are the average of three minutes recording. Preliminary analysis indicates that flux appears to be lower in varicose veins in comparison with flux in the normal vein wall.

However the variability of results and technical problems in flux measurements indicate the need of a larger measurement sample before confirming the observation of a decreased perfusion of the varicose venous wall.

OXYGEN TENSION IN THE WALL OF VARICOSE AND NORMAL VEINS

A. TACCOEN*, C. LEBARD**, J.C. POULLAIN***,
I. GERENTES*, F. ZUCCARELLI**
* Laboratoires NEGMA, Toussus-Le-Noble, France
** Hôpital Saint Michel, Paris, France
*** Clinique de Noisy le Sec, France

Objective : To evaluate the oxygen tension of the venous wall in normal and varicose human saphenous veins.

Design : In vivo comparative study of site-matched saphenous veins from patients undergoing surgery.

Patients : Patients undergoing varicose veins surgery and controls undergoing femoro popliteal by-pass.

Measurements : Measurement of venous wall oxygen tension was performed by a polarographic needle probe moved through the three layers owing to a stepwise micromanipulator (Eppendorf, Sigma). All the data were recorded in a microprocessor file.

Results : Oxygen profiles followed the same pattern in all the veins. A dramatic decrease was showed in the central media of the venous wall in both varicose and normal saphenous veins. It seems that varicose vein oxygen tension was reduced compared to normal saphenous vein.

Conclusion : For the first time, the media of the human venous wall was found in vivo to be exposed to critically oxygen supply. These findings support the view that insufficient vasa vasorum supply could lead to histological varicose changes in the vein wall.

LOCALIZATION OF TROXERUTIN IN THE VENOUS WALL, MEASURED USING A SCANNING LASER MICROSCOPE

K. CARLSSON*, A. PATWARDHAN*, A. TACCOEN**, I. GERENTES**,
J.C. POULLAIN***
* Physics IV, The Royal Institute of Technology, Stockholm , Sweden
** Laboratoires NEGMA, Toussus-Le-Noble, France
*** Clinique de Noisy le Sec, France

The uptake and localization of troxerutin, a tri-hydroxy-ethyl-rutoside, in the venous wall have been studied in patients undergoing long saphenous vein surgery. Troxerutin, an autofluorescent drug, is currently used to relieve oedema and subjective symptoms in patients with chronic venous insufficiency. In order to determine the localization of the troxerutin, a confocal scanning laser microscope has been used to record the fluorescence from vein cross sections. The quantified fluorescence was used as a measure of the local concentration of troxerutin. In order to reduce the effects of local variation, several images have been scanned from each specimen. Then the recorded data have been analysed to see how the fluorescence varies in the radial direction within the venous wall. Results showed that troxerutin was significantly accumulated in both inner and outer parts of the venous wall. Whereas inner wall troxerutin uptake resulted from direct diffusion through the lumen, the outer wall uptake proceeded likely from the vasa vasorum circulation.

Satellite Symposia

THUASNE
Compression and Therapy
A Discussion of Recent Research from Around the World

Phlebology '95, D. Negus et al. (eds.). Phlebology (1995) Suppl. 1: 1134-1137

The Physiology of Compression: Clinical Consequences, Precautions and Contraindications

F. Vin

Paris, France

Our ancestors knew that a well-applied bandage was able to reduce varicose veins and ease the pain they caused. The Greeks and the Romans used compression to treat ulcers. The compression method was relaunched in the 20th Century, following the work of Unna who developed the zinc paste boot in 1885. In 1910, Fischer demonstrated that it was possible to treat thrombophlebitis with a combination of bandaging and bed rest. It was necessary to wait until the end of the century for progress in the textile industry to enable us to carry out elastic compression of different strengths, exerting relatively standard pressures with efficacy and comfort. The mode of action of elastic compression had been hypothesised but never proven. New non-invasive techniques, such as plethysmography, radioisotope studies and the use of echodoppler, have enabled its efficacy to be demonstrated.

CLINICAL CONSEQUENCES

1. Action on the superficial venous system and the deep venous system

Elastic compression is transmitted to the venous system via the intermediary of tissue pressure which causes a reduction in the calibre, a more exact closing of the valves when they are not damaged, and consequently a reduction in reflux disorders. A study by Emter [1] showed a reduction of 31% of the intravascular volume in subjects presenting with varicose veins which were treated with elastic compression.

Coleridge Smith observed by echo doppler studies that wearing an anti-thrombotic stocking caused a decrease in the diameter of communicating veins from 2.6 to 1.6 mm.

Sarin et al [2], confirmed that there was restoration of valvular function in a certain number of cases in the same patients.

Van Cleef [3] argued that in view of the oval cross-section of the vein, and the presence of a commissural gap, compression does not completely prevent venous reflux.

2. Action on venous return

The reduction in the calibre of the veins by compression causes an increase in the velocity of venous return even if the flowrate remains unchanged. According to Partsch [4], elastic compression accelerates venous return just like movement of the foot. On the other hand, in recumbent subjects, there is no significant difference in the speed of venous return between patients with compression and those without, when they carry out foot dorsiflexion exercises. A study by Emter [5] using bidimentional echodoppler showed that treatment with compression accelerates the speed of the blood flow in the venous system. This study confirms the results of other studies carried out by Bollinger, Wuppermann and Sigel. There is always an improvement in the function of the musculo-venous pump during exercise. In normal subjects during exercise, whether it be volume or pressure, the values at rest (90 mmHg for pressure) fall to a minimum value of 20 to 30 mgHg. Using either venous blood pressure or plethysmography, the quality of the sural pump is assessed by the drop in volume, the minimum pressure during the exercise and the time of filling and half-filling. In the presence of chronic venous insufficiency, there is a reduction in the fall in volume during exercise. This reduction may be linked to obstruction or to reflux. Numerous studies have shown a significant increase in the drop in volume on exercise with medium or strong compression stockings.

In most cases, the filling time with elastic compression is increased in the presence of superficial venous insufficiency. Conversely, in the presence of deep venous insufficiency, there seems to be little change in the filling time except with strong compression.

3. Action on blood volume

The blood volume of the lower limb depends on the position of the subject. The volume doubles from the sitting to the lying position. It is three times greater in subjects with chronic venous insufficiency. Compression bandaging reduces the volume by 45% in the lying position and by 62% in the standing position, and right cardiac filling is also improved. In patients with varicose veins, thoracic electric impedance is reduced when wearing a class 1 elastic stocking, which reflects the increase in the central blood volume.

4. Action on tissues

The external pressure increases the tissue pressure until the effective oncotic pressure exceeds the hydrostatic pressure, thus enabling the resorption of liquid in the venous compartment. This has been evaluated by the clearance of ^{24}Na following sub-cutaneous injection of 0.1 ml of labelled saline.
Partsch et al [4] measured the reduction in oedema by a radioisotope method. The effect of compression is also seen in the rate of isotope clearance from sub-cutaneous tissue.

Christopoulos [6] observed a 45% reduction in the cutaneous flow rate in 32 varicose limbs after 30 minutes of wearing a 25 mmHg elastic stocking. The transcutaneous O_2 pressure ($TcPO_2$) is reduced at the level of trophic disorders in varicose patients. It is increased under the effect of compression without, however, being completely normalised.

5. Action on coagulation

There is no consensus at present on the action of elastic compression on the different coagulation factors. Some studies seem to have suggested an increase in fibrinolysis induced by intermittent pneumatic compression.

Decousus et al [7] demonstrated the absence of effect of elastic compression on fibrinolysis by carrying out measurements of euglobulin clot lysis test, antigen TPA antigen, PAI 1 activity and TPA-PAII complexes.

PRECAUTIONS FOR USE

As with all therapies, there are indications for the use of elastic compression, precautions in its use, and contraindications.

Compression should be adapted to the patient and the limb treated.

It should not be too strong (difficult to tolerate and uncomfortable) or too weak (ineffective). Suitably adapted compression should conform to the dimensions of the limb. Depending on the clinical condition, the choice needs to be made between elastic bandage, knee-length stockings, and thigh stockings or tights.

Cutaneous tolerability should be acceptable. A study carried out by Bak Christensen, after elimination of patients with arteriopathy, demonstrated echymoses and redness of the skin in 17 out of the 117 patients treated with compression [8].

In other cases, intolerance with an allergic basis can be the cause of pruritis, erythema or friction burns.

CONTRAINDICATIONS

Bilateral compression therapy of the lower limbs causes a rise in right and left ventricular filling pressure [9]. Because of these pressure rises, cardiac decompensation may be precipitated in subjects suffering from heart disease.

According to Emter [10], cardiac insufficiency is a reason for not using elastic compression. Arteriopathy of the lower limbs remains a contraindication for the use of elastic compression. For Becker [11], there is no absolute contraindication unless the index of residual pressure measured by doppler is less than 0.55 and the arterial disorder is of sufficient severity with a sub-ischaemic condition, to reduce tissue perfusion. These data have been confirmed by Emter who gave a reminder of the harmful role of elastic compression when lying down in arteriopaths.

Many elderly patients with osteoarthritis of the hip or knee, or even the arms, find it difficult to put on a compression stocking. The prescription of elastic compression in this type of patient is not contraindicated but compliance may be poor because of the physical difficulties encountered.

CONCLUSION

Elastic compression has been used for several centuries and is of proven efficacy.

Its mode of action is still not completely understood. It can be used at all stages of the disease. The more advanced the disease, the stronger should be the force of compression. The use of non-removable bandages is reserved for the acute stage of the disease. It should rapidly be replaced by removable compression at the chronic stage.

Scientific studies are needed to confirm the efficacy of elastic compression which at present is considered to be unreplaceable.

REFERENCES
1.	Emeter M, Pret Schner DP. Etude des variations du volume sanguin et du volume des oedèmes des membres inférieurs par des méthodes de médicine nucléaire. Phlébologie 1991; 44 (2): 473-476.
2.	Sarrin S, Scurr JH, Coleridge-Smith PD. Mechanism of action of external compression in venous disease. Phlébologie 1992; P Raymond-Martimbeau, R Prescott M Zummo Eds, John Libbey Eurotext, Paris.
3.	van Cleef JF. Valves in varicose veins and external compression studied by angioscopy. Phlébologie 1993; 8: 116-119.
4.	Partsch H. Preuves de l'efficacité de la compression par des méthodes de médicine nucléaire, la pléthysmographie et la mesure de pression veineuse. Phlébologie 1979; 32: 179.
5.	Emeter M. Modifications du flus sanguin dans les veines des membres inférieurs aprés compression. Phlébologie 1991; 44 (2): 481-484.
6.	Christopoulos D, Nicolaides AN, Belgaro G. The long-term effect of elastic compression on the venous haemodynamics of the leg. Phlebology 1991; 6: 85-96.
7.	Decousus H, et coll. Etude de la méthode compressive sur la fibrinolyse chez le volontaire sain. Traitement compressif en phlébologie. John Libbey Ed Paris 1992: 47-48.
8.	Bak-Christensen A. Cutaneous reactions in relation to the use of 'ted' stockings. The Lancet Dec 1989: 1346.
9.	Dereppe H, et coll. Répercussions hémodynamiques de la pressotherapie. J Mal Vasc 1990; 15: 267-269.
10.	Emeter M, et coll. Blood shifting patients with chronic venous insufficiency using compression therapy. Phlébologie 1989; A Davy, R Stemmer Eds, John Libbey Eurotext Ltd: 878-880.
11.	Becker F, Mollard JM. Contention élastique et artériopathic des membres inférieurs. Phlébologie 1995; 48 (1): 83-85.

Phlebology '95, D. Negus et al. (eds.). Phlebology (1995) Suppl. 1: 1138-1149

Haemodynamic Modifications Induced by Elastic Compression Therapy in CVI Evaluated by Microlymphography

C. Allegra, E. Oliva, M. Bartolo Jr. and R. Sarcinella

Department of Angiology, S. Giovanni Hospital, Rome, Italy

Nowadays the use of compression bandages is the treatment of choice for lower limb oedema, since 75% of venous and lymphatic disorders can be treated successfully with elastic stockings [38].

It is generally known that the physical principles underlying the use of compression are governed by Laplace's law. According to this law, the pressure exerted by an elestic bandage is proportional to its tension and is inversely proportional to the radius of the curved surface which is being treated.

The knowledge of these parameters has enabled us to produce the various types of bandages currently marketed, as well as to classify the various procedures involved in bandaging and compression, and to specify its duration on the basis of the grade of venous pathology [50].

In chronic venous insufficiency (CVI) in particular, the venular hypertension is associated with dynamic lymphatic incompetence due to overloading of the lymphatics induced by reduced venous return.

This will overload the most superficial lymphatics because of the increased interstitial pressure [49].

The unbalanced metabolic changes at the level of the capillary bed caused by loss of local self-regulation underlies the clinical features of CVI (dermohypodermitis, liposclerosis, atrophie blanche, oedema, etc).

The correction of passive venous hypertension, which is greatest at the level of the ankle, is achieved by using "heavy" elastic compression of between 30 and 50 mmHg, applied by means of inelastic or short stretch bandages. This kind of compression acts at the level of the deep venous system, promoting centripetal drainage of oedema by the compression of collateral varices and the veins in which reflux is occurring [29]. This type of compression also exerts an influence on distal valves, permitting the restoration of blood flow in the direction of the heart [31].

The effectiveness of elastic compression on lower limb oedema has been studied by many authors using various methods such as ultrasonography, echo-doppler imaging, echotomography, radioisotopic studies, plethysmography, oximetry, microscopic and histopathological techniques [9,11,12,20,22,24,28,29,36,44,45,47,52,53,55].

From these studies the following conclusions may be drawn:

A) Compressive action on venous and lymphatic microcirculation of the lower limbs

1 Reduction of the calibre of deep and superficial veins [Emter 1989]
2 Reduction of pathological reflux by up to 30 to 40% [Sarin 1992]
3 Overloading of the valve cusps, mainly in the deep venous system [Partsch 1979]
4 Increase of the velocity of venous flow [Emter 1992]
5 Increase in fibronolytic activity [Altenkamper 1979]
6 Acceleration of lymphatic transport [Stoberl 1989]

B) Compressive action on the tissues at the microvascular level

1 Decrease of capillary-venous ectasia [Curri 1989]
2 Reactive thickening of the basement membrane [Curri 1989]
3 Decrease in interstitial oedema [Stemmer 1984]
4 Improvement of skin oxygenation [Bollinger 1993, Rashid 1992]

Hitherto in vivo evaluation of the structural changes in the microcirculation in CVI has been achieved using non-quantitative microscopic pictures of the areas of the limb in question showing the greatest clinical changes, using videocapillary microscopy with an optic probe. The morphological findings in the microcirculation of the skin were capillary-venular ectasia, microaneurisms, capillary kinking, the phenomenon of sludging, a reduction of capillary density and narrowing of the microcirculation [21]. Fagrell himself maintains that the number of capillaries is often reduced, to such an extent that it is apparent to the naked eye [26].

According to recent research, the more advanced stages of CVI are associated with signs and symptoms of injury to lymphatic vessels [19].

A strong relationship does in fact exist between the veins and the lymphatic vessels at the level of the microcirculation. When the blood flows from the capillaries towards the venules, the lymphatic vessels play the role of returning the fluid and proteins of endovascular and extravascular origin, which have been filtered out of the capillary bed because of the pressure difference between the capillaries and the venules, to the venous circulation.

This function of the lymphatic vascular system provides a component of active protection against microcirculatory stasis. During the initial stages of venous insufficiency, the lymphatics get overloaded because of the increased interstitial filtration.

The frequency and the amplitude of lymphatic constriction are influenced by the quantity of fluid entering them. The lymphatics have an important intrinsic mechanism which governs the removal of fluid from the tissues on the basis of the increase in the interstitial pressure. In CVI the increase in interstitial pressure is followed by an increase in oncotic pressure because of the passage of macromolecules out of the capillary into the institium. In addition, the capacity of the lymphatics is increased because they are stretched by their anchoring fibres when the connective tissues are put under pressure. As a result, the lymphatic system acts as an alternative route for reabsorption and circulatory return acting independently from the venous end of the capillary system. The shortcomings of the venous system stimulate a lymphatic counterbalance [46].

During the past few years, it has also been possible to investigate the cutaneous microcirculatory network in a quantitative manner, and to verify the haemorheological changes, and the variation in capillary tension and in the tension in the lymphatics and the interstitial tissues as well.

The microlymphatic system of the skin can be studied using Bollinger's methology [14,15] as modified by Allegra [6,7,10].

By a subepidermal injection of high molecular weight dextran, we can visualise the cutaneous lymphatic network and we have the opportunity to study its structural and functional parameters: ie, the features of its micronetwork, the diameters of the lymphatics, the permeability of microvessels using the measurement of escape of fluorescent material, and the endolymphatic and interstitial pressures.

Using the similar method described by Allegra, it is possible to record the interstitial pressure changes close to the lymphatic microvessel in order to calculate the pressure balance between the interstitium and the lymphatic network which is a direct expression of reabsorption itself.

MATERIALS AND METHODS

Nine patients were examined: 6 affected by stage III CVI classified according to Widmer [54] (3 males and 3 females; average age 38.5 years), and 3 healthy subjects (1 male and 2 females; average age 32.8 years), who acted as a control.

All the patients were suffering from stable oedema affecting a third of the lower limb at the medial side and all had dermohypodermitis. None of the patients had ulcers at the time.

The extent of the oedema was evaluated clinically by detailed measurement in centimetres. Measurements were taken starting from the lower margin of the patella and measuring the diameters of the limb every 10 cm proximally towards the top of the thigh and every 5 cm distally towards the malleolar region including the dorsum of the foot.

Measurements were made using the following instruments:

1 Doppler CW. phlebotensiometry in the standing position evaluated by placing the cuff of the sphigmomanometer exactly one third of the way up the lower part of the leg, measuring from the medial malleolus, and inflating it to a pressure a little greater than the expected venous pressure. The tibial vein was found by placing the probe behind the posterior tibial artery; the saphenous vein was found by moving the probe 3 cm from the medial malleolus onto the instep of the foot.

Compression was carried out for as short a time as possible and the cuff was deflated quickly. A sound like a gust of wind indicated the appearance of venous reflux and thus indicated the venous pressure value.

2 The microlymphographic study was carried out using a moving arm with a fluorescence videomicroscope [Wild Leitz] mounted on it. At a magnification of 1.0 X we visualised the microlymphatic network, stained by a subepidermal injection of 0.01 FICT dextran 150,000 25%, given 5 cm above the medial malleolus under microscopic control [14].

The microscopic pictures were filmed using a video camera (Ikegami ITC-410). The video images were stored in digital form using a video recorder (Sony SLV-415) and they were also displayed in real time on two or more monitors.

Each recording lasted for at least 15 minutes.

From the images we are able to analyse:

a) microlymphatic network morphological characters;
b) the features of the microlymphatic network;
c) the average diameter of the microlymphatic vessels evaluated by computerised morphometric measurement in microns using data from the ten best stained networks;
d) the extension of fluorescence evaluated in millimetres, indicative of the spread of dye in the network. This can be considered to be an index of the receptiveness of the lymphatic endothelium for the stain.

We used a servo nulling method to make direct pressure measurements. The microscope was used at a magnification of 3.2 X and the pressure measurements were made using a micropipette and micromanipolator connected to the servo nulling system (Mod 5A), a pressure transductor (Mod 915) and a video signal control (515).

a) the lymphatic pressure was measured by introducing a 7-9 μm micropipette into the lymphatic which took up the stain the most strongly using the micromanipolator, and then connecting the pipette to the servo nulling system to measure the pressure within the selected vessel over a period of at least one minute. The data were analysed by computer to obtain lower, mean and higher values for the microlymphatic pressure.
b) the interstitial tissue pressure was obtained by moving the same pipette into the surrounding tissue, using the micropipette vessel chosen for pressure recording and the capillary used for dextran diffusion as reference points.

3 Dynamic fluorescence capillaroscopy was carried out following the intravenous injection of 1-2 ml of 20% NaF [9,17]. In this study we focused on relative haematocrit (HCT) and velocimetric values (rCVB) from amongst the many parameters which can be evaluated using this method.

a) HCT was measured in at least three capillaries in each subject. The value obtained was relative because it was deduced from the continuous recording by a videodensitometric system (Capiflow) of a window located on the capillary in relation to a window located in the pericapillary tissue. The purpose of this reference window was to record variations in optical density between the tissue surrounding the capillary and the inside of the capillary, taking as the zero haematocrit the signal given when the window on the capillary recorded a moment of absence of erythrocytes.

b) the rCVB was always calculated from at least three capillaries using the technique of simplified cross-correlation modified by a computerised photometric analysis.

At D0 and at D28 the patients were studied using the methods described above, and a clinical examination was performed.

At the initial assessment patients were allocated to a stocking therapy treatment which was performed as follows:
- Daily application of a removable short stretch bandage to the limb affected by CVI.
- Wearing of stocking for at least 12 hours/day
- Recommending patients to carry on their usual daily activities with their bandages on.
Patients were given instructions by the physicians who saw them on how to apply the bandage correctly.

RESULTS

The results of our study are summarised in tables 1, 2, 3, 4 and 5.

At D28 all the patients were found to have experienced the disappearance of oedema from their limbs. The mean diameters of the oedematous leg were reduced significantly (Table 1).

The results for venous tensiometry showed that it decreased significantly in relation to the assessment time (Tables 2, 3) [29].

Using microlymphographic methods it has been shown that the lymphatic network is destroyed in CVI; its network was fragmented and dilated and the vessels showed increased permeability to FICT dextran in comparison with controls [30].

At the end of the study the microlymphatic network appeared to have a more uniform structure and the abnormal features were reduced (Table 4).

Based on nine microlymphographic studies, the spread of the dye through the lymphatic vessels was reduced in proportion to the abnormal features of the stained network [16].

The abnormal lymphatic pressures detected in CVI provide evidence of a special functional lymphatic microangiopathy suggesting an additional lymphatic component in the formation of oedema [3,24,38]. The decrease in endolymphatic pressure after compression therapy has demonstrated its ability to restore the microcirculatory pressure balance through the rearrangement of macrocirculatory haemodynamics (Table 4).

In addition, we observed a decrease in interstitial pressure at the end of treatment (Table 4).

The capillaroscopic data showed greater velocimetric values and lower haematocrit values following compression, by comparison to baseline, although normal values were not reached (Table 5).

CONCLUSIONS

It is common knowledge that the aim of elastic compression therapy, in the various stages of venous insufficiency, is the reduction of the diameter of the vascular lumen to restore the physiological pressure gradients between Superficial Venous Circulation and Deep Venous Circulation.

This occurs because the bandage exerts its action mostly on the muscle-venous pump of the calf both at rest and under tension during exercise [34].

In this respect, it is necessary for the tension of an inelastic bandage to maintain a pressure higher than the deep venous system pressure so that blood flows from the superficial veins to the deep veins, which is the normal physiological situation [49].

The reduction of reflux from the proximal to the distal part of the limb slows down the production of oedema and thus of stasis, the common denominator of the trophic complications of CVI.

Indeed, stasis is really a result of flooding of the microcirculatory interstitium, even though it is due to macrocirculatory haemodynamic decompensation [1,2,4,8].

The arterialisation of the veins to decrease intraluminal venular pressure, carried out by arterio-venous anastomoses, aims to avoid an increasing capillary hydrostatic pressure [40,41,42]. This phenomenon causes vasomotion modifications upstream at the arteriolar level, and flow modification in the capillary network [32]. Such changes express themselves firstly by promoting the prevalence of the closing periods of precapillary tissue fluid excess and secondly by causing the associated phenomenon of capillary haemoconcentration.

When this defence mechanism is stressed, both the flow pressure and the tissue pressure are exceeded.

The prolonged haemoconcentration causes capillary obstruction by leukocyte trapping. Leukocyte activation injures the continuity of the endothelial barriers and produces the escape of blood cells into the interstitium [23].

In this pathological condition, the blood and tissue defence mechanisms give rise to the reversible formation of a fibrin cuff which restricts diffusion across the wall of the capillary loop.

In this complication of CVI, alterations of the capillary endothelium are produced as a results of modifications of capillary function and haemodynamics.

This has been confirmed by dynamic capillaroscopy which shows a decrease in rCVB and an increase in relative HCT.

The increase in rCVB and the decrease in HCT during therapy (either a physical treatment or a pharmacological one), is an expression of the natural resolution of capillary stasis, although there is a quantitative discrepancy between these parameters. In fact, in the capillary circulation the strong relationship between velocity and viscosity, and therefore haematocrit, no longer exists [27].

However, viscosity and haematocrit are an expression of the deformability of red blood cells and haematocrit varies in different areas of the same subject and in the different phases of the development of CVI.

Furthermore, the fibrin cuff represents the final reaction of the overburdened interstitium and also results in tissue hypoxia. This accounts for the ischaemic origin of the phlebostatic ulcers [3]. Indeed, the transcutaneous tension is reduced in proportion to the microangiopathy observed in the superficial nutrient capillaries [5,26,35].

Several studies have shown that treatments aimed at improving the microangiopathy in CVI result in an increase in the skin $TcPO_2$ [39], by the reduction in pericapillary fibrin [48] or an improvement in the physiological changes which result in white cell accumulation [18]. However, it has also been suggested that the reduction in $TcPO_2$ is a direct result of oedema [37].

When the haemodynamic events which produce the initial pathology of CVI are not resolved, the consequence is the flooding of the alternative routes for drainage (interstitial connective tissue and initial lymphatic network). The methodology most suitable for studying in vivo the lymphatic overloading observed in CVI is microlymphography [6,7,16,30].

COMMENTS

Elastic compression, by decreasing stasis, reduces its microcirculatory consequences. Christopoulos has demonstrated that as in CVI, compression produces a reduction of skin hyperaemia due to the local vasoparalysis that follows VAR impairment [22]. At the same time Belcaro, using Laser-Dopper methods, has recorded a reduciton of resting flow and standing flow after elastic compression. It must be remembered that Laser-Dopper detects flow in deeper non nutrient skin vessels which are congested in CVI. This explains the increase in the Laser-Doppler signal in routine examination of the skin in severe cases of venous disease [12]. In attempting to restore the impaired balance of pressure gradients in CVI, both at rest and on exercise, the compression pressure provided by the application of a bandage should be aimed so as to avoid pressures which are too low or too high [13,33,43,51]. This fact would explain both the failures and the complications of bandages which are applied irrationally.

It is difficult to believe that elastic compression exerts a direct action on the microcirculatory unit. If it did, compressive force would have to be regulated to match changes in intracapillary pressure, interstitial pressure and microlymphatic pressure, all of which show considerable variability between subjects and between adjacent areas [25].

From this point of view our study is entirely speculative in its nature. It has been possible to demonstrate the action of bandaging on the microcirculation as an extension of the normal behaviour of the microcirculation. In this sense, pharmacological therapy can be seen as being complementary to compression therapy but it has effects when the patient is standing as well as when he exercises.

Table 1

Mean diameters of the oedematous limb before and after compression therapy (cm)

		PRE	POST p<0.01	CONTROL
thigh	30	62.6	59.6	53.3
	20	58.4	55.9	47.4
	10	50.9	48.6	42.3
patella	0	42.8	42.0	36
	5	43	41.2	38.5
	10	37.3	35.5	30.7
	15	33.2	30.6	27.6
	20	28.9	27.2	25.3
malleolus	25	23.2	22.3	21.4

Table 2

Venous pressure values in the deep and superficial venous circulation before and after compression therapy - chronic venous incompetence

Mean Superficial Pressure		Mean Deep Pressure	
Before	After	Before	After
95.83 ± 14.27	80 ± 11.67	105 ± 8.7	82.5 ± 19
	p<0.05		p<0.019

Table 3

Venous pressure values in the deep and superficial venous circulation before and after compression therapy - healthy controls

Mean Superficial Pressure		Mean Deep Pressure	
Before	After	Before	After
50 ± 5	40 ± 5	60 ± 5	45 ± 8
	p<0.01		p<0.01

Table 4

Microlymphatic parameters before and after compression therapy

	D 0	D 28	Controls
Meshes features	14.7 ± 7	10 ± 4 (n.s.)	6.6 ± 5
Diameters	80.5 ± 3	61.6 ± 18 (p<0.01)	54
Spread	9.3 ± 2	5 ± 2 (n.s.)	3 ± 1
Endolymphatic pressure	7.2 ± 2	5.89 ± 1 (p<0.05)	4.19 ± 1
Interstitial pressure	5.3 ± 1	3.5 ± 1.7 (p<0.01)	0.62 ± 1

Table 5

Dynamic capillaroscopic parameters before and after elastic compression therapy

	Before	After	Control
HCT rel	57%	48%	30%
rCVB	0.25 mm/sec	0.30 mm/sec	0.38 mm/sec

REFERENCES
1.   Allegra C. Fino a che punto la stasi venulare è un fenumeno reversibile senza sequele? 5th National Congress of the Italian Clinical and Experimental Phlebology Society, Palermo Dec 1988; Monduzzi Pubbl.
2.   Allegra C. Flebopatie e microcircolo: concetto di stasi. Microcirc Oggi 1988; anno V: 1-3.
3.   Allegra C. The role of the microcirculation in venous ulcers. Phlebolinphology. Les laboratoires Servier 1994; 2: 5-8.
4.   Allegra C. Endotelio come organo. Pragma Ed Milano March 1981.
5.   Allegra C, Carlizza A. Microcirculatation in CVI. XI Cong Of U.I.L Budapest Sept 1993; 165.
6.   Allegra C, e coll. Mycrolymphatic diameters in mild and severe chronic venous insufficiency. 18th European Congress on Microcirculation Roma Sept 1994.
7.   Allegra C, e coll. Lymphatic capillary pressures in human skin of patients with chronic venous insufficiency. 18th European Congress on Microcirculation Roma Sept 1994.
8.   Allegra C. The microcirculation in venous disease. Medicografia 1994; 16 (2): 50-54.
9.   Allegra C, et al. CVI and capillary perfusion after pharmacological stimulation. XI Cong of U.I.L Budapest Sept 1993; 164.
10.   Allegra C. Approccio al malato flebologico. Servier Roma Ed 1995.
11.   Altenkamper H. Effects de la compression forte intermittente sue les activateurs du plasminogene dans la saphene interne. Acta World Congress of U.I.P Bruxelles Maggio 1983; 489-491.
12.   Belcaro G, et al. Evaluation of the effects of elastic compression in patients with post-phlebitic limbs by Laser-Doppler Flowmetry. Phlebologie Nov-Dec 1988; 41 (4): 797-802.
13.   Boivin P, et al. Bas élastique, unique ou superposés, comparaison de leurs effects hémodynamiques artériels. Phlebologie 1989; A Davy and R Stemmer Eds: 865-867.
14.   Bollinger A. Fluorescence microlymphography. Circulation 1981; 64: 1195-1200.
15.   Bollinger A, Junger M, Jager K. Fluroescence video microscopy techniques for the evaluation of human skin microcirculation. Prog Appl Microcirc 1986; 11: 77-79.
16.   Bollinger A, e coll. Lymphatic capillary pressure and network extension in patients with lymphoedema before and after combined physical therapy. 18th Conference on Microcirculation Roma Sept 1994.
17.   Bollinger A, Fagrell B. Clinical capillaroscopy. Hogrefe e Huber Publ 1990.
18.   Coleridge-Smith PD, et al. Causes of venous ulceration: a new hypothesis. Br Med J 1988; 1727-1727.
19.   Cossio Jimenez JA. Los linfáticos en la insufficiencia venosa crònica. Progresos en linfologia Ed Jarpyo Madrid 1987.
20.   Curri SB, et al. Changes of cutaneous microcirculation from elasto-compression in chronic venous insufficiency. X World Congress of U.I.P. Strasburg 1989; 852-854.
21.   Curri SB. Anatomia del microcirculo cutaneo: nuove acquisizioni morfofunzionali sulla microangiotettonica distrettuale delle diverse regioni della superficie cutanea indagate con video-Capillaroscopia a Sonda Ottica (VCSO). Flebologia 1992; 3: 247-259.
22.   Cristopoulos DC, et al. Venous hypertensive microangiopathy in relation to clinical severity and effect of elastic compression. J. Dermatol Surg Oncol Oct 1991; 17 (10): 809-813.
23.   Dormandy J, Thomas P. The role of leukocytes in chronic venous insufficiency and venous leg ulceration. Phlébologie 1989; Stemmer Ed John Libbey Eurotext Ltd: 113-115.
24.   Emter M, et coll. Venous flow in the lower limb with compression therapy study with the Duplex Scanner. Phlébologie 1989; A Davy and R Stemmer Eds: 868-870.
25.   Emter M, et coll. Changes of microcircolo in the skin in patients with chronic venous insufficiency in various positions and with compression therapy. Phlébologie 1989; A Davy and R Stemmer Eds: 871-872.
26.   Fagrell B. Local microcirculation in chronic venous incompetence and leg ulcers. Vasc Surg 1979; 13: 217-225.

1148

27.   Fagrell B, Intaglietta M, Ostergren J. Relative haematocrit in human skin capillaries and its relation to capillary blood flow velocity. Microvasc Res 1980; 20: 327-335.
28.   Fischer H. Action de la compression sur les vines. Phlébologie 1979; 32: 171-178.
29.   Flamini FO, De Angelis V. Controllo flebotensiometricodella terapia elastocompressiva nella patologia venosa degli arti inferiori. Corso di Aggiornamento e Simposio Internazionale Varici degli arti inferiori. Cortona Sept 1981.
30.   Franzeck UK, et al. Microangiopathy of cutaneous blood and lymphatic capillaries in chronic venous insufficiency (CVI). Yale J Biol Med Jan-Feb 1993; 66 (1): 37-46.
31.   Hach W. L'insuffisance veineuse chronique sévère et son traitement.   Traitement compressif en phlébologie 1992; John Libbey Eurotext Paris: 67-68.
32.   Intaglietta M, Allegra C. Vasomotion and flowmotion. Min Med 1992; 17 (2 suppl 2).
33.   Johnson G. Compression of the lower extremity. Phlébologie 1989; A Davy and R Stemmer Eds: 849-851.
34.   Junger M, e coll. Physical exercise training as therapy for patients with chronic venous incompetence. XIth World Congress de l'U.I.P. Montrèal Sept 1992.
35.   Leu AJ, et al. Microangiopathies in chronic venous insufficiency (CVI). Ther Umsch Oct 1991; 48 (10): 715-721.
36.   Mancini S, e coll. Compression of the lower limbs by elastic stocking: a morphological study of the peripheral veins with TAC. XIth World Congress of U.I.P. Montreal Sept 1992.
37.   Mani R, et al. Tissue oxygenation, venous ulcers and phibrin cuffs. J Roy Soc Med 1989; 82: 345.
38.   Marmasse J. La Méthode compressive à travers les ages. Phlébologie 1979; 32/2: 119-131.
39.   McMullin GM, et al. Efficacy of fibrinolytic enhancement with Stanzolol in the treatment of venous insufficiency. Aust NZ J Surg 1991; 61: 306-309.
40.   Merlen JF. Relations histo-angéiques en phlébologie. Phlébologie 1974; 27 (4): 427-431.
41.   Merlen JF. Les pressions tissulaires au niveau de la jambe. Phlébologie 1979; 32: 133-137.
42.   Merlen JF. Les modalités réactionnelles à l'étage du lit vasculaire.   Congrés Anesthésiologie Evian 1967.
43.   Mollard JM. Compression et troubles trophiques. Traitement compressif en phlébologie 1992; John Libbey Eurotext Paris: 69-75.
44.   Partsch H. Amélioration du rendement de la pompe veineuse dans l'insuffisance veineuse chronique par la compression en fonction de la pression exercée et du matériel utilisé. Vasa 1984; 13: 58-64.
45.   Rashid P, et al. The effects of using high compression elastic stockings on oedema and skin oxygenation. Phlébologie 1992; P Raymound-Martimbeau Ed: 882-884.
46.   Rehinarez D. L'insuffisance circolatoire lymphatique. Veines, lymphatiques, interstitium 1987; Boots-Dacour Ed:44-48.
47.   Sarin S. Mechanism of action of external compression in venous disease. Phlébologie 1992; P Raymond-Martimbeau Ed: 879-880.
48.   Stacey MC, et al. Transcutaneous oxygen tensions in assessing the treatment of healed venous ulcers. Br J Surg 1990; 77: 1050-1054.
49.   Stemmer R. Starling'sche hypothese und venose oedeme der unteren extremitat. Zentralbl Phlebologie 1967; 3/3: 36-44.
50.   Stemmer R, Marescaux J, Furderer C. Il trattamento compressivo degli arti inferiori, in particolare mediante calze e collant di contenimento. Der Hautartzt, Springer-Verlag 1980; Centro Documentazione Pabish (Milano).
51.   Stemmer R. Perspectives de la compression. Phlébologie 1989; A Davy and R Stemmer Eds: 856-858.
52.   Stoberl C, et al. Nuclear medicine and compression therapy. Phlébologie 1989; A Davy and R Stemmer Eds: 855.

53.   Strejcek J.   Objectivisation of the long term effect of various types of compression bandages with Digital Photoplethysmography.   XIth World Congress of U.I.P. Montreal Sept 1992.
54.   Widmer LK.   Peripheral venous disorders.   Basle Study III 1978; Huber, Bern.
55.   Wienert V, Streuf S.   The effect of elastic stockings on the venous capacity and the venous outflow.   Phlébologie 1989; A Davy and R Stemmer Eds: 859-861.

Phlebology '95, D. Negus et al. (eds.). Phlebology (1995) Suppl. 1: 1150-1152

Compression Bandages

Elbert Einarsson

The art of compression bandage therapy has been known since long before the time of Christ and probably no-one today can dispute its benefit. An enormous number of references in the literature aim to elucidate the effect of compression therapy but it is obvious from studying this literature that the mechanism of action remains unresolved, and may be somewhat theoretical despite the results.

First I would like to stress the importance of using the correct nomenclature. In its 'Product News' one manufacturer defines its short-stretch bandage as 'elasticity 60%'. Such statements are very confusing and in order to understand the science of bandaging it is necessary to use the correct definitions.

The first important property of a bandage is the *extensibility* or stretch. This is the change in length of the bandage when it is subjected to an extending force and is usually expressed as a percentage of the unstretched length.

Elasticity, on the other hand, is the ability of the bandage to counteract a stretching force and resist any change in length, and also its ability to return to its unstretched length when the force is removed. This means that there is *tension* in the bandage which is proportional to the stretching force.

The *compression* (P) exerted on the leg from a bandage depends on the tension (T), the radius of the leg (r), the width of the bandage (W) and the number of layers of bandage (n) according to Laplace's law $P = Tn/rW$. It is obvious that it is the tension and not the extensibility that produces the pressure.

Bandages are usually classed as either non-elastic or elastic. Non-elastic bandages have no extensibility and no elastic tension in the material. The pressure they exert depends entirely on how tightly they are applied to the leg. In the literature, elastic bandages are divided into short-stretch (extensibility < 70%), medium-stretch (70 - 140%) and long-stretch. It is, however, important to realise that different bandages may have equal extensile properties but quite different tension at the same stretch. This depends on the kind of elastic material that is woven into the textile material; this can be either natural rubber, latex, or synthetic threads. Elasticity is also dependent on the thickness and the characteristics after washing; g) it should be comfortable, not prevent activity, and should allow shoes to be worn and, most important, h) it should have a high patient compliance. No compression bandage can fulfil all these criteria for every patient, but the correct bandage should be selected for each individual patient.

In principle there are three kinds of bandages: unprepared pure textile bandages, adhesive bandages, and cohesive bandages.

There is one randomised study, comparing adhesive with non-adhesive bandages, which showed that a non-adhesive bandage will retain its pressure less than 24 hours compared to one week for the adhesive bandage. Another non-randomised study showed that a cohesive bandage is effective for up to 6 days compared to less than 24 hours for a non-adhesive elastic bandage.

There are numerous ways of using a compression bandage. It may be applied in a single or multiple layers, upwards or downwards on the leg, in spiral fashion or in figures of eight. Different kinds of bandage materials may be used on top of each other (ie double bandages, Unna's boot). The most important thing is that the final bandage gives a graduated compression decreasing upwards from the ankle. It is obvious from Laplace's law that if a bandage is applied with the same tension all the way along the limb, the pressure will decrease with the increasing radius of the limb. In a conical leg, graduated pressure in proximal direction is automatically achieved except around the knee area. The foot should be included in the bandage. It seems to be sufficient to bandage only the leg below the knee in most cases, except when treating oedema involving the whole length of the leg.

One randomised study compared a one layer bandage with a triple layer bandage. No difference was found in efficacy.

Arnoldi stated at one time that every phlebologist, in time, develops a method for compression treatment that suits him, thereby achieving good results. This means that the bandage should always be applied by an experienced and trained person.

What is the correct compression to use in different situations? It is theoretically claimed that the higher the ambulatory venous hypertension, the higher the bandage pressure needed. After reviewing a large number of papers in the literature I am, however, surprised that there is still almost no good randomised study that shows which type of bandage, material or bandage technique or what compression pressure is needed, or which is the best in different clinical situations. Some authors advocate inelastic bandaging to enhance venous return and control oedema, and others claim this to have no benefit compared to bandages with a higher degree of elasticity. This, however, seems to be empirical rather than based on real scientific fact. Good randomised clinical studies are urged for the future and hopefully the results will help us to design and select more effective regimens for each patient and clinical indication.

number of elastic threads per surface unit. It is stated in the literature that different bandages have different effects in the static situation compared with the dynamic situation. In the static situation it is only the tension in the material that exerts pressure on the tissues; when the patient is contracting the muscles of the leg, however, the bandage will act as an outer fascia against which the muscles press during contraction. This will give a swinging working pressure in the veins and tissues. A so-called short-stretch bandage with low to moderate tensile properties will give low resting, but high working pressure. In contrast, a more 'elastic' bandage with higher tension and higher extensibility will give higher resting, and relatively lower working pressure because of its extensibility. The degree of pressure depends both on how tightly the bandage is applied to the leg, and on how much it is stretched during use. Thus it is possible to select the type of bandage depending on the patient's disease and mobility.

It has been pointed out that there is no uniformity among manufacturers or phycisists in describing the properties of extensibility and tension. So far there is no agreed international standard. There is some overlap between so-called short-stretch and medium-stretch bandages, and the tension is almost never given. Serious efforts should be made to achieve a consensus for bandages, as has already been started for compression hosiery. Different bandages could then be accurately compared.

An important finding in chronic venous insufficiency is ambulatory venous hypertension. The effect of compression on venous pressure, however, shows contradictory results in the literature. Some authors find no difference in ambulatory venous hypertension or venous refilling time with outer compression, and others find that these parameters are improved. The peak systolic pressure seems to be reduced. There is agreement that the resting pressure does not change with compression. Several authors, using different methods of recording venous flow, found that deep venous flow is increased during compression. There are some indications that non-elastic bandages are better at increasing deep venous flow in mobile patients.

Compression has been shown to reduce venous volume. In some studies the volume expelled during muscular contraction has also been shown to be improved. It has also been shown that a reduction in venous diameter is possible and it has been claimed that this may help to regain venous valvular competence. An increase in venous tone may also influence blood flow. It has been shown that with a compression pressure of 25 mmHg the mean arterial flow was reduced, as was the skin blood flow. In contrast, another study has shown that a pressure of 40-50 mmHg increased the skin blood flow and the oxygen tension in the skin. It has also been stated that transcutaneous PO_2 in liposclerotic tissue was reduced despite hyperaemia.

Measurements of the tissue pressure in the epifascial compartment have shown that non-elastic bandages produced higher pressure during exercise and on standing than elastic bandages. The pressure naturally varies directly with the applied bandage pressure.

The ideal compression bandage should fulfil the following criteria. a) it should provide a reproducible and effective level of compression; b) it should provide graduated compression; c) it should retain consistent compression; d) it should stay in position and not slip down; e) it should not be affected by dampness or exudate, and compression should remain adequate even in the presence of a wound dressing; f) it should retain its

Phlebology '95, D. Negus et al. (eds.). Phlebology (1995) Suppl. 1: 1153-1157

The Use of Medical Elastic Compression Hosiery in Phlebology

H.A.M. Neumann and J.C.J.M. Veraart

Department of Dermatology, Akademisch Ziekenhuis Maastricht, Maastricht, The Netherlands

Most authors agree that compression therapy has a central role in the treatment of venous diseases. Compression therapy can be divided into elastic and nonelastic compression. Compression using hosiery is always elastic compression therapy. Recently the different aspects of compression therapy have been reviewed by Neumann and Tazelaar [1].

Chronic venous insufficiency (CVI) is characterised by the delayed and disturbed return of venous blood to the heart. In most cases the venous (calf) muscle pump is not able to reduce the venous pressure during walking (due to reflux in the venous system). The capillaries are unable to remain resistant to this long-standing high pressure and become insufficient [2]. The visible (skin) signs of CVI correlate with the disturbance of the microcirculation. Oxygen becomes less available to the tissue and finally a leg ulcer develops [2,3,4,5].

Not only the high WVP but also the linked venous refill time influence the venous system. Veins with valvular insufficiency fill more easily due to the effect of gravity compared with physiologically normal veins when blood drains from the tissues. Compression therapy itself has little or no influence on the pressure profile during walking. Thus the high WVP will remain elevated even with adequate compression therapy. However, the venous refill time is improved and sometimes becomes normal using compression.

The beneficial effects of compression can be further explained by the following:
- reduction of oedema with recovery of the Starling equilibrium
- reduction of the venous volume
- increase of blood transmission time in the leg
- increase of arterial influx
- increase of lymphatic flow with reduction of dermal back flow

Due to all the abovementioned effects of compression on the total circulation of the lower leg, the therapy treats and prevents venous leg ulcers. It is, however, essential to obtain sufficient compression to achieve this aim. For long-term compression it is preferable to use medical compression hosiery.

Due to the use of modern materials such as Spandex, the cosmetic appearance of hosiery, and with it patient compliance, have made great progress. The methods of knitting are variable. Discussion continues among the manufacturers concerning whether an elastic inlaid thread[1] is essential for the quality of the hosiery. For the German and French industry norm (DIN, AINOR) it is considered essential, but for the British norm (BSI) it is not. However, there are good indications that comfort and durability are increased with elastic inlaid thread, especially in the higher compression classes.

Two main types of compression hosiery can be distinguished: 1) flat knitted and 2) round knitted. Flat knitted compression hosiery can be tailor-made for size.

To prescribe hosiery correctly it is essential to observe the leg carefully. The manufacturers use a specific code for standardised measuring points. For standard size hosiery each manufacturer uses its own size table. If the leg being measured does not fit into this table, custom-made hosiery is required [6].

Medical compression hosiery is used to exert a known pressure on the skin and the underlying tissue. To avoid congestion it is essential for the pressure to decrease gradually from the distal to the proximal end by at least as much as the natural fall in the venous standing pressure under the influence of gravity.

The medical effectiveness of the hosiery depends on the amount of compression and the slope or stiffness value [2] of the elastic materials used. In general, compression is divided into four classes. The European Committee for Standardisation (CEN) has, up to now, not reached a European consensus about these classes. However, it is wise to refer to CEN document CEN/TC 205 N 354 which proposes a standardised compression class table [7].
It is not only the degree of compression, but also the characteristics of the elastic material which determine the medical qualities of compression hosiery. In about 90% of cases in venous patients AD hosiery will be sufficient.

The extent to which the intended effects of compression are achieved depends largely on the pressure of the elastic materials [8]. This pressure (P) is directly correlated with the tension (S) and indirectly with the radius of the leg. This known as Laplace's law: $P=S/R$. Thus the pressure on the leg will vary according to the different surface curvatures. The risk of exceptional high pressures and of pressure necrosis, exists at areas with a small radius, such as the malleolus, Achilles tendon, and the sharp edge of the tibia. On the other hand, pressure may be insufficient in the retromalleolar space and other places with low convex curvature. Pads or padding can be used to fill in these areas.

The pressure exerted by the hosiery changes during walking. The characteristics of the materials used make a highly significant contribution to these pressure changes [9,10]. Less elastic hosiery, that is, hosiery with a high slope value, will produce large pressure differences during walking, thus improving the muscle pump function and providing a strong anti-oedema effect [11,12,13].

In the supine position, due to the absence of the effect of gravity, elastic hosiery can cause ischaemia, particularly when arterial flow is impaired. Hosiery with a pressure of more than 25 mmHg must be removed at night [14,15].

The prescriber has to choose between ready-made hosiery and custom-made hosiery. Ready-made hosiery will not fit:
1. when there is a difference between the A and B values,
2. when the D value is equal or higher than the C value [20].

The indications for hosiery are more or less the same as for compression therapy in general. However, in many cases it is not convenient to use hosiery during active leg ulcer treatment. The main difference between hosiery and compression therapy with bandages is that hosiery is not suitable for reducing oedema, only for the prevention of the formation of oedema. When cure is not possible, as in the post-thrombotic syndrome or angiodysplasia, compression hosiery is the treatment of choice [16,17].

The key to good maintenance of compression is thorough education of the patient. Very often the hosiery is poorly fitting, inconvenient, or regarded by the patient as ugly. Half of the hosiery prescribed in the Netherlands is not worn by the patient [17]. The importance of wearing "effective" compression hosiery (often of a higher class), rather than stockings that do not achieve good clinical results, should not be forgotten. The hosiery must maintain its effective pressure for at least 6 months [18]. After 6-12 months the pressure exerted usually falls [10,19]. Therefore it is advisable to replace the hosiery every six months. For proper hygiene it is advisable to prescribe at least two sets of hosiery at a time for each leg.

There are no good objective parameters available to determine the effectiveness of compression other than the clinical sign of oedema formation. For this reason patients treated with compression hosiery should ideally make their visit to the physician late in the afternoon. In cases where oedema forms, compression must be increased. The following steps are recommended:
1. Choose hosiery from a higher compression class.
2. Choose hosiery from the same compression class, but with a higher slope value.
3. Wear two stockings, one over the other. As the pressure exerted is additive, two 25 mmHg stockings will result in the same pressure as one 50 mmHg stocking. In some patients, so-called anti-thrombotic hosiery with a non-graduated pressure profile (13-17mmHg) can be used under medical compression hosiery. In this case the pressure is at every level increased by 13-17 mmHg.

Only a well-motivated patient together with an experienced physician are able to ensure the ongoing success of this therapy. If either of these two factors is inadequate, treatment with medical elastic compression hosiery will produce disappointing results [21].

In the supine position, due to the absence of the effect of gravity, elastic hosiery can cause ischaemia, particularly when arterial flow is impaired. Hosiery with a pressure of more than 25 mmHg must be removed at night [14,15].

The prescriber has to choose between ready-made hosiery and custom-made hosiery. Ready-made hosiery will not fit:
1. when there is a difference between the A and B values,
2. when the D value is equal or higher than the C value [20].

The indications for hosiery are more or less the same as for compression therapy in general. However, in many cases it is not convenient to use hosiery during active leg ulcer treatment. The main difference between hosiery and compression therapy with bandages is that hosiery is not suitable for reducing oedema, only for the prevention of the formation of oedema. When cure is not possible, as in the post-thrombotic syndrome or angiodysplasia, compression hosiery is the treatment of choice [16,17].

The key to good maintenance of compression is thorough education of the patient. Very often the hosiery is poorly fitting, inconvenient, or regarded by the patient as ugly. Half of the hosiery prescribed in the Netherlands is not worn by the patient [17]. The importance of wearing "effective" compression hosiery (often of a higher class), rather than stockings that do not achieve good clinical results, should not be forgotten. The hosiery must maintain its effective pressure for at least 6 months [18]. After 6-12 months the pressure exerted usually falls [10,19]. Therefore it is advisable to replace the hosiery every six months. For proper hygiene it is advisable to prescribe at least two sets of hosiery at a time for each leg.

There are no good objective parameters available to determine the effectiveness of compression other than the clinical sign of oedema formation. For this reason patients treated with compression hosiery should ideally make their visit to the physician late in the afternoon. In cases where oedema forms, compression must be increased. The following steps are recommended:
1. Choose hosiery from a higher compression class.
2. Choose hosiery from the same compression class, but with a higher slope value.
3. Wear two stockings, one over the other. As the pressure exerted is additive, two 25 mmHg stockings will result in the same pressure as one 50 mmHg stocking. In some patients, so-called anti-thrombotic hosiery with a non-graduated pressure profile (13-17mmHg) can be used under medical compression hosiery. In this case the pressure is at every level increased by 13-17 mmHg.

Only a well-motivated patient together with an experienced physician are able to ensure the ongoing success of this therapy. If either of these two factors is inadequate, treatment with medical elastic compression hosiery will produce disappointing results [21].

REFERENCES
1.   Neumann HAM, Tazelaar DJ. Compression therapy. Varicose veins and telcangiectasias - diagnosis and treatment. Quality Medical Publishing Inc 1993; JJ Bergan and MP Goldman Eds St Louis Missouri: 103-122.

2.   Neumann HAM, Brock van den MJTB.   Evaluation of O-(B-hydroxyethyl)-rutosides in chronic venous insufficiency by means of non-invasive techniques. Phlebology 1990; 5: 13-20.

3.   Neumann HAM, Leeuwen van M, Broek van den MJTB, Berretty PJM. Transcutaneous oxygen tension in chronic venous insufficiency syndrome. VASA 1984; 13: 213-219.

4.   Franzeck UK. Sauerstoffpartialdruck und kapillarmorphologic bei patienten mit chronisch-venoeser insuffizienz (CVI). Phlebol u Proktol 1993; 12: 149-160.

5.   Vanscheidt W, Stengele K, Wokalek H, Schoepf E. Perikapillaere fibrinmanschetten - ein O2-Diffusionsblock? VASA 1991; 20: 142-146.

6.   Hohlbaum GG. Masz - oder konfektionsstrumpf. Phlebol Proktol 1982; 11: 42-49.

7.   Document CEN/TC 205 N354. European Committee for Standardisation Brussels 1994.

8.   Molen van de H, Kuiper J. Mesure de la compression en therapeutique phleboloque et notament de la pression permanente efficace a près reduction de le oedeme. Phlébologie 1960; 13: 21.

9.   Stemmer R. Konzentrische und exzentrische kompression. Phebol Proktol 1984; 13: 53-57.

10.   Gregory von R. Eigenschaften elastischer binden. Phlebol Proktol 1978; 7: 171-182.

11.   Hargens AR, Millard RW, Petterson K, Johansen K. Gravitation haemodynamics and oedema prevention in the giraffe. Nature 1987; 329: 59-60.

12.   Wupperman TH, Pretschner DP, Holm I, Emter M. Nuklearmedizinische messung des intravasal-und xtravasalraumes an wade und fuss beim gehen und sitzen zum vergleich zweier arten der kompressionstherapie. Phlebol Proktol 1987; 16: 175-183.

13.   Ohlert P, Wienert V. Zum wirkungsnachweis von kompression onversbänden. VASA 1988; 17: 262-266.

14.   Berg van den F, Wupperman TH. Plethysmographische ermittlung des andruckes elastischer kompressionsstrümpfe - "Anti-thrombose strümpfe". Swiss Med 1980; 2: 4a.

15.   Callam MJ, Haiart D, Farouk M, Brown D, Prescott RJ, Ruckley CV. Effect of time and posture on pressure profiles obtained by three different types of compression. Phlebology 1991; 6: 79-84.

16.   Somerville JJF, Brow GO, Byrne PJ, Quill RD, Fegan WG. The effect of clastic stockings on superficial venous pressures in patients with venous insufficiency. Brit J Surg 1974; 61: 979-981.

17.   Korstanje MJ, Newumann HAM. Compressietherapie door middel can elastische kousen. Ned Tijdschr Geneesk 1990; 134: 799-802.

18.   Bernink BP. Elastische strümpfe und ihre qualitäts beurteilung. Mcdita 1978; 8: 152-157.

19.   Stemmer R. Vorschläge zur verbesscrung der kompressionsstrümpfe. Phlebol Proktol 1980; 9: 129-137.

20.   Olsen G. Zur praxis der versorgung von beinkranken mit gumistrümpfen. Fortschr Med 1965; 83: 697-699.

21.   Ellerbrock U. Arzt und kompressionsstrümpfverordnung. Therapiewoche 1976; 26: 2376.

Phlebology '95, D. Negus et al. (eds.). Phlebology (1995) Suppl. 1: 1158-1161

Intermittent Compression Therapy in Australia and How We Compare with the Rest of the World

Peter Conrad FRCS, FRCS(Ed), FRACS, FACS(US)

Chairman, Department of Surgery, Nepean Hospital, Sydney
A teaching hospital, University of Sydney

INTRODUCTION

Intermittent compression therapy using external pneumatic compression (EPC) devices has increased in use and popularity in Australia over the last decade. Especially over the last five years, EPC devices have become more widely available in hospitals and better and more efficient models are now smaller and more portable.

EPC in Australia is now used for three purposes:

1 Prevention of postoperative deep vein thrombosis (DVT) and pulmonary embolism (PE).
2 The treatment of lymphoedema.
3 The treatment of venous ulcers.

EPC devices reverse two out of the three factors in Virchow's Triad. EPC activates fibrinolysis in the blood and reduces venous stasis.

PREVENTION OF POSTOPERATIVE DVT AND PE

In Australia the initial thrust of postoperative DVT and PE prophylaxis in the past, especially in the 1980's, has relied on low dose Heparin (LDH). This was the case especially in general surgery where based on the literature it was feld LDH significantly reduced DVT and PE [1-3]. There was no concerted effort to identify major risk factors.

In the 1990's, with the advent of more extensive orthopaedic procedures such as joint replacement with its increased risk of DVT, surgeons have realised that LDH alone is insufficient. There has been a move to identify high risk patients.

Over the past five years there has been a move to use EPC devices more and more. In the higher risk patients and higher risk operations the EPC is used peri operatively and often in the postoperative period for the first 24 - 48 hours. The benefit of this in reducing DVT is well supported in the literature [5-7].

LDH is still used extensively however in the highest risk patient is being replaced by the newer low molecular weight Heparins (LMWH). This is used usually in combination with EPC and often postoperative compression hosiery (POCH).

Although no comprehensive studies have been performed in Australia, anecdotal evidence now is that in most hospitals there is increasing use of EPC devices both peri operatively and postoperatively.

In the highest risk patients, such as those undergoing major orthopaedic surgery, EPC devices are very widely used usually in combination with LMWH and POCH. This agrees with the recommendations of Caprini et al [4].

In moderate risk patients especially now with laparoscopic surgery, EPC devices are used more and more often in combination with LDH (although in the future this may be replaced with LMWH) and POCH.

In fit young patients undergoing lesser surgical procedures where early mobilisation is anticipated, EPC does not appear to be used widely.

Over the last five years in Australia there has been a concerted effort to identify both the patients at high risk of DVT and PE and also to identify the high risk operations.

The high risks in patients include older age groups, immobility, obesity, smoking, malignancy, previous DVT or PE, myocardial infarction, dehydration, sepsis, thrombophilia, contraceptive pill and pregnancy.

The high risk operations include in orthopaedics hip and knee surgery, surgery on major fractures in the legs and leg amputation. In general surgery, abdominal laparoscopic procedures, bowel resection and surgery for malignancy. Major urology operations, especially on the prostate and bladder, major gynaecological operations especially for carcinoma of the uterus and major heart, lung and neurosurgical operations.

THE TREATMENT OF LYMPHOEDEMA

There is no doubt that in established lymphoedema EPC devices have a place alongside other established modalities such as massage techniques and pharmacological treatments.

In Australia generally physiotherapists specialising in lymphoedema treatment use EPC on an outpatient basis.

THE TREATMENT OF VENOUS ULCER

This is a new concept and EPC devices have been shown to be of benefit in the treatment of resistant venous ulcers [8].

In Australia there are only a handful of surgeons interested in ulcer treatment and testing this technique but no results are yet to hand.

CONCLUSION

This use of EPC devices has increased dramatically over the last five years in Australia. Its major use in hospitals has been in the peri operative and postoperative prevention of DVT and PE and here it has been combined with the use of LDH and LMWH as well as POCH. On an anecdotal basis, there is now an increase in the use of these devices throughout Australia. In particular, identification of high risk patients and high risk operations has taken place.

The plan for prophylaxis in high risk patients has been to use EPC devices peri operatively and 48 hours postoperatively, Heparin with increasing moves to low molecular weight Heparins peri operatively and five days postoperatively, and the use of compression stockings postoperatively.

By way of comparison with the rest of the world we find that in Australia EPC is widely used combined with Heparin and stockings in high risk patients. In the rest of the world EPC is used more widely in the USA and Heparin is more widely used in Europe.

In Australia with EPC devices, thigh compression has only been recently introduced. In Australia, EPC is only used 48 hours postoperatively whereas in Europe reliance is put more on using these devices for up to seven to ten days. In Australia, EPC is rarely used in medical cases whereas in the rest of the world there is a tendency to use these in the prophylaxis of DVT and PE in myocardial infarct, stroke and general immobility cases.

Its use in lymphoedema and venous ulcer treatment is in specialised hands at the moment but no doubt as more data becomes available its place in the treatment of these diseases will be more clear cut.

REFERENCES
1.   Colditz GA, Tuden RL, Oster G.   Rates of venous thrombosis after general surgery. Lancet 1986;2: 143-146.
2.   Collings R, Scrimgeur A, Yusus S, Peto R.   Reduction in fatal pulmonary embolism and venous thrombosis by peri operative administration of subcutaneous heparin.   N Ingl J Med 1988; 318: 1162-1173.
3.   Clagett GP, Reisch JS.   Prevention of venous thrombo embolism in general surgical patients. Annals of Surgery 1988; 208: 227-240.
4.   Caprini JA, Arcelus JI, Traverso CI, Hasty JH.   Low molecular weight heparins and esxternal pneumatic compression as options for venous thrombo embolism prophylaxis: A surgeon's perspective. Seminars in Thrombosis and Haemostatis 1991; 17 (4).
5.   Hull RD, Raskob GE, Gent M, Mcloughlin D, Julian D, Smith FC, et al.   Effectiveness of intermittent pneumatic leg compression for preventing deep vein thrombosis after total hip replacement. JAMA 1990; 263 (17).
6.   Millard JA, Hill BB, Cook PS, Fenoglio ME, Sthlgren LH.   Intermittent sequential pneumatic compression in prevention of venous stasis associated with pneumo peritoneum during laparoscopic cholecystectomy. Arch Surg 1993; 128: 914-919.

7.   Pidala MJ, Donovan DL, Kepley RF. A prospective study of intermittent pneumatic compression in the prevention of deep vein thrombosis in patients undergoing total hip or total knee replacement. Surgery Gynaecology and Obstectrics 1992; 175: 47-51.

8.   Coleridge-Smith PD, Sarin SA, Wilson LA, Scurr JH.   Intermittent pneumatic compression improves venous ulcer healing. Phlebologie 1989; Davy A, Stemmer R Eds John Libbey Eurotext : 1146-1148.

Phlebology '95, D. Negus et al. (eds.). Phlebology (1995) Suppl. 1: 1162-1165

Compression Therapy in Venous Ulcers

H. Partsch

Department of Dermatology, Wilhelminenhospital, A-1171 Vienna, Austria

INTRODUCTION

About 70% of leg ulcers are of venous origin. This is true both for people living in the community [1:Nelzen] and for patients attending the outpatient department of a hospital [2:Mayer].

Compresssion therapy is the basis of treatment of venous ulcers [3: Breddin]. Its influence on healing is much greater than that of local dressings, as has been demonstrated by various comparative studies [4:Kikta, 5:Rubin, 6:Stacey]. (Table 1).

PATHOLOGY

Venous reflux due to valvular incompetence reaching down into the skin area of the distal lower leg is the main trigger for local changes in the microcirculation. The resulting inflammation, oedema and lymphatic involvement ultimately lead to tissue breakdown (Table 2).

Several factors with a negative effect on the healing rate of venous ulcers are summarised in Table 3 [7:Skene, 2:Mayer].

EFFECTS OF COMPRESSION

Compression therapy not only influences venous macro-haemodynamics but also has major effects on the microcirculation. Reflux is reduced by compression of the large, superficial (varicose) veins and, if strong enough, also of the perforators and the incompetent deep venous system. This can be shown by Duplex [8:Mayberry] and by air plethysmography (APG) [9:Christopoulos]. By APG we found a more marked reduction of venous volume and of venous filling index with short stretch bandages compared with elastic stockings [10:Horakova, 11:Partsch WMW].

Conflicting results have been reported concerning ambulatory venous hypertension which certainly is the most significant functional parameter in triggering venous ulceration [8:Mayberry, 12:Horner, 13:Partsch, VASA]. Measurement of the venous pressure in a dorsal foot vein during exercise is affected in different ways by short and long stretch material exerting the same resting pressure. We have observed a statistically significant decrease of ambulatory venous hypertension with short stretch bandages but not with elastic compression stockings [13:Partsch].

Only recently the different mechanisms of the action of compression were shown in the compromised microcirculation [14:Own, Coleridge Smith]. The disturbance in lymphatic drainage in the area surrounding venous ulcers can be improved by compression [15:Partsch].

Despite all these new insights into the mode of action of good compression, much work still remains to be done in this field.

TYPES OF COMPRESSION

Table 4 presents a list of different compression modalities and Table 5 shows the important characteristics of an ideal bandaging system for venous ulcers [16:Ruckley].

Local pressure on venous ulcers and on incompetent perforators can be increased by using special rubber pads, based on Laplace's law. Pneumatic pressure devices have been shown to enhance the healing rate of ulcers [17:Coleridge-Smith].

Fixed bandages, mainly using short stretch material, are changed every few days whereas long stretch bandages are removed before going to bed.

Some of the specifications of short and long stretch bandages are summarised in Table 6. It should be emphasised that the use of short stretch material requires training since it should be put on using a much higher pressure than an elastic bandage. Elastic bandages maintain the pressure much more effectively than non-elastic compression and show a significantly smaller decrease in pressure on lying down [16:Ruckley, 10:Horakowa]. The loss of pressure of the non-elastic compression is proof of its therapeutic effect which consists of reduction in oedema. In this case short stretch bandages have to be changed.

We have advocated the use of "inelastic", short stretching, fixed bandages for the therapy-phase until the ulcers heal and then changing to long stretch bandages or compression stockings for maintenance [15:Partsch JDSO]. However, it has been shown that satisfactory results can also be obtained by using compression stockings [17:Samson] especially when local pressure on the ulcer is increased by using special pads [10:Horakova]. One knee-length class III stocking or one class II stocking worn on top of a class I stocking may be recommended.

COMPRESSION PRESSURE

Graduated pressure is recommended with resting values on the distal lower leg of between 30 and 40 mmHg. Table 7 shows the corresponding compression classes of stockings as recommended by the European Committee for Standardisation. During walking the so-called "working pressure" rises up to about 50 mmHg using elastic bandages and stockings and to 60 mmHg during muscle systole using non-elastic short stretch material [15:Partsch JDSO].

HEALING RATES

With good compression therapy 60-70% of ulcers should heal within 12 weeks (Table 8). Moffat and co-workers report a healing rate of 69% in 3 months with their four layer bandage [18:Moffat]. Callam et al [19] achieved better results with elastic compared to non-elastic material which may have been because the short stretch bandages had been applied at too low a pressure and by inadequately trained staff. This would explain how our own group achieved much better healing rates using Unna's boot which consists of completely rigid material [2:Mayer].

The extremely favourable results of Horakova [10] using elastic stockings can in the main be explained by positive selection of ulcer-patients in this group. In a randomised study Coleridge-Smith reported very poor healing rates with elastic stockings alone but impressively better results in the group treated with sequential compression [17]. This finding again underlines the importance of adequate compression pressure.

Better training of doctors and nurses is required to improve the therapeutical results in the continually neglected field of ulcer-therapy.

RECURRENCES AND LONG-TERM COMPRESSION

In our experience the recurrence rate of a healed ulcer in the first year is about 30%, mainly due to non-compliance of the use of long-term compression [2:Mayer]. Harper and co-workers were able to show much better results with 15% recurrence using high compression pressure and 24% recurrence using low compression stockings [20:Harper].

The non-compliance of patients ranges between 11% [8:Mayberry] and 63% [16:Ruckley] (Table 9).

"CONSENSUS"

Most authors agree that compression is the most effective treatment modality for venous ulcers. Local dressings are less important.

Disagreement exists about the use of bandages in patients with non-venous ulcers, for example in mixed cases with peripheral arterial occlusions and in diabetics.

Still under discussion are the issues of optimal compression material (short-stretch versus long-stretch), the use of compression stockings for active venous ulcers and the various mechanisms of action.

REFERENCES
1. Nelzen O, Bergqvist D, Lindhagen A. Leg ulcer etiology: A cross sectional population study. J Vasc Surg 1991; 557-564.
2. Mayer W, Jochmann W, Partsch H. Ulcus cruris: Abheilung unter konservativer therapie. Eine propspektive studie. Wein Med Wochenschr 1994; 144: 250-252.
3. The Alexander House Group. Consensus on paper on venous leg ulcers. Phlebology 1992; 7: 48-58.
4. Kikta MJ, Schuler JJ, Meyer JP, Durham JR, Eldrup-Jorgensen J, Schwarcz TH, Flanigan DP. A prospective, randomised trial of Unna's Boots versus hydroactive dressing in the treatment of venous stasis ulcers. J Vasc Surg.
5. Rubin JR, Alexander J, Plecha EJ, Marman C. Unna's boot versus polyurethane foam dressings for the treatment of venous ulceration. Arch Surg 1990; 125: 489-490.
6. Stacey MC, Jopp-McKay A, Raschid P, Hoskin S. The influence of dressing on venous ulcers healing. Phlébologie 1992; P Raymond-Martimbeau, R Prescott, M Zummo Eds, John Libbey, Paris 1992; 1318-1320.
7. Skene AL, Smith JM, Dore CJ, Charlett A, Lewis JD. Venous leg ulcers: a prognastic index to predict time to healing. BMJ 1992; 305: 1119-1121.
8. Mayberry JC, Moneta GL, Taylor LM Jr, Porter JM. Fifteen-year results of ambulatory compression therapy for chronic venous ulcers. Surgery 1991; 109: 575-581.
9. Christopoulos DG, Nicolaides AN, Szendro G, Irvine AT, Bull M, Eastcott HHG. Air-plethysmography and the effect of elastic compression on venous haemodynamics of the legs. J Vasc Surg 1987; 5: 148-159.
10. Horakova MA, Partsch H. Ulcères de jambe d'origine veineuse: indications pour les bas de compression? Phlébologie 1994; 47: 53-57.
11. Partsch H, Horakova MA. Kompressionsstrümpfe zur behandlung venöser unterschenkelgeschwüre. Wein Med Wochenschr 1994; 144: 242-249.
12. Horner J, Fernandes e Fernandes J, Nicolaides AN. Value of graduated compression stockings in deep venous insufficiency. BMJ 1980.
13. Partsch H. Besserung der venösen pumpleistung bei chronischer veneninsuffizienz durch kompression in Abhängigkeit von Andruck un Material. VASA 1984; 13: 58-64.
14. Own AA, Scurr JH, Coleridge-Smith PD. Effets des bas de contention sur la microcirculation cutanée. Phlébologie 1993; 46: 671-672.
15. Partsch H. Compression therapy of the legs. J Dermatol Surg Oncol 1991; 17: 799-805.
16. Ruckley CV. Treatment of venous ulceration. Compression therapy. Phlebology 1992; suppl 1: 22-26.
17. Coleridge-Smith PD, Sarin S, Hasty J, Scurr JH. Sequential gradient pneumatic compression enhances venous ulcer healing: a randomised trial. Surgery 1990; 108: 871-875.
18. Samson RH. Compression stockings and non-continuous use of polyurethane foam dressings for the treatment of venous ulceration. A pilot study. J Dermatol Surg Oncol 1993; 19: 68-72.
19. Moffatt CJ, Franks PJ, Oldroyd M, Bonsaquet N, Brown P, Greenhalgh RM, McCollum CN. Community clinics for leg ulcers and impact of healing. BMJ 1992; 305: 1389-1392.
20. Callam MJ, Harper DR, Dale JJ, Brown D, Gibson B, Prescott RJ, Ruckley CV. Lothian and Fort Valley leg ulcer healing trial, part 1: elastic versus non-elastic bandaging in the treatment of chronic leg ulceration. Phlebology 1992; 7: 136-141.
21. Harper DR, Ruckley CV, Dale JJ, Callam Mc, Allan P, Brown D, Gibson B, Nelson A, Prescott RJ. Prevention of recurrence of chronic leg ulcer: a randomised trial of different degrees of compression. Phlébologie 1992; P Raymond-Martimbeau, R Prescott, M Zummo Eds, John Libbey Eurotext, Paris: 902-903.

Phlebology '95, D. Negus et al. (eds.). Phlebology (1995) Suppl. 1: 1166-1168

Graduated Compression Stockings in the Prophylaxis Against Deep Venous Thrombosis

S.K. Shami and J.H. Scurr

Department of Surgery, University College London Medical School, London, UK

INTRODUCTION

Deep venous thrombosis (DVT) is a common post-operative event if prophylaxis to prevent it is not undertaken. DVT in the short term may result in pulmonary embolism with its high morbidity and mortality. In the long term about 40 to 70% of patients with DVT develop the post-thrombotic syndrome and its associated manifestations of oedema, skin changes (lipodermatosclerosis) and venous ulceration. The incidence of clinical DVT in the population is estimated at 0.1% per year, though it is likely that twice as many people are having asymptomatic DVTs. Reviews of the literature in the early 1980's suggested that without prophylaxis as many as 30% of patients after a general surgical procedure suffered a DVT and that the figure was even higher for patients undergoing pelvic and hip operations. Without prophylaxis the incidence of fatal pulmonary embolism has been estimated as between 0.4 and 1.6%. All patients within a hospital are at risk, including patients who have suffered myocardial infarcts or strokes where the incidence of DVT is 20 to 60%.

The incidence of DVT may be reduced by a number of methods including drugs such as heparin and dextran and physical means such as compression stockings and intermittent pneumatic compression as well as a combination of these coupled with early ambulation. The purpose of this paper is to examine the role of graduated compression stockings in the prevention of DVT.

GRADUATED COMPRESSION STOCKINGS IN DVT PROPHYLAXIS

Graduated compression stockings have been evaluated in many clinical studies and their efficacy in the prevention of deep vein thrombosis is well established. Using the fibrinogen uptake test to make the initial diagnosis of deep vein thrombosis in general surgical patients, the incidence of deep vein thrombosis in the untreated group ranges from 49% to 4% with a mean of 32%, and from 23% to 3.6% in the treated group, with a mean of 9%. In a postmortem study, it was shown that patients wearing graduated compression stockings had a reduced incidence of fatal pulmonary embolism. All studies using graduated compression stockings have shown a beneficial effect in reducing the incidence of deep vein thrombosis. Compression stockings are simple, safe and effective and are recommended for use in low risk patients, and in combination and other prophylactic modalities, for moderate to high risk patients. By producing graduated compression stockings of differing sizes, it is possible to fit 95% of the population with a stocking offering the correct compression profile.

MODE OF ACTION

The mode of action of compression stockings remains uncertain. Virchow in 1856 proposed that stasis and vein wall damage may promote the formation of deep vein thrombosis. Venous distension has been shown to occur in the upper limb veins and lower limb veins during surgery and it has been proposed that venous distension may cause vein wall injury, thereby contributing to the development of DVT. It has been shown that venous distention in patients undergoing surgery is associated with an increase in the incidence of DVT. Early studies suggested that compression stockings increased venous flow velocity. By increasing and decreasing the amount of graduated compression, it is possible to establish the maximum possible percentage increase in femoral vein blood velocity, and this profile was used to develop the graduated compression stocking. The prevention of venous stasis and increase of blood flow, through the deeper veins, is thought to be important in the prevention of deep vein thrombosis. However, other studies failed to show a deep venous haemodynamic effect using compression stockings. It is probable that the graduated compression stocking exerts at least some of its effect by the prevention of venous distension. The significance of venous distension relates in part to venous pooling, but also in part to an alteration in the nature of the vein wall. As the veins are stretched, gaps appear between the endothelial cells, collagen is exposed, and a site for thrombosis started. Whether it is necessary to compress the whole leg or just calf, has not been studied.

GRADUATED COMPRESSION STOCKINGS AND INTERMITTENT PNEUMATIC COMPRESSION

Compression stockings may be used on their own or in combination with other prophylactic measures When looking at the effectiveness of ermittent pneumatic compression on the leg, used in combination with a graduated compression stocking, it was noted that the presence of a compression stocking increased the effectiveness of external pneumatic compression. The graduated compression stocking prevented venous distension during the relaxation phase of the pneumatic compression cycle. There have also been preliminary reports suggesting that foot pumping using a special slipper incorporating an expanding chamber connected to a pump may be effective in prophylaxis against DVT. This has been shown to be effective in patients undergoing total knee arthroplasty and total hip arthroplasty. It has been shown that the combined use of footpumps and compression stockings increases venous blood flow and velocity without a corresponding increase in vein diameter. In addition, combined use of the two methods is more effective in increasing flow velocity and volumetric flow compared to the effects of compression stockings alone. However it is not clear whether the combined use of the footpump and compression stockings is likely to offer increased protection from DVT.

GRADUATED COMPRESSION STOCKINGS AND SUBCUTANEOUS HEPARIN

Graduated compression stockings have been combined with low-dose heparin in the prevention of DVT. Using subcutaneous heparin and graduated compression stocking on alternate legs, it was shown that the incidence of DVT in the non-stockinged leg was 12%, compared to 4% in the stocking leg. In a controlled study, it was demonstrated that the incidence of DVT was 12% in patients receiving subcutaneous heparin alone, compared to 2% in those patients receiving both subcutaneous heparin and graduated compression stockings.

CONCLUSION

In order to reduce the incidence and avoid the complications of DVT, it is necessary to have an efficacious policy for its prevention. This policy should take into account identification of patients at risk, selection of an effective method of prophylaxis and ensuring that the protocol is clear and simple enough to be followed by junior medical and nursing staff.

There is now good evidence that graduated compression stockings are effective in the prevention of deep venous thrombosis. The mechanism by which these stockings exert their effect is uncertain. It may be by promoting blood flow or by preventing venous distension . Graduated compression stockings used alone are effective in the prevention of deep vein thrombosis in low-risk patients. In combination with intermittent pneumatic compression or subcutaneous heparin, they are effective in moderate and high-risk patients. Graduated compression stockings are relatively free of complications, although care should be taken if using these stockings on patients with peripheral vascular disease.

The prophylactic measures should be continued at least until the patient is fully mobile and in most cases until discharge from hospital. A recent study suggested that patients remain at risk of developing pulmonary emboli even after discharge from hospital and in some units, the patient is advised to continue wearing the compression stockings for a few weeks after discharge.

Phlebology '95, D. Negus et al. (eds.). Phlebology (1995) Suppl. 1: 1169-1173

Compression Therapy of Deep Vein Thrombosis

W. Blättler

Current treatment of deep vein thrombosis: heparin and immobilisation

The aim of treatment in acute deep vein thrombosis (DVT) is to achieve adequate anticoagulation in order to prevent potentially life-threatening pulmonary embolism (PE). Except for the rare patients who are treated by thrombolysis, every patient with a confirmed diagnosis of DVT will receive heparin initially and subsequently oral anticoagulants. All too often, symptomatic patients are treated alike despite lack of proof of DVT or PE. For decades, heparin was administered intravenously which necessitated hospital admission of all patients. The fear of PE, which undoubtedly did occur frequently before the availability of heparin, was another reason to admit patients to hospital. Clinicians who worked during the time before the general use of thromboprophylaxis and before the availability of early diagnostic testing of symptomatic patients remember that PE often followed sudden leg movements and using the toilet. Such memorable events contributed to the widespread custom of strictly immobilising all affected patients. Bed rest with leg elevation obviously leads to rapid relief of pain and regression of oedema. Thus the therapeutic approach of using heparin, immobilisation and in-patient supervision was established without being tested in clinical trials.

A treatment that has not (yet) made its mark: compression therapy

Compression stockings and intermittent pneumatic compression are effective in the prevention of postoperative DVT. The usefulness of compression therapy (CT) in established DVT is however unknown. During the time before the use of heparin therapy, a few phlebologists in various countries treated patients with suspected DVT using firm compression bandages and active mobilisation [1-4]. They even challenged the need for hospital admission and blamed immobilisation as being counterproductive and dangerous. Unfortunately, instead of producing convincing clinical data, theories on the pathophysiologic effect of compression were discussed and complicated techniques of bandage application were described. The idea proposed was that compression would fix the free-floating tip of the thrombus to the vessel wall and thus prevent embolisation. It would also speed up blood flow through the deep veins which in turn might result in thrombus breakdown, lysis and anticoagulation. The necessity for using heparin and anticoagulants was questioned by some early supporters of compression therapy [5] which may have cast doubt on their seriousness and jeopardised their otherwise sound views. CT and mobilisation, although appreciated by patients, found widespread acceptance only among phlebologists, and not because of published data but because each phlebologist made his own, notably positive observations.

Changing perception of DVT

In recent years it has been learned that PE is not just a rare and dangerous complication of DVT, but that the two clinical entities, together with superficial thrombophlebitis, regularly coexist as variations of the same disease process. It has also been shown that the relatively poor prognosis in patients with DVT is not due to the thromboembolic disease itself, but to the underlying medical condition. Indeed, further PE in adequately treated patients seems to be an infrequent short-term sequel, although a lifelong tendency for further episodes of thromboembolism occurs in many patients. These clinical experiences removed much of the dispute about acute DVT and prompted a shift of interest from mortality endpoints towards phlebology endpoints. The incidence, the conditions causing the occurrence of DVT, and the possibility of prevention of the postthrombotic syndrome gained more attention. The numerous studies of use of anticoagulation were only recently supplemented by a controlled clinical trial of compression therapy. This showed, not unexpectedly, that early and persistent use of elastic stockings can prevent the postthrombotic syndrome.

Heparin therapy made easy

Therapy with conventional heparin became easier when it was demonstrated in clinical trials that therapeutic concentrations could be achieved by subcutaneous injection and its use limited to five days. Anticoagulant therapy was also made easier when fractionated, low molecular weight heparins (LMWH) were shown to be at least as efficacious as standard heparin. LMWH is dosed according to body weight, does not require laboratory control and can be administered once daily. These simplifications, together with the changing concept of the nature of the disease, fostered interest in ambulatory management of acute DVT [6,7].

Management of symptoms: immobilisation versus CT and ambulation

Some patients with acute DVT may have few symptoms, but the great majority experience severe pain which results from congestion of the muscles and deep conduction veins with blood. The pain is worse in the upright position and during the first few steps taken when walking. Oedema, cyanosis and prominent superficial veins accompany the pain. Many patients feel the need to rest and keep the affected leg elevated. Prompt relief from symptoms is of paramount importance if mobilisation is to be achieved. Fortunately, compression therapy and mobilisation work efficiently and even faster than leg elevation and have a more lasting effect [8,9]. Informing the patient early and throroughly improves compliance. Obviously, knowledge of the action and indication for the different types of compression, skill in bandage application and training in the selection of hosiery is essential.

Agreements on CT in DVT

In the light of the slowly changing concepts of DVT and its therapy, and despite the lack of evidence from controlled trials in many areas, most physicians would agree to the following statements:
- A definite diagnosis is required in order to consider appropriate treatment. The risk and related factors, the age and extent of the thrombus, likely complications, and potential contraindications to treatment need to be known.
- Heparin is to be given to every patient unless contraindicated, followed by oral anticoagulants, irrespective of any other measures taken.
- CT should be used in hospitalised patients when mobilisation begins. Subsequently, assessment of the function and morphology of the venous system determines the need for continued use of CT and the duration of its use.
- In suitable patients CT and deliberate mobilisation is a valid alternative to immobilisation. It provides rapid relief from symptoms and is essential if therapy is to take place on an outpatient basis.
- Patients treated by CT and mobilisation should not receive less care than those treated by immobilisation. This is particularly important if outpatient management is undertaken.
- CT in DVT requires knowledge and skills that are not self-evident, but have to be obtained by adequate training. Physicians and staff should be familiar with the modalities of CT and observe the contraindications.
- CT and mobilisation save costs when carried out on an outpatient basis.

Disagreements concerning CT in DVT

So far, few centres have been involved in systematic studies of CT and mobilisation of patients with extensive DVT. When they reported their results, concerned participants regularly put forward their arguments concerning areas of disagreement. Although most statements were motivated by fear rather than personal experience, these issues are unlikely to be cleared up in the near future. Among them are:
- CT and mobilisation in DVT are not proven to be safe. Indeed, this proof is not at hand and large controlled studies are not under way. However, the studies that have been undertaken so far show that the results of CT and mobilisation are comparable to those expected with immobilisation [8-10].
- The possibility of extension of thrombosis, which might permit or preclude the use of CT and mobilisation, is debated. There is evidence that proximal DVT more frequently causes PE, and therefore should be treated by immobilisation. Objective data from patients with pelvic DVT, however, demonstrate the same frequency of new pulmonary embolism as is known to occur with bedrest [11].
- The presence of free-floating thrombi is considered a risk factor for embolisation. This fear is neither substantiated by personal experience nor by later studies [12].
- The modalities of CT are discussed. Most phlebologists assume that compression with inelastic bandages should be used. Indeed, phlebology lore and tradition point in this direction, but our own experience has taught us that compression stockings are also suitable in most cases [9].

Issues that cannot be settled at the moment

A review article recently published in the New England Journal of Medicine [13] makes no mention at all of CT in established DVT. On the other hand, an article in the French journal Phlébologie [2] assumes CT to be a generally accepted form of therapy of DVT. This discrepancy shows a large communication gap between the academic and the phlebology community. The question is how can this be bridged.

What we do not know with certainty at present is whether CT and mobilisation is as effective, or more or less effective, than immobilisation, and whether it is practicable other than in phlebology centres. Unfortunately, the odds are that we will not get the answers quickly, or from the desirable controlled trials. This is because hospital physicians seem reluctant to withhold bed rest in a symptomatic patient, and are not able to provide adequate CT, while phlebologists are not inclined to admit a patient to a hospital bed knowing that outpatient treatment with CT and ambulation is as effective and much less expensive. We experienced these difficulties when trying to recruit centres for participation in a randomised trial of the two treatment strategies.

In our own clinic, we faced another unexpected problem: most of the fully informed patients declined randomisation and expressed their own preferences. The minority, mostly women and people living alone, with a known diagnosis of cancer or other severe illness, or with abrupt onset of symptoms, chose hospital admission and bed rest, whereas the majority, typically men who had experienced a previous DVT, had risk factors other than cancer and symptoms of longer duration opted for ambulant treatment and CT [14].

Thus it seems that we have to continue to live with unresolved issues. Extremists on one side will continue to claim that lives are put at risk, while extremists on the other side will still deplore the costs and problems which result from unnecessary measures. Reconciliation may be achieved by physicians who initially treat limited or older DVTs with CT and mobilisation and subsequently, with greater experience, gradually extend the indications. To accept this pragmatic approach is probably more reasonable than to keep suggesting large scale controlled trials which seem impossible to organise, at least for the time being.

REFERENCES
1.   Partsch H. Compression therapy of legs. J Dermatol Surg Oncol 1991; 17: 799-805.
2.   Vin F. Compression et thrombose veineuse profonde. Phlébologie 1994; 47: 35-39.
3.   Haid-Fischer F, Haid H, Venenerkrankungen. Phlebologie für Klinik und Praxis 1985; Georg Thieme, Stuttgart.
4.   Wuppermann T. Varizen, Ulcus cruris und Thrombose 1986; Springer-Verlag, Berlin.
5.   Tournay R. Priorité et supériorité par rapport aux anticoagulants du bandage élastocompressif et de l'ambulation immédiate dans la prévention et le traitement des thromboses veineuses des membres inférieurs. Phlébologie 1955; 4: 147-156.
6.   Bakker M, Dekker P-J, Knot EAR, et al. Home treatment for deep venous thrombosis with low-molecular weight heparin. Lancet 1988; 2: 1142.
7.   Salzman EW. Low-molecular weight heparin and other new antithrombotic drugs. N Engl J Med 1992; 326: 1017-1019.

8.   Lofferer O, Mostbeck A, Partsch H, Tham B.   Die ambulante therapie der teifen beinvenenthrombosen mit kompressionsverbänden (möglichkeiten und grenzen).   Ehringer H ed. Akute teife Becken-und Beinvenenthrombosen; Bern, Hans Huber 1977:184-192.

9.   Blättler W.   Ambulatory care for ambulant patients with deep vein thrombosis.   J Mal Vasc 1991; 16: 137-141.

10.   Nielson HK, Husted SE, Krusell L, et al.   Anticoagulant therapy in deep vein thrombosis. A randomised controlled study.   Thromb Haemostas 1985; 54: 233 (abstr.).

11.   Partsch H, Oberger K, Mostbeck A, König B, Köhn H.   Frequency of pulmonary embolism in ambulant patients with pelvic vein thrombosis: A prospective study.   J Vasc Surg 1992; 16: 715-722.

12.   Baldridge ED, Martin MA, Welling RE.   Clinical significance of free-floating venous thrombi.   J Vasc Surg 1990; 11: 62-69.

13.   Weinmann EE, Salzman EW.   Deep-vein thrombosis.   N Engl J Med 1994; 331: 1630-1641.

14.   Blättler W, Frick E.   In-hospital versus outpatient treatment of acute deep vein thrombosis: the patients' preferences.   XVth Congr Int Soc Thomb Haemostas 1995; 1627 (abstr.).

Phlebology '95, D. Negus et al. (eds.). Phlebology (1995) Suppl. 1: 1174-1176

Compression and Sclerotherapy

Pauline Raymond-Martimbeau

INTRODUCTION

The role of compression in the sclerotherapy of venous disease continues to be a subject of debate, but not enough significant scientific studies have been performed to allow objective standards to be determined. A review of the recent literature confirms the existence of two major schools, as described by Stemmer [1]. The maximalist school, represented by Sigg and Fegan, holds that compression is essential after each sclerotherapy session, even for telangiectasias, and that compression should be continued for up to 6 weeks. In contrast, the minimalists, whose treatment strategy proceeds from the highest to the lowest point of reflux and from the largest varices to the smallest, contend that this sequential approach reduces the need for strong compression [1,2]. They advocate medium or mild compression, for as little as 24 hours in some cases, or no compression at all. Other practitioners occupy a middle ground, prescribing compression only under special circumstances. Some experts maintain that, when the immediate sclerotherapeutic outcome is doubtful, compression is useful because it minimises an increase in venous pressure that can result from treatment distal to points of reflux [1,2].

EXTENT OF COMPRESSION

Goldman et al [3,4] maintain that compression sclerotherapy is the standard practice for the treatment of all veins, whether telangiectatic or varicose. These researchers believe that, when adequate, compression results in direct apposition of the treated vein walls, thereby producing more effective fibrosis; it decreases the risk of recanalisation, ankle oedema, postsclerotherapeutic pigmentation, and telangiectatic matting; and it improves the function of the calf muscle pump and provides external support for untreated large veins. In treating leg telangiectasias with 3-day, medium-strength compression, Goldman et al [4] found that veins in the distal leg and/or veins larger than 0.5 mm in diameter underwent greater clinical resolution.

Likewise, Fernandini [5] uses compression in all cases. Bisacci et al [6] and Santos-Gaston [7] maintain that compression plays an important role in achieving aesthetic results, particularly in treating angiomatosis associated with pregnancy [7]. In contrast, Stemmer [1] uses compression discriminately, depending on a varicose vein's diameter and location. He prescribes compression for large veins, more often in the legs than the thigh, and asserts that it is mandatory in the presence of skin changes or potential complications.

Several authors [1,6,8] maintain that the compression regimen may vary according to the phlebologist's experience. They use compression discriminately [1,8]. We believe that, if treatment is performed at the highest point of reflux, according to a sound protocol [8], and if closure of this point allows normalisation of the distal pressure, strong compression may impede venous return. Therefore, we prescribe compression ranging from 12 to 20 mmHg for asymptomatic patients without presclerotherapeutic skin changes and leg oedema, and we prescribe compression ranging from 20-30, 30-40 mmHg for patients with mild (stage 2) or severe (stage 3) presclerotherapeutic chronic venous insufficiency.

TYPE OF COMPRESSION

According to Stemmer [1], "A bandage obtains a result and the stocking maintains it". Goldman et al [3,4] believe that use of a medium-strength compression stocking optimises patient acceptability and compliance. Shouler and Runchman [9] maintain that bandaging is not required if a high-compression stocking is used. These physicians found that a stocking alone slips down more frequently than a combined bandage/stocking but is more comfortable for the patient and, therefore, is left in place more often. Bernbach [10] recommends strong compression, obtained by means of reduced-elasticity elastic bandages worn during the day for 2 to 4 weeks after therapy. Afterward, an elastic stocking is worn for the same length of time.

CONCOMITANT TREATMENT

Queral et al [11] advocate sclerotherapy of adjacent venous channels as an adjunct to the use of Unna's compressive boot for treating ankle ulcers. Doneiger [12] believes that, in patients without leg oedema, the combination of sclerotherapy, electrodessication, and elastic bandages (24 hours a day for 1 week; then during waking hours for 4 additional weeks) produces more clinical improvement than each of these treatments separately. He does not specify the size of veins for which he uses this approach.

CONCLUSION

Although one approach involves strong compression, maintained for up to 6 weeks, current practice varies widely and often involves more moderate, short-term compression or none at all. A review of the foregoing references reveals a need for controlled clinical trials in order to develop scientifically based standards of care regarding postsclerotherapeutic compression. For these studies to be meaningful, however, they must be based on standardised protocols that allow comparison of research data from many centres.

REFERENCES

1. Stemmer R. Sclérose des varices et compression. Phlébologie 1991; 44: 49-67.
2. Raymond-Martimbeau P. Sclerotherapy techniques - video text. Phlebologia 1991: 249-253.
3. Goldman MP. Compression in the treatment of leg telangiectasia: theoretical considerations. J Dermatol Surg Oncol 1989; 15: 184-188.
4. Goldman M, Beaudoing D, Marley W, Lopez L, Butie A. Compression in the treatment of leg telangiectasia: a preliminary report. J Dermatol Surg Oncol 1990; 16: 322-325.
5. Fernandini VG. Nécessité d'utiliser le traitement compressif aprés sclérothéropie? Traitement compressif en phlébologie 1992; John Libbey Eurotext Paris: 35-37.
6. Bisacci R, Colasanti A, Genovese G. La compression immédiate en sclérothérapie, un nouvel instrument. Traitement compressif en phlébologie 1992; John Libbey Eurotext Paris: 39-42.
7. Santos-Gaston M. Importance de la compression aprés sclérothérapie. Traitement compressif en phlébologie 1992; John Libbey Eurotext Paris: 43-44.
8. Raymond-Martimbeau P. Role of sclerotherapy in greater saphenous vein incompetence. Varicose Veins and Telangiectasias St Louis Quality Medical Publishing 1993; Bergan J, Goldman M Eds: 226-258.
9. Shouler PJ, Runchman PC. Varicose veins: optimum compression after surgery and slcerotherapy. Ann R Coll Surg Eng 1989; 71: 402-404.
10. Bernbach HR. Le traitement sclérosant selon Sigg. Phlébologie 1991; 44: 31-36.
11. Queral LA, Criado FJ, Lilly MP, Rudolphi D. The role of sclerotherapy as an adjunct to Unna's boot for treating venous ulcers: a prospective study. J Vasc Surg 1990; 11: 572-575.
12. Doneiger E. Thérapie scléro-électro-compressive: traitement médical des varices des membres inférieurs. Phlébologie 1989; 42: 617-621.

Phlebology '95, D. Negus et al. (eds.). Phlebology (1995) Suppl. 1: 1177-1179

Compression and Dermatology

E. Rabe

Department of Dermatology, University of Bonn, Germany

INTRODUCTION

Many skin changes in the lower limbs are influenced or even caused by a disturbance of the circulation.

Therefore, compression therapy is a well established part of dermatologic therapy in these diseases.

SKIN MICROCIRCULATION

Most authors agree that compression therapy leads to an improvement in skin microcirculation [9,16]. The pathologic venoarteriolar response can be improved in patients with diabetic microangiopathy as shown by Belcaro using laser-Doppler-flowmetry [3].

In these patients PO_2 measured transcutaneously increased and capillary permeability decreased [3]. The pathological increas in skin blood flow in patients with diabetic microangiopathy was decreased using compression as well [3] as in patients with chronic venous diseases as demonstrated by Christopoulos [8].

In contrast to the results in diabetic microangiopathy Empter and Rhitalia demonstrated a reduction of $TcPO_2$ values using compression in patients with chronic venous insufficiency [10,19].

Gniadecki was able to show that the venoarteriolar response in healthy volunteers was reversed by compression therapy [11].

SKIN CHANGES DUE TO CHRONIC VENOUS INSUFFICIENCY (CVI)

Most authors consider the treatment of skin changes due to chronic venous insufficiency (CVI), such as lipodermatoslerosis, ulceration and atrophie blanche, with compression bandages, stockings or intermittent pneumatic compression, to be a basic and well accepted therapy. The beneficial effect in lipodermatosclerosis was demonstrated by Belcaro, Walloios and many other authors [1,2,6,12,13,15,16,18,22] in recent years whereas literature concerning atrophie blanche is less recent [14].

SKIN DISEASES PROVOKED BY VENOUS STASIS

Skin-diseases such as psoriasis and Lichen planus may be exacerbated in the area of chronic venous insufficiency by means of a Koebner phenomenon. In these cases, as well as in dermatologic diseases in which venous insufficiency plays a role in the cause, such as leucocytoclastic vasculitis, compression therapy is used to compensate the vascular component. Publications about this therapeutic concept however are uncommon. In addition, the beneficial effect of compression therapy for some skin diseases has been reported. This, for instance, relates to necrobiosis lipoidica and pretibial mucinosis, as demonstrated by Zabel [23] and Schleicher [20].

DIABETES MICROANGIOPATHY

A beneficial effect of compression therapy was reported in diabetic microangiopathy in improving the parameters of disturbed microcirculation as mentioned above by two working groups. Belcaro et al in Italy [2,4,5,7] and Boulton et al in Manchester [17,21].

CONCLUSION

In conclusion most authors agree that there is an improvement of the disturbed microcirulation using compression therapy [3,8,9,10,11,16,19].

Most authors also agree that skin changes such as lipodermatosclerosis and atrophie blanche caused by chronic venous insufficiency should be treated by compression [1,2,6,12,13,14,15,16,18,22].

Most authors in the available literature agree about the benefit of compression therapy in patients with diabetic microangiopathy [3,4,5,7,17,21].

The beneficial effect of compression in several other skin diseases such as necrobiosis lipoidica and pretibial mucinosis is still under discussion [20,23].

REFERENCES
1.   Belcaro G, Marelli C. Treatment of venous lipodermatosclerosis and ulceration in venous hypertension by elastic compression and fibrinolytic enhancement with defibrotide. Phlebology 1989; 4: 91-106.
2.   Belcaro G, Marelli C, Laurora G, Cesarone MR, Errichi BM. Treatment of venous lipodermatosclerosis and ulceration by fibrinolytic enhancement and elastic compression with defibrotide. Phlebology 1989; A Davy and R Stemmer Eds, Libbey Eurotext 1989:1152-1153.
3.   Belcaro G, Chrostopoulos A, Nicolaides AN. Diabetic microangiopathy treated with elastic compression - A microcirculatory evaluation using Laser-Doppler Flowmetry, transcutaneous PO_2/PCO_2 and capillary permeability measurements. VASA 1990; 19: 247-251.
4.   Belcaro G, Laurora G, Cesarone MR, Pomante P. Elastic stockings in diabetic microangiopathy. VASA 1992; 21: 193-197.

5.   Belcaro G, Laurora G, Cesarone R, de Sanctis MT, Incandela L. Microcirculatory effects of elastic stockings in diabetic microangiopathy: A 24 week study. J Cardiovasc Surg 1993; 34: 478-482.

6.   Blaauw GHM, Neumann HAM, Berretty PJM. La lipodermatosclérose et l'épaisseur demale, étude préliminaire. Phlébologie 1993; 46: 25-31.

7.   Cesarone MR, Christopoulos D, Laurora G, de Sanctis MT, Belcaro G. La compressione elastica nel trattamento della microangiopatia diabetica. Minerva Angiol 1991; 16: 507-512.

8.   Christopoulos D, Nicolaides AN, Belcaro G, Kalodiki E. Venous hypertensive microangiopathy in relation to clinical severity and effect of elastic compression. J Dermatol Surg Oncol 1991; 17: 809-813.

9.   Curri SB, Annoni F, Pabisch S, de Stefano A, Montorsi W. Changes of cutaneous microcirculation from elasto-compression in chronic venous insufficiency. Phlébologie 1989; A Davy, R Stemmer Eds, Libbey Eurotext: 852-854.

10.   Emter M, Bewermeier H, Breitenbach C, Alexander A. Changes of microcirculation in the skin in patients with chronic venous insufficiency in various positions and with compression-therapy. Phlébologie 1989; A Davy, R Stemmer Eds, Libbey Eurotext: 871-872.

11.   Gniadecki R, Gniadecki M, Kotowski R, Serup J. Alterations of skin microcirculatory rhythmic oscillations in different positions of the lower extremity. Acta Derm Venereol (Stockh) 1992; 72: 259-260.

12.   Grondin L. Mercury pressotherapy in the treatment of lipodermatosclerosis. J Dermatolo Surg Oncol 1992; 18: 140-141.

13.   Kirsner RS, Pardes JB, Eaglstein WH, Falanga V.   The clinical spectrum of lipodermatosclerosis. J Am Acad Dermatol 1993; 28: 623-627.

14.   Metz J, Sturm G. Atrophie blanche (sog. Capillaritis alba). Hautarzt 1974; 25: 105-109.

15.   Milleret R. Opération de vigoni modifiée dans le traitement des hypodermites scléreuses. J des Maladies Vasculaires 1992; 17: 121-122.

16.   Mollard JM. Compression et troubles trophiques. John Libbey Eurotext, Paris, 1992: 69-75.

17.   Murray HJ, Veves A, Young MJ, Richie DH, Boulton AJM. Role of experimental socks in the care of the high-risk diabetic foot. Diabetes Care 1993; 8: 1190-1192.

18.   Ouvry PA, Ouvry PAG. Traitement médical des hypodermites scléreuses. Phlébologie 1991; 44: 819-825.

19.   Rithalia SVS, Consalkorale M, Edwards J. Effect of intermittent pneumatic compression on lower limb skin perfusion. Angiology 1989; 40: 249-254.

20.   Schleicher SM, Milstein HJ. Treatment of pretibial mucinosis with gradient pneumatic compression. Arch Dermatol 1994; 130: 842-844.

21.   Veves A, Masson EA, Fernando DJS, Boulton AJM. Studies of experimental hosiery in diabetic neuropathic patients with high foot pressures. Diabetic Medicine 1990; 7: 324-326.

22.   Wallois P. La compression traitement actuel des hyperdermites aigues. Phlébologie 1991; 44: 815-818.

23.   Zabel M, Lindscheid KR.   Zur kompressionstherapie der necrobiosis lipodica (diabeticorum). Phlebol u Proktol 1989; 18: 245-248.

Phlebology '95, D. Negus et al. (eds.). Phlebology (1995) Suppl. 1: 1180-1183

Analysis of the Published Works on Elastic Compression and Orthopaedics Between 1989 and 1995

Eugenio Oscar Brizzio

Vascular Peripheral Laboratory, 965 San Martin Street, 1st Floor, Buenos Aires, Argentina
Argentine School of Phlebology AMA, 1171 Santa Fe Avenue, Buenos Aires, Argentina

INTRODUCTION

On reviewing the papers, they can be separated into three groups: the first group deals with deep vein thromboprophylaxis in orthopaedic surgery, the second group comprises studies relating to the range of mobility of the ankle joint, and the third group refers to studies of the physiology and physiopathology of venous flow.

DEEP VEIN THROMBOPROPHYLAXIS IN ORTHOPAEDIC SURGERY

Effects of anaesthetic methods
Jorgensen (1991) [1] discusses continuous extradural analgesia.
Sharrock (1993) [2] discusses extradural anaesthesia with aspirin and compression stockings.

Intermittent pneumatic compression
Woolson (1991) [3] and Pidala (1992) [4] suggest the use of intermittent pneumatic compression.
Francis (1992) [5] compares the results of warfarin for thromboprophylaxis with those of intermittent pneumatic compression.
Kraay (1993) [6] discusses intermittent pneumatic compression, low-dose warfarin, the Continuous Passive Motion device and early mobilisation.

Preventive equipment
Hübner (1990) [7] developed the **Pedomat** device with a view to mobilising the lower limbs in a seated working position.

Autogenic exercises
Köstler (1990) [8] suggests auto-exercises for ulcers occurring in equinus deformity of the foot.

Ankle pump
Used by Grotenhuis (1993) [9] (**vortrag**). Bonnaire (1993) [10].

Mechanic plantar pump
Used by Fordyce (1992) [11] Scurr, Coleridge-Smith (1993) [12].
Santori (1994) [13] compares the results of heparin with those of the mechanic plantar pump.

Drugs
Benson (1992) [14] discusses the use of non-fractionated heparin.
Feldman (1992) [15] discusses the use of aspirin and dextran.
Imperiale (1994) [16] discusses the use of low-molecular-weight heparin and elastic stockings.

STUDY OF THE ANGLE OF MOBILITY OF THE ANKLE JOINT

Schmeller (1990) [17] concluded that:
a) as age advances, the range of mobility of the ankle joint is reduced,
b) in patients with venous disorders there is evidence of reduced dorsiflexion compared to patients without varicose veins,
c) women have less dorsiflexion than men, and
d) when comparing both legs, the left side shows less dorsiflexion.

STUDY OF THE PHYSIOLOGY AND PHYSIOPATHOLOGY OF VENOUS FLOW

Emter (1989) [18] tested flow velocity with compression stockings and confirmed that it was increased.

Claeys (1990) [19] studied electrical impulses during muscle activity. In the standing position, the leg muscles showed no intermittent activity; standing on the tip of the toes, the activity of the calf muscles was maximum; while walking or pedalling, muscular contraction was intermittent.

Nehler (1993) [20] studied the effects of elastic compression stockings on the pressure produced in the perimalleolar subcutaneous tissue. He found that in patients with chronic venous insufficiency the effects of elastic compression stockings were due to an increase in subcutaneous pressure which may contribute to increasing the efficiency of absorption of perimalleolar extracellular fluid.

Chiappara (1993) [21] described the process and made a breakdown of its components.

Brizzio (1994) [22]. Studied the haemodynamic effects of elastic compression stockings in chronic venous insufficiency. Confirmed:
a) an increase in venous flow velocity,
b) the beneficial effects of a well-adapted shoe and the negative effects of an unadapted shoe in legs with compression stockings,
c) a decrease in proximal and distal venous reflux.

Petermans (1994) [23] studied the muscle-venous pump in an elderly population, and concluded that old age in itself does not alter the venous system.

CONCLUSION

With reference to the first item, thromboprophylaxis is the aim in total hip replacement and total knee arthroplasty. We agree with the following papers: 1, 2, 3, 5, 4, 6, 7, 8, 10, 9, 11, 12, 13, 14, 16.

We agree to differ on the following points:
1. The thromboprophylactic effects of the combination of aspirin and dextran [7].
2. Although we agree with the papers mentioned, we would like to see discussion of the effectiveness of mechanical devices compared with one another, but not the comparative effectiveness of drugs, which has already been discussed.
3. We would also like to see discussion of the effect of the use of drugs and mechanical devices together.
4. The systematic use of medical compression stockings.
5. A universally validated method for the correct diagnosis of thrombosis.
6. Minimum amount of time for postoperative control.

With reference to the second item, mobility of the ankle joint, we agree with this paper [17].

With reference to the third item, physiology and pathophysiology of venous flow, we agree with [18], [19], [20] and [23].

In addition we point out that our paper [22] studies the incidence of the effectiveness of compression stockings in relation to the footwear used.

REFERENCES
1.   Jorgensen IN, Rasmussen IS, Nielsen PT, Leffers A, Albrecht-Beste E. Antithrombotic efficacy of continuous analgesia extradural after knee replacement. British Journal of Anaesthesia 1991; 66: 8-12.
2.   Sharrock NE, Hargett MJ, Urquhart B, Peterson MGE, Ranawat C, Insall J, et al. Factors affecting deep vein thrombosis rate following total knee arthroplasty under epidural anaesthesia. The Journal of Arthroplasty 1993; 8 (2).
3.   Woolson ST, Watt JM. Intermittent pneumatic compression to prevent proximal deep venous thrombosis during and after total hip replacement. The Journal of Bone and Joint Surgery 1991; 73-a (4).
4. Pidala MJ, Donovan DI, Kepley RF. A prospective study on intermittent pneumatic compression in the prevention of deep vein thrombosis in patients undergoing total hip or total knee replacement surgery. Gynaecology y Obstetrics July 1992; 175: 47-51.
5.   Francis CW, Pellegrini VD, Marder VJ, Totterman S, Harris CM, Ruben K, et al. Comparison of Warfarin and external pneumatic compression in prevention of venous thrombosis after total hip replacement. JAMA June 1992; 267 (21).
6.   Kraay M, Goldemberg VM, Herbener TE. Vascular ultrasonography for deep venous thrombosis after total knee arthroplasty. Clinical Orthopaedics and Related Research Jan 1993.
7.   Hübner K. Pedomat. Ein neues gerät zur verbsserung der venosen 1990; 19: 29-32.

8.   Köstler H, Heede G. Spitzfuß und autogene Sprunggelenkmobilisierung. Phlebol Proktol 1990; 19: 80-83.

9.   Grotenhuis JA. Eine Sprunggelenkpumpe mit automatischer Einstellung. Phlebol 1993; 22: 262-263.

10.   Bonnaire F, Brandt R, Raedecke J, Bonk A. Mechanische sprunggelenkpumpe zur thromboseprophylaxe. Phlebol 1993; 22: 272-275.

11.   Fordyce MJF, Ling RSM. A venous foot pump reduces thrombosis after total hip replacement. The Journal of Bone and Joint Surgery Jan 1992; 74-b (1).

12.   Scurr JH, Coleridge-Smith P. La pompe muculaire du pied: Importance physiologique et clinique. Phlébologie 1993; 46 (2): 209-216.

13.   Santori FS, Vitullo A, Stopponi M, Santori N, Ghera S. Prophylaxis against deep vein thrombosis in total hip replacement. The Journal of Bone and Joint Surgery July 1994; 76-b (4).

14.   Besson L, Petit PY, Banssillon V. . Bénéfices et risques de l'héparine non fractionnée en orthopédie. Ann Fr Annesth Réanim 1992; 11: 307-313.

15.   Feldman DS, Zuckerman JD, Walters Y, Sakales SR. Clinical efficacy of Aspirin and Dextran for thromboprophylaxis in geriatric hip fracture patients. Journal of Orthopaedic Trauma; 7 (1): 1-5.

16.   Imperiale TF, Speroff T. A meta-analysis of methods to prevent venous thrombo-embolism following total hip replacement. JAMA June 1994; 271 (22).

17.   Schmeller W. Uber den bewegungsumfang im oberen sprunggelenk bei venengesunden und venen kraken. Ein beitrag zum arthrogenen stauungssyndrom phlebol proktol 1990; 19: 100-110.

18.   Emter M, Alexander K. Venous flow in the lower limb with compression therapy study with the duplex-scanner. Phlébologie 1989; A Davy, R Stemmer Eds John Libbey Eurotext Ltd: 868-870.

19.   Claeys R. Activités de la musculature jambiére dans la vie courante. Phlébologie 1990; 43 (1): 55-62.

20.   Nehler MR, Moneta GL, Woodars DM, Defrang RD, Harker CT, Taylor LM, et al. Perimaleolar subcutaneous tissue pressure affects of elastic compression stockings. Journal of Vascular Surgery Nov 1993; 18 (5).

21.   Chiappara P, Dagnino G, Gulino MT, Giacche P. Phlébologie et podologie. Phlébologie 1993; 46 (2): 272-286.

22.   Brizzio EO, Stemmer R, de Simone J, Salvia C. Effets hémodynamiques des bas médicaux de compression sur le retour veineux. Phléologie 1994; 47 (1): 12-17.

23.   Petermans J, Zicot M. La pompe musculo-veineuse de la personne agée. Journal des Maladies Vasculaires (Paris) Masson 1994; 19: 115-118.

Phlebology '95, D. Negus et al. (eds.). Phlebology (1995) Suppl. 1: 1184-1186

Lymphoedema and Compressive Treatment

Professor J.A. Jimènez Cossio

Department of Angiology and Vascular Surgery, Hospital "La Paz" Madrid, Spain

The purpose of the vast vascular network which constitutes the lymphatic system and is widely distributed throughout the body, is to absorb proteins from the capillary filter and also to transport excess interstitial fluid back to the blood stream. It is important to remember the role played by lymphocytes and lymphoid tissue in immunity and tumour growth.

Olszewski established the principal functions of the lymphatic system:

- Maintain the composition, integrity and function of the interstitial fluid and the fundamental substance.
- Transportation of the substances made by the cells.
- Removal of damaged cells from the organism.
- Elimination of foreign substances from the organism.

Anatomical knowledge of the lymphatic flow, as established by Caplan and Ciucci, is essential in the application of, and indication for, treatment. However, even if initially compression treatments are similar, lymphoedema presents specific characteristics as far as type of lymphoedema, grade of compression and type of application are concerned.

In 90% of patients, the treatment of lymphoedemas is based on conservative measures, with surgical treatment (lymphovenous anastomoses) being carried out in only 10%, when conservative measures have failed. The therapeutic armamentarium consists of manual lymph drainage, drugs which act on the lymphatics, mechanical compression therapy, bandages and elastic stockings.

The classification of lymphoedema as established by the 'Club de Linfologia', distinguishes:

- Aetiological classification: Primary and secondary lymphoedema.
- Clinical classification: Grades I to IV.

- Topographical classification: Lymphoedema affecting upper limbs, lower limbs and genitalia.

Depending on the type of disease and the length of time over which it has evolved, various therapeutic possibilities are available; in the decompression phase we suggest mechanical compression therapy and manual lymph drainage, and then maintaining and securing the decrease in volume of the limb by using different types of bandages. Finally, a maintenance phase is achieved by using elastic hosiery.

We consider that compression treatment is indicated in primary and secondary lymphoedema, in phlebolymphoedema, as well as in angiodisplasia with demonstrable lymphatic involvement.

It is very important to know the type of elastic compression to use in relation to the grade of the lymphoedema: In Grade I, type II would be sufficient; in Grade II, types III or IV and possibly IV, remembering to take into consideration that in certain circumstances made-to-measure stockings will be required, as may happen in severe cases of elephantiasis, lymphoedema in children, and in postmastectomy lymphoedema with marked involvement of the hand.

In the majority of cases, the tolerability of bandages and elastic hosiery is usually excellent, but one must take into consideration the fact that in certain circumstances this therapy may be unsuitable, for example in the presence of an erysipelas crisis or initially in lymphangitis. Skin problems, infectious exudate, and allergy to certain types of fibres may interfere with treatment.

The application of the compression treatment, particularly when using bandages, must be carried out by highly qualified staff. Measures such as protection using cotton or soft foam, or using padded latex or silicone are indispensable in managing certain types of lymphoedema.

The treatment protocol followed by our group is as follows:

- Manual lymph drainage + padded bandages in layers (4 weeks)
- Elastic bandages (4 weeks)
- Elastic hosiery. Compression III-IV (lifetime)

In considering postmastectomy lymphoedema, many types of elastic sleeves, bracelets, gloves, etc, are available. The essential common requirements of these is limitation of the number of stitches as far as possible to avoid friction and pressure areas, to avoid localised compression at the shoulder, and the elasticity must be adequate.

In general, it is helpful to recall some basic premises in relation to elastic hosiery:

- Symptoms must always be evaluated by a specialist.
- The limb must be measured at different levels before treatment.
- The stocking used must be a recognised make.
- The maximum durability of the stocking should be between 6 and 12 months.

- The patient must have at least two pairs of stockings.
- In the case of children and in patients with elephantiasis, stockings must be made to measure.

In conclusion:

- Compression treatment is one of the main breakthroughs in the treatment of lymphoedema.
- Compression treatment must always be initiated by a specialist.
- Compression must always be carried out by highly qualified staff.

REFERENCES
1.   Alliot F, Ghabboun S, Cluzan RV. La compression dans le traittement de lymphoedemes des membres. Phlébologie 1994; 47: 47-52.
2.   Földi M, Casley-Smith JR. Lymphangiology. FK Schattauer Verlag Stuttgart 1983.
3.   Jimènez Cossìo JA.   Diagnostico y tratamiento de loslinfedemas.   Ed Centro de Documentacion Uriach Madrid 1987.
4.   Jimènez Cossio JA. Fisiopatologa del sistema linfàtico. Patologia Vascular 1995; 1: 69-73.
5.   Olszewski WL. Lymph stasis: pathophysiology, diagnostic and treatment. CRS Press Boca Raton 1991.
6.   Stemmer R. Le bas mèdical de compresion dans le trainement du lymphoedema des membres. Journa de Maladies Vasculaires 1990; 15: 285-286.

Author Index